Understanding Pulmonary Hypertension

Understanding Pulmonary Hypertension

Editor: Carter Moore

FOSTER ACADEMICS
www.fosteracademics.com

www.fosteracademics.com

FOSTER ACADEMICS

Cataloging-in-Publication Data

Understanding pulmonary hypertension / edited by Carter Moore.
p. cm.
Includes bibliographical references and index.
ISBN 978-1-63242-801-1
1. Pulmonary hypertension. 2. Hypertension. 3. Pulmonary circulation. 4. Lungs--Diseases.
5. Respiratory organs--Diseases. 6. Respiratory infections. I. Moore, Carter.
RC776.P87 U53 2019
616.24--dc23

Foster Academics,
118-35 Queens Blvd., Suite 400,
Forest Hills, NY 11375, USA

ISBN 978-1-63242-801-1 (Hardback)

Printed and bound in China.

Contents

Preface

This book aims to highlight the current researches and provides a platform to further the scope of innovations in this area. This book is a product of the combined efforts of many researchers and scientists, after going through thorough studies and analysis from different parts of the world. The objective of this book is to provide the readers with the latest information of the field.

The condition of high blood pressure within the arteries of the lungs is known as pulmonary hypertension. Chest pain, tiredness, fast heartbeat, syncope, shortness of breath and swelling of the legs are some of its most common symptoms. The causes of pulmonary hypertension are not completely known. However, some of the risk factors include a family history of pulmonary hypertension, sickle cell disease, sleep apnea, HIV/AIDS, blood clots in the lungs and problems with the mitral valve. Physical examination, electrocardiography, chest X-rays, pulmonary function tests and computed tomography scans are some of the common techniques of diagnosing pulmonary hypertension. Treatment methods include atrial septostomy, lung transplantation and pulmonary thromboendarterectomy. The topics included in this book on pulmonary hypertension are of utmost significance and bound to provide incredible insights to readers. It presents researches and studies performed by experts across the globe. The extensive content of this book provides the readers with a thorough understanding of the subject.

I would like to express my sincere thanks to the authors for their dedicated efforts in the completion of this book. I acknowledge the efforts of the publisher for providing constant support. Lastly, I would like to thank my family for their support in all academic endeavors.

Editor

1

Recombinant Human Interferon Alpha 2b Prevents and Reverses Experimental Pulmonary Hypertension

Eileen M. Bauer[1,2]*, Han Zheng[1], Michael T. Lotze[1,2], Philip M. Bauer[1,3,4]

1 Department of Surgery, University of Pittsburgh School of Medicine, Pittsburgh, Pennsylvania, United States of America, **2** University of Pittsburgh Cancer Institute, University of Pittsburgh School of Medicine, Pittsburgh, Pennsylvania, United States of America, **3** Department of Pharmacology and Chemical Biology, University of Pittsburgh School of Medicine, Pittsburgh, Pennsylvania, United States of America, **4** Vascular Medicine Institute, University of Pittsburgh School of Medicine, Pittsburgh, Pennsylvania, United States of America

Abstract

Pulmonary hypertension (PH) is a progressive and fatal disease with no cure. Vascular remodeling in PH involves intraluminal growth of endothelial and smooth muscle cells, leading to obliterative vascular lesions. Cell growth in these lesions is quasi-neoplastic, with evidence of monoclonality, apoptosis resistance and cancer-like metabolic derangements. Herein we tested the effect of human interferon alpha 2b (IFNα), a pleiotropic cytokine and anti-cancer therapeutic, on the development and progression of PH in the rat SU5416/hypoxia (SUH) model and mouse hypoxia model of the disease. In both models IFNα attenuated the development of PH and reversed established PH as assessed by measuring right ventricular systolic pressure and right ventricular hypertrophy. The effect of IFNα was dependent on the type I interferon receptor (IFNAR) since mice lacking a subunit of the IFNAR were not protected by IFNα. Morphometric analysis of pulmonary aterioles from hypoxic mice or SUH rats showed that IFNα inhibited pulmonary vascular remodeling in both models and that IFNα reversed remodeling in SUH rats with established disease. Immunohistochemical staining revealed that IFNα decreased the number of PCNA and Tunel positive cells in the wall of pulmonary arterioles. *In vitro*, IFNα inhibited proliferation of human pulmonary artery smooth muscle cells and as well as human pulmonary artery endothelial cell proliferation and apoptosis. Together these findings demonstrate that IFNα reverses established experimental PH and provide a rationale for further exploration of the use of IFNα and other immunotherpies in PH.

Editor: You-Yang Zhao, University of Illinois College of Medicine, United States of America

Funding: NIH R01 HL085134 to PM Bauer. The funders had no role in study design, data collection and analysis, decision to publish, or preparation of the manuscript.

* E-mail: bauerpm@upmc.edu

Introduction

Pulmonary Hypertension (PH) is a devastating disease characterized by increased pulmonary artery pressure, right ventricular (RV) failure and death. Although the natural history of the disease is incompletely understood, the traditional view is that endothelial dysfunction and upregulation of pulmonary vasoconstrictors leads to pulmonary vasoconstriction and increased pulmonary artery (PA) pressure. In addition, several pulmonary vasoconstrictors are also smooth muscle cell (SMC) mitogens [1] and prolonged exposure to these vasoconstrictors results in hypertrophy and proliferation of medial SMC [2].

In severe disease the PAs of PH patients exhibit invasive growth of endothelial cells (EC) into the vessel lumen resulting in luminal obstruction by clusters of ECs known as plexiform lesions. EC growth in plexiform lesions is aberrant with some areas containing a solid core of ECs and others exhibiting various stages of angiogenesis [3]. In addition, there is evidence of EC monoclonality [4], resistance of ECs to apoptosis [5], and a cancer-like shift to glycolysis [6] within plexiform lesions. Thus, the vascular lesions in PH exhibit several hallmarks of cancer [7]. These findings represent a major paradigm shift in PH research, which has relied on models of hypoxic vasoconstriction, and indicate that concepts derived from the cancer field should be considered when developing PH therapeutics [4].

Type I interferons (IFN), were identified in 1957 by Isaacs and Lindenmann based on the ability to inhibit viral replication [8,9]. The type I IFN family of at least 15 subtypes includes the IFNα family of 13 functional subtypes of IFNα, IFN-β, and IFNω [10]. The individual IFNα subtypes share the same receptor and exhibit similar biological activities [10]. Type I interferons exhibit a variety of biological effects in addition to those on viral replication, including antitumor activity, anti-angiogenic activity, and utility in multiple sclerosis [11]. Today, IFNα is the most widely used therapeutic cytokine in patients.

Little is known about the effect of IFNα on the pathogenesis of pulmonary hypertension. There are case studies of patients receiving IFNα therapy for the treatment of hepatitis C or chronic myelogenous leukemia developing reversible or irreversible PH [12–14]. On the other hand IFNα has been used to treat PH associated with pulmonary capillary hemangiomatosis [15,16]. In several instances IFNα stabilized or caused regression of pulmonary capillary hemangiomatosis associated PH.

The goal of the present study was to evaluate the effect of IFNα on experimental PH. Based on the case studies demonstrating IFNα-induced PH, and our data showing activation of interferon

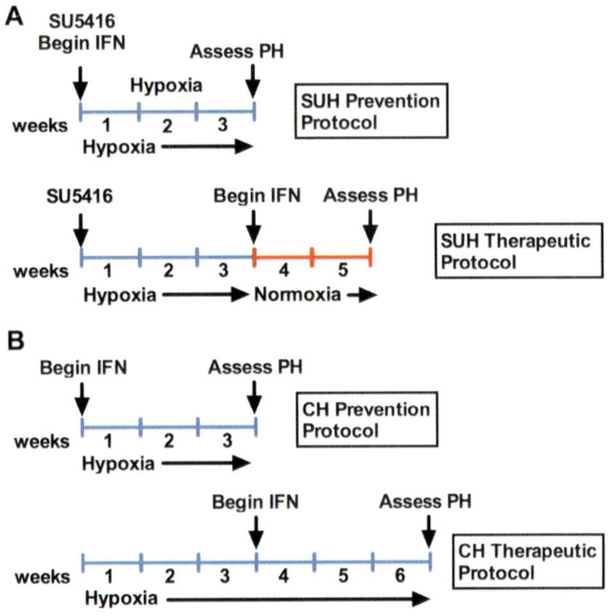

Figure 1. Schema of IFNα treatment protocols. (A) Schema of prevention and therapeutic protocols for IFNα treatment in SU5416/hypoxia-induced PH in rats. (B) Schema of prevention and therapeutic protocols for IFNα treatment in hypoxia-induced PH in mice.

response factor-3 in PH our original hypothesis was that IFNα would exacerbate experimental PH. Instead, we found that, in both the mouse model of chronic hypoxia and the rat model of SU5416 plus chronic hypoxia, IFNα not only attenuated the development of PH, but also reversed established disease.

Methods

Human IPAH cells and serum samples were obtained in compliance with University of Pittsburgh Institutional Review Board (IRB) guidelines **and the studies were approved by the University of Pittsburgh IRB. All** patients gave written consent. Animal studies were approved by the University of Pittsburgh Institutional Animal Care and Use Committee (University of Pittsburgh Animal Assurance # A3187–01).

Animal Use

C57BL/6J mice were purchased from The Jackson Laboratory (Bar Harbor, ME) and 129S6/SvEvTac WT mice were purchased from Taconic Farms (Watertown, NY). IFNAR-deficient mice (IFN-IR−/−129S6) were a kind gift of Akiko Iwasaki (Yale University, New Haven, CT) [17]. Age-matched 8- to 12-wk-old male mice were used for the studies. 225–250 g Sprague Dawley rats purchased from Charles Rivers were used for the studies.

Chronic Hypoxia Mouse Model

Eight to ten week old male mice were placed into a partially ventilated Plexiglas chamber (Biospherix,) and exposed to chronic hypoxia (FIO2 = 0.10, 90% nitrogen) for 21 or 42 days under normobaric conditions. Mice maintained in room air served as normoxic controls. For all mouse studies mice were treated with daily subcutaneous injections of 10^4 IU human recombinant interferon alpha 2b (Intron A; Schering Corporation, Kenilworth, NJ). The dose of interferon alpha 2b was chosen based on a search of the literature [18,19]. The interferon was reconstituted using sterile water for injection, USP provided by the manufacturer and was stored at 4°C after reconstitution per the manufacturer's instructions.

Rat SU5416/Hypoxia Model

225–250 g male Sprague Dawley Rats were injected with a single dose of 20 mg/kg s.c. SU-5416 (A VEGF receptor inhibitor) or vehicle and were placed into a partially ventilated Plexiglas chamber (Biospherix,) and exposed to chronic hypoxia (FIO2 = 0.10, 90% nitrogen) for 21 days under normobaric conditions. Rats maintained in room air served as controls. Some Rats were returned to room air on day 22, and maintained in normoxia for an additional 14 days. For rat studies animals were treated with daily subcutaneous injections of 10^5 IU human recombinant interferon alpha 2b. This dose was chosen to approximately match the dose given to mice. The interferon was prepared and stored as described above for the chronic hypoxia mouse model.

Right Ventricular Systolic Pressure

Right ventricular systolic pressure (RVSP) was measured essentially as described [20]. Briefly, mice or rats were anesthetized with sodium pentobarbital (60 mg/kg i.p. mice; 40 mg/kg i.p. rats) and ventilated via tracheotomy with room air. Body temperature was monitored and regulated with a rectal temperature probe and heating pad. RVSP was determined by placing a 1 F solid-state pressure-transducing catheter (Millar Instruments, Houston, TX, USA) directly into the right ventricle (RV). Data were acquired using a PowerLab data acquisition system and LabChart Pro software (AD Instruments).

Right Ventricular Hypertrophy

Following hemodynamic measurements the vasculature was flushed with PBS, the heart was excised and right heart hypertrophy was determined by the ratio of the weight of the RV to the left ventricle (LV) plus septum (Fulton index) or the ration of weight of the RV to body weight. The right lung was tied off, dissected and flash frozen, and the left lung was perfused with paraformaldehyde (4%) for embedding in paraffin.

Assessment of Pulmonary Vascular Remodeling

For mice, pulmonary vascular remodeling was assessed by counting the number of partially and fully muscularized peripheral arterioles (35–100 mm) per high-power field (200× total magnification). For each mouse, at least 20 high-power fields were analyzed in multiple lung sections. Wall thickness % was determined by measuring the thickness at four points on pulmonary arterioles using the Java-based image-processing program ImageJ (National Institutes of Health, Bethesda, MD, USA). Vascular occlusion was assessed in a blinded fashion by grading at least 50 small (<50 μm) pulmonary arterioles in at least 3 lung tissue samples per group.

Serum IFNα.

Serum IFNα was measured using commercially available ELISA kits ((R&D Systems, Minneapolis, MN).

Immunohistochemistry

Paraffin-embedded lung sections (5 μm) were baked 60 min at 55°C, deparaffinized in xylenes and rehydrated through decreasing alcohol concentrations (three xylenes, 2×100%, 1×95%, 1×90%, 1×70% ethanol, 1×PBS, for 3 min each) followed by antigen retrieval citrate buffer by using a microwave. Smooth

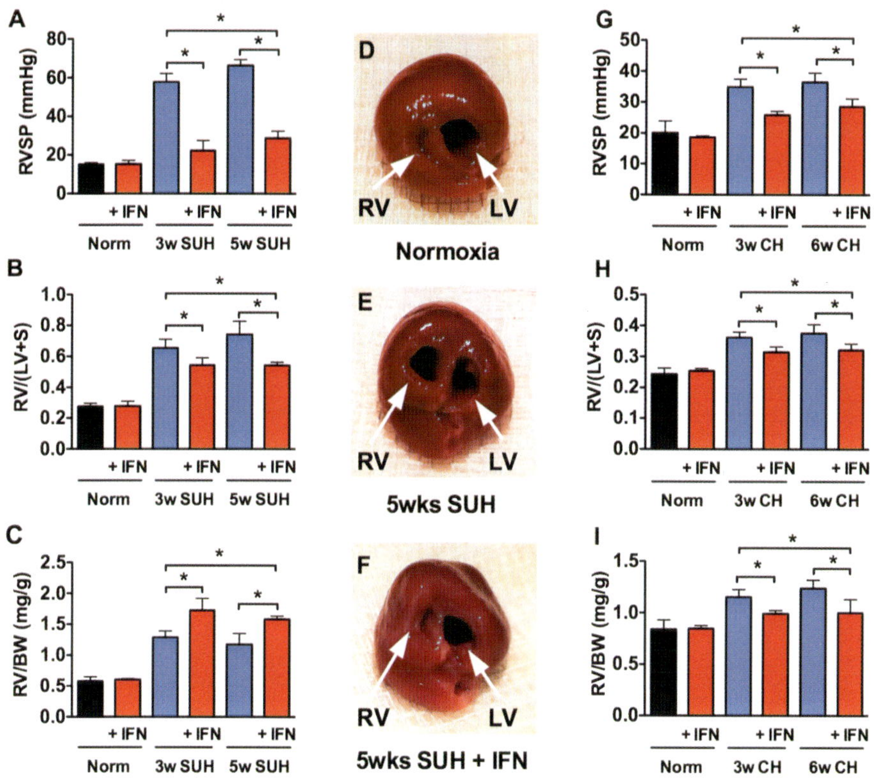

Figure 2. IFNα prevents and reverses experimental PH. (A) Effect of IFNα on RVSP and (B, C) RVH in SUH rats treated with IFNα or vehicle (n = 6 rats per group). (D–F) Representative Images of hearts from normoxic, 5 week SUH, and 5 week SUH rats treated with IFNα. Effect of IFNα on (G) RVSP and (H–I) RVH in hypoxic mice treated with IFNα or vehicle (n = 8 mice per group). Analysis of variance $^*P<0.05$.

muscle α-actin staining was performed as described [21]. TUNNEL staining was performed using the Chemicon kit (S7100) using AEC (Vector) as color reagent and slides were counterstained using hematoxylin. PCNA (sc-7907, Santa Cruz) staining was done using the Elite Vectastain ABC kit (rabbit igG PK-6101) with DAB to obtain a color reaction.

Cultured Cells

Control Human pulmonary artery endothelial cells (HPAECs) and human pulmonary artery smooth muscle cells (HPASMC) were from Lonza. Control and IPAH HPAEC were cultured in EBM2 media and HPASMC were cultured in SBM2 (Lonza) containing the recommended serum and growth factors. Cells were used between passages 4 and 9.

Cell Proliferation

Briefly, HPAEC or HPASMC were serum-starved for 24 h in 12-well plates and treated with the indicated doses of IFNα with or without VEGF (50 ng/ml) or platelet-derived growth factor (PDGF) (10 ng/mL, Sigma P4056) for 24 h in the presence 0.2 μCi [3H] thymidine. Cell Proliferation was then determined by measuring [3H] incorporation as previously described [21].

Western Blotting

30 μg of cell lysate was separated by SDS-PAGE and transferred to nitrocellulose membranes. Membranes were blocked in TBST (Tris-buffered saline, 0.1% Tween 20), 5% nonfat dry milk for 30 min, followed by incubation in primary antibody overnight. Membranes were washed in TBST before incubation for 1 h with horseradish peroxidase conjugated secondary antibodies. Membranes were washed and developed using enhanced chemiluminescence substrate (Pierce). Blots were probed against p21 (#sc-397 Santa Cruz), stat3 (#9132 Cell Signaling), phospho-Stat3 (9131 Cell Signaling), Stat1 (sc-98783 Santa Cruz), phospho-Stat1 (7649 Cell Signaling), Phospho-Akt (9271 Cell Signaling), Akt (61086 BD Transduction Laboratories), β-actin (4967 Cell Signaling).

Statistical Analysis

Statistical analyses were performed by using Graphpad Prism software. Data were analyzed by one-way ANOVA and Tukey's post hoc tests. P values of <0.05 were considered significant.

Results

Treatment with IFNα improves hemodynamics in two animal models of PH

To examine the effect of IFNα on experimental PH we employed the rat model of SU5416/Hypoxia-induced PH (SUH). SUH rats were randomly assigned to a 3-week "prevention protocol" or a 5 week "therapeutic protocol" (**Fig. 1A**). In the prevention protocol, rats received a single injection of SU5416 (20 mg/kg s.c.) and were placed in hypoxia for 3 weeks (10% O_2). These rats received daily injections of IFNα (10^5 IU/day, s.c.) or sterile saline (vehicle) for the duration of the experiment. For the therapeutic protocol, the SUH rats were given a single injection of SU5416, exposed to 3-weeks of hypoxia and then returned to normoxia for 2 weeks. These rats were given daily injections IFNα (10^5 IU/day, s.c.) or vehicle during the 2 week normoxic period. Rats maintained

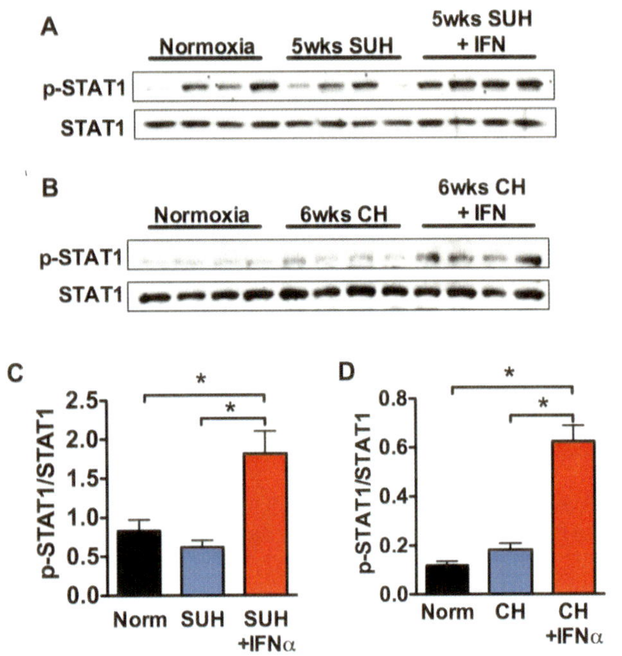

Figure 3. Human IFNα stimulates STAT1 phosphorylation in mice and rats. WB analysis of STAT1, phospho-STAT1 in whole lung homogenates from: (A) normoxic rats, 5 week SUH rats, and 5 week SUH rats treated with IFNα (n = 4 rats per group); or (B) normoxic mice, 6 week hypoxic mice, and 6 week hypoxic mice treated with IFNα. Densitometric ratio of phospho-STAT1 to STAT1 and phospho-STAT3 to STAT3 in lung tissue of different treatment groups in (C) SUH rats and (D) hypoxic mice.

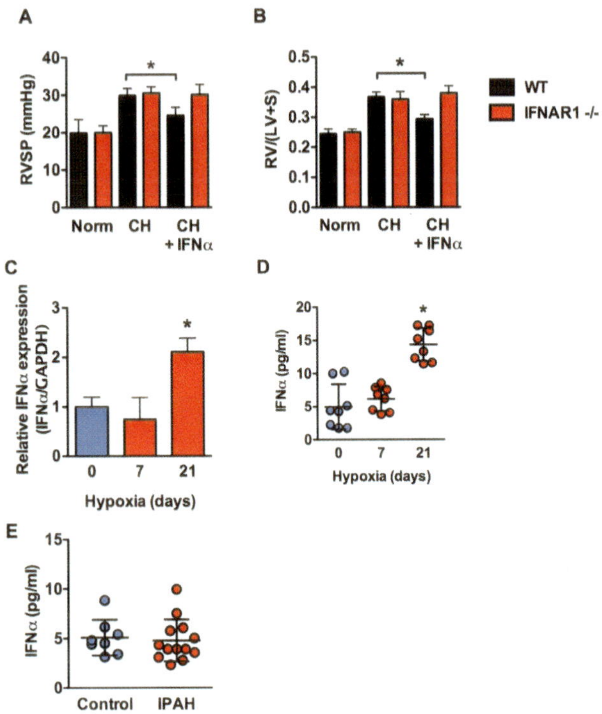

Figure 4. Human IFNα attenuates PH in mice in a IFNAR-dependent fashion. Effect of IFNα on (A) RVSP and (B) RVH in normoxic and hypoxic WT or IFNAR1 −/− mice (n = 6 mice per group). (C) Relative expression of IFNα (normalized to GAPDH) in total lung from C57BL/6J mice exposed to 0, 7, or 21 days of CH as determined by qRT-PCR. (D) Serum concentration of IFNα in C57BL/6J mice exposed to 0, 7, or 21 days CH as determined by ELISA. n = 8 animals per group. Analysis of variance *P<0.05. (E) Serum concentration of IFNα in control vs. IPAH human serum as determined by ELISA.

in normoxia served as controls. Treatment of SUH rats with IFNα using the prevention protocol attenuated the development of PH, as evidenced by decreased right ventricular systolic pressure (RVSP) and decreased right ventricular hypertrophy (RVH) compared to vehicle treated animals (**Fig. 2A–1C**). More importantly, IFNα treatment of SUH rats with established PH (therapeutic protocol) decreased RVSP and RVH compared with untreated SUH rats assessed for PH at 3 or 5 weeks (**Fig. 2A–1C**). Visual inspection of hearts from SUH rats further suggests that the hearts from 5-week SUH rats demonstrate increased RV dilatation compared with hearts from 3-weeks SUH rats, which was prevented by therapeutic IFNα (**Fig. 2D–F**).

To further explore the effect of IFNα in PH we also utilized the mouse model of hypoxia-induced PH. Mice were exposed to hypoxia for 3 weeks with or without concomitant IFNα (10^4 I.U./day, s.c.). To establish the efficacy of IFNα on established disease, mice were exposed to 6 weeks of hypoxia and treated daily with IFNα (10^4 I.U./day, s.c.) from week 4 through week 6 (**Figure 1B**). Mice maintained in normoxia served as controls. Treatment of mice with IFNα using the prevention or therapeutic protocol resulted in decreased disease severity as assessed by measuring RVSP and RVH (**Fig. 2G–I**). Importantly, in the therapeutic protocol, IFNα treated mice exhibited improvement when compared with the 3-week hypoxic mice demonstrating disease reversal.

Exogenous IFNα acts via the type I interferon receptor

Human recombinant IFNα exhibits reduced activity in rodents. To demonstrate that our results were not due to off-target effects of IFNα but occur via activation of the type I interferon receptor (IFNAR) we examined whether 1) human IFNα could elicit a typical type I interferon signaling response in rats and mice and 2) whether genetic deletion of a subunit of the type I interferon receptor could prevent the effect of IFNα in hypoxic mice. As expected of a type I IFN response, IFNα increased phosphorylation of STAT1 in both SUH rats (**Fig. 3A, C**) and hypoxic mice (**Fig. 3B, D**).

We next explored the effect of deleting the IFNAR1 subunit of the type I interferon receptor on the effect of IFNα in hypoxic mice. Deletion of this subunit abrogates type I interferon signaling in response to mouse IFNα. Exposure of WT or IFNAR1 −/− mice to 3-weeks hypoxia led to increased RVSP and RVH compared with normoxic controls (**Fig. 4A, B**). However, while treatment of WT mice with IFNα resulted in decreased RVSP and RVH, IFNα had no effect in IFNAR1 −/− mice demonstrating that human IFNα requires the type I interferon receptor in mice (**Fig. 4A, B**). These findings further demonstrate that endogenous IFNα does not affect disease development or progression in this model since there was no effect of IFNAR1 deletion on RVSP or RVH in hypoxic IFNAR1 −/− mice. This was despite the fact that IFNα mRNA in lung and circulating IFNα was elevated in CH mice after 21 days. We also determined the circulating levels of IFNα in control human (n = 8) vs. IPAH patient (n = 13) serum and found no difference.

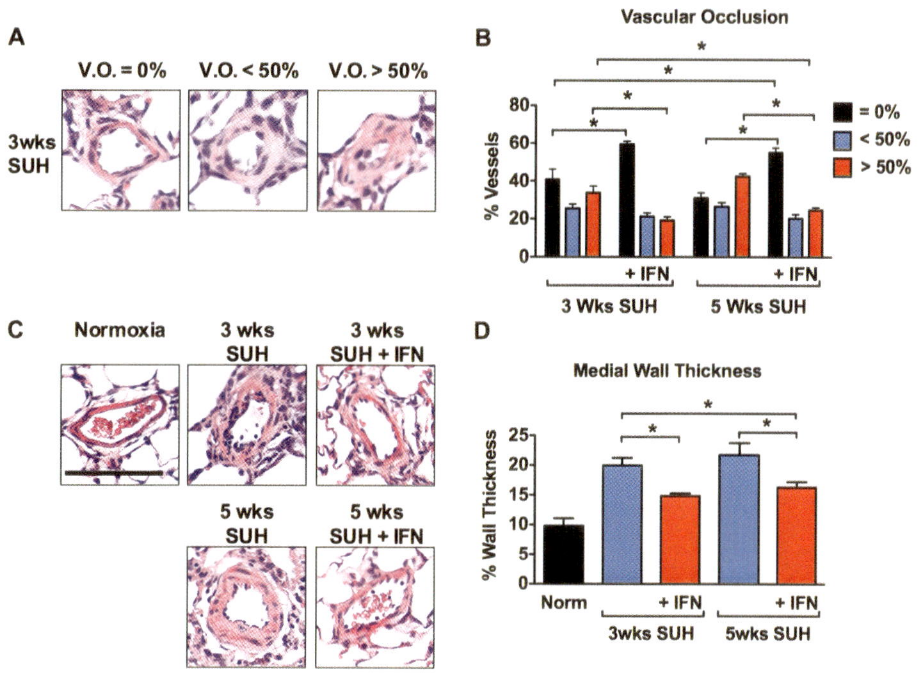

Figure 5. IFNα prevents and reverses pulmonary vascular remodeling in SUH rats. (A) Representative photomicrographs of small pulmonary arterioles (≤50 μm) from an SUH rat with vascular occlusion (V.O.) of 0%, <50%, and >50%. (B) Percent of small pulmonary arterioles (≤ 50 μm) with V.O. 0%, <50%, or >50% in SUH treatment groups (50 arterioles per animal, n = 4 animals per group). (C) Representative photomicrographs of pulmonary arterioles (≤100 μm) from SUH treatment groups demonstrating differences in wall thickness. (D) % Wall thickness in pulmonary arterioles (≤100 μm) from SUH treatment groups (20 arterioles per animal, n = 4 animals per group).

Treatment with IFNα regresses pulmonary vascular remodeling

SU5416 with concurrent hypoxic exposure for 3 weeks caused severe PH with occlusive lesions in rats, which progressed in animals that were returned to normoxia for an additional two weeks. The proportion of vessels (≤50 um) that were occluded greater than 50% was less in the 3-week SUH or 5-week SUH treated with IFNα compared with untreated SUH rats (**Fig. 5A, B**). The 5-week SUH rats treated with IFNα also had a lower proportion of vessels that were occluded more than 50% when compared to 3-week SUH rats. This was associated with an increase in non-occluded vessels in IFNα treated vs. untreated SUH rats. Likewise, medial wall thickness of pulmonary arterioles (≤100 um) was less in the IFNα treated SUH rats and demonstrated reverse remodeling when comparing IFNα treated 5-week SUH rats to untreated 3-week SUH rats (**Fig. 5C, 3D**).

IFNα inhibits vascular cell proliferation *in vivo* and *in vitro*

Pulmonary vascular remodeling in SUH rats is characterized by increased proliferation of vascular smooth muscle and endothelial cells. Thus, we observed increased expression of proliferating cell nuclear antigen (PCNA) in the vessel wall of both 3 week and 5 week SUH rats. Consistent with the anti-proliferative effects of IFNα we observed less PCNA staining in the wall of pulmonary arterioles from SUH rats treated with IFNα (**Fig. 6A–D**). WB analysis confirmed the finding of increased PCNA in SUH rats and suppression of PCNA expression by IFNα (**Fig. 6E–F**). Furthermore, expression of the cyclin dependent kinase inhibitor p21 was decreased in SUH rats and IFNα increased p21 expression in SUH rats (**Fig. 6E–F**). Consistent with our finding of decreased number of proliferating cells in IFNα treated rats, IFNα dose-dependently inhibited the proliferation of human pulmonary artery smooth muscle cells (HPASMC) and human pulmonary artery endothelial cells (HPAEC) **(Fig. 6G–H) from both control and IPAH patients**.

Decreased apoptotic cells in the pulmonary vascular wall of SUH rats treated with IFNα

Because decreased proliferation can not fully explain our observation of reverse remodeling in IFNα treated SUH rats, we were interested in the effect of IFNα on pulmonary vascular cell apoptosis. There was increased number of TUNEL positive cells in the vessel wall of both 3 wk and 5 wk SUH rats when compared with normoxic controls. Treatment of SUH rats with IFNα caused a striking decrease in the number of TUNEL positive cells in the vessel wall using both the prevention and therapeutic protocol (**Fig. 7A–I**). Increased apoptosis in SUH rats was associated with decreased anti-apoptotic signaling as indicated by decreased AKT phosphorylation, which was reversed by IFNα treatment (**Fig. 7J**). In cultured cells, we found no effect of IFNα on HPASMC apoptosis (**Fig. 7K–L**) whereas IFNα potently inhibited apoptosis of control HPAEC, but not IPAH HPAEC, in response to serum starvation or the combination of cycloheximide and hydrogen peroxide (**Fig. 7M–N**).

Discussion

IFNα belongs to a family of cytokines participating in innate immunity against viruses and other pathogens. IFNα also has anti-tumor activities due to its anti-proliferative, anti-angiogenic and immune-regulatory properties [22,23]. Two isoforms of IFNα, IFNα 2a and IFNα 2b (used in this study), are used clinically for the treatment of Hepatitis B and C as well as various cancers. The seminal finding of this study is that IFNα

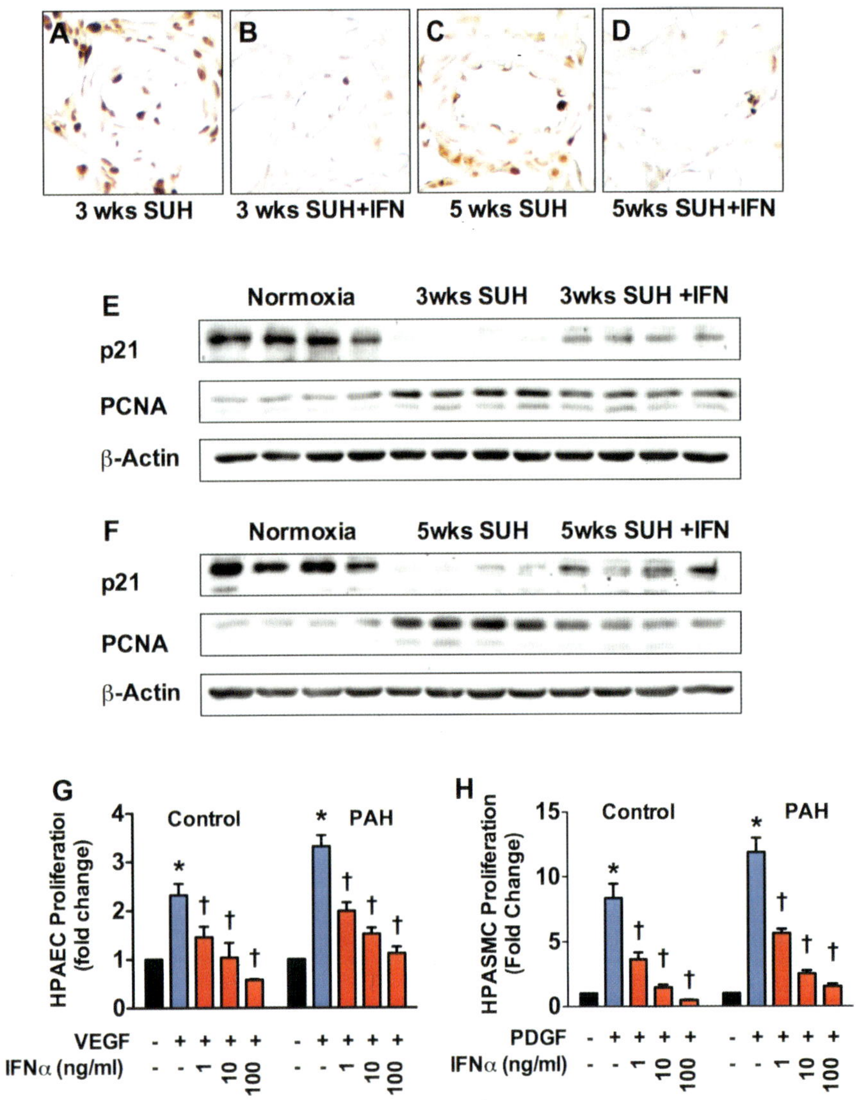

Figure 6. IFNα inhibits pulmonary vascular cell proliferation. (A–D) Representative 40x images of lung sections from 3 week SUH rat, 3 week SUH rat + IFNα, 5 weeks SUH rat, and 5 week SUH rats+ IFNα stained for PCNA (brown) as an indicator of proliferating cells. WB analysis for PCNA and p21 in whole lung lysates from (E) 3-week SUH rats or (F) 5-week SUH rats with or without IFNα (n = 4 animals per group). (G) Control or IPAH HPASMC were serum starved 24 h and then stimulated with PDGF (10 ng/ml) with or without increasing IFNα for 24 hours. (H) Control or IPAH HPAEC were serum starved overnight and then stimulated with VEGF (50 ng/ml) with or without increasing IFNα for 24 hours. Proliferation was assessed by measuring [H3]-thymidine incorporation. Analysis of variance *$P<0.05$.

2b attenuates the onset of PH and more excitingly causes regression of established PH in two experimental animal models of the disease. Of particular interest are our findings that IFNα can cause regression of established PH in SUH rats since the resulting hemodynamic and histopathologic changes in this model most closely mimic those in human PH [24,25].

In this study we demonstrate that, in two rodent models of PH, IFNα significantly reduced RVSP and RVH compared with vehicle-treated animals. Importantly, we also demonstrate that SUH rats or hypoxic mice treated with IFNα using our therapeutic protocol showed significant improvements in RVSP and RVH when compared with the 3 week control animals demonstrating reversal of established disease. The positive changes in hemodynamics and RVH were accompanied by decreased pulmonary vascular remodeling and perivascular inflammation. In the rat SUH model, treatment with IFNα led to a decrease in the number of occlusive lesions in both treated groups compared with vehicle. Importantly, in 5-week SUH rats we found less occlusive lesions when compared with SUH 3-week control animals. Similarly, we observed a decrease in medial wall thickness of SUH rats treated with IFNα, again with evidence of reverse remodeling in the 5-week SUH rats.

The effect of IFNα on pulmonary vascular remodeling was accompanied by reduced numbers of PCNA-positive cells in pulmonary arterioles from IFNα treated animals demonstrating decreased pulmonary vascular cell proliferation *in vivo*. *In vitro* experiments further demonstrated that IFNα directly inhibits proliferation of both HPAEC and HPASMC from control or IPAH patients. While the anti-proliferative effect of IFNα is sufficient to explain the suppression of pulmonary vascular remodeling in prevention groups, it cannot completely explain reverse remodeling in the SUH therapeutic groups.

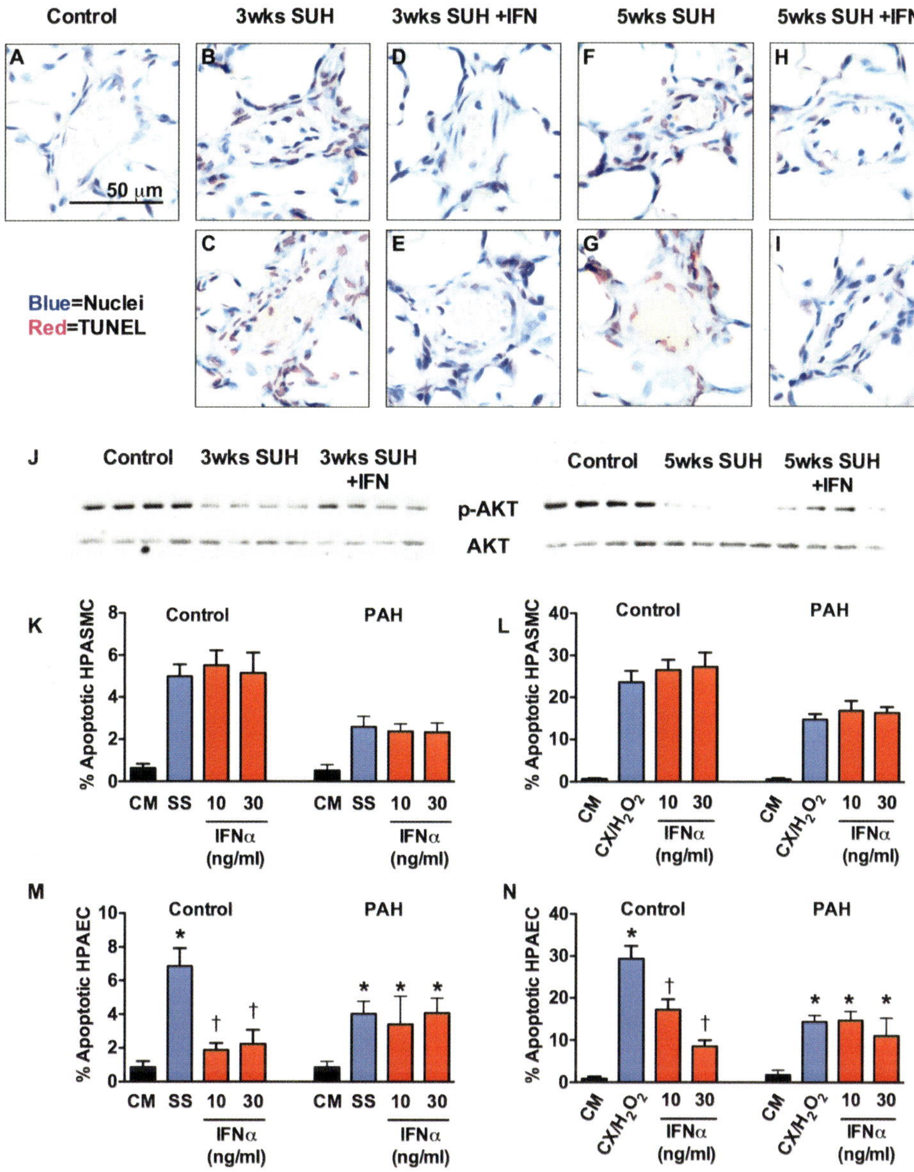

Figure 7. IFNα reduces the number of TUNEL positive cells in the pulmonary arterioles of SUH rats and inhibits HPAEC apoptosis. Representative photomicrographs of pulmonary arterioles stained for TUNEL (red) and nuclei (blue) in (A) normoxic control rats; (B, C) 3 week SUH rats; (D, E) 3 week SUH rats treated with IFNα; (F, G) 5 week SUH rats; and (H, I) 5 week SUH rats treated with IFNα. Photomicrographs are representative of 4–6 animals per group. (J) WB analysis for total AKT and phospho-AKT in whole lung lysates from 3-week SUH rats or 5-week SUH rats with or without IFNα (n = 4 animals per group). Control or IPAH HPASMC were grown in complete media and apoptosis was induced by (K) serum starvation or (L) cycloheximide plus hydrogen peroxide with or without IFNα. Control or IPAH HPAEC were grown in complete media and apoptosis was induced by (M) serum starvation or (N) cycloheximide plus hydrogen peroxide. Percent apoptotic cells was assessed by the ratio of TUNEL positive nuclei to total nuclei.

This led us to explore the effect of IFNα on apoptosis. In our *in vitro* studies we found that while IFNα had no effect on control or IPAH HPASMC, IFNα inhibited apoptosis in control HPAEC but not in ECs from IPAH patients. As was previously demonstrated the IPAH HPAEC were somewhat resistant to apoptosis as compared to control [26], which may partially explain why IFNα had no effect on these cells. These results suggest that IFNα may prevent or attenuate apoptosis of healthy endothelium helping to preserve normal endothelial function. Despite these *in vitro* results demonstrating decreased EC apoptosis, it was somewhat surprising to find a striking decrease in TUNEL positive cells in the pulmonary vascular wall of SUH rats treated with IFNα. We had anticipated that reverse remodeling requires increased apoptosis. There are several possible explanations for these observations. Studies demonstrate that EC apoptosis contributes to pathologic remodeling in the SUH model of pulmonary hypertension and that caspase inhibition ameliorates PH in this model [27]. Thus, direct inhibition of EC apoptosis is likely to play a role in the therapeutic effects observed in response to IFNα. We also cannot rule out the possibility that in the therapeutic model there was an early increase in apoptosis in response to IFNα that resolved before endpoint measurements were made.

Another interesting possibility is the idea that phagocytosis of apoptotic cells (efferocytosis) is impaired in the SUH model and that IFNα stimulates efferocytosis. The number of apoptotic cells in a tissue is affected both by the rate of apoptosis and the rate of efferocytosis by macrophages and resident cells. Apoptotic cells that are not cleared become necrotic causing release of pro-inflammatory molecules [28]. Impaired efferocytosis is linked to the pathogenesis of chronic vascular and pulmonary inflammatory diseases including atherosclerosis [29], systemic lupus erythematosus, chronic obstructive pulmonary disease (COPD) [30,31], cystic fibrosis [32] and asthma [33,34]. Interestingly, in a 2006 review article Vandivier et al. reported that efferocytosis is impaired in a SU5416 model of COPD [28]. In addition, we recently demonstrated a role for high mobility group box 1 in the pathogenesis of PH [35,36], and high mobility group box 1 inhibits efferocytosis [37–39]. In contrast, efferocytosis suppresses innate immunity and promotes its resolution by suppressing the expression of inflammatory mediators [40]. To that end, IFNα increases phagocytosis by macrophages [41,42] suggesting that the effect of IFNα in SUH rats may be partially attributable to stimulation of efferocytosis. Additional studies are needed to address the role of apoptosis and efferocytosis in the effect of IFNα on PH and in the pathogenesis of the disease itself.

IFNα is a pleiotropic cytokine that affects many cell types. Thus, it is likely that other cell types beyond those explored in this study are involved in the effect of IFNα in these models of PH. Of interest is the possibility that the effects of IFNα may be mediated by activation of natural killer cells. Ormiston et al. recently demonstrated impairment of natural killer cell phenotype and function in PH patients, hypoxia-induced PH in mice, and monocrotaline-induced PH in rats [43]. In contrast, IFNα augments natural killer cell cytotoxicity and up-regulates expression of cytolytic effectors Fas-L and perforin [44,45]. It is tempting to hypothesize that the effect IFNα has on pulmonary vascular remodeling is partly due to increased natural killer cell function.

Despite our finding that IFNα prevents and reverses experimental pulmonary hypertension in 2 distinct models, chronic treatment with IFNα for hepatitis C or chronic myelogenous leukemia was associated with the onset of PH in humans and the Food and Drug Administration has labeled IFNα with a warning about the risk of PH with its use. Recently, Dhillon et al. [12] reported four cases of PH in hepatitis C patients treated with IFN-α. Two of the patients were non-cirrhotic and two were post-liver transplant. Other causes of PH including portopulmonary hypertension and were ruled out. The authors suggest the acceleration of a previously subclinical phenomenon caused by factors such as human herpes virus 8, hepatitis C virus, or genetic predisposition [12] as potential mechanisms. Another case report described reversible PH in a chronic myelogenous leukemia patient treated with IFNα. Interestingly, there are several case reports of chronic myelogenous leukemia patients developing PH after treatment with the tyrosine kinase inhibitor dasatinib [46–48] and, like IFNα, dasatinib has been shown to reverse experimental PH [49]. The fact that these two unrelated drugs lead to the development of PH in chronic myelogenous leukemia, but reverse experimental PH suggests that some feature of chronic myelogenous leukemia renders a fraction of these patients susceptible to PH. In either case, PH remains a rare complication of these drugs suggesting individual and/or disease-related susceptibility to PH.

In terms of a role for endogenous IFNα in the development of PH we found that despite a slight elevation in circulating levels of IFNα in mice after 21 days of CH that deletion of IFNAR1 subunit of the type I interferon receptor had no effect on the progression of PH. Interestingly this is different from what was recently reported by George et al. where they found that deletion of this subunit protected mice from the development of chronic hypoxia-induced PH. In this study they also report that IFNAR1 is upregulated in Systemic Sclerosis patients with PH and that Interferon Regulated Protein 10 (IP10) correlated positively with pulmonary hemodynamics and serum brain natriuretic peptide and negatively with 6-minute walk test and cardiac index [50]. The correlation of IP10 with PH in SSC patients has also been shown by another group, however, that group and another failed to find a direct correlation between circulating IFNα and PH in SSC patients [51,52]. We also found no evidence for increased circulating IFNα in a limited number of IPAH patients.

To our knowledge this is only the second demonstration of disease reversal in the SUH rat model of PH. While case studies suggest that IFNα therapy may cause pulmonary hypertension, our data raise legitimate questions as to the role of IFNα in this process. IFNα is a pleiotropic cytokine that mediates a wide range of biological effects including, anti-proliferative, anti-angiogenic and anti-tumor activities, which theoretically could provide benefit to PH patients. The reversal of PH with an immunotherapeutic modality is novel and provides proof of principle that immunotherapy can have a positive impact on PH progression. While evidence of IFNα-induced PH in humans might mean that IFNα will never be used to treat human PH our results warrant further investigation of IFNα and other immunotherapeutics in PH.

Acknowledgments

Human recombinant interferon alpha 2b was a kind gift from John Kirkwood, M.D. The HPASMC and HPAEC from IPAH patients as well as the control and IPAH serum were from the Pulmonary Hypertension Breakthrough Initiative of the Cardiovascular Medicine Research Fund.

Author Contributions

Conceived and designed the experiments: EMB PMB MTL. Performed the experiments: EMB HZ. Analyzed the data: EMB PMB. Contributed reagents/materials/analysis tools: MTL. Wrote the paper: EMB PMB.

References

1. Voelkel NF, Tuder RM (1995) Cellular and molecular mechanisms in the pathogenesis of severe pulmonary hypertension. Eur Respir J 8: 2129–2138.
2. Voelkel NF, Tuder RM (2000) Hypoxia-induced pulmonary vascular remodeling: a model for what human disease? J Clin Invest 106: 733–738.
3. Tuder RM, Groves B, Badesch DB, Voelkel NF (1994) Exuberant endothelial cell growth and elements of inflammation are present in plexiform lesions of pulmonary hypertension. Am J Pathol 144: 275–285.
4. Lee SD, Shroyer KR, Markham NE, Cool CD, Voelkel NF, et al. (1998) Monoclonal endothelial cell proliferation is present in primary but not secondary pulmonary hypertension. J Clin Invest 101: 927–934.
5. Masri FA, Xu W, Comhair SA, Asosingh K, Koo M, et al. (2007) Hyperproliferative apoptosis-resistant endothelial cells in idiopathic pulmonary arterial hypertension. Am J Physiol Lung Cell Mol Physiol 293: L548–554.
6. Fijalkowska I, Xu W, Comhair SA, Janocha AJ, Mavrakis LA, et al. (2010) Hypoxia inducible-factor1alpha regulates the metabolic shift of pulmonary hypertensive endothelial cells. Am J Pathol 176: 1130–1138.
7. Hanahan D, Weinberg RA (2011) Hallmarks of cancer: the next generation. Cell 144: 646–674.
8. Isaacs A, Lindenmann J, Valentine RC (1957) Virus interference. II. Some properties of interferon. Proc R Soc Lond B Biol Sci 147: 268–273.
9. Isaacs A, Lindenmann J (1957) Virus interference. I. The interferon. Proc R Soc Lond B Biol Sci 147: 258–267.
10. Mogensen KE, Lewerenz M, Reboul J, Lutfalla G, Uze G (1999) The type I interferon receptor: structure, function, and evolution of a family business. J Interferon Cytokine Res 19: 1069–1098.
11. Pfeffer LM, Dinarello CA, Herberman RB, Williams BR, Borden EC, et al. (1998) Biological properties of recombinant alpha-interferons: 40th anniversary of the discovery of interferons. Cancer Res 58: 2489–2499.

12. Dhillon S, Kaker A, Dosanjh A, Japra D, Vanthiel DH (2010) Irreversible pulmonary hypertension associated with the use of interferon alpha for chronic hepatitis C. Dig Dis Sci 55: 1785–1790.
13. Jochmann N, Kiecker F, Borges AC, Hofmann MA, Eddicks S, et al. (2005) Long-term therapy of interferon-alpha induced pulmonary arterial hypertension with different PDE-5 inhibitors: a case report. Cardiovasc Ultrasound 3: 26.
14. Fruehauf S, Steiger S, Topaly J, Ho AD (2001) Pulmonary artery hypertension during interferon-alpha therapy for chronic myelogenous leukemia. Ann Hematol 80: 308–310.
15. Olin J, Abman S, Grady R, Ivy D, Lovell M, et al. (2011) A 7-year-old with pulmonary hypertension. BMJ Case Rep 2011: bcr0220113843.
16. Almagro P, Julia J, Sanjaume M, Gonzalez G, Casalots J, et al. (2002) Pulmonary capillary hemangiomatosis associated with primary pulmonary hypertension: report of 2 new cases and review of 35 cases from the literature. Medicine (Baltimore) 81: 417–424.
17. Muller U, Steinhoff U, Reis LF, Hemmi S, Pavlovic J, et al. (1994) Functional role of type I and type II interferons in antiviral defense. Science 264: 1918–1921.
18. Siddegowda NK, Kumar Rao NS, Andrade C (2011) Development of a murine animal model of depression for repeated dosing with human interferon alpha. Indian J Psychiatry 53: 239–243.
19. Cao B, Chen XP, Zhu P, Ding L, Guan J, et al. (2008) Inhibitory effect of interferon-alpha-2b on expression of cyclooxygenase-2 and vascular endothelial growth factor in human hepatocellular carcinoma inoculated in nude mice. World J Gastroenterol 14: 6802–6807.
20. Cruz JA, Bauer EM, Rodriguez AI, Gangopadhyay A, Zeineh NS, et al. (2012) Chronic hypoxia induces right heart failure in caveolin-1 −/− mice. Am J Physiol Heart Circ Physiol 302: H2518–2527.
21. Bauer EM, Zheng H, Comhair S, Erzurum S, Billiar TR, et al. (2011) Complement C3 deficiency attenuates chronic hypoxia-induced pulmonary hypertension in mice. PLoS One 6: e28578.
22. Ezekowitz RA, Mulliken JB, Folkman J (1992) Interferon alfa-2a therapy for life-threatening hemangiomas of infancy. N Engl J Med 326: 1456–1463.
23. Tarhini AA, Gogas H, Kirkwood JM (2012) IFN-alpha in the treatment of melanoma. J Immunol 189: 3789–3793.
24. Abe K, Toba M, Alzoubi A, Ito M, Fagan KA, et al. (2010) Formation of plexiform lesions in experimental severe pulmonary arterial hypertension. Circulation 121: 2747–2754.
25. Nicolls MR, Mizuno S, Taraseviciene-Stewart L, Farkas L, Drake JI, et al. (2012) New models of pulmonary hypertension based on VEGF receptor blockade-induced endothelial cell apoptosis. Pulm Circ 2: 434–442.
26. Sakao S, Taraseviciene-Stewart L, Lee JD, Wood K, Cool CD, et al. (2005) Initial apoptosis is followed by increased proliferation of apoptosis-resistant endothelial cells. FASEB J 19: 1178–1180.
27. Taraseviciene-Stewart L, Kasahara Y, Alger L, Hirth P, Mc Mahon G, et al. (2001) Inhibition of the VEGF receptor 2 combined with chronic hypoxia causes cell death-dependent pulmonary endothelial cell proliferation and severe pulmonary hypertension. FASEB J 15: 427–438.
28. Vandivier RW, Henson PM, Douglas IS (2006) Burying the dead: the impact of failed apoptotic cell removal (efferocytosis) on chronic inflammatory lung disease. Chest 129: 1673–1682.
29. Van Vre EA, Ait-Oufella H, Tedgui A, Mallat Z (2012) Apoptotic cell death and efferocytosis in atherosclerosis. Arterioscler Thromb Vasc Biol 32: 887–893.
30. Hodge S, Hodge G, Scicchitano R, Reynolds PN, Holmes M (2003) Alveolar macrophages from subjects with chronic obstructive pulmonary disease are deficient in their ability to phagocytose apoptotic airway epithelial cells. Immunol Cell Biol 81: 289–296.
31. Vandivier RW, Ogden CA, Fadok VA, Hoffmann PR, Brown KK, et al. (2002) Role of surfactant proteins A, D, and C1q in the clearance of apoptotic cells in vivo and in vitro: calreticulin and CD91 as a common collectin receptor complex. J Immunol 169: 3978–3986.
32. Vandivier RW, Fadok VA, Ogden CA, Hoffmann PR, Brain JD, et al. (2002) Impaired clearance of apoptotic cells from cystic fibrosis airways. Chest 121: 89S.
33. Simpson JL, Gibson PG, Yang IA, Upham J, James A, et al. (2013) Impaired macrophage phagocytosis in non-eosinophilic asthma. Clin Exp Allergy 43: 29–35.
34. Fernandez-Boyanapalli R, Goleva E, Kolakowski C, Min E, Day B, et al. (2012) Obesity impairs apoptotic cell clearance in asthma. J Allergy Clin Immunol 131: 1041–1047.
35. Bauer EM, Shapiro R, Zheng H, Ahmad F, Ishizawar D, et al. (2013) High Mobility Group Box 1 Contributes to the Pathogenesis of Experimental Pulmonary Hypertension via Activation of Toll-like Receptor 4. Mol Med 18: 1509–1518.
36. Bauer EM, Shapiro R, Billiar TR, Bauer PM (2013) High mobility group Box 1 inhibits human pulmonary artery endothelial cell migration via a Toll-like receptor 4- and interferon response factor 3-dependent mechanism(s). J Biol Chem 288: 1365–1373.
37. Friggeri A, Yang Y, Banerjee S, Park YJ, Liu G, et al. (2010) HMGB1 inhibits macrophage activity in efferocytosis through binding to the alphavbeta3-integrin. Am J Physiol Cell Physiol 299: C1267–1276.
38. Banerjee S, Friggeri A, Liu G, Abraham E (2010) The C-terminal acidic tail is responsible for the inhibitory effects of HMGB1 on efferocytosis. J Leukoc Biol 88: 973–979.
39. Liu G, Wang J, Park YJ, Tsuruta Y, Lorne EF, et al. (2008) High mobility group protein-1 inhibits phagocytosis of apoptotic neutrophils through binding to phosphatidylserine. J Immunol 181: 4240–4246.
40. Henson PM, Bratton DL, Fadok VA (2001) Apoptotic cell removal. Curr Biol 11: R795–805.
41. Chen BD, Najor F (1987) Macrophage activation by interferon alpha + beta is associated with a loss of proliferative capacity: role of interferon alpha + beta in the regulation of macrophage proliferation and function. Cell Immunol 106: 343–354.
42. Rollag H, Degre M, Sonnenfeld G (1984) Effects of interferon-alpha/beta and interferon-gamma preparations on phagocytosis by mouse peritoneal macrophages. Scand J Immunol 20: 149–155.
43. Ormiston ML, Chang C, Long LL, Soon E, Jones D, et al. (2012) Impaired natural killer cell phenotype and function in idiopathic and heritable pulmonary arterial hypertension. Circulation 126: 1099–1109.
44. Hervas-Stubbs S, Perez-Gracia JL, Rouzaut A, Sanmamed MF, Le Bon A, et al. (2011) Direct effects of type I interferons on cells of the immune system. Clin Cancer Res 17: 2619–2627.
45. Liang S, Wei H, Sun R, Tian Z (2003) IFNalpha regulates NK cell cytotoxicity through STAT1 pathway. Cytokine 23: 190–199.
46. Mattei D, Feola M, Orzan F, Mordini N, Rapezzi D, et al. (2009) Reversible dasatinib-induced pulmonary arterial hypertension and right ventricle failure in a previously allografted CML patient. Bone Marrow Transplant 43: 967–968.
47. Rasheed W, Flaim B, Seymour JF (2009) Reversible severe pulmonary hypertension secondary to dasatinib in a patient with chronic myeloid leukemia. Leuk Res 33: 861–864.
48. Dumitrescu D, Seck C, ten Freyhaus H, Gerhardt F, Erdmann E, et al. (2011) Fully reversible pulmonary arterial hypertension associated with dasatinib treatment for chronic myeloid leukaemia. Eur Respir J 38: 218–220.
49. Pullamsetti SS, Berghausen EM, Dabral S, Tretyn A, Butrous E, et al. (2012) Role of Src tyrosine kinases in experimental pulmonary hypertension. Arterioscler Thromb Vasc Biol 32: 1354–1365.
50. George PM, Oliver E, Dorfmuller P, Dubois OD, Reed DM, et al. (2014) Evidence for the involvement of type I interferon in pulmonary arterial hypertension. Circ Res 114: 677–688.
51. Wuttge DM, Lood C, Tufvesson E, Scheja A, Truedsson L, et al. (2013) Increased serum type I interferon activity in early systemic sclerosis patients is associated with antibodies against Sjogren's syndrome antigens and nuclear ribonucleoprotein antigens. Scand J Rheumatol 42: 235–240.
52. Eloranta ML, Franck-Larsson K, Lovgren T, Kalamajski S, Ronnblom A, et al. (2010) Type I interferon system activation and association with disease manifestations in systemic sclerosis. Ann Rheum Dis 69: 1396–1402.

2

Notch Signaling Change in Pulmonary Vascular Remodeling in Rats with Pulmonary Hypertension and its Implication for Therapeutic Intervention

Lina Qiao[1,2]*, Liang Xie[1,2], Kun Shi[3], Tongfu Zhou[1,2], Yimin Hua[1,2], Hanmin Liu[1,2]

1 Department of Pediatric Cardiology, West China Second University Hospital, Sichuan University, Chengdu, China, **2** Key Laboratory of Obstetric & Gynecologic and Pediatric Diseases and Birth Defects of Ministry of Education, West China Second University Hospital, Sichuan University, Chengdu, China, **3** Department of Cardiology, Chengdu Women & Children Center Hospital, Chengdu, China

Abstract

Pulmonary hypertension (PH) is a fatal disease that lacks an effective therapy. Notch signaling pathway plays a crucial role in the angiogenesis and vascular remodeling. However, its roles in vascular remodeling in PH have not been well studied. In the current study, using hypoxia-induced PH model in rat, we examined the expression of Notch and its downstream factors. Then, we used vessel strip culture system and γ-secretase inhibitor DAPT, a Notch signaling inhibitor to determine the effect of Notch signaling in vascular remodeling and its potential therapeutic value. Our results indicated that Notch 1–4 were detected in the lung tissue with variable levels in different cell types such as smooth muscle cells and endothelial cells of pulmonary artery, bronchia, and alveoli. In addition, following the PH induction, all of Notch1, Notch3, Notch4 receptor, and downstream factor, HERP1 in pulmonary arteries, mRNA expressions were increased with a peak at 1–2 weeks. Furthermore, the vessel wall thickness from rats with hypoxia treatment increased after cultured for 8 days, which could be decreased approximately 30% by DAPT, accompanied with significant increase of expression level of apoptotic factors (caspase-3 and Bax) and transformation of vascular smooth muscle cell (VSMC) phenotype from synthetic towards contractile. In conclusion, the current study suggested Notch pathway plays an important role in pulmonary vascular remodeling in PH and targeting Notch signaling pathway could be a valuable approach to design new therapy for PH.

Editor: James West, Vanderbilt University Medical Center, United States of America

Funding: This research was supported by National Natural Science Foundation of China (30700913) and Program for Changjiang Scholars and Innovative Research Team in University "PCSIRT" (IRT0935). The funders had no role in study design, data collection and analysis, decision to publish, or preparation of the manuscript.

Competing Interests: The authors have declared that no competing interests exist.

* E-mail: iaqiao@163.com

Introduction

Pulmonary hypertension (PH) is a fatal clinical diseases that can be idiopathic or secondary to heart, pulmonary, and vascular diseases. Importantly, PH is one of the important factors determining the prognosis of patients with congenital heart defects. Currently, there is no effective treatment for severe PH patients, who usually have low quality of life and poor prognosis. Pulmonary vascular remodeling is a common feature of severe PH regardless of primary cause, suggesting that intervention of pulmonary vascular remodeling may be valuable for pulmonary hypertension, which was supported by animal studies and evidence-based studies [1,2].

The most important characteristic of pulmonary vascular remodeling is the thickening of the vascular intima, media, and adventitia, which is generally thought to result from cell hypertrophy, proliferation, migration, and extracellular matrix deposition. This process involves many cell types, including endothelial cells, smooth muscle cells, fibroblasts, inflammatory cells, and platelets. These cells produce and respond to a variety of factors, such as endothelin, angiotensin II, transforming growth factor beta (TGF-β), platelet-derived growth factor (PDGF), fibroblast growth factor (FGF), vascular endothelial growth factor (VEGF), serotonin, and angiopoietin as well as intracellular signaling molecules such as tyrosine kinases, mitogen-activated protein kinases (MAPKs), protein kinase C (PKC), and phosphatidylinositol 3-kinase (PI3K), Rho kinases, SMAD and calcium ion channels [3,4,5,6,7]. However, because of the complicated process of PH, the potentially effective molecular targets remain to be defined [1,2,3,4,5,6,7]. In the past decades, extensive investigation have been conducted to study whether angiogensis and vascular remodeling factors involved in the development of mammal embryos could be targeted for the intervention of PH. For example, VEGF, TGF-β, PDGF, Angiopoietin/Tie, FGF, and Ephrin/Eph signal pathways have been determined and reported in the literature [8,9,10,11,12]. One of the major finding is that Notch signaling pathway plays a crucial role in the angiogensis and vascular remodeling [8,9,10,11,12,13,14,15,16,17,18].

The Notch system is highly conservative in evolution and plays an important role in cell proliferation, differentiation, and apoptosis. To date, four Notch receptors (Notch1, Notch 2, Notch 3, and Notch 4), and five ligands (Jagged1, Jagged 2, Delta-like 1, Delta-like 2, and Delta-like 3) have been determined [19,20,21]. Owing to the transmembrane domain of the Notch ligands and receptors, the signal transduction of Notch system is primarily based on cell-to-cell contact [19,20,21,22]. It has been found that

Notch receptors 1, 3 and 4 and ligands Dll4, Jagged1 and 2 are mainly expressed in the arterial system in human and critical for maintenance of normal vascular structure, angiogenesis, and vascular remodeling in both physiological and pathological conditions [9,10,13,16,17,18]. The indispensable roles of Notch system have been supported by the fetal lethality of Notch signaling deficiency. For example, either knockout of Notch1, Notch1 plus Notch4, HERP1 plus HERP2, Jagged1, DLL4, presenillin-1, or constant expression of Notch4 results in embryonic death due to vascular remodeling defects [9,10,13,16,17,20,23]. In addition, gene mutation of Notch system has been observed in human diseases with involvement of artery, such as Algille Syndrome, which is associated with Jagged1 gene mutations and narrowing of small pulmonary arteries, as well as CADASIL Syndrome, which results from mutations of Notch3 gene and progressive degeneration of the vascular smooth muscle cells (VSMCs) [9,10,13,16,17,20]. However, its role in vascular remodeling in PH has not been well elucidated. To date, there were about three studies focusing on the effect of Notch signaling pathway in vascular remodeling of PH. [24,25,26] Li etc found that overexpression of NOTCH3 existed in the lungs of humans and rodents with pulmonary hypertension, knock-out mice with homozygous deletion of Notch3 did not develop pulmonary hypertension in response to hypoxic stimulation and pulmonary hypertension could be successfully treated in mice by administration of N-[N-(3,5-difluorophenacetyl)-L-alanyl]-S-phenylglycine t-butyl ester (DAPT), a γ-secretase inhibitor [24]. Also, our previous work found that DAPT could inhibit pulmonary vascular remodeling induced by angiotensin II and PDGF ex vivo [25,26]. However, Notch signaling pathway is very complicated. The mechanism of the effects of this pathway on PH is still unclear. In this study, we examined the expression of Notch 1–4 receptors and downstream factors during the development of PH and tried to determine the role of Notch signaling in vascular remodeling of PH by using DAPT as an inhibitor of Notch signaling pathway.

Materials and Methods

Ethical Statements

All these cleaning laboratory Wistar rats were obtained from Experimental Animal Center of West China Medical Center in Sichuan University. The Committee on the Ethics of Animal Experiments of Sichuan University approved all protocols related to the animal experiments in this study and the study was carried out in accordance with the National Institute of Health guideline for the Care and Use of Laboratory Animals.

Hypoxia Experiments

Thirty-five adult Wistar rats (average age: 8 weeks; weight: 200–220 g) were divided into seven groups and received hypoxia treatment for designated duration of time: 0, 1, and 3 days, or 1, 2, 3 and 4 week, respectively. Accordingly, the experimental groups were named as control, hypoxia-one-day, hypoxia-three-day, hypoxia-one-week, hypoxia-two-week, hypoxia-three-week, hypoxia-four-week.

For one-day treatment, rats stayed in a hypoxia chamber with 10%±1% oxygen, less than 3% carbon dioxide, and normal atmospheric pressure for 8 hours everyday. The concentrations of oxygen and carbon dioxide were monitored every 10–15 minutes. Food and water were provided normally. The control rats were kept in the same conditions except hypoxia. The remaining treatment regiments are the expansion of this one-day treatment according to the designated time duration. Following designated hypoxia treatment, rats were anaesthetized at 0.5–1 hour after leaving the hypoxia chamber by 10% chloral hydrate (400 mg/kg, i.p). The pressures were measured in right ventricle and pulmonary artery via right external jugular vein intubation. The heart and lungs were isolated after cervical dislocation. Fulton index was calculated as RV/(LV+S). The left lungs were dissected for isolating pulmonary arteries: fixing the left pulmonary artery by a pair of forceps and dissecting the lung tissue as far as possible by ophthalmic scissors. These pulmonary arteries were kept in liquid nitrogen immediately for mRNA extraction. And the right lungs were fixed in formalin and embedded in paraffin for Hematoxylin-eosin (HE) and immunohistochemistry (IHC) staining.

Pulmonary Artery Vascular Strips Culture

24 pulmonary artery strips were collected from rats following hypoxia treatment for 28 days by isolating and cutting open the pulmonary arteries via vertical axis. 700 µl rat rail collagen, 100 µl M199, 200 µl sterile $NaHCO_3$ (11.76 mg/ml) were mixed on ice and spread in 35 mm petri dishes. The strips were put in the dishes with endothelium on the top and incubated at 37°C with 5% CO2 for 15 minutes. Then, 1.5 ml M199 medium with 5% FBS and 100 U/ml streptomycin and penicillin were added to the dishes and dish was returned to the incubator. The culture medium was replaced with fresh medium every day for seven days. Each time the renewed culture medium was added by 3 µl M199, 3 µl DMSO, 3 µl 0.5 mmol/l DAPT (N-[N-(3,5-Difluorophenacetyl)-L-alaryl]-S-phenylalycine t-butyl ester, C23H26F2N2O4, Sigma D5942), and 3 µl 5 mmol/l DAPT respectively according to the different experimental groups. On the ninth day of the culture, the strips were cut into two parts, one part was kept in liquid nitrogen for extraction of mRNA and the other was fixed in formalin and embedded in paraffin for HE and IHC staining.

RT-PCR

Total RNA was isolated using Trizol (MRC, U.S.A). cDNA was synthesized by the RevertAid™ First Strand cDNA Synthesis Kit (MBI, Lithuania). Real-time PCR was performed by SYBR Green I (Roche, Switzerland) method. The reaction included cDNA, primers (table 1, Takara, China), dNTP (Promega, U.S.A), and Taq DNA polymerase (BioDev, China). The PCR procedure was as follows: pre-denaturing at 94°C for 2 minutes, and 45 cycles of denaturing at 94°C for 20 seconds, annealing at 52°C for 30 seconds, elongation at 72°C for 40 seconds. $2^{-\Delta\Delta Ct}$ method was applied for relative quantification of the target genes. The $2^{-\Delta\Delta Ct}$ value of RT-PCR was in a skew distribution and were logarithmically transformed for further analyses.

Measurement of the Thickness of Vessel Wall

The thickness of vessel wall in strips was measured by Verhoeff iron hematocylin stain method. The elastic fiber was black or dark blue after staining. The results were scanned and analyzed using Image-Pro Plus software. Four fields were selected randomly for one strip. The distance between inner and outer elastic fibers was measured for three times in one field. The average of the twelve distance values was used as the thickness of vessel wall in this strip.

Immunohistochemistry

The IHC was conducted following the manufacture instruction for kits SP-9001, SP-9002, and SP-9003 (Zhong Shan -Golden Bridge Biological Technology CO., LTD, Beijing). The following antibodies were used: Notch1 (sc-6014, Santa Cruz Biotechnology, Inc.), Notch2 (sc-7423, Santa Cruz Biotechnology, Inc.), Notch3

Table 1. The sequences of primers used in this study.

Gene Name	*Primers*	*Product Size (bp)*
Notch1	Forward: 5′-TCTCAACTGCCAGAACCTTGT-3′ Reverse: 5′-ATGCCTCGCTTCTGTGCAG-3′	171
Notch2	Forward: 5′-CACTGAGAGCTCCTGTTTCAA-3′ Reverse: 5′-CAGGCCATCAACACACGTTC-3′	160
Notch3	Forward: 5′-ATGGCAGGCTTCACAGGAAC-3′ Reverse: 5′-TGCAGCTGAAGCCATTGACT-3′	109
Notch4	Forward: 5′-AGTGTCTCCCAGGCTTTGAA-3′ Reverse: 5′-GAAGATCAAGGCAGCTGGCT-3′	96
HERP1	Forward: 5′-GATGCTCCAGGCAACAGG-3′ Reverse: 5′-GTGGGTCCGAAGGGTCAA-3′	143
HERP2	Forward: 5′-CCAACCACATCGTCCCA-3′ Reverse: 5′-CTAGCTTCGCAGATCCCTG-3′	145
SM-MHC	Forward: 5′-ATGCTGGGAAGGTGGACTAT-3′ Reverse: 5′-CGGTCCACATCCTTCCACA-3′	133
SM22α	Forward: 5′-TCTGAGCAAGTTGGTGAACA-3′ Reverse: 5′-GAGGTCAACAGTCTGGAACAT-3′	169
MGP	Forward: 5′-GCCCTGTGCTATGAATCTCA-3′ Reverse: 5′-GCGTGCCATCTCTGCTGA-3′	107
OPN	Forward: 5′-CACTCAGATGCTGTAGCCACTT-3′ Reverse: 5′-GTTGCTTGGAAGAGTTTCTTGCT-3′	126
Bcl-Xl	Forward: 5′-CCTTCATAAGAGCCACAAAGA-3′ Reverse: 5′-ATGGGCTCAACCAGTCCATT-3′	130
BAX	Forward: 5′-GTTTCATCCAGGATCGAGCA-3′ Reverse: 5′-CAATCATCCTCTGCAGCTCC-3′	156
GAPDH	Forward: 5′-CCTCAAGATTGTCAGCAAT-3′ Reverse: 5′-CCATCCACAGTCTTCTGAGT-3′	141

(sc-7424, Santa Cruz Biotechnology, Inc.), Notch4 (sc-8646, Santa Cruz Biotechnology, Inc.), PCNA (Neomarker, MS-106-P, Lab Vision Co.), and Caspase-3 (Neomarker, MS-1121-P, Lab Vision Co.). PCNA and caspase-3 positive cells were counted from five random fields (×400) of one strip. The positive rate was calculated by dividing the number of all positive cells by the total number of cells in the five fields.

Statistics

The SPSS program software (version 13.0, SPSS Inc., USA) was used for statistical analysis. Quantitative data were expressed as mean ± s.e.m. One-way or repeated-measure ANOVA was used to analyze the difference among groups. LSD for homogeneity of variances, or Tamhane's T2 for heterogeneity of variances was used for the multiple comparisons of the means of each group. The differences were considered significant when $p<0.05$.

Results

Validation of Rat PH Model Induced by Hypoxia

Body weight, mean pulmonary artery pressure (mPAP) and the Fulton index of rat have been obtained to validate the successful induction of PH. As shown in Figure 1A, the body weight of hypoxia rats is significantly lower than that of normoxia rats ($p<0.001$). The curve of weight changes in control rats was nearly a straight line, whereas the curve in model rats was nearly a quadratic function curve. The changes of the mPAP and the Fulton index of the hypoxia rats are shown in Figure 1B. The mPAP increased and reached the peak at the second week since the initiation of hypoxia treatment. The Fulton index progressively increased, suggesting the right ventricle thickening continuously progressed. The HE staining for lung tissues are shown in Figure 2. The increased thickness of pulmonary arterioles in the hypoxia rats indicated the progressive worsening of pulmonary vascular remodeling. Collectively, it was suggested that PH has been successfully induced with the hypoxia treatment.

The Gene Expression of Notch Receptors and their Downstream Effectors in PH Rats

Next, using IHC, we examined Notch receptor expression following the induction of PH. Our results revealed that the positions where each of these four Notch receptors located in PH rats were the same as the positions in normal rats. Notch1 located in cell membrane and cytoplasm, Notch 2 and Notch 4 located in cell membrane, whereas Notch 3 located in nucleus in rat lung tissues (Figure 3). In addition, Notch1 was detected in smooth muscle cells and endothelial cells of pulmonary artery, smooth muscle cells, epithelial cells, and macrophages of bronchia. Notch2 expressed in epithelial cells of bronchia and alveoli. Notch3 was observed in smooth muscle cells of pulmonary artery and epithelial cells of bronchia. Notch4 was present in endothelial cells of pulmonary artery and epithelial cells of bronchia, little in smooth muscle cells of pulmonary artery.

Regarding the change of mRNA levels, Notch1, Notch3, Notch4 receptor expression exhibited different patterns along the course of hypoxia treatments (Figure 4A). The peak of Notch3 was 1 week, and 2 weeks for Notch1 and Notch4. Compared to the control, Notch3 mRNA level was increased two folds, 4 folds for Notch1, and 5 folds for Notch4. Then they returned to the baseline level. The gene expression changes of Notch downstream genes, HERP1 and HERP2, were also changed (Figure 4B). While HERP1 reached the peak at the second week and gradually dropped to the base level, HERP2 declined quickly at the first day of hypoxia and maintained at the low level.

The Wall Thickness Changes of Vascular Strip in Culture

In the extended culture study, we measured the changes of vascular strip wall thickness in culture. As shown in Figure 5, the thickness of vascular wall of the strips of four groups were different significantly ($p<0.05$). The thickness of vascular media of the hypoxia rats increased significantly, it was about 30%, when PH occurred. Of note, there was no significant difference between the strips of the normoxia rats before and after culturing ($p>0.20$). In contrast, the strips of the hypoxia-treated rats were significantly thicker after culturing than before, increasing about 30 μm, nearly 30%. It was suggested that vascular strips from PH rats have a prolonged proliferative trait in culture.

The Impact of DAPT on Notch Signaling in Vascular Strips from PH Rats

In the classic Notch signal transduction, following the binding of ligands to Notch receptors, two steps of enzymolysis occurs. As the

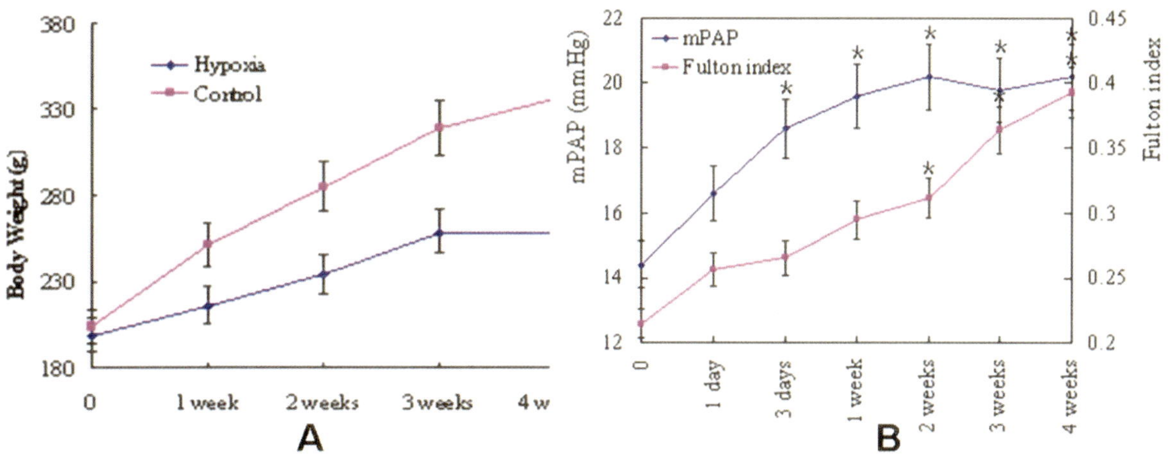

Figure 1. Validation of rat PH model induced by hypoxia. (A) weight changes in the course of hypoxia treatment. The results of F test showed that there were significant differences between the weights of experimental and control groups at each time points. The curve of weight changes in control rats is nearly a straight line, whereas the curve in model rats is nearly a quadratic function curve. (B) the changes of mean pulmonary artery pressures (mPAP) and the Fulton index in PH rats. ANOVA analyses revealed that mPAP and the Fulton index were significantly different in each points. With the increase of hypoxia duration, the mPAP in hypoxia rats increased with a peak at the second week, and maintained a high level until the end point. The continuous increase of Fulton index suggested progressive hypertrophy of rat right ventricle. (*, $P<0.05$ compared to control group, Data are expressed as means ± s.e.m.)

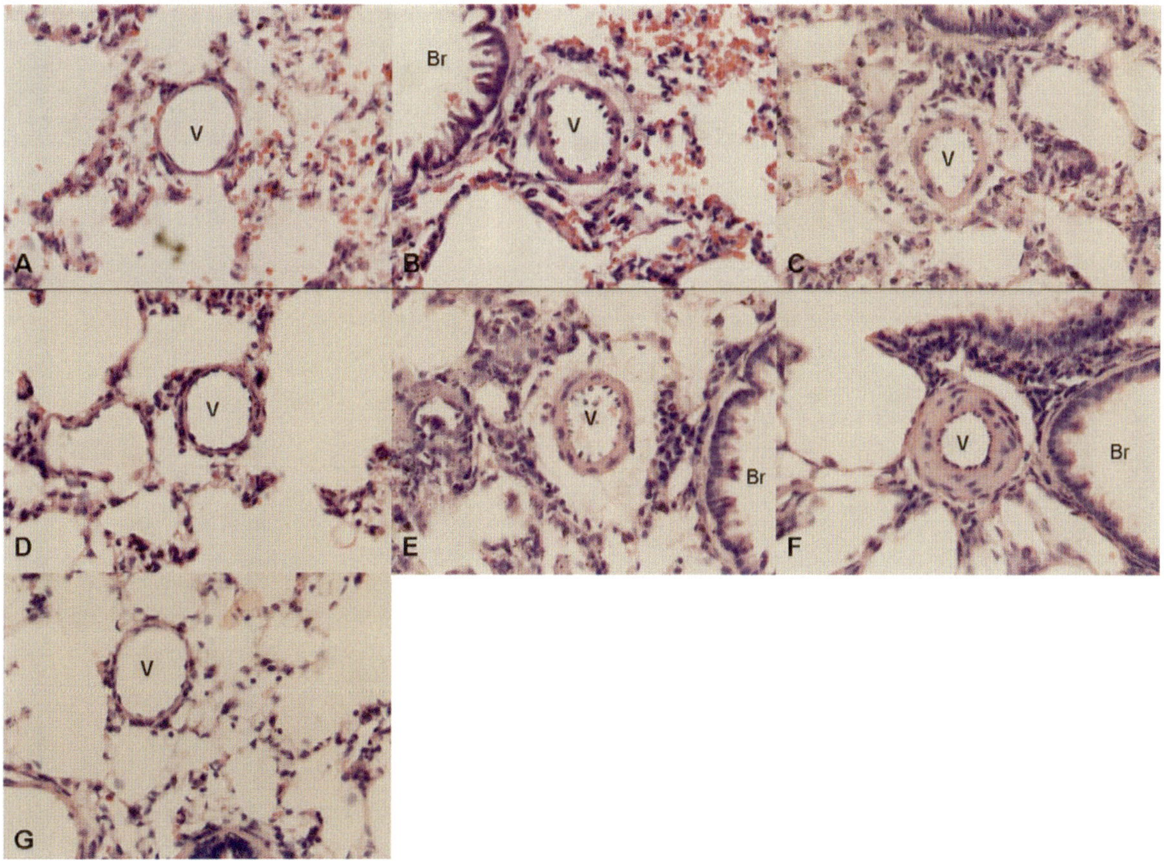

Figure 2. Hematoxylin-eosin staining of rat lung tissue. (A–G) HE staining of lung tissues of hypoxia rats for 1, 3 days, and 1, 2, 3, 4 weeks, and normal rats, respectively. (×400) V: Vessel; Br: Bronchium.

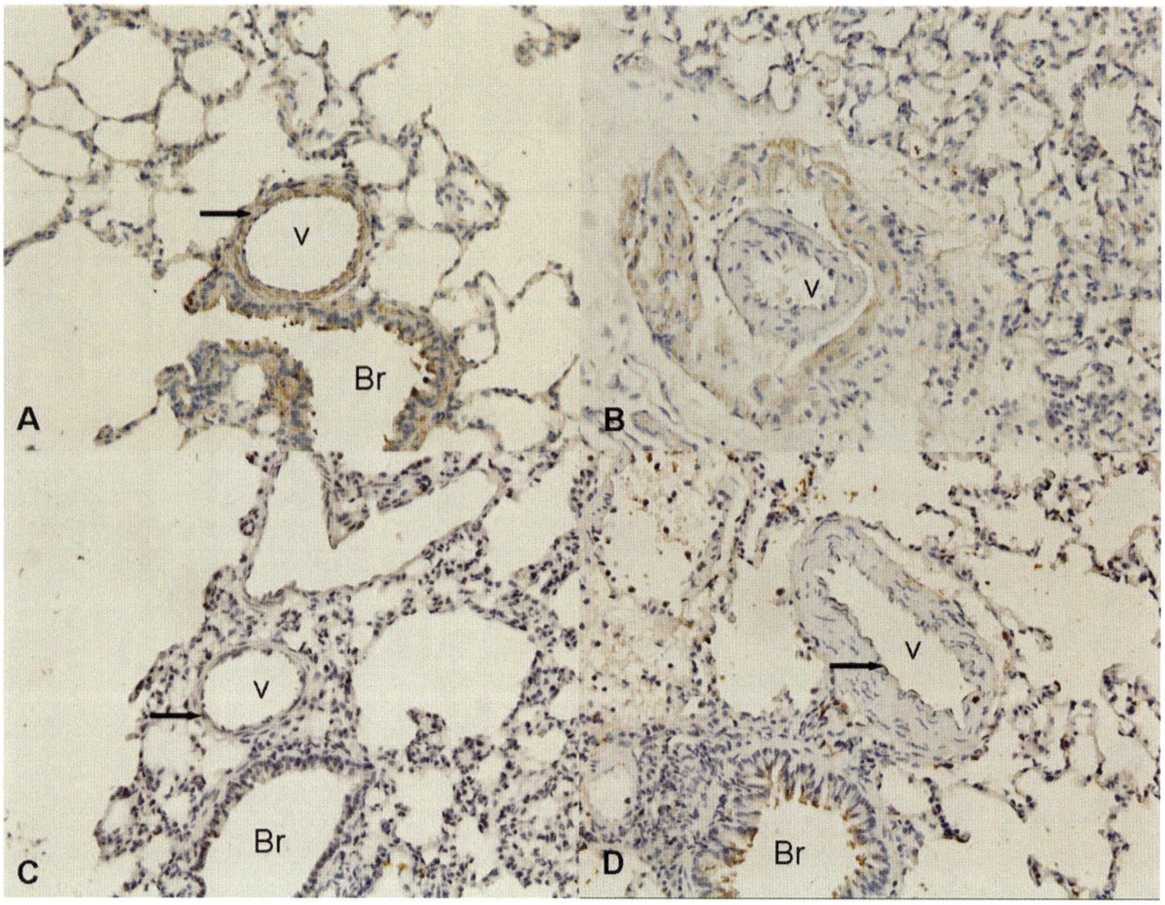

Figure 3. Immunohistochemistry staining of Notch1-4 receptors in rat lung tissues. (A–D) immunohistochemistry staining of Notch1-4 receptors in pulmonary artery of normal rats, respectively. (×400) V: Vessel; Br: Bronchium; Arrow: positive staining.

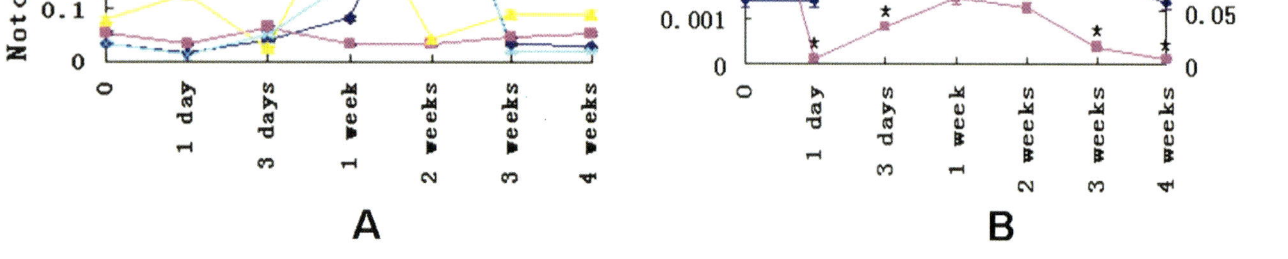

Figure 4. The gene expression of Notch receptors and their downstream effectors in PH rats. (A) the change of mRNA levels of Notch1-4 receptors in lung tissues of hypoxia rats. Notch3 mRNA level reached the peak at 1 week, whereas Notch1 and Notch4 did at 2 weeks. Compared to the baseline, the increase of Notch3 mRNA level was two folds, Notch1 four folds, and Notch4 five folds. All of them returned to the baseline by 3 weeks. (B) the change of mRNA levels of HERP1 and HERP2 in lung tissues of hypoxia rats. The mRNA level of HERP1 reached the peak at the second week and returned to basa level at the following days. The mRNA level of HERP2 decreased at the first day and maintained a low level in the following days. (*, $P<0.05$ compared to control group, Data were normalized to GAPDH and expressed as means ± s.e.m.)

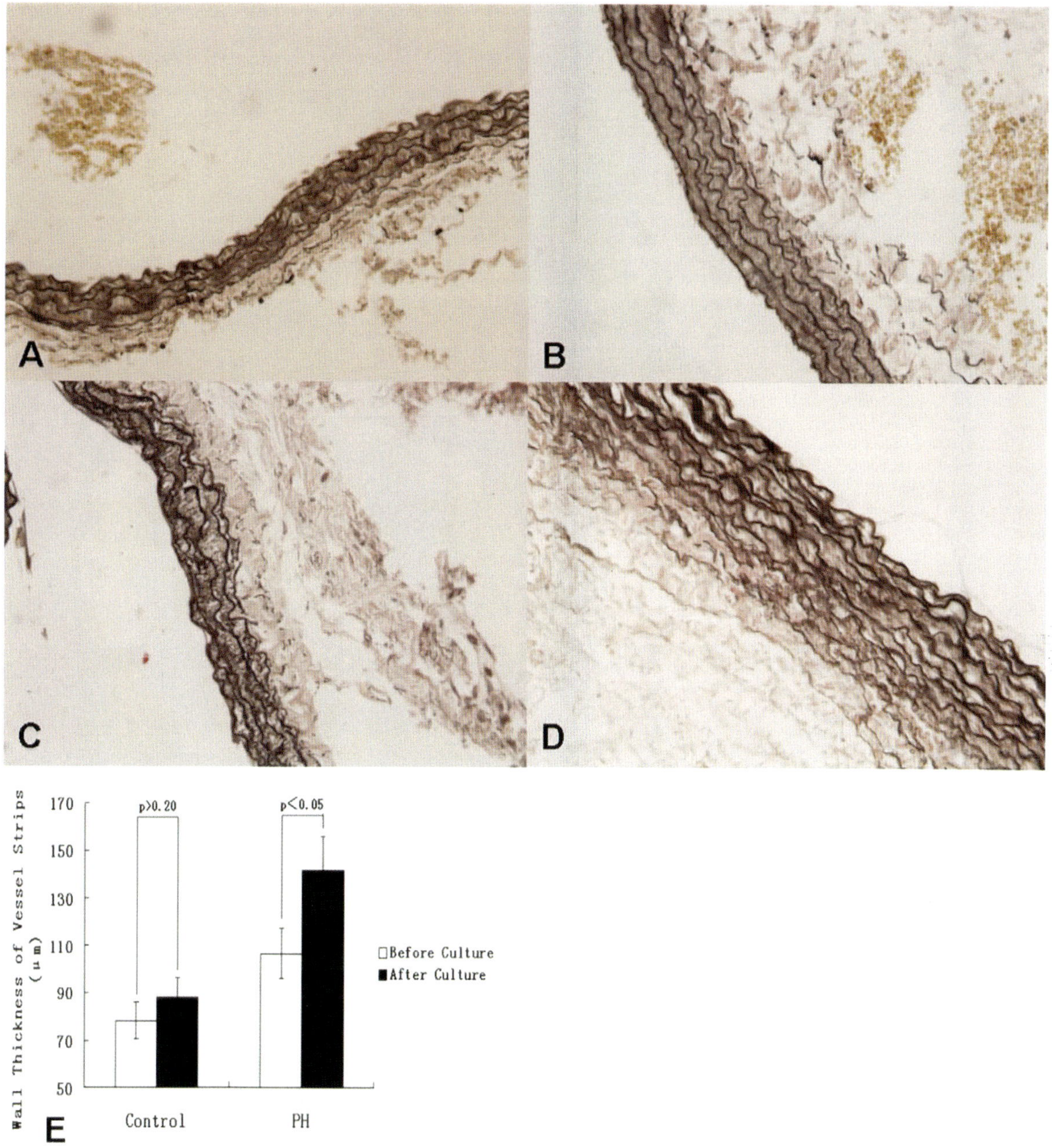

Figure 5. The wall thickness changes of vascular strips in culture. (A–D) Verhoeff iron hematocylin staining of Pulmonary artery vascular strips (×400): (A) pulmonary artery of control rat; (B) pulmonary artery of rat with 4-week-hypoxia; (C) pulmonary artery of control rat cultured for 8 days; (D) pulmonary artery of rat with 4-week-hypoxia cultured for 8 days. (E) the change of wall thickness of vessel strips in control and PH groups. Compared to the control, the thickness of vascular media of the hypoxia rats was significantly increased. While there was no significant difference between the strips of the control rats before and after culturing ($p>0.20$), the wall thickness of the strips from the hypoxia rats after culturing were significantly thicker than those before culturing, increasing about 30 μm. (*, $P<0.05$ compared to control group. Data are expressed as means ± s.e.m.)

result, the Notch intracellular domain (NICD) will be released, which then translocate to nucleus and activate the Notch signaling. The second enzymolysis is mediated by presenilin-dependent γ-secretase. DAPT is a specific inhibitor of γ-secretase that inhibits the hydrolysis of Notch protein. Accordingly, we determined whether the administration of DAPT influence the expression of Notch system. It was found that none of 4 Notch receptor mRNA levels showed significant differences following DAPT treatment when compared to the control (Figure 6A). However, the expressions of HERP-1 and HERP-2 genes were significantly inhibited in DAPT-low and DAPT-high groups, comparing with blank and DMSO control groups (Figure 6B, $p<0.05$).

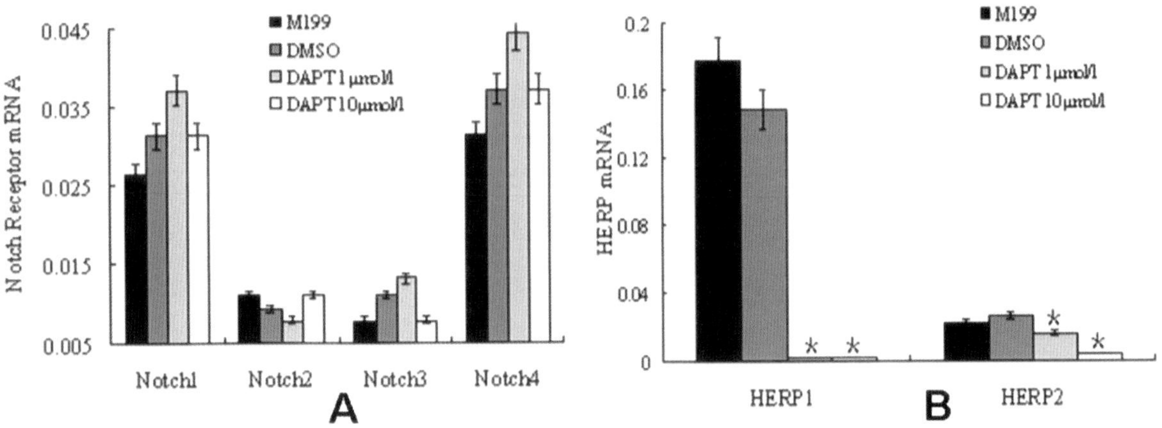

Figure 6. The impact of DAPT on Notch signaling in vascular strips from PH rats. (A) the effects of DAPT on the mRNA level of Notch receptors in vessel strips of hypoxia rats. No significant differences of Notch receptors mRNA levels among experimental groups were detected by ANOVA. (B) the effects of DAPT on the mRNA levels of HERP1 and HERP2 in vessel strips of hypoxia rats. The mRNA levels of HERP1 and HERP2 were significantly lower In both low and high dosage of DAPT groups than in blank and DMSO control groups. However, there were no significant differences between blank and DMSO control groups, or between DAPT-low and DAPT-high groups. (*, $P<0.05$ compared to control group. Data were normalized to GAPDH and expressed as means ± s.e.m.)

DAPT Inhibits the Increase of Wall Thickness in Cultured Vascular Strips from PH Rats

Next, we determined the thickness of vascular wall in presence of DAPT in the culture. As shown in Figures 5&7, in the absence of DAPT, the thickness of vascular wall in rats of hypoxia treatment increased significantly ($p<0.05$). However, DAPT treatment decreased the thickness of vascular strips when compared to blank and DMSO controls.

PCNA is a co-factor of DNA polymerase δ involved in DNA synthesis and associated with cell proliferation. To understand the DAPT-mediated inhibition of vascular wall thickening, we determined the presence status of PCNA among different culture conditions. It was found that PCNA positive rates in blank control and DMSO control groups were higher than in DAPT-low and DAPT-high groups. There were no significant differences between blank and DMSO control groups, or between DAPT-low and DAPT-high groups (Figure 8), suggesting DAPT mediated an effect of anti-proliferation.

The Effects of DAPT on the Phenotype of Vascular Smooth Muscle Cells (VSMCs) in Culturing Strips from PH Rats

According to the structure and function difference, two phenotypes of VSMCs have been defined: contractile and synthetic. The contractile VSMCs are full of muscle fibers with less cell organelles such as rough endoplasmic reticulum and Golgi apparatus, and express some specific proteins such as SM-MHC and SM22α, and the former is the most reliable marker of the mature contractile VSMCs [27]. The synthetic VSMCs are lack of muscle fibers but contain rich cell organelles such as rough endoplasmic reticulum, ribosome, and Golgi apparatus, Synthetic VSMCs proliferate actively, and synthesize matrix proteins, such as matrix Gla protein (MGP) and osteopontin which are considered as the specific markers of the synthetic VSMCs [28]. In the current study, to determine the impact of Notch signaling on VSMC phenotypes, we measured the mRNA levels of SM-MHC, SM22α, MGP, and osteopontin in cultured strips in the absence or presence of DAPT. Our results revealed that the mRNA levels of SM-MHC and SM22α were significantly lower in blank and DMSO control groups than in DAPT-low and DAPT-high groups ($p<0.05$). There were no significant differences of the mRNA levels of SM-MHC and SM22α either between blank control and DMSO control groups, or between DAPT-low and DAPT-high groups. Furthermore, there were no significant differences of the mRNA levels of MGP and osteopontin among blank control, DMSO control, DAPT-low, and DAPT-high groups (Figure 9). These results suggested that inhibition of Notch signaling by DAPT, promoted the expression of contract proteins in pulmonary arterial smooth muscle cells and facilitated the development of contractile phenotype.

The Effects of DAPT on Apoptosis of VSMCs in Culturing Strips from PH Rats

Caspase-3 is an effect factor in caspase-mediated apoptosis, which plays an indispensable role in apoptosis. The expression of caspase-3 is widely used for estimation of apoptosis. Therefore, the percentages of caspase-3 positive cells were measured in the present study and they were significantly higher in DAPT-low and DAPT-high groups than blank control and DMSO control groups. There were no significant differences between blank control and DMSO control groups, or between DAPT-low and DAPT-high groups. (Figure 10).

Bax promotes apoptosis, whereas Bcl-xl promotes cell survival. When the ratio of Bax to Bcl-xl is high, the cell is more prone to apoptosis, or vice versa. Our results indicated that DAPT treatment led to an increase of Bax mRNA level, and decrease of Bcl-xl level in vascular strips, resulting in a significant increase of Bax/Bcl-xl ratio and apoptosis (Figure 11). Collectively, we postulated that DAPT may attenuate PH by inhibiting proliferation and inducing apoptosis through regulating caspase-3, Bax, and Bcl-xl expression.

As to the culturing strips from normal rats, DAPT could also impact on Notch signaling (Figure S1). However, DAPT did not effect on the wall thickness (Figure S2). Meanwhile, there were no significant changes of PCNA positive rate, VSMCs' phenotype, and the expressions of caspase 3 and Bax in normal pulmonary arterial strips treated by DAPT (data not shown). These results suggested that the inhibition of Notch signaling by DAPT in normal pulmonary arteries would not change the biological traits of these arteries.

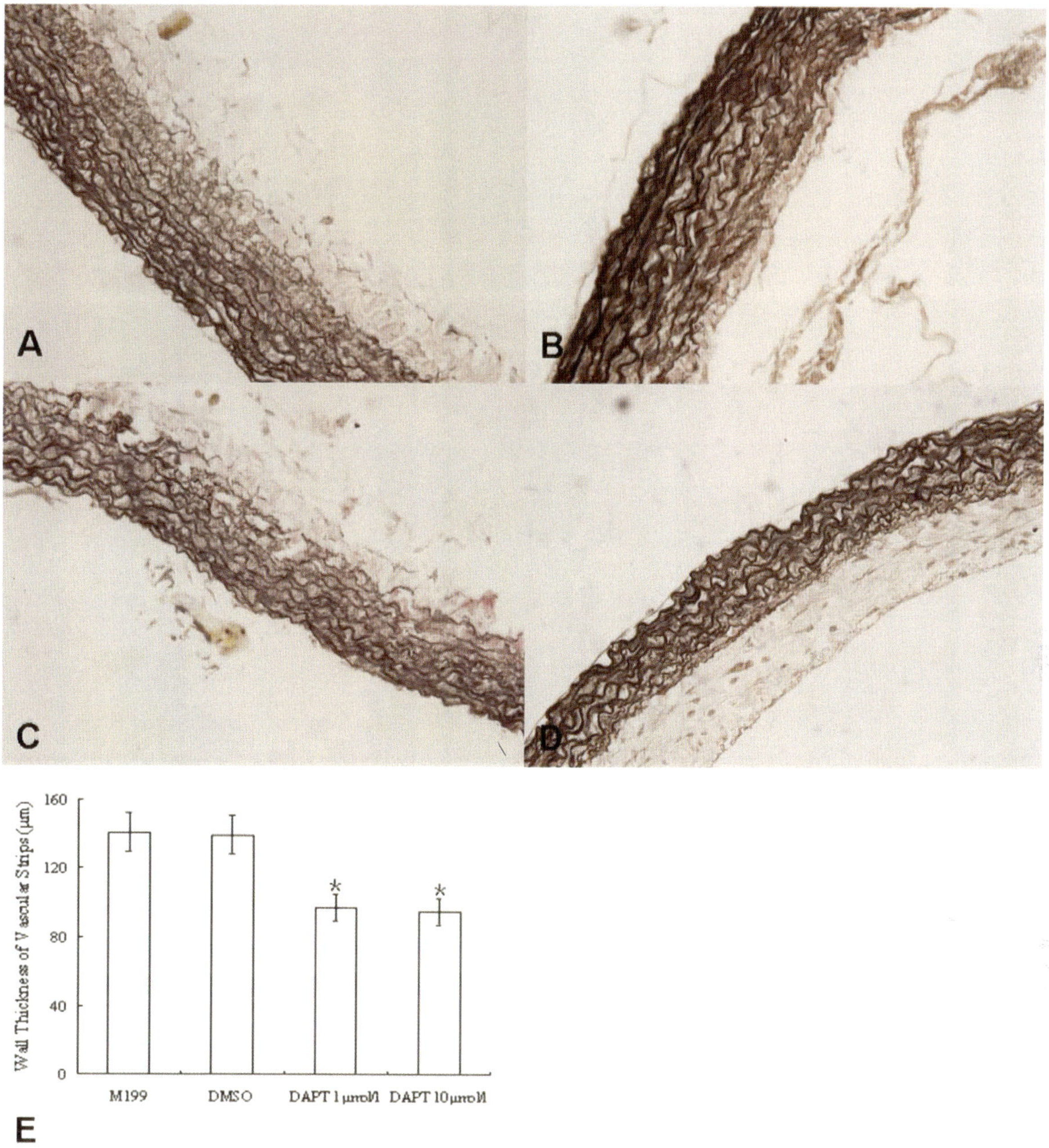

Figure 7. DAPT inhibits the increase of wall thickness in cultured vascular strips from PH rats. (A–D) Verhoeff iron hematocylin staining of Pulmonary artery vascular strips (×400): (A) pulmonary artery in culturing lung tissue strip treated with additional equivalent M199; (B) pulmonary artery in culturing lung tissue strip treated with DMSO; (C) pulmonary artery in culturing lung tissue strip treated with DAPT (1 μmol/l); (D) pulmonary artery in culturing lung tissue strip treated with DAPT (10 μmol/l). (E) the change of vascular media thickness of hypoxia rats with or without DAPT treating. The vascular media of hypoxia rats treated with DAPT were significantly thinner than those treated with M199 or DMSO. (*, $P<0.05$ compared to control group. Data are expressed as means ± s.e.m.)

Discussion

The rat model of PH inducted by hypoxia is one of the most successful models in the studies of PH. When rats stay in hypoxia environment, the initial contraction of pulmonary arteriole leads to a temporary increase of pulmonary arterial pressure. As the hypoxia persists, the pulmonary arterial remodeling occurs, including thickening of the vessel wall, decreasing the vessel lumen and compliance, and increasing the pulmonary arterial pressure and vascular resistance, ultimately the hypertrophy of right ventricle [3]. In this study, this hypoxia-induced PH was utilized and validated with the body weight decrease and pulmonary arterial pressure increase which reached the peak at 14 days. Consistently, with the prolongation of the hypoxia condition, Fulton index increased in rats. Therefore, the rat model of PH in this study was valid for the evaluation of the roles of Notch system in the pathogenesis of PH.

To date, four Notch receptors (Notch1, Notch2, Notch3, and Notch4) have been defined in mammals. Among them, Notch1,

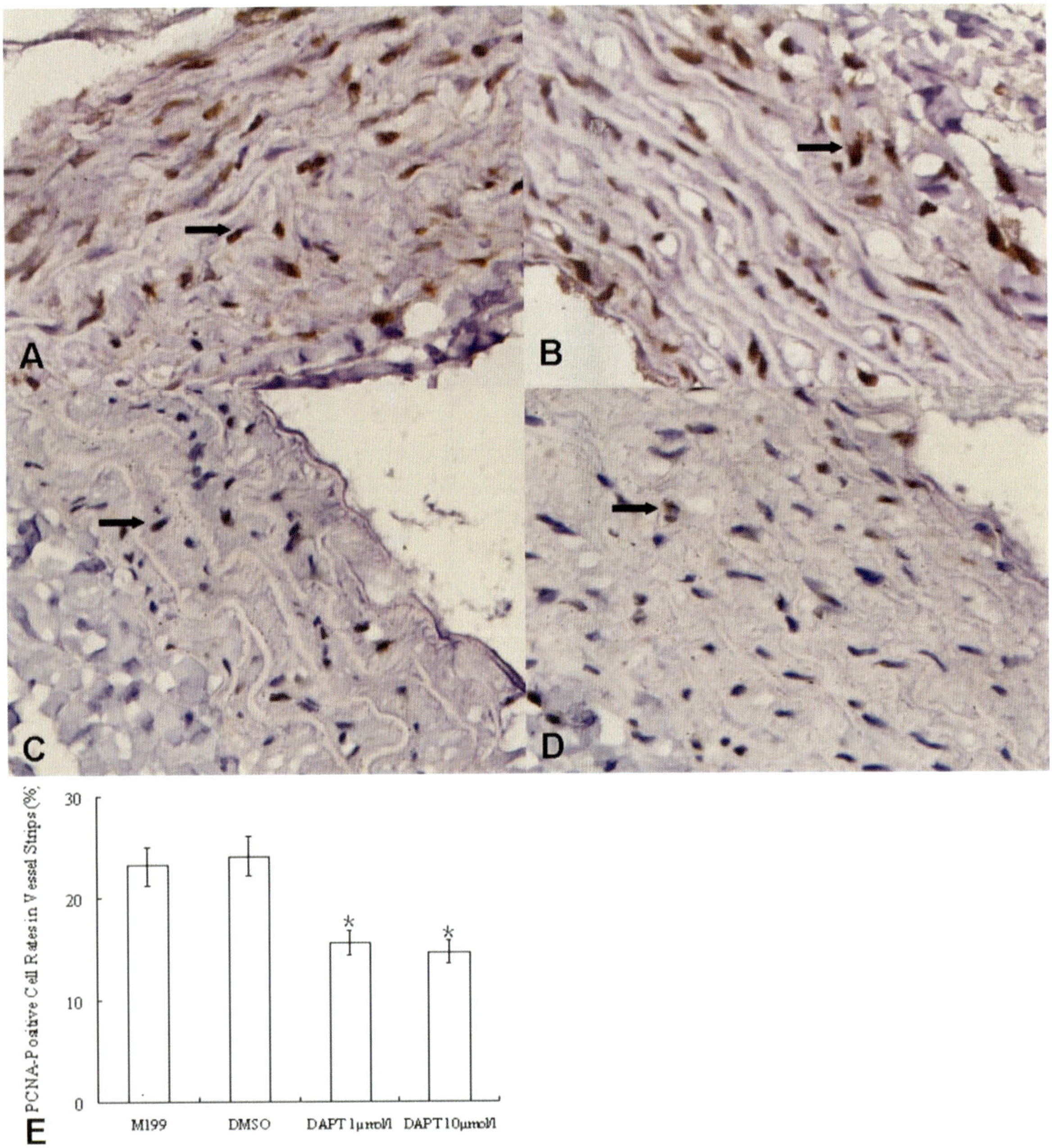

Figure 8. DAPT inhibits the proliferation of cultured vascular strips from PH rats. (A–D) PCNA immunohistochemistry staining in pulmonary artery strips (×400, nuclear staining): (A) pulmonary artery in culturing lung tissue strip treated with additional equivalent M199; (B) pulmonary artery in culturing lung tissue strip treated with DMSO; (C) pulmonary artery in culturing lung tissue strip treated with DAPT (1 μmol/l); (D) pulmonary artery in culturing lung tissue strip treated with DAPT (10 μmol/l). (E) the change of PCNA-positive cell rate in vessel strips from hypoxia rats with or without DAPT treatment. The PCNA-positive cell rates in vessel strips from hypoxia rats treated with DAPT were significantly lower than those of blank and DMSO control hypoxia rats. However, the PCNA-positive cell rates between the two DAPT treating groups or between the blank and DMSO control groups were not significantly different. (*, $P<0.05$ compared to control group. Data are expressed as means ± s.e.m.) Arrow: positive staining.

Notch3, and Notch4 exist in blood vessels. In addition, three downstream effectors (HERP1, HERP2, and HERP3) of Notch signaling are mainly present in arteries. In the current study, we examined the localization of Notch receptors in the rat PH model and the results were consistent with previous studies in other conditions: Notch4 is mainly expressed in arterial endothelial cells and occasionally in arterial smooth muscle cells; Notch3 is mainly expressed in arterial smooth muscle cells; Notch1 is expressed in both arterial endothelial cells and smooth muscle cells [9,13,14,16,17,18,21]. However, the expression levels of Notch1, Notch3, Notch4, and the downstream target genes HERP1 and HERP2 all have been changed in pulmonary arteries in the condition of PH. Among them, the mRNA levels of Notch1, Notch3, Notch 4, and HERP1 progressively increased with a peak at one week for Notch 3 and at two weeks for Notch1, Notch 4, and HERP1. The mRNA levels of the four proteins gradually

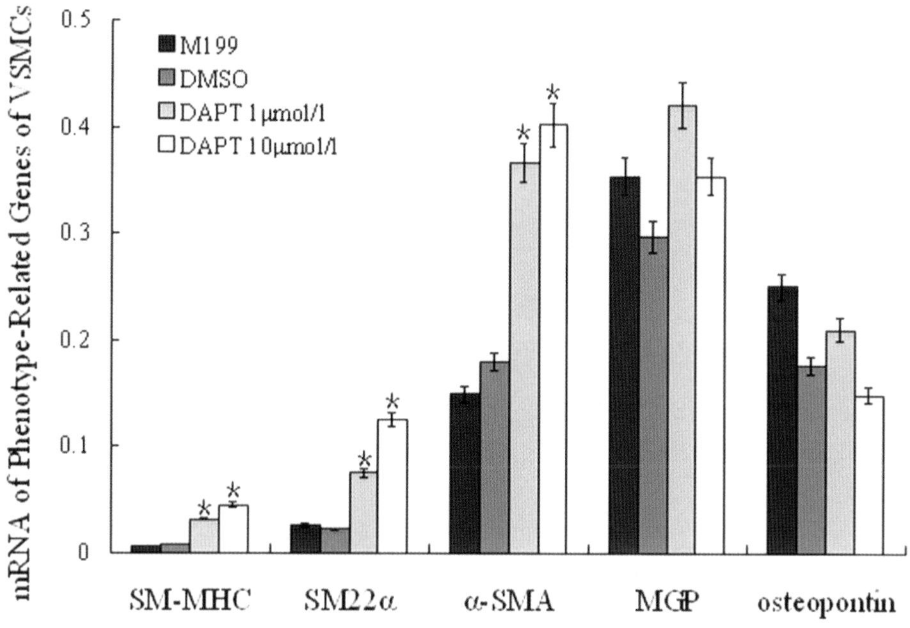

Figure 9. The effect of DAPT on the expression of phenotype-related genes of VSMCs from hypoxia rats. Compared to blank and DMSO control groups, the expressions of SM-MHC and SM22α in both low- and high- dosage of DAPT groups were significantly increased ($p<0.05$). There were no significant differences of expression of these two genes between low- and high- dosage of DAPT groups, or between blank and DMSO control groups, respectively ($p>0.2$). The expressions of MGP and osteopontin were not significantly different in the four groups ($p>0.2$). (*, $P<0.05$ compared to control group. Data were normalized to GAPDH and expressed as means ± s.e.m.)

decreased. The time of peaks of mRNA levels were coincident with the time of fastest increase of PH. The results suggested that Notch signaling pathway, especially those factors involved in vascular remodeling, contributed to the development of PH induced by hypoxia. To date, the role that Notch signaling plays in the development of hypoxia induced PH has not been clearly elucidated. But in the studies of neural precursor cells, glioblastoma stem cells, medulloblastoma stem cell, and myogenic cell, it has been found that hypoxia-inducible factor-1α (HIF-1α), an intracellular mediator of oxygen sensing, could interact and stabilize NICD, and activate Notch signaling pathway, to preserve these cell viability and expansion under hypoxic conditions [29,30,31,32]. In addition, HIF-1α and VEGF regulate Notch signaling to accelerate choroidal neovascularization angiogenesis [33]. Thus, NICD is at the convergence point of HIF-1α, which has been implicated in the development of PH. Recently, integration between Notch and BMP signaling pathways has been found in several organs and cell types, while BMPR2 mutations have been found to be associated with the development of familial human PAH [2,3,4,5,34,35,36,37]. It might be one of the mechanisms that Notch signaling pathway functioned in the development of PH. Especially, as to Notch 3, Li et al showed that the mRNA and protein levels of Notch3 continually increased along with the development of PH in the lungs of idiopathic PH patients as well as in hypoxia-induced PH mice and in monocrotaline-induced PH rats [24]. However, in this study, the mRNA level of Notch 3 reached the peak at one week after hypoxia. This difference may be attributed to the distinct tissues where total RNA were isolated.

In the classic Notch pathway, there are two consecutive protein enzymolysis processes after the conjunction of Notch receptors and ligands. The second enzymolysis involves presenilin-dependent γ-secretase. A similar γ-secretase was found in the transmembrane domain of APP, which is important in the last step of amyloid-β protein production, which is thought to contribute to the pathogenesis of Alzheimer's disease. DAPT, a small molecular specific inhibitor of γ-secretase, has been shown to have potential therapeutic value for Alzheimer's disease [38,39,40]. Recent studies showed that DAPT could inhibit Notch signaling in Drosophila and cultured cells, such as neuron, nephron cell, and myocardial cell. Furthermore, DAPT can inhibit the translocation of NICD [38,39,40]. Because the transduction of Notch signaling is restricted to interaction of ligands and receptors of Notch from cell-to-cell contact, which can be greatly affected by interactions of cells and cellular microenvironments [20,21]. In the current study, we used an organ culture system containing rat tail collagen [41] to imitate the in vivo environment for vascular adventitia [42,43]. Of note, because the rat tail collagen is the same vascular extracellular matrix for the pulmonary strip in the culture, it is one key component for successful culturing artery strip to maintain the endothelium, smooth muscle, fibroblasts, and extracellular matrix of the vessel in a similar environment in vivo. Using this system of organ culture, we found the thickness of vascular wall of PH rats decreased 30% after treating with DAPT to the cultured vascular strips of PH rats by hypoxia, as well as the expression level of apoptotic factors (caspase-3 and Bax) increased significantly. The results suggested that DAPT treating could inhibit cellular proliferation and promote apoptosis, which was consistent with previous study [24]. Notably, our results highlighted the bax/caspase-3 pathway in the apoptosis induced by DAPT treating. In addition, while DAPT did not change the mRNA level of Notch receptors of the vascular strips, the mRNA levels of downstream effectors, HERP1 and HERP2, decreased significantly in the presence of DAPT, suggesting that DAPT mediated inhibition of intracellular Notch signaling pathway without impacting on the expression of Notch receptors. At the same time, the mRNA levels of SM-MHC and SM22α increased significantly by DAPT, suggesting a conversion of VSMC phenotype.

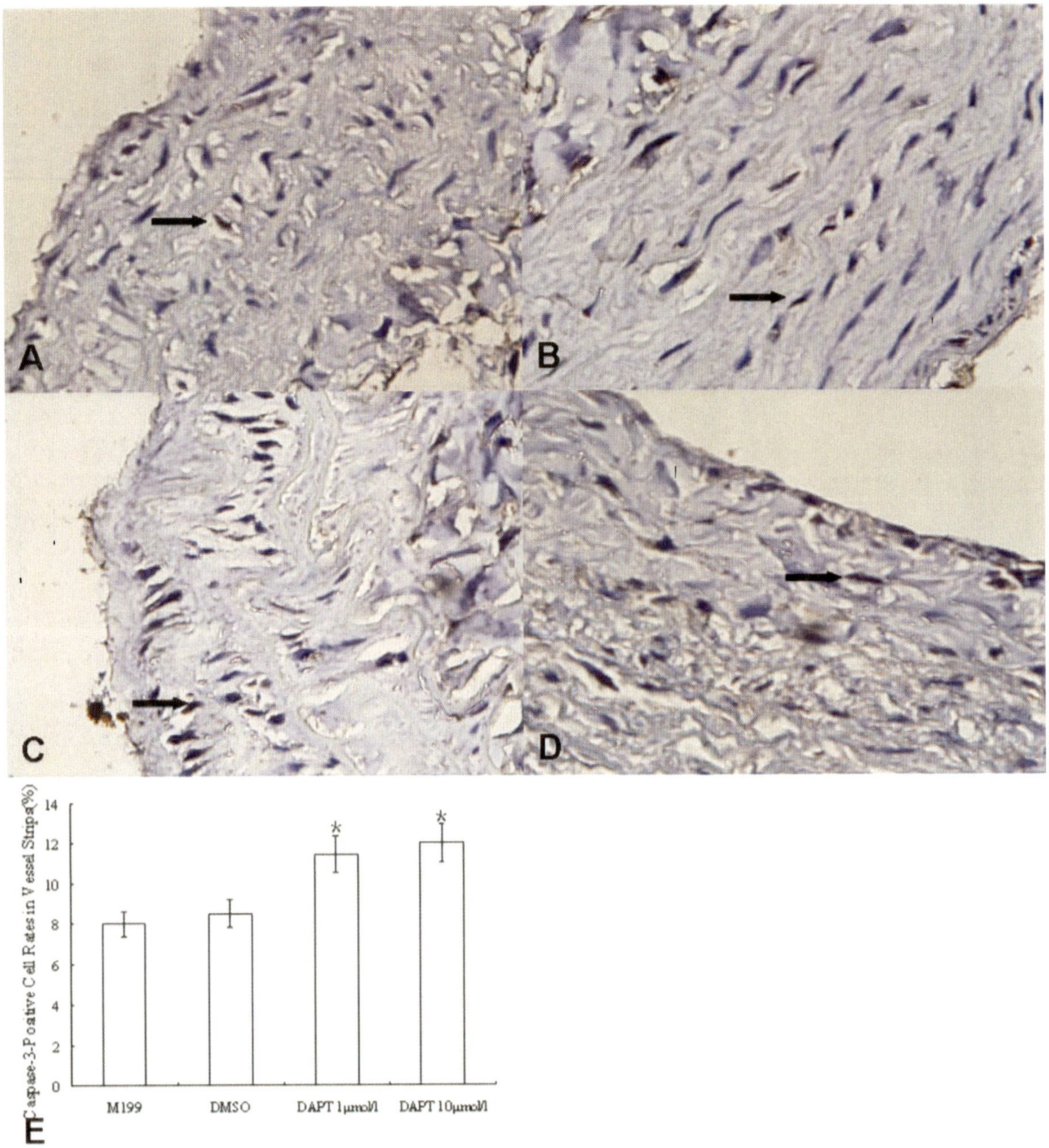

Figure 10. The change of caspase-3-positive rates of vascular wall cells from hypoxia rats with or without DAPT treating. (A–D) Caspase-3 immunohistochemistry staining in pulmonary artery strips (×400, cytoplasmic staining): (A) pulmonary artery in culturing lung tissue strip treated with additional equivalent M199; (B) pulmonary artery in culturing lung tissue strip treated with DMSO; (C) pulmonary artery in culturing lung tissue strip treated with DAPT (1 μmol/l); (D) pulmonary artery in culturing lung tissue strip treated with DAPT (10 μmol/l). (E) The change of caspase-3-positive rate of vascular wall cells from hypoxia rats with or without DAPT treating. The caspase-3-positive cell rates in vessel strips from hypoxia rats treated with DAPT (1 μmol/l) or (10 μmol/l) were significantly higher than those treated with M199 (blank control)or DMSO($p<0.05$). However, the caspase-3-positive cell rates between the two DAPT treatment groups or between the blank and DMSO control groups were not significantly different. (*, $P<0.05$ compared to control group. Data are expressed as means ± s.e.m.) Arrow: positive staining.

Our results suggested an important role of Notch signaling pathway in vascular remodeling in PH, not only Notch3 but also Notch1 and 4. However, this pathway functions differently depending on time, environment, and cell types. Notch system in arterial system is delicately regulated by regulatory factors involved in development and growth factor released following vascular injury [33,34,35]. It has been shown that Notch 1 and Notch 3 promoted the proliferation, migration and aggregation of VSMCs, disinhibited cell cycle arrest, inhibited apoptosis of VSMCs, and facilitated the conversion of endothelial cells and fibroblasts to smooth muscle cells [24,27,44,45,46,47,48,49,50,51,52,53,54,55,56,57,58,59,60,61,62-,63]. These potential mechanisms may include: 1) inhibiting the transcription of p27kip1 and p21cip1, prompting VSMCs to

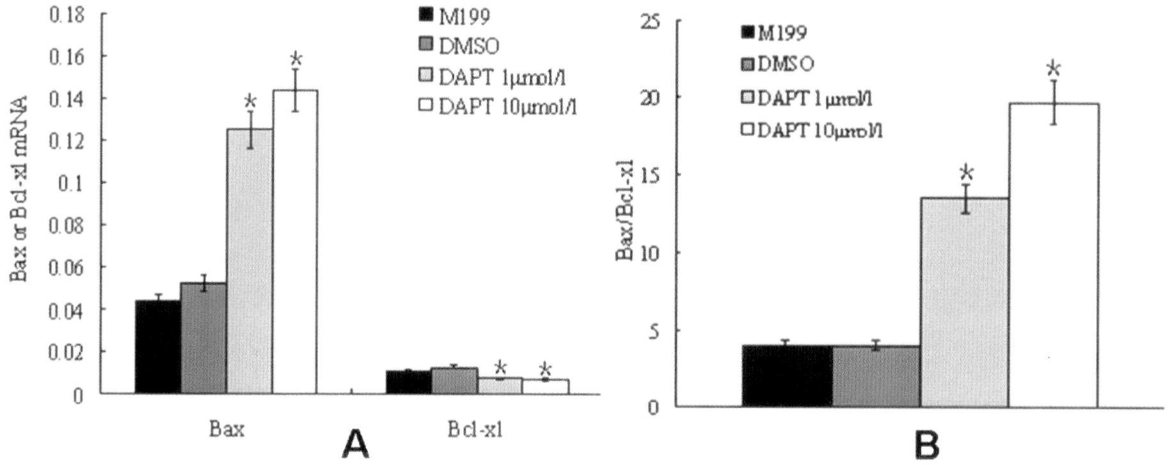

Figure 11. The effect of DAPT on Bax and Bcl-xl mRNA expressions in pulmonary artery strips from hypoxia rats. The mRNA level of Bax increased while the mRNA level of Bcl-xl decreased after DAPT treatment. The ratio of Bax mRNA to Bcl-xl mRNA significantly increased after DAPT treating. (*, P<0.05 compared to control group. Data were normalized to GAPDH and expressed as means ± s.e.m.)

enter S phase, and causing the proliferation of VSMCs; 2) promoting the transcription of Guanine exchange factor of Rac and Sos1, and leading to increasing activity of Rac1 and proliferation, migration, and aggregation of VSMCs; 3) promoting the expression of C-FLIP, activating Akt, increasing the expression of Bcl-xl and decreasing the expression of Bax, and inhibiting the apoptosis of VSMCs; 4) activating the promoter of Smooth muscle α-actin (SMA) gene, increasing the expression of SMA, and prompting VSMCs to transform to synthetic phenotype and EMT; 5) inhibiting the expressions and activities of various marker genes of VSMCs under certain circumstances, preventing the combination of serum response factor (SRF) and CArG box and differentiation of VSMCs, and prompting VSMCs to transform to synthetic phenotype [24,27,44,45,46,47,48,49,50,51,52,53,54,55,56,57,58,59,60,61,62-,63]. In the mean time, Notch 1 and Notch 4 inhibit the proliferation, migration, and apoptosis of endothelial cells, maintain the "quiescence" phenotype of the cells, and keep vascular endothelium stable [64,65,66,67,68,69,70,71,72,73,74]. Notch 1 regulates endothelial progenitor cell activity [75,76] and impedes the appearance of endothelial teloblasts and the budding/growth of blood vessels [77]. In summary, the function of Notch pathway in vascular remodeling is complicated. We found that the expressions of Notch1, Notch 3, and Notch4 changed in a time dependent pattern following the development of PH and the inhibition of Notch signaling by DAPT could reverse the biological traits of VSMCs in PH rats, including the decreasing proliferation, the increasing apoptosis, and the phenotypic transformation of VSMCs, finally inhibiting the pulmonary vascular remodeling. Therefore, further investigation is needed to dissect the specific function of each Notch factors, especially Notch1 and 4, in different types of cell and different stages of vascular remodeling in PH.

In conclusion, the current study suggested Notch pathway play an important role in pulmonary vascular remodeling in PH and targeting Notch signaling pathway could be a valuable approach to design new therapy for PH.

Supporting Information

Figure S1 The impact of DAPT on Notch signal in vascular strips of normal rats. (A) the effects of DAPT on the mRNA level of Notch receptors in vessel strips of normal rats. No significant differences of Notch receptors mRNA levels among experimental groups were detected by ANOVA. (B) the effects of DAPT on the mRNA levels of HERP1 and HERP2 in vessel strips of normal rats. The mRNA levels of HERP1 and HERP2 were significantly lower in both low and high dosage of DAPT groups than in blank and DMSO control groups. However, there were no significant differences between blank and DMSO control groups, or between DAPT-low and DAPT-high groups. (*, P<0.05 compared to control group. Data were normalized to GAPDH and expressed as means ± s.e.m.)
(TIF)

Figure S2 DAPT does not decrease wall thickness in cultured vascular strips from normal rats. (A-D) Verhoeff iron hematocylin staining of Pulmonary artery vascular strips (×400): (A) pulmonary artery in culturing lung tissue strip treated with additional equivalent M199; (B) pulmonary artery in culturing lung tissue strip treated with DMSO; (C) pulmonary artery in culturing lung tissue strip treated with DAPT (1 μmol/l); (D) pulmonary artery in culturing lung tissue strip treated with DAPT (10 μmol/l). (E) the change of vascular media thickness of hypoxia rats with or without DAPT treating. The vascular media of hypoxia rats treated with DAPT were not significantly different to those treated with M199 or DMSO. (*, P<0.05 compared to control group. Data are expressed as means ± s.e.m.)
(TIF)

Acknowledgments

We thank Drs. Bangliang Xiao, Lixing Yuan, Qianping Tang, and Weibo Chen for the expert technical assistance. We acknowledge Drs. Wendong Wang and Qin Huang for conducting immunohistochemistry experiments. We also thank Dr. Qiongying Li, for providing lab space to conduct some experiments in the present study.

Author Contributions

Conceived and designed the experiments: LNQ TFZ. Performed the experiments: LNQ KS YMH HML. Analyzed the data: LNQ LX. Contributed reagents/materials/analysis tools: LNQ LX KS TFZ YMH HML. Wrote the paper: LNQ LX TFZ.

References

1. Stenmark KR, Fagan KA, Frid MG (2006) Hypoxia-induced pulmonary vascular remodeling: cellular and molecular mechanisms. Circ Res 99: 675–691.
2. Chan SY, Loscalzo J (2008) Pathogenic mechanisms of pulmonary arterial hypertension. J Mol Cell Cardiol 44: 14–30.
3. Humbert M, Morrell NW, Archer SL, Stenmark KR, MacLean MR, et al. (2004) Cellular and molecular pathobiology of pulmonary arterial hypertension. J Am Coll Cardiol 43: 13S–24S.
4. Yildiz P (2009) Molecular mechanisms of pulmonary hypertension. Clin Chim Acta 403: 9–16.
5. Morrell NW, Adnot S, Archer SL, Dupuis J, Jones PL, et al. (2009) Cellular and molecular basis of pulmonary arterial hypertension. J Am Coll Cardiol 54: S20–31.
6. Agarwal R, Gomberg-Maitland M (2011) Current therapeutics and practical management strategies for pulmonary arterial hypertension. American Heart Journal 162: 201–213.
7. McLaughlin VV (2011) Looking to the future: a new decade of pulmonary arterial hypertension therapy. Eur Respir Rev 20: 262–269.
8. Ahmed Z, Bicknell R (2009) Angiogenic signalling pathways. Methods Mol Biol 467: 3–24.
9. Gridley T (2010) Notch signaling in the vasculature. Curr Top Dev Biol 92: 277–309.
10. Li JL, Harris AL (2005) Notch signaling from tumor cells: a new mechanism of angiogenesis. Cancer Cell 8: 1–3.
11. Swift MR, Weinstein BM (2009) Arterial-venous specification during development. Circ Res 104: 576–588.
12. Hirashima M (2009) Regulation of endothelial cell differentiation and arterial specification by VEGF and Notch signaling. Anat Sci Int 84: 95–101.
13. Kume T (2010) Specification of arterial, venous, and lymphatic endothelial cells during embryonic development. Histol Histopathol 25: 637–646.
14. Corada M, Nyqvist D, Orsenigo F, Caprini A, Giampietro C, et al. (2010) The Wnt/beta-catenin pathway modulates vascular remodeling and specification by upregulating Dll4/Notch signaling. Dev Cell 18: 938–949.
15. Holderfield MT, Hughes CC (2008) Crosstalk between vascular endothelial growth factor, notch, and transforming growth factor-beta in vascular morphogenesis. Circ Res 102: 637–652.
16. Gridley T (2007) Notch signaling in vascular development and physiology. Development 134: 2709–2718.
17. Roca C, Adams RH (2007) Regulation of vascular morphogenesis by Notch signaling. Genes Dev 21: 2511–2524.
18. Hofmann JJ, Iruela-Arispe ML (2007) Notch signaling in blood vessels: who is talking to whom about what? Circ Res 100: 1556–1568.
19. Yamamizu K, Matsunaga T, Uosaki H, Fukushima H, Katayama S, et al. (2010) Convergence of Notch and beta-catenin signaling induces arterial fate in vascular progenitors. J Cell Biol 189: 325–338.
20. Miele L (2006) Notch signaling. Clin Cancer Res 12: 1074–1079.
21. Ehebauer M, Hayward P, Arias AM (2006) Notch, a universal arbiter of cell fate decisions. Science 314: 1414–1415.
22. Sprinzak D, Lakhanpal A, LeBon L, Santat LA, Fontes ME, et al. (2010) Cis-interactions between Notch and Delta generate mutually exclusive signalling states. Nature 465: 86-U95.
23. Miniati D, Jelin EB, Ng J, Wu JF, Carlson TR, et al. (2010) Constitutively active endothelial Notch4 causes lung arteriovenous shunts in mice. American Journal of Physiology-Lung Cellular and Molecular Physiology 298: L169–L177.
24. Li X, Zhang X, Leathers R, Makino A, Huang C, et al. (2009) Notch3 signaling promotes the development of pulmonary arterial hypertension. Nat Med 15: 1289–1297.
25. Qiao LN, Wang XM, Liu ZQ, Wang XQ, Zhou TF, et al. (2011) [The influence of inhibiting notch signal on pulmonary vascular remodeling induced by PDGF]. Sichuan Da Xue Xue Bao Yi Xue Ban 42: 766–70. Chinese.
26. Qiao LN, Xu HB, Shi K, Zhou TF, Hua YM, et al. (2011) [Effect of inhibition of Notch signal on pulmonary vascular remodeling induced by angiotensin II]. Zhongguo Dang Dai Er Ke Za Zhi 13: 503–8. Chinese.
27. Doi H, Iso T, Sato H, Yamazaki M, Matsui H, et al. (2006) Jagged1-selective notch signaling induces smooth muscle differentiation via a RBP-Jkappa-dependent pathway. J Biol Chem 281: 28555–28564.
28. Yamamoto M, Aoyagi M, Azuma H, Yamamoto K (1997) Changes in osteopontin mRNA expression during phenotypic transition of rabbit arterial smooth muscle cells. Histochem Cell Biol 107: 279–287.
29. Mutoh T, Sanosaka T, Ito K, Nakashima K (2012) Oxygen levels epigenetically regulate fate switching of neural precursor cells via hypoxia-inducible factor 1α-notch signal interaction in the developing brain. Stem Cells 30: 561–9.
30. Qiang L, Wu T, Zhang HW, Lu N, Hu R, et al. (2012) HIF-1α is critical for hypoxia-mediated maintenance of glioblastoma stem cells by activating Notch signaling pathway. Cell Death Differ 19: 284–94.
31. Pistollato F, Rampazzo E, Persano L, Abbadi S, Frasson C, et al. (2010) Interaction of hypoxia-inducible factor-1α and Notch signaling regulates medulloblastoma precursor proliferation and fate. Stem Cells 28: 1918–29.
32. Zheng X, Linke S, Dias JM, Zheng X, Gradin K, et al. (2008) Interaction with factor inhibiting HIF-1 defines an additional mode of cross-coupling between the Notch and hypoxia signaling pathways. Proc Natl Acad Sci U S A 105: 3368–73.
33. Dong X, Wang YS, Dou GR, Hou HY, Shi YY, et al. (2011) Influence of Dll4 via HIF-1α-VEGF signaling on the angiogenesis of choroidal neovascularization under hypoxic conditions. PLoS One 6: e18481.
34. Bordonaro M, Tewari S, Atamna W, Lazarova DL (2011) The Notch ligand Delta-like 1 integrates inputs from TGFbeta/Activin and Wnt pathways. Exp Cell Res 317: 1368–81.
35. Tang Y, Urs S, Boucher J, Bernaiche T, Venkatesh D, et al. (2010) Notch and transforming growth factor-beta (TGFbeta) signaling pathways cooperatively regulate vascular smooth muscle cell differentiation. J Biol Chem 285: 17556–63.
36. Zhang Y, Zhang J, Navrazhina K, Argaw AT, Zameer A, et al. (2010) TGFbeta1 induces Jagged1 expression in astrocytes via ALK5 and Smad3 and regulates the balance between oligodendrocyte progenitor proliferation and differentiation. Glia 58: 964–74.
37. Blokzijl A, Dahlqvist C, Reissmann E, Falk A, Moliner A, et al. (2003) Cross-talk between the Notch and TGF-beta signaling pathways mediated by interaction of the Notch intracellular domain with Smad3. J Cell Biol 163: 723–8.
38. Micchelli CA, Esler WP, Kimberly WT, Jack C, Berezovska O, et al. (2003) Gamma-secretase/presenilin inhibitors for Alzheimer's disease phenocopy Notch mutations in Drosophila. FASEB J 17: 79–81.
39. Morohashi Y, Kan T, Tominari Y, Fuwa H, Okamura Y, et al. (2006) C-terminal fragment of presenilin is the molecular target of a dipeptidic gamma-secretase-specific inhibitor DAPT (N-[N-(3,5-difluorophenacetyl)-L-alanyl]-S-phenylglycine t-butyl ester). J Biol Chem 281: 14670–14676.
40. Nelson BR, Hartman BH, Georgi SA, Lan MS, Reh TA (2007) Transient inactivation of Notch signaling synchronizes differentiation of neural progenitor cells. Dev Biol 304: 479–498.
41. Montesano R, Orci L (1985) Tumor-promoting phorbol esters induce angiogenesis in vitro. Cell 42: 469–477.
42. Cowan KN, Jones PL, Rabinovitch M (1999) Regression of hypertrophied rat pulmonary arteries in organ culture is associated with suppression of proteolytic activity, inhibition of tenascin-C, and smooth muscle cell apoptosis. Circ Res 84: 1223–1233.
43. Merklinger SL, Jones PL, Martinez EC, Rabinovitch M (2005) Epidermal growth factor receptor blockade mediates smooth muscle cell apoptosis and improves survival in rats with pulmonary hypertension. Circulation 112: 423–431.
44. Sakata Y, Xiang F, Chen Z, Kiriyama Y, Kamei CN, et al. (2004) Transcription factor CHF1/Hey2 regulates neointimal formation in vivo and vascular smooth muscle proliferation and migration in vitro. Arterioscler Thromb Vasc Biol 24: 2069–2074.
45. Lindner V, Booth C, Prudovsky I, Small D, Maciag T, et al. (2001) Members of the Jagged/Notch gene families are expressed in injured arteries and regulate cell phenotype via alterations in cell matrix and cell-cell interaction. Am J Pathol 159: 875–883.
46. Doi H, Iso T, Yamazaki M, Akiyama H, Kanai H, et al. (2005) HERP1 inhibits myocardin-induced vascular smooth muscle cell differentiation by interfering with SRF binding to CArG box. Arterioscler Thromb Vasc Biol 25: 2328–2334.
47. Noseda M, Fu YX, Niessen K, Wong F, Chang L, et al. (2006) Smooth muscle alpha-actin is a direct target of Notch/CSL. Circulation Research 98: 1468–1470.
48. Havrda MC, Johnson MJ, O'Neill CF, Liaw L (2006) A novel mechanism of transcriptional repression of p27kip1 through Notch/HRT2 signaling in vascular smooth muscle cells. Thromb Haemost 96: 361–370.
49. Wang Q, Zhao N, Kennard S, Lilly B (2012) Notch2 and notch3 function together to regulate vascular smooth muscle development. PLoS One 7: e37365.
50. Proweller A, Pear WS, Parmacek MS (2005) Notch signaling represses myocardin-induced smooth muscle cell differentiation. J Biol Chem 280: 8994–9004.
51. Morrow D, Sweeney C, Birney YA, Cummins PM, Walls D, et al. (2005) Cyclic strain inhibits Notch receptor signaling in vascular smooth muscle cells in vitro. Circ Res 96: 567–575.
52. Morrow D, Scheller A, Birney YA, Sweeney C, Guha S, et al. (2005) Notch-mediated CBF-1/RBP-J{kappa}-dependent regulation of human vascular smooth muscle cell phenotype in vitro. Am J Physiol Cell Physiol 289: C1188–1196.
53. Sweeney C, Morrow D, Birney YA, Coyle S, Hennessy C, et al. (2004) Notch 1 and 3 receptor signaling modulates vascular smooth muscle cell growth, apoptosis, and migration via a CBF-1/RBP-Jk dependent pathway. FASEB J 18: 1421–1423.
54. Noseda M, McLean G, Niessen K, Chang L, Pollet I, et al. (2004) Notch activation results in phenotypic and functional changes consistent with endothelial-to-mesenchymal transformation. Circ Res 94: 910–917.
55. Domenga V, Fardoux P, Lacombe P, Monet M, Maciazek J, et al. (2004) Notch3 is required for arterial identity and maturation of vascular smooth muscle cells. Genes Dev 18: 2730–2735.
56. Wang W, Prince CZ, Hu X, Pollman MJ (2003) HRT1 modulates vascular smooth muscle cell proliferation and apoptosis. Biochem Biophys Res Commun 308: 596–601.
57. Wang W, Prince CZ, Mou Y, Pollman MJ (2002) Notch3 signaling in vascular smooth muscle cells induces c-FLIP expression via ERK/MAPK activation. Resistance to Fas ligand-induced apoptosis. J Biol Chem 277: 21723–21729.

58. Wang W, Campos AH, Prince CZ, Mou Y, Pollman MJ (2002) Coordinate Notch3-hairy-related transcription factor pathway regulation in response to arterial injury. Mediator role of platelet-derived growth factor and ERK. J Biol Chem 277: 23165–23171.
59. Campos AH, Wang W, Pollman MJ, Gibbons GH (2002) Determinants of Notch-3 receptor expression and signaling in vascular smooth muscle cells: implications in cell-cycle regulation. Circ Res 91: 999–1006.
60. Tang Y, Urs S, Boucher J, Bernaiche T, Venkatesh D, et al. (2010) Notch and transforming growth factor-beta (TGFbeta) signaling pathways cooperatively regulate vascular smooth muscle cell differentiation. J Biol Chem 285: 17556–17563.
61. Liu H, Zhang W, Kennard S, Caldwell RB, Lilly B (2010) Notch3 is critical for proper angiogenesis and mural cell investment. Circ Res 107: 860–870.
62. Morrow D, Sweeney C, Birney YA, Guha S, Collins N, et al. (2007) Biomechanical regulation of hedgehog signaling in vascular smooth muscle cells in vitro and in vivo. Am J Physiol Cell Physiol 292: C488–496.
63. Boucher J, Gridley T, Liaw L (2012) Molecular pathways of notch signaling in vascular smooth muscle cells. Front Physiol 3: 81.
64. Zhang J, Fukuhara S, Sako K, Takenouchi T, Kitani H, et al. (2011) Angiopoietin-1/Tie2 signal augments basal Notch signal controlling vascular quiescence by inducing delta-like 4 expression through AKT-mediated activation of beta-catenin. J Biol Chem 286: 8055–8066.
65. Yan M, Callahan CA, Beyer JC, Allamneni KP, Zhang G, et al. (2010) Chronic DLL4 blockade induces vascular neoplasms. Nature 463: E6–7.
66. Sainson RC, Aoto J, Nakatsu MN, Holderfield M, Conn E, et al. (2005) Cell-autonomous notch signaling regulates endothelial cell branching and proliferation during vascular tubulogenesis. FASEB J 19: 1027–1029.
67. Patel NS, Li JL, Generali D, Poulsom R, Cranston DW, et al. (2005) Up-regulation of delta-like 4 ligand in human tumor vasculature and the role of basal expression in endothelial cell function. Cancer Res 65: 8690–8697.
68. Noseda M, Niessen K, McLean G, Chang L, Karsan A (2005) Notch-dependent cell cycle arrest is associated with downregulation of minichromosome maintenance proteins. Circ Res 97: 102–104.
69. Limbourg FP, Takeshita K, Radtke F, Bronson RT, Chin MT, et al. (2005) Essential role of endothelial Notch1 in angiogenesis. Circulation 111: 1826–1832.
70. Noseda M, Chang L, McLean G, Grim JE, Clurman BE, et al. (2004) Notch activation induces endothelial cell cycle arrest and participates in contact inhibition: role of p21Cip1 repression. Mol Cell Biol 24: 8813–8822.
71. MacKenzie F, Duriez P, Wong F, Noseda M, Karsan A (2004) Notch4 inhibits endothelial apoptosis via RBP-Jkappa-dependent and -independent pathways. J Biol Chem 279: 11657–11663.
72. Itoh F, Itoh S, Goumans MJ, Valdimarsdottir G, Iso T, et al. (2004) Synergy and antagonism between Notch and BMP receptor signaling pathways in endothelial cells. EMBO J 23: 541–551.
73. Liu ZJ, Shirakawa T, Li Y, Soma A, Oka M, et al. (2003) Regulation of Notch1 and Dll4 by vascular endothelial growth factor in arterial endothelial cells: implications for modulating arteriogenesis and angiogenesis. Mol Cell Biol 23: 14–25.
74. Leong KG, Hu X, Li L, Noseda M, Larrivee B, et al. (2002) Activated Notch4 inhibits angiogenesis: role of beta 1-integrin activation. Mol Cell Biol 22: 2830–2841.
75. Ii M, Takeshita K, Ibusuki K, Luedemann C, Wecker A, et al. (2010) Notch signaling regulates endothelial progenitor cell activity during recovery from arterial injury in hypercholesterolemic mice. Circulation 121: 1104–1112.
76. Wang L, Wang YC, Hu XB, Zhang BF, Dou GR, et al. (2009) Notch-RBP-J signaling regulates the mobilization and function of endothelial progenitor cells by dynamic modulation of CXCR4 expression in mice. PLoS One 4: e7572.
77. Hellstrom M, Phng LK, Hofmann JJ, Wallgard E, Coultas L, et al. (2007) Dll4 signalling through Notch1 regulates formation of tip cells during angiogenesis. Nature 445: 776–780.

3

Cardiovascular Agents Affect the Tone of Pulmonary Arteries and Veins in Precision-Cut Lung Slices

Annette D. Rieg[1,2*], Rolf Rossaint[1], Stefan Uhlig[2], Christian Martin[2]

1 Department of Anaesthesiology, Institute of Pharmacology and Toxicology, Medical Faculty Aachen, RWTH-Aachen, Aachen, Germany, **2** Institute of Pharmacology and Toxicology, Medical Faculty Aachen, RWTH-Aachen, Aachen, Germany

Abstract

Introduction: Cardiovascular agents are pivotal in the therapy of heart failure. Apart from their action on ventricular contractility and systemic afterload, they affect pulmonary arteries and veins. Although these effects are crucial in heart failure with coexisting pulmonary hypertension or lung oedema, they are poorly defined, especially in pulmonary veins. Therefore, we investigated the pulmonary vascular effects of adrenoceptor agonists, vasopressin and angiotensin II in the model of precision-cut lung slices that allows simultaneous studies of pulmonary arteries and veins.

Materials and Methods: Precision-cut lung slices were prepared from guinea pigs and imaged by videomicroscopy. Concentration-response curves of cardiovascular drugs were analysed in pulmonary arteries and veins.

Results: Pulmonary veins responded stronger than arteries to α_1-agonists (contraction) and β_2-agonists (relaxation). Notably, inhibition of β_2-adrenoceptors unmasked the α_1-mimetic effect of norepinephrine and epinephrine in pulmonary veins. Vasopressin and angiotensin II contracted pulmonary veins via V_{1a} and AT_1 receptors, respectively, without affecting pulmonary arteries.

Discussion: Vasopressin and (nor)epinephrine in combination with β_2-inhibition caused pulmonary venoconstriction. If applicable in humans, these treatments would enhance capillary hydrostatic pressures and lung oedema, suggesting their cautious use in left heart failure. Vice versa, the prevention of pulmonary venoconstriction by AT_1 receptor antagonists might contribute to their beneficial effects seen in left heart failure. Further, α_1-mimetic agents might exacerbate pulmonary hypertension and right ventricular failure by contracting pulmonary arteries, whereas vasopressin might not.

Editor: Martin R. J. Kolb, McMaster University, Canada

Funding: These authors have no support or funding to report.

Competing Interests: The authors have declared that no competing interests exist.

* E-mail: arieg@ukaachen.de

Introduction

Treatment of acute and chronic heart failure is based on the therapy with cardiovascular agents that aim at improved ventricular contractility, enhanced coronary perfusion and reduced myocardial oxygen consumption. Importantly however, cardiovascular agents interact with the pulmonary vascular bed and thereby also influence myocardial function: First, contraction of pulmonary arteries (PAs) enhances right ventricular afterload and worsens right ventricular failure. Second, contraction of pulmonary veins (PVs) increases pulmonary capillary pressure and causes hydrostatic pulmonary oedema and deterioration of gas exchange. Thus, it is clinically important how PAs and PVs respond to cardiovascular agents. However, the differential effects of cardiovascular drugs along the pulmonary vascular bed are only incompletely defined. Most previous studies focused on PAs [1–5], probably due to their central role in pulmonary hypertension and right ventricular failure. Recently, PVs are receiving growing attention and their relevance in the regulation of total pulmonary vascular resistance is becoming evident [6]. Therefore, and due to completely different responses of PAs and PVs [7], simultaneous studies of both vessels are of great clinical interest; however, they are rare [4]. Further, pulmonary vessels differ from systemic vessels in their response to hypoxia, hypercapnia and acidosis [8], thus results from systemic vessels may not be applicable to the low pressure pulmonary vascular bed.

The aim of this study was to investigate the effects of adrenoceptor agonists, vasopressin and angiotensin II on PAs and PVs. We have chosen the model of precision-cut lung slices (PCLS), because it permits simultaneous studies of PAs and PVs. Further, guinea pigs (GPs) were chosen, because previous studies on airway pharmacology suggest that GPs may be a reasonable proxy of human lung tissue [9]. Our results indicate that GPs' PAs and PVs respond significantly different to adrenoceptor agonists, vasopressin and angiotension II. These findings suggest that differential effects of cardiovascular drugs along the pulmonary vascular tree might influence the success of heart failure therapy.

Materials and Methods

Guinea pigs (GPs)

Female Dunkin Hartley GPs (400±50 g) were obtained from Charles River (Sulzfeld, Germany) and held under standard conditions. All animal care and experimental procedures were performed according to the rules of the University Hospital Aachen (Aachen, Germany) and the Directive 2010/63/EU of the European Parliament. They were approved by the Landesamt für Natur, Umwelt und Verbraucherschutz Nordrhein-Westfalen (LANUV, approval-ID: 8.87–51.05.20.10.245).

Precision-cut lung slices (PCLS)

PCLS from GPs (n = 39) were prepared as described before [9]. In brief, intraperitoneal anaesthesia was performed with 95 mg kg^{-1} pentobarbital (Narcoren; Garbsen, Germany) and its depth was monitored by missing reflexes. Afterwards, the abdomen was opened and the GP exsanguinated. Further, the trachea was cannulated, the diaphragm opened and the lungs filled with low melting point agarose (final concentration: 1.5%), containing 1 μM isoproterenol. To solidify the agarose, the lungs were covered with ice. The lobes were removed; tissue cores prepared and cut into 300 μm thick slices with a Krumdieck tissue slicer (Alabama Research & Development, Munford, AL, USA). Afterwards, PCLS were incubated at 37°C in a humid atmosphere in minimal essential medium (MEM), containing $CaCl_2$ (1.8 mM), $MgSO_4$ (0.8 mM), KCl (5.4 mM), NaCl (116.4 mM), glucose (16.7 mM), $NaHCO_3$ (26.1 mM), Hepes (25.17 mM), sodium pyruvate, amino acids, vitamins and glutamine. To wash out the agarose from the slices, the MEM was changed every half hour during the first 2 h and every hour during the next 2 h. For overnight culture, MEM was completed with penicillin and streptomycin and changed every 24 h.

Identification of the vessels, histology

Pulmonary vessels were identified using the following criteria: PAs accompany the airways and PVs lie aside. After staining with haematoxylin and eosin (HE) PAs show a wrinkled inner lining and a thick media wall [7], as it is illustrated in Fig. 1A–D. Thus, after termination of the experiments PCLS were fixed in 4% formalin and embedded in paraffin. Sections (4 μM) were cut and HE-stained. Images were taken by a microscope (Leica, DM 600 B).

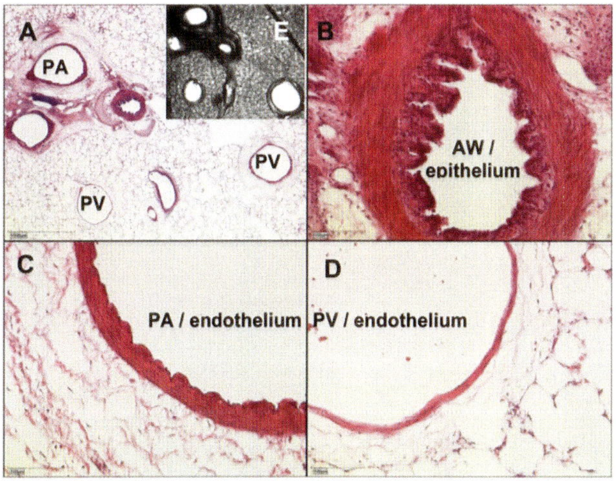

Figure 1. Identification of pulmonary vessels. A) A representative PCLS after staining with haematoxylin and eosin. **B**) epithelium of an airway (AW) **C**) Pulmonary artery (PA): endothelium with typical wrinkled inner lining and thick media **D**) Pulmonary vein (PV): endothelium without wrinkled inner lining and thin media **E**) corresponding unstained PCLS.

Measurements and Imaging

At the beginning of the study, all agents were investigated with regard to the onset of their maximal contractile or relaxant effect. According to these results, the duration of exposure was defined for all agents, i.e. for (nor)epinephrine, isoproterenol, phenylephrine, procaterol, denopamine, CL 316243 and A 61603 3 minutes, for vasopressin 5 minutes and for angiotensin 10 minutes. The slices were exposed to different drugs on day one and two after preparation. Concentration-response curves were performed on pulmonary arteries and veins and cross sectional area of the vessels was calculated. Control experiments were performed on consecutive sections. Pulmonary vessels were imaged and digitised using a digital video camera (Leica Viscam 1280 or Leica DFC 280). The images were analysed with Optimas 6.5 (Media Cybernetics, Bothell, WA).

Agents

All agents were purchased from Sigma-Aldrich (Steinheim, Germany), except CGP 20712 A, procaterol and CL 316243, which were from Tocris Bioscience (Ellisville, Missouri, USA).

Statistics

Statistics was conducted using SAS software version 9.1 (SAS Institute, Cary, North Carolina, USA) and GraphPad Prism version 5.0 (GraphPad Software, La Jolla, USA). Homoscedasticity of values was evaluated. Changes of the vessel area are expressed as percentage of its initial area. All values are shown as mean ± SEM. Paired observations were analysed using the one sample t-test or the Wilcoxon signed rank test. Unpaired observations were compared using the Mann-Whitney Test. When the effect of increasing concentrations on the vessels was roughly linear, data were analysed using a linear mixed model analysis (LMM). In case of sigmoidal concentration-response curves; the standard logistic regression model was used to calculate and compare EC_{50} values. For LMM and logistic regression the AIC-criterion was used to select the preferred model. All p-values were adjusted for multiple comparisons by the false discovery rate [10]. P-values <0.05 were considered as significant. For all experiments, (n) indicates the numbers of animals.

Results

Stimulation of α- and β-receptors in PAs and PVs

The endogenous vasoactive compounds norepinephrine and epinephrine [(nor)epinephrine] represent cardiovascular agents, that are worldwide most commonly used to restore circulation in cardiac failure and shock.

In PAs, (nor)epinephrine induced maximal contraction at 1 μM, though epinephrine was more potent. Above 1 μM this difference disappeared, suggesting the additional activation of β_2-adrenoceptors by epinephrine (Fig. 2A). Pre-treatment of PAs with the α_1-antagonist prazosine (100 nM) prevented (nor)epinephrine-induced contraction (Fig. 2A). Comparable to norepinephrine, the α_1-agonist phenylephrine induced only slight contraction in PAs (Fig. 2B). Similar results were obtained for the α_1-agonist A 61603, whereas the α_2-agonist clonidine had no effect (not shown). Pre-treatment of PAs with the selective β_2-antagonist ICI 118551 (100 nM) enhanced norepinephrine-induced contraction and 10 μM ICI 118551 had an even stronger effect (Fig. 2C). However, ICI 118551 at 100 nM (Fig. 2D) or 10 μM (not shown) did not alter the effect of epinephrine. The $\beta_{1/2}$-agonist isoproterenol had no effect in PAs (Fig. 2C), whereas the pure β_2-agonist procaterol relaxed them (Fig. 2D). Further, procaterol completely abolished contraction due to (nor)epinephrine (Fig. 2C/

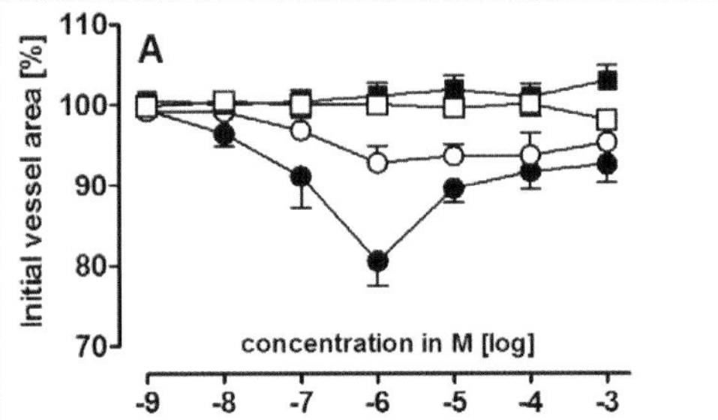

A: ● epinephrine, n=7; ○ norepinephrine, n=5; ■ prazosine (100 nM), epinephrine, n=7; □ prazosine (100 nM), norepinephrine, n=4

agents	effect	p-level	statistics
● 1 nM *vs.* ● 1 μM	constriction	**	linear mixed model
● 1 μM *vs.* ● 1 mM	partial relaxation	**	linear mixed model
○ 1 nM *vs.* ○ 1 μM	constriction	*	linear mixed model
● 1 μM *vs.* ○ 1 μM	constriction	*	linear mixed model
● 1 μM *vs.* ■ 1 μM	constriction	**	linear mixed model
○ 1 μM *vs.* □ 1 μM	constriction	**	linear mixed model

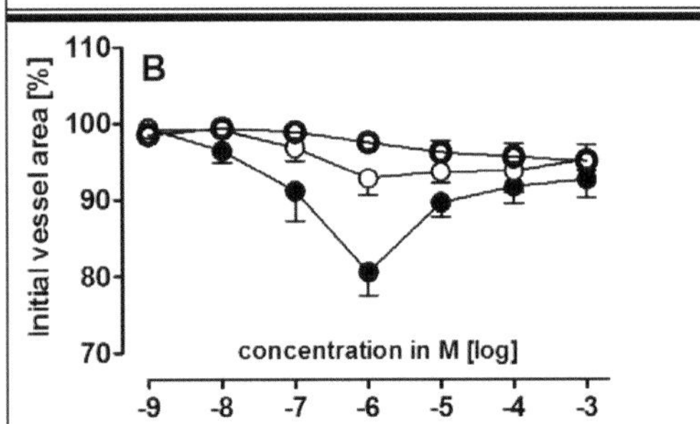

B: ● epinephrine, n=7; ○ norepinephrine, n=5; **o** phenylephrine, n=5

agents	effect	p-level	statistics
○ 1 μM *vs.* **o** 1mM	constriction	ns	Mann-Whitney-Test (observations are not paired)

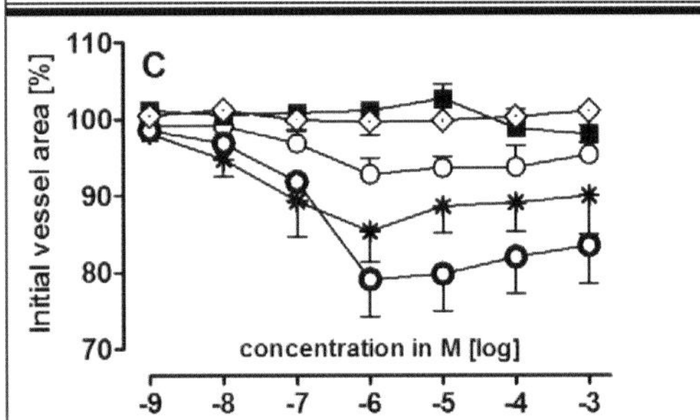

C: ○ norepinephrine, n=5; ✱ ICI 118551 (100 nM), norepinephrine, n=5; **o** ICI 118551 (10 μM), norepinephrine, n=6; ■ isoproterenol, n=5; ◇ norepinephrine / procaterol, n=4

agents	effect	p-level	statistics
○ 1 μM *vs.* ✱ 1 μM	constriction	*	linear mixed model
○ 1 μM *vs.* **o** 1 μM	constriction	**	linear mixed model
○ 1 μM *vs.* ◇ 1 μM	constriction	**	linear mixed model

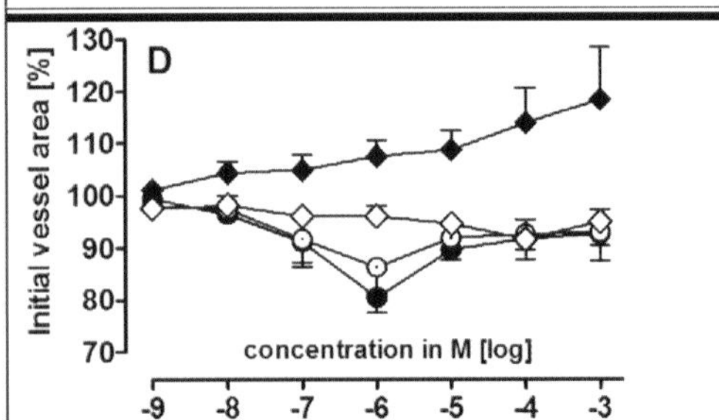

D: ● epinephrine, n=7; ⊙ ICI 118551 (100 nM) / epinephrine, n=5; ◆ procaterol, n=7; ◇ epinephrine / procaterol, n=5

agents	effect	p-level	statistics
● 1 μM *vs.* ⊙ 1 μM	constriction	ns	linear mixed model
● 1 μM *vs.* ◇ 1 μM	constriction	**	linear mixed model
◇ 1nM *vs.* ◇ 10 μM	constriction	ns	linear mixed model
◆ 1 nM *vs.* ◆ 1 mM	relaxation	*	linear mixed model

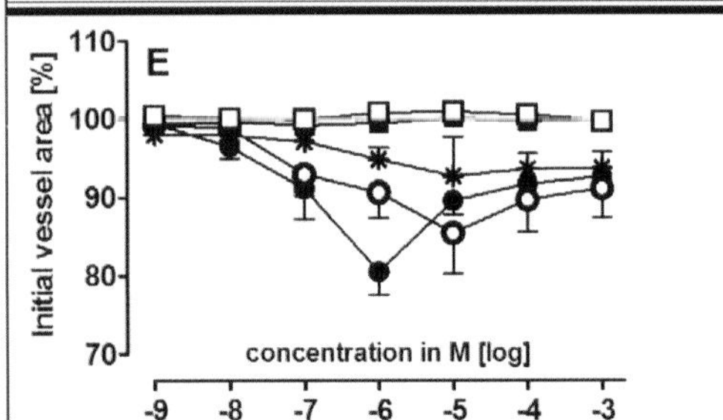

E: ● epinephrine, n=7; **o** propanolol (1 μM), epinephrine, n=7; ✱ CGP 20712 A (100 nM), epinephrine, n=4; ■ denopamine, n=3; □ CL 316243, n=3

agents	effect	p-level	statistics
● 1 μM *vs.* **o** 1 μM	constriction	*	linear mixed model
● 1 μM *vs.* **o** 10 μM	constriction	ns	linear mixed model
● 1 μM *vs.* ✱ 1 μM	constriction	**	linear mixed model
● 1 μM *vs.* ✱ 10 μM	constriction	**	linear mixed model
✱ 1 nM vs. ✱ 1mM	constriction	ns	linear mixed model

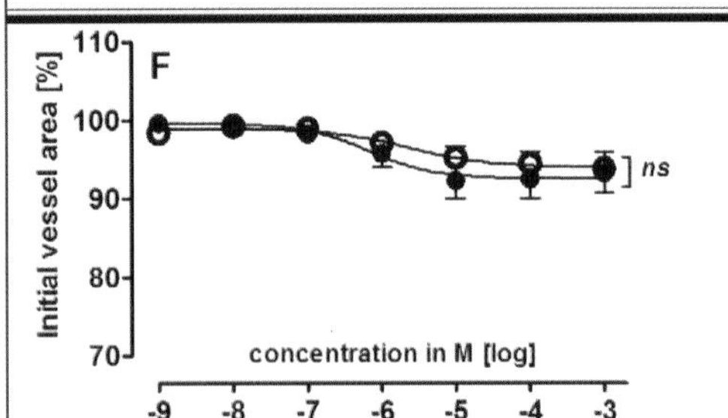

F: **o** phenylephrine, n=6; ● denopamine (1 μM), phenylephrine, n=6

agents	effect	p-level	statistics
o EC_{50} *vs.* ● EC_{50}	constriction	ns	EC_{50} comparison

Figure 2. Responses of pulmonary arteries (PAs) to increasing dosages of adrenergic agents. A-F) Pre-treatment concentrations were fixed. P<0.05 are considered as statistical significant and are indicated as followed * p<0.05, ** p<0.01 and *** p<0.001.

D). Pre-treatment of PAs with the $\beta_{1/2}$-antagonist propanolol (1 µM) shifted epinephrine-induced contraction rightwards, without altering its maximal effect (Fig. 2E). Pre-treatment with the β_1-antagonist CGP 20712A (100 nM) abolished epinephrine-induced contraction (Fig. 2E). However, the β_1-agonist denopamine had no effect on PAs. Further, denopamine given as pre-treatment prior to increasing concentrations of phenylephrine did not enhance phenylephrine-induced contraction (Fig. 2F). Also the β_3-agonist CL 316243 had no effect (Fig. 2E). Finally, the tone of PAs was not affected by prazosine, CGP 20712A, ICI 118551 and propanolol (Table 1).

In PVs, isoproterenol, procaterol, norepinephrine and epinephrine caused relaxation, with the following EC_{50} values: isoproterenol 0.26 µM, procaterol 0.12 µM, norepinephrine 30 µM and epinephrine 1 µM (Fig. 3A). Simultaneous treatment with epinephrine and the pure β_2-agonist procaterol did not enhance epinephrine-induced relaxation (Fig. 3B). Further, combined treatment with norepinephrine and procaterol did not alter the maximal relaxant effect of norepinephrine; however EC_{50} values were shifted leftwards to lower concentrations, i.e. EC_{50} values were 8.6 nM for simultaneous treatment with procaterol and norepinephrine instead of 30 µM for norepinephrine alone. Pre-treatment with 100 nM prazosine had no effect alone (Table 1) or on epinephrine-induced relaxation (Fig. 3B), but enhanced the effect of norepinephrine (Fig. 3C). When PVs were pre-treated with the β_2-antagonist ICI 118551 (10 µM or 100 nM) the effect of (nor)epinephrine was reversed and it became contractile (Fig. 3B/C). At 1 mM epinephrine showed some relaxation despite the presence of ICI 118551 (Fig. 3B). Similar results were obtained for (nor)epinephrine after pre-treatment with 1 µM propanolol (not shown). Neither ICI 118551 nor propanolol did affect the basal tone of PVs (Table 1). The α_1-agonist A 61603 contracted PVs, whereas the α_1-agonist phenylephrine had only a slight contractile effect at 10 µM that was reversed at higher concentrations (Fig. 3D). However, after pre-treatment with 100 nM ICI 118551 PVs responded to phenylephrine comparable to A 61603 (Fig. 3D). In addition, the α_2-agonist clonidine, the β_1-agonist denopamine and the β_3-agonst CL 316243 had no effects in PVs (not shown).

Effects of vasopressin on PAs and PVs

The neurohypophyseal peptide vasopressin contracts vascular smooth muscles via binding to V_{1a} receptors. PVs, but not PAs, contracted to vasopressin (EC_{50}: 2 pM, Fig. 4A/B). The cyclooxygenase inhibitor indomethacin (10 µM) attenuated vasopressin-induced contraction. Conversely, the NO synthase inhibitor N-nitro-L-arginine methyl ester (L-NAME, 100 µM) showed a trend towards enhancement (Fig. 4B). However, neither L-NAME nor indomethacin changed the vascular responses of PAs to vasopressin (Fig. 4A). Pre-treatment of PVs with the V_{1a} antagonist SR 49059 (10 nM) showed no effect alone (Table 1), but abolished contraction due to vasopressin (Fig. 4B). Further, the NO-donor S-Nitroso-N-acetyl-DL-penicillamine (SNAP) partly reversed vasopressin-induced contraction in PVs (Fig. 4B). Indomethacin slightly contracted PVs (Table 1) and L-NAME induced time-dependent contraction (Fig. 5A), which was reversed by SNAP. Further, native PVs also relaxed to SNAP (Fig. 5B), whereas PAs did not react to L-NAME or SNAP (Fig. 5A/B).

Effects of angiotensin II on PAs and PVs

Angiotensin II induces vasoconstriction via the G-protein coupled AT_1 receptor. Angiotensin II contracted PVs (EC_{50}: 0.1 nM; Fig. 6B–D), but not PAs (Fig. 6A). Pre-treatment with indomethacin (10 µM) or L-NAME (100 µM) did not alter the response of pulmonary vessels to angiotensin II (Fig. 6A–C). In order to analyse, whether angiotensin-induced contraction is specific to AT_1 binding, PCLS were pre-treated with the AT_1 antagonist losartan. Losartan (1 µM) had no effect alone, but abolished the effect of angiotensin II (Fig. 6D, Table 1).

Discussion

(Nor)epinephrine and vasopressin are clinically relevant cardiovascular agents that are daily applied in the treatment of acute haemodynamic instability. Further, angiotensin-converting enzyme inhibitors and AT_1 antagonists are used to treat chronic heart failure. Commonly, their effects on systemic circulation are well controlled; whereas their pulmonary vascular effects are rarely assessed, especially in PVs. However this entity is of relevance, especially in pulmonary hypertension and right heart failure. This study compared the pulmonary vascular effects of (nor)epinephrine, vasopressin and angiotensin II in PCLS of GPs. Adrenergic agonists contracted PAs and PVs, but their contractile effect on PVs was unmasked only in the presence of β_2-inhibition. Vasopressin and angiotensin II only contracted PVs.

Table 1. Influence of various antagonists and inhibitors on the initial vessel area.

agents	PA mean (%)	n	SEM	p-value	PV mean (%)	n	SEM	p-value
prazosine 100 nM	102	8	3.7	0.64	103	8	3.2	0.33
CGP 20712 A 100 nM	101	5	1.3	0.81	102	5	1.5	0.31
ICI 188551 10 µM	101	6	1.2	1	95	9	5.5	0.34
ICI 188551 100 nM	100	10	1.2	0.7	97	10	3.5	0.38
propanolol 1 µM	97	8	1.2	0.06	93	9	4.7	0.16
indomethacin 10 µM	98	7	0.9	0.15	95	9	1.1	0.001
SR 49059 10 nM	102	3	3.2	1	101	3	1.4	1
losartan 1 µM	100	4	2.4	1	98	4	1.2	0.25

Observations were paired, thus statistics was conducted using the One sample t-test or the Wilcoxon Test. P<0.05 are considered as statistical significant.

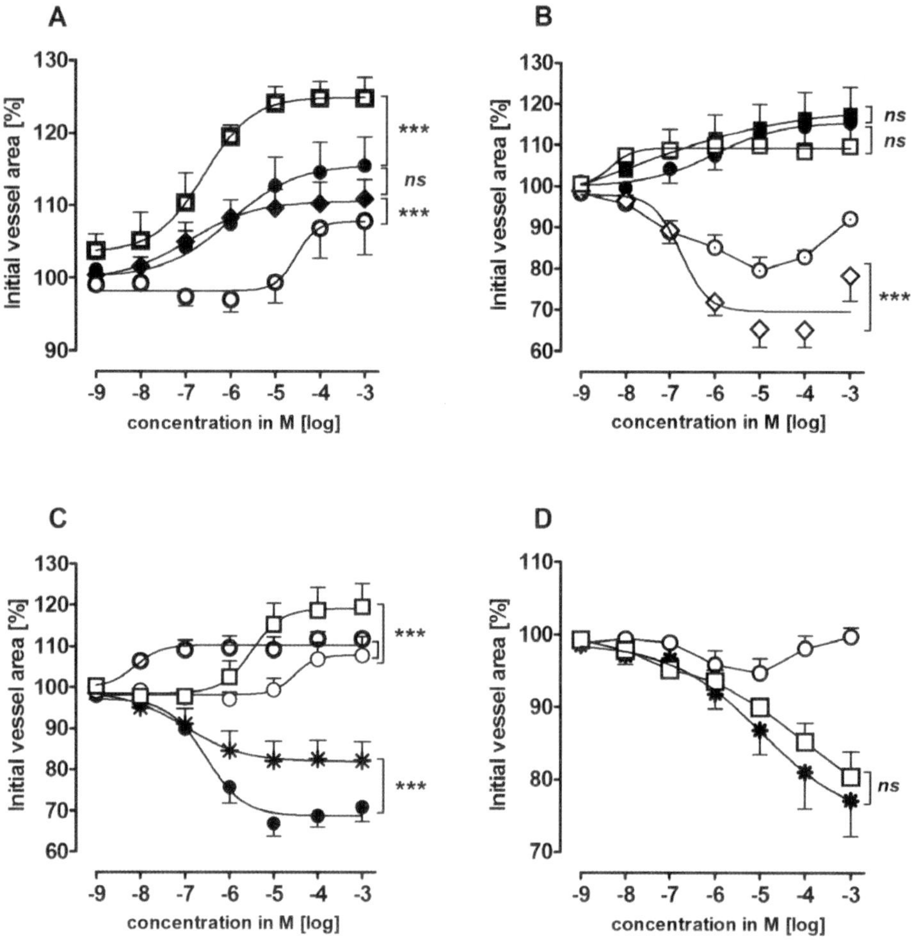

Figure 3. Responses of pulmonary veins (PV) to adrenergic agents. **A)** (◘) isoproterenol (n = 5); (●) epinephrine (n = 6); (◆) procaterol (n = 7); (**O**) norepinephrine (n = 6); **B)** (●) epinephrine (n = 6); (■) prazosine (100 nM), epinephrine (n = 6); (⊙) ICI 118551 (100 nM), epinephrine (n = 5); (◇) ICI 118551 (10 μM), epinephrine (n = 5); (◘) procaterol, epinephrine (n = 4); **C)** (○) norepinephrine (n = 6); (□) prazosine (100 nM), norepinephrine (n = 3); (✱) ICI 118551 (100 nM), norepinephrine (n = 9); (●) ICI 118551 (10 μM), norepinephrine (n = 6); (**O**) procaterol, norepinephrine (n = 4); **D)** (○) phenylephrine (n = 6); (✱) A 61603 (n = 5), (□) ICI 118551 (100 nM), phenylephrine (n = 5). Asterics indicate different EC_{50}-values of the various curves. $P<0.05$ are considered as statistical significant and are indicated as followed * $p<0.05$, ** $p<0.01$ and *** $p<0.001$.

Alpha - and β-adrenergic stimulation

(Nor)epinephrine interacted with $\alpha_1/\beta_{1/2}$-adrenoceptors of PAs and PVs. (Nor)epinephrine-related contraction of PAs was inhibited by prazosine and thus most likely caused by activation of α_1-adrenoceptors. In addition, inhibition of β_1-adrenoceptors abolished epinephrine-induced contraction, suggesting their involvement in α_1-mediated contraction. This somewhat surprising conclusion is supported by two findings: First, $\alpha_1/\beta_{1/2}$-agonists such as (nor)epinephrine contracted PAs stronger than phenylephrine and A 61603, which selectively act on α_1-adrenoceptors in PAs. Second, the selective β_2-agonist procaterol relaxed PAs, whereas the $\beta_{1/2}$-agonist isoproterenol did not, suggesting neutralization of β_1-mediated contraction by β_2-mediated relaxation. Concurrent activation of α_1/β_1-adrenoceptors was before reported in PVs [11], albeit with regard to ectopic activity. Previously, isoproterenol that binds stronger on β_1-adrenoceptors than on β_2-adrenoceptors [12] was observed to contract vessels [13]. Of note, the β_1-agonist denopamine failed to contract PAs or to enhance phenylephrine-induced contraction. These findings suggest a complex and indirect activation of β_1-adrenoceptors by epinephrine that remains to be further elucidated.

Interestingly, the contractile potency of epinephrine decreased above 1 μM indicating the additional activation of β_2-adrenoceptors and subsequent vasorelaxation. This conclusion is supported by the effects of procaterol that relaxed PAs and prevented epinephrine- and norepinephrine-induced contraction. Further, treatment of PAs with ICI 118551 enhanced norepinephrine-related contraction. Thus, vasoconstriction appears to be partially masked by stimulation of β_2-adrenoceptors. In contrast, ICI 118551 did not alter epinephrine-induced contraction. Possibly, epinephrine at 1 μM mainly acts as a relatively pure α_1-agonist, whereas above 1 μM it competes with ICI 118551 for β_2-adrenoceptors.

Thus, adrenergic agents interact in a complex manner with $\alpha_1/\beta_{1/2}$-adrenoceptors of PAs (Table 2). Contraction is mainly mediated by α_1-adrenoceptors, but is antagonised by β_2-adrenoceptors and aggravated by β_1-adrenoceptors.

The pulmonary venous vascular bed contributes up to 40% to total pulmonary vascular resistance [6]. In PVs, β_2-adrenoceptors appear to be dominant and mask the activation of α_1-adrenoceptors (Table 2). This is concluded from the observation that PVs contracted to (nor)epinephrine and phenylephrine only in

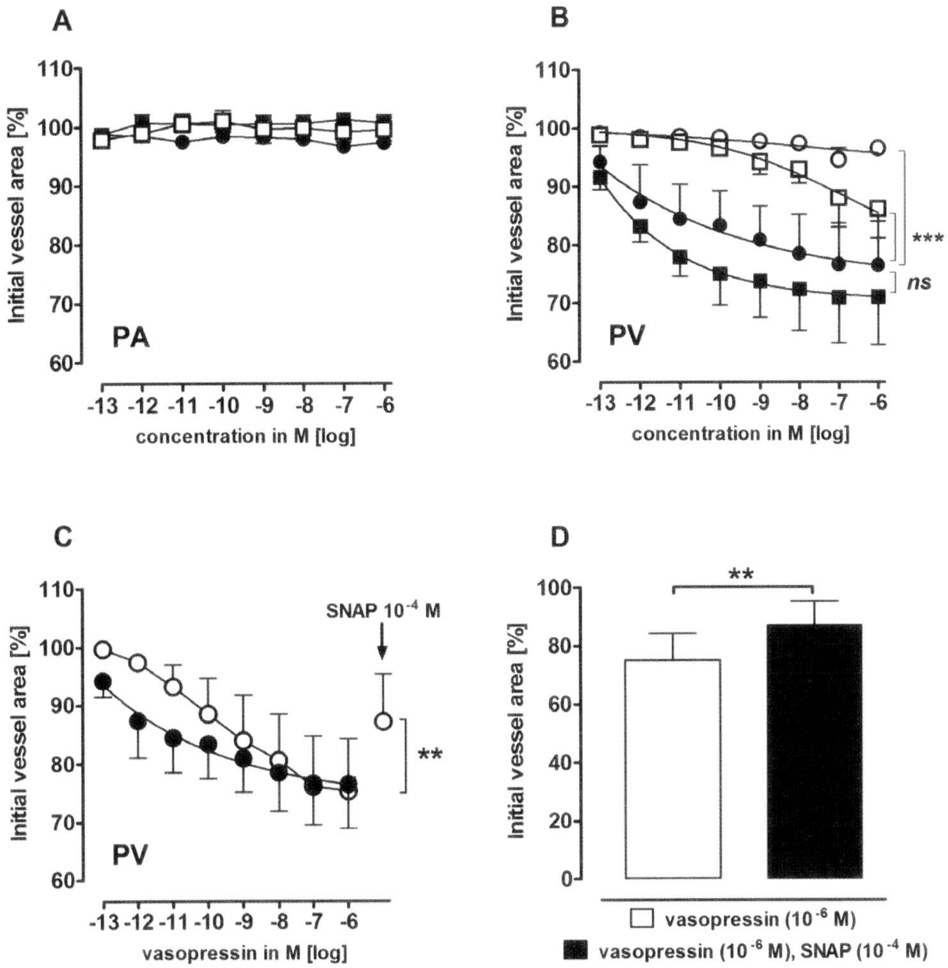

Figure 4. Responses of pulmonary arteries (PAs) and pulmonary veins (PVs) to vasopressin. **A**) PA: (●) vasopressin (n = 6); (□) indomethacin (10 μM), vasopressin (n = 4); (■) L-NAME (100 μM), vasopressin (n = 5) **B**) PV: (●) vasopressin (n = 5); (□) indomethacin (10 μM), vasopressin (n = 4); (■) L-NAME (100 μM), vasopressin (n = 5); (○) SR 49059 (10 nM), vasopressin (n = 3). **C**) PV: (●) vasopressin (n = 5); (○) vasopressin, SNAP (n = 7). **D**) PV: vasopressin, SNAP (n = 7). **B**) Asterics indicate different EC_{50}.values of the various curves. **C–D**) Statistics was performed using the Wilcoxon test. For all: $P<0.05$ are considered as statistical significant and are indicated as followed * $p<0.05$, ** $p<0.01$ and *** $p<0.001$.

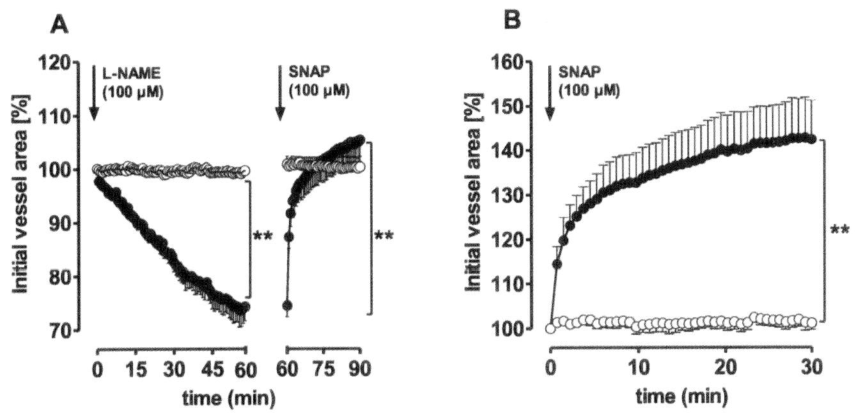

Figure 5. Responses of pulmonary arteries (PAs) and pulmonary veins (PVs) to L-NAME and SNAP. **A**) (●) PV (n = 3); (○) PA (n = 3). **B**) (●) PV (n = 3); (○) PA (n = 3). Statistics was conducted using a linear mixed model analysis. P-values were adjusted for multiple comparisons by the false discovery rate. $P<0.05$ are considered as statistical significant and indicated as followed * $p<0.05$, ** $p<0.01$ and *** $p<0.001$.

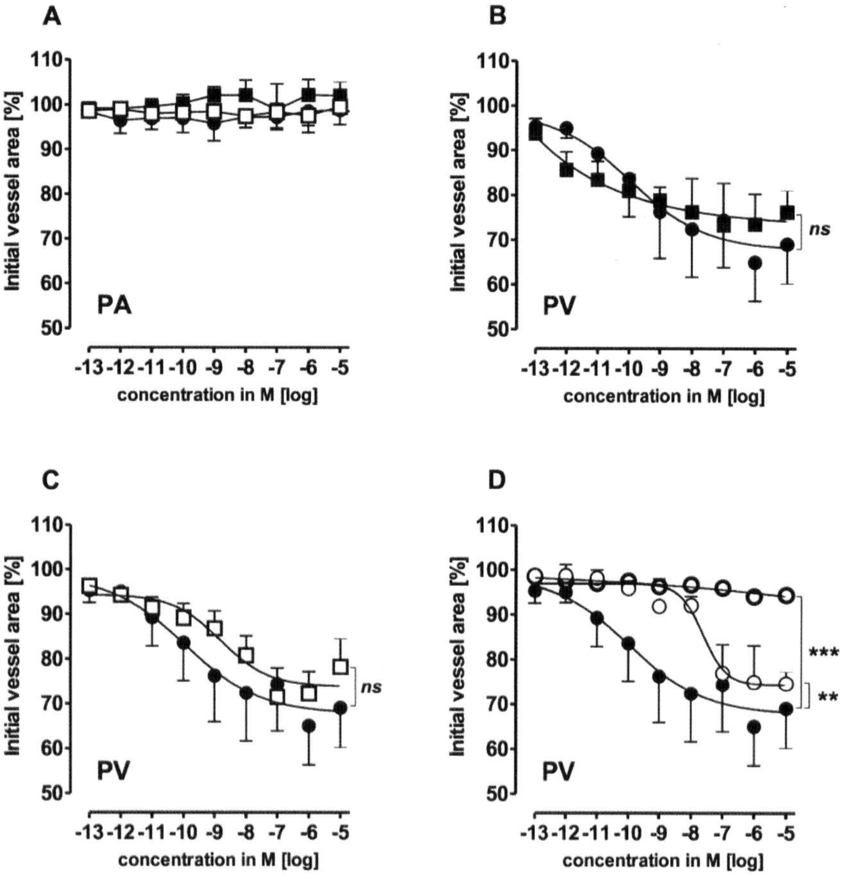

Figure 6. Responses of pulmonary arteries (PAs) and pulmonary veins (PVs) to angiotensin II. A) PA: (●) angiotensin II (n = 6); (□) indomethacin (10 μM), angiotensin II (n = 5); (■) L-NAME (100 μM), angiotensin II (n = 5) **B**) PV: (●) angiotensin II (n = 5); (■) L-NAME (100 μM), angiotensin II (n = 5) **C**) PV: (●) angiotensin II (n = 5); (□) indomethacin (10 μM), angiotensin II (n = 5) **D**) PV: (●) angiotensin II (n = 5); (**○**) losartan (1 μM), angiotensin II (n = 3); (○) losartan (10 nM), angiotensin II (n = 3). Asterics indicate different EC_{50}.values of the various curves. $P<0.05$ are considered as statistical significant and are indicated as followed * $p<0.05$, ** $p<0.01$ and *** $p<0.001$.

the presence of β_2-blockers. Given alone, (nor)epinephrine was relaxant, whereas phenylephrine was not, which is in line with its weak β_2-affinity. Pre-treatment with prazosine only enhanced the relaxant effect of norepinephrine. Probably, maximal relaxation of epinephrine was already reached, as it stimulates β_2-adrenoceptors more potently than norepinephrine [12]. Further, combined treatment with procaterol and epinephrine did not alter epinephrine-induced relaxation in PVs, probably due to similar binding affinities in respect of the β_2-receptor [14]. However, as expected, simultaneous treatment with procaterol and norepi-

Table 2. Overview of cardiovascular agents and their receptor-mediated vascular effects.

agents	PA/contraction	PA/relaxation	PV/contraction	PV/relaxation
epinephrine 1 μM	α_1 (β_1)		(α_1)	β_2
norepinephrine 1 μM	α_1		(α_1)	β_2
epinephrine 1 mM	α_1	β_2	(α_1)	β_2
norepinephrine 1 mM	(α_1)	(β_2)	(α_1)	β_2
phenylephrine	α_1		(α_1)	(β_2)
A 61603	α_1		α_1	
procaterol	–	β_2	–	β_2
>1 pM vasopressin	–	–	V_{1a}	–
angiotensin II	–	–	AT_1	–
NO	–	–	–	NO

Masked effects are expressed with ().

nephrine was superior compared to norepinephrine alone and is in line with the high binding affinity of procaterol to the β_2-receptor [14].

Our results may help to put previous findings into perspective. In perfused feline lung lobes, norepinephrine and phenylephrine enhanced pulmonary vascular resistance; while epinephrine and isoproterenol had the opposite effect [15]. These results might reflect the net effect of α_1-dependent pulmonary arterial contraction versus β_2-dependent pulmonary venous relaxation. Though, in perfused rat lungs norepinephrine and phenylephrine reduced the pulmonary perfusion pressure [5], likely due to β_2-mediated relaxation [16].

Beta$_2$-mediated pulmonary venous relaxation is of clinical interest, as mixed $\beta_{1/2}$-blockers are widely-used. Commonly, α_1/$\beta_{1/2}$-agonists, such as (nor)epinephrine are applied in heart failure or shock. However, if these patients are pre-treated with mixed $\beta_{1/2}$-blockers, circulation support with (nor)epinephrine might worsen gas exchange, due to pulmonary venoconstriction, as (nor)epinephrine mainly activate α_1-adrenoceptors, while β_2-adrenoceptors are still blocked. In pulmonary hypertension, (nor)epinephrine might increase right ventricular afterload and aggravate right ventricular failure. If these findings could be confirmed in humans, this should be considered in the therapy of heart failure.

Vasopressin

Vasopressin has various physiological functions, including V_{1a} receptor-mediated regulation of blood pressure and V_2 receptor-mediated control of body water [17]. Further, its relevance in resuscitation is increasingly discussed. Here, vasopressin only contracted PVs. Inhibition of endothelial NO-synthase (eNOS) tended to enhance this contractile effect and the NO-donor SNAP reversed it in part. Further, L-NAME given alone also contracted PVs. This indicates the critical role of eNOS in PVs as opposed to arteries, similar to observations in human [18] and porcine PVs [19]. Moreover, indomethacin attenuated the effect of vasopressin, indicating its partial action through the release of contractile prostanoids such as thromboxane.

In contrast to our results, vasopressin relaxed PAs in isolated perfused rat lungs [3] and isolated canine pulmonary vessels in dependence to eNOS [1,4]. In dogs, it contracted PAs [2]. Vasopressin contracts vessels via V_{1a} receptor-mediated phospholipase C activation and IP_3-signalling [17] and opposing to our results, the involvement of relaxant prostaglandins was shown [20]. Thus, the effect of vasopressin in pulmonary vessels may strongly depend on the studied species [21]. Best to our knowledge, pulmonary venous contraction due to vasopressin was not yet reported.

Interestingly, human data indirectly support our results [22]: application of vasopressin led to enhanced pulmonary capillary wedge pressures (PCWP). Vice versa, application of the $V_{1a/2}$ antagonist conivaptan decreased PCWP [23], whereas the V_2 antagonist tolvaptan did not, but increased vasopressin plasma levels [24]. Thus, vasopressin antagonists that do not block V_{1a} receptors might be problematic. In patients with heart failure, vasopressin plasma levels are increased up to 0.28 nM [25], concentrations that contracted PVs in our *in vitro* model. Hence, vasopressin-related contraction of PVs might enhance pulmonary hydrostatic pressures, left ventricular preload and wall stress. Taken together, our findings suggest that V_{1a} antagonists might reduce pulmonary complications in heart failure and further, that vasopressin might not worsen right ventricular afterload (Table 2).

Angiotensin II

Angiotensin II is the key peptide of the renin-angiotensin system and mainly produced in the pulmonary arterial vascular bed [26]. In the present study, angiotensin II only contracted the PVs; neither inhibition of NO- nor prostanoid synthesis altered this response.

In contrast to our results, angiotensin contracted endothelium denuded, isolated PAs of GPs and dogs [4,27,28], whereas canine PVs relaxed [4] or failed to respond [28]. Moreover, indomethacin enhanced the contractile effect of angiotensin in PAs [4]. In line with our results, angiotensin contracted rat PVs [29]. Further, in patients with atrial and ventricular septum defects, angiotensin increased left atrial and pulmonary venous pressures, but did not alter the pulmonary arterial resistance [30]. In addition, only the extent of left to right shunts increased. According to our results, pulmonary venoconstriction might be a reasonable explanation for these observations. Prevention of pulmonary venous contraction by AT_1 antagonists or ACE-inhibitors might contribute to their beneficial effect in heart failure.

PCLS from GPs

Thus, our findings are in line with clinical studies and suggest that PCLS from GPs resemble human pulmonary vascular pharmacology reasonably well, as already indicated for airway pharmacology [9]. This study was performed *in vitro* and thus excludes factors that affect vascular responses *in vivo* such as shear stress or embolism. *In vivo*, the PA can be accessed by catheterization, whereas the access of PVs is more difficult. The PCWP relates to left atrial pressure and to large PVs, but small PVs are not reflected [31]. Further, vascular pressure represents a product of vascular tone and filling. Hence, it is influenced by ventricular contractility. Complementary to *in vivo* studies, PCLS allow exclusively studying the vascular tone of pulmonary vessels.

For the first time, this study systematically compared the effects of clinically relevant cardiovascular agents simultaneously on PAs and PVs. Our results indicate that PAs and PVs are contracted by α_1-agonists, while relaxation, which occurs predominantly in PVs, is mediated by β_2-adrenoceptors. Of note, β_1-adrenoceptors contribute to adrenergic contraction in PAs. Further, vasopressin and angiotensin target predominantly PVs and thus raise the hypothesis that activation of V_{1a} receptors and AT_1 receptors favours pulmonary oedema. Thus, clinically, the application of vasopressin in left heart failure should be faced with caution and conversely suggests a beneficial role of V_{1a} and AT_1 antagonists. In contrast to vasopressin, (nor)epinephrine may increase right ventricular afterload, but not pulmonary oedema, except in patients pre-treated with $\beta_{1/2}$-inhibitors. Taken together, both vascular beds exhibit important differences in their responses to cardiovascular drugs. In conclusion, successful restoration of circulation in heart failure and shock should take into account the differential effects of cardiovascular agents on PAs and PVs.

Acknowledgments

The authors gratefully acknowledge Hanna Czajkowska and Xhina Schneider for technical assistance, the facility for immunohistochemistry of the IZKF Aachen for performance of histology and Eva Verjans, MD for critical reading of the manuscript.

Author Contributions

Conceived and designed the experiments: ADR CM SU RR. Performed the experiments: ADR. Analyzed the data: ADR CM SU. Contributed reagents/materials/analysis tools: ADR CM SU RR. Wrote the paper: ADR CM SU RR.

References

1. Evora P, Pearson P, Schaff H (1993) Arginine vasopressin induces endothelium-dependent vasodilatation of the pulmonary artery. V1-receptor-mediated production of nitric oxide. Chest 103: 1241–1245.
2. Leather H, Segers P, Berends N, Vandermeersch E, Wouters P (2002) Effects of vasopressin on right ventricular function in an experimental model of acute pulmonary hypertension. Crit Care Med 30: 2548–2552.
3. Russ R, Resta T, Walker B (1992) Pulmonary vasodilatory response to neurohypophyseal peptides in the rat. J Appl Physiol 73: 473–478.
4. Sai Y, Okamura T, Amakata Y, Toda N (1995) Comparison of responses of canine pulmonary artery and vein to angiotensin II, bradykinin and vasopressin. Eur J Pharmacol 282: 235–241.
5. Uma S, Tuncer M (1988) Beta-adrenoceptor stimulating effects of phenylephrine and noradrenaline in the rat pulmonary vascular bed. J Pharm Pharmacol 40: 219–220.
6. Gao Y, Raj J (2005) Role of veins in regulation of pulmonary circulation. Am J Physiol Lung Cell Mol Physiol 288: L213–L226.
7. Shi W, Wang C, Dandurand R, Eidelman D, Michel R (1998) Differential responses of pulmonary arteries and veins to histamine and 5-HT in lung explants of guinea-pigs. Br J Pharmacol 123: 1525–1532.
8. Evans A, Hardie D, Peers C, Mahmoud A (2011) Hypoxic pulmonary vasoconstriction: mechanisms of oxygen-sensing. Curr Opin Anaesthesiol 24: 13–20.
9. Ressmeyer A, Larsson A, Vollmer E, Dahlen S, Uhlig S, et al. (2006) Characterisation of guinea pig precision-cut lung slices: comparison with human tissues. Eur Respir J 28: 603–611.
10. Curran-Everett D (2000) Multiple comparisons: philosophies and illustrations. Am J Physiol Regul Integr Comp Physiol 279: R1–R8.
11. Maupoil V, Bronquard C, Freslon J, Cosnay P, Findlay I (2007) Ectopic activity in the rat pulmonary vein can arise from simultaneous activation of alpha1- and beta1-adrenoceptors. Br J Pharmacol 150: 899–905.
12. Hoffmann C, Leitz M, Oberdorf-Maass S, Lohse M, Klotz K (2004) Comparative pharmacology of human beta-adrenergic receptor subtypes--characterization of stably transfected receptors in CHO cells. Naunyn Schmiedebergs Arch Pharmacol 369: 151–159.
13. Ferrell W, Khoshbaten A (1989) Adrenoceptor profile of blood vessels in the knee joint of the rabbit. J Physiol 414: 377–383.
14. Baker JG (2010) The selectivity of beta-adrenoceptor agonists at human beta1-, beta2- and beta3-adrenoceptors. Br J Pharmacol 160: 1048–1061.
15. Hyman A, Nandiwada P, Knight D, Kadowitz P (1981) Pulmonary vasodilator responses to catecholamines and sympathetic nerve stimulation in the cat. Evidence that vascular beta-2 adrenoreceptors are innervated. Circ Res 48: 407–415.
16. Gao Y, Tolsa J, Botello M, Raj J (1998) Developmental change in isoproterenol-mediated relaxation of pulmonary veins of fetal and newborn lambs. J Appl Physiol 84: 1535–1539.
17. Vincent J, Su F (2008) Physiology and pathophysiology of the vasopressinergic system. Best Pract Res Clin Anaesthesiol 22: 243–252.
18. Norel X, Walch L, Gascard J, deMontpreville V, Brink C (2004) Prostacyclin release and receptor activation: differential control of human pulmonary venous and arterial tone. Br J Pharmacol 142: 788–796.
19. Back M, Walch L, Norel X, Gascard J, Mazmanian G, et al. (2002) Modulation of vascular tone and reactivity by nitric oxide in porcine pulmonary arteries and veins. Acta Physiol Scand 174: 9–15.
20. Aldasoro M, Mauricio M, Serna E, Cortina B, Segarra G, et al. (2008) Effects of aspirin, nimesulide, and SC-560 on vasopressin-induced contraction of human gastroepiploic artery and saphenous vein. Crit Care Med 36: 193–197.
21. Pettibone D, Kishel M, Woyden C, Clineschmidt B, Bock M, et al. (1992) Radioligand binding studies reveal marked species differences in the vasopressin V1 receptor of rat, rhesus and human tissues. Life Sci 50: 1953–1958.
22. Goldsmith S, Francis G, Cowley AJ, Goldenberg I, Cohn J (1986) Hemodynamic effects of infused arginine vasopressin in congestive heart failure. J Am Coll Cardiol 8: 779–783.
23. Udelson J, Smith W, Hendrix G, Painchaud C, Ghazzi M, et al. (2001) Acute hemodynamic effects of conivaptan, a dual V(1A) and V(2) vasopressin receptor antagonist, in patients with advanced heart failure. Circulation 104: 2417–2423.
24. Konstam M, Gheorghiade M, Burnett JJ, Grinfeld L, Maggioni A, et al. (2007) Effects of oral tolvaptan in patients hospitalized for worsening heart failure: the EVEREST Outcome Trial. JAMA 297: 1319–1331.
25. Novella S, Martinez A, Pagan R, Hernandez M, Garcia-Sacristan A, et al. (2007) Plasma levels and vascular effects of vasopressin in patients undergoing coronary artery bypass grafting. Eur J Cardiothorac Surg 32: 69–76.
26. Dzau V, Bernstein K, Celermajer D, Cohen J, Dahlof B, et al. (2001) The relevance of tissue angiotensin-converting enzyme: manifestations in mechanistic and endpoint data. Am J Cardiol 88: 1L–20L.
27. Camarda V, Rizzi A, Calo G, Gendron G, Perron S, et al. (2002) Effects of human urotensin II in isolated vessels of various species; comparison with other vasoactive agents. Naunyn Schmiedebergs Arch Pharmacol 365: 141–149.
28. Hyman A (1969) The direct effect of norepinephrine of angiotensin on the pulmonary veins of intact dogs. J Pharmacol Exp Ther 165: 87–96.
29. Bronquard C, Maupoil V, Arbeille B, Fetissof F, Findlay I, et al. (2007) Contractile and relaxant properties of rat-isolated pulmonary veins related to localization and histology. Fundam Clin Pharmacol 21: 55–65.
30. Cumming G (1963) Acute hemodynamic effects of angiotensin II. Preliminary report. Can Med Assoc J 88: 827–832.
31. Montani D, Price L, Dorfmuller P, Achouh L, Jais X, et al. (2009) Pulmonary veno-occlusive disease. Eur Respir J 33: 189–200.

Smooth Muscle Myosin Inhibition: A Novel Therapeutic Approach for Pulmonary Hypertension

David Ho[2]❡, Li Chen[2]❡, Xin Zhao[2], Nicquanna Durham[3], Malar Pannirselvam[3], Dorothy E. Vatner[2], David J. Morgans[3], Fady I. Malik[3], Stephen F. Vatner[1,2]*, You-Tang Shen[1,2]

1 CV Dynamics, Inc., North Brunswick, New Jersey, United States of America, **2** Cardiovascular Research Institute, University of Medicine and Dentistry of New Jersey, New Jersey Medical School, Newark, New Jersey, United States of America, **3** Cytokinetics, Inc., South San Francisco, California, United States of America

Abstract

Objective: Pulmonary hypertension remains a major clinical problem despite current therapies. In this study, we examine for the first time a novel pharmacological target, smooth muscle myosin, and determine if the smooth muscle myosin inhibitor, CK-2019165 (CK-165) ameliorates pulmonary hypertension.

Materials and Methods: Six domestic female pigs were surgically instrumented to measure pulmonary blood flow and systemic and pulmonary vascular dynamics. Pulmonary hypertension was induced by hypoxia, or infusion of the thromboxane analog (U-46619, 0.1 µg/kg/min, i.v.). In rats, chronic pulmonary hypertension was induced by monocrotaline.

Results: CK-165 (4 mg/kg, i.v.) reduced pulmonary vascular resistance by 22±3 and 28±6% from baseline in hypoxia and thromboxane pig models, respectively ($p<0.01$ and 0.01), while mean arterial pressure also fell and heart rate rose slightly. When CK-165 was delivered via inhalation in the hypoxia model, pulmonary vascular resistance fell by 17±6% ($p<0.05$) while mean arterial pressure and heart rate were unchanged. In the monocrotaline model of chronic pulmonary hypertension, inhaled CK-165 resulted in a similar (18.0±3.8%) reduction in right ventricular systolic pressure as compared with sildenafil (20.3±4.5%).

Conclusion: Inhibition of smooth muscle myosin may be a novel therapeutic target for treatment of pulmonary hypertension.

Editor: Martin Gerbert Frasch, Université de Montréal, Canada

Funding: This study was funded by National Institutes of Health (grants HL033107-27, HL069020-10, HL101420-01, HL093481-02, HL102472-01, HL069752-08, AG027211-04), and a grant from Cytokinetics and CV Dynamics. The funders had no role in study design, data collection and analysis, decision to publish, or preparation of the manuscript.

Competing Interests: FIM and DJM are employees and stockholders of Cytokinetics, Inc. SFV and YTS are employees and stockholders of CV Dynamics, Inc. Cytokinetics holds the patent of the smooth muscle myosin inhibitor CK-2019165 (U.S. Patent publication 2009-0275537 A1). At the current time, there are no products related to this work in clinical development or on the market to declare. CV Dynamics has no patent rights or financial interest in product development.

* E-mail: vatnersf@umdnj.edu

❡ These authors contributed equally to this work.

Introduction

Pulmonary artery hypertension is a serious and progressive disease of varied etiologies including genetic and environmental factors that also may be associated with other chronic medical conditions [1]. Regardless of the underlying condition, a progressive rise in pulmonary artery pressure and vascular resistance leads to right heart dysfunction and eventual right heart failure, exercise intolerance and ultimately death [2]. Prostacyclin and prostaglandin analogues (e.g., epoprostenol, iloprost, treprostinil), endothelin receptor antagonists (e.g., bosentan, ambrisentan) and phosphodiesterase inhibitors (e.g., sildenafil, tadalafil) are the three major classes of medications currently approved for treatment of pulmonary artery hypertension [1,3–5]. Despite the number of currently available therapeutic options, three year mortality remains high and survival has been estimated at 87%, 76%, and 67% for years 1, 2 and 3 respectively [6]. Accordingly, there remains a continued need for novel therapeutic options to treat pulmonary hypertension. The rationale for this study is to elucidate, for the first time, a novel pharmacological target, pulmonary arterial smooth muscle myosin.

Smooth muscle myosin is responsible for vascular contraction and maintenance of vascular tone [7,8]; current pulmonary vasodilating mechanisms indirectly inhibit smooth muscle myosin function by acting through second messenger signaling cascades. The relationship between vascular tone and intravascular pressure has been well established. Since the mechanical force generated through the hydrolysis of ATP by smooth muscle myosin is needed for the generation of vascular tone [8,9], it follows that all regulatory pathways of vascular tone and intravascular pressure ultimately converge at smooth muscle myosin. Recently, selective direct smooth muscle myosin inhibitors capable of blocking ATP hydrolysis and relaxing vascular smooth muscle have been developed and we have reported the efficacy of one such inhibitor,

CK-2018448, in a model of systemic hypertension [10]. These smooth muscle myosin inhibitors relax vascular smooth muscle by binding to the myosin enzymatic domain and inhibiting ATP turnover, leaving smooth muscle myosin in a weak actin binding state. However, it is unknown whether smooth muscle myosin inhibitors are able to reduce pulmonary vascular tone in the setting of pulmonary hypertension. In the current study, we examined the therapeutic potential of the smooth muscle myosin inhibitor, CK-2019165 (CK-165, US Patent Application No. 20098/0275537), delivered either as an intravenous infusion or by inhalation of a nebulized solution, in porcine and rodent models of acute pulmonary hypertension. We also compared the effects of pulmonary vascular smooth muscle myosin inhibition with the nitric oxide donor, sodium nitroprusside, the prostacyclin analog, treprostinil, and the phosphodiesterase 5 inhibitor, sildenafil. We also compared the efficacy of CK-165 to sildenafil in a rat model of chronic pulmonary arterial hypertension induced by monocrotaline.

Results

Models of Acute Pulmonary Artery Hypertension in Pigs

Hypoxia model. Hypoxia was achieved by continuous monitoring and titration of the fraction of inspired oxygen to 10%. This resulted in non-significant increases in heart rate and in pulmonary blood flow with a significant 26±1% reduction in mean arterial pressure ($p<0.01$), a 63±8% increase ($p<0.01$) in mean pulmonary arterial pressure as well as a 104±20% ($p<0.01$) increase in pulmonary vascular resistance (Figure 1, Table 1).

Thromboxane model. Thromboxane infusion in anesthetized pigs resulted in non-significant changes in mean arterial pressure, heart rate and pulmonary blood flow with a significant 88±8% increase ($p<0.01$) in mean pulmonary arterial pressure, and a 125±18% increase in pulmonary vascular resistance ($p<0.05$) (Figure 1, Table 2).

Antihypertensive Effects of CK-165 Compared with Nitroprusside

Hypoxia Model of Pulmonary Hypertension. Intravenous delivery of the smooth muscle myosin inhibitor CK-165 (4 mg/kg) in anesthetized pigs, compared with nitroprusside (2 µg/kg) resulted in a lesser peak reduction in mean arterial pressure of 11±3% vs. 26±3% ($p<0.01$), but with similar peak reductions in mean pulmonary arterial pressure (3.7±1 mmHg vs. 5.8±0.7 mmHg, $p=0.056$) and pulmonary vascular resistance (22±3 vs. 15±5%). These results suggest that similar pulmonary vascular effects were obtained with the two drugs, with a lower risk of systemic hypotension with CK-165. Furthermore, a greater increase in peak pulmonary blood flow was seen with CK-165 (9±1%) as compared to nitroprusside (4±2%) ($p<0.01$) along with a more sustained effect as compared to nitroprusside. (Figure 2, Table 1).

When CK-165 (10 mg/ml) and nitroprusside (4 mg/ml) were delivered via inhalation in the hypoxia model of pulmonary artery hypertension in anesthetized pigs, they resulted in relatively minor effects on mean arterial pressure, and similar, but modest effects on pulmonary artery pressure and vascular resistance (Figure 3), suggesting that when delivered via inhalation, CK-165 and nitroprusside have similar effects on pulmonary hypertension.

Thromboxane Model of Pulmonary Hypertension. In anesthetized pigs, intravenous delivery of CK-165 resulted in a significantly greater maximal reduction in mean arterial pressure of 25±3% vs. 14±4% ($p<0.05$) compared with nitroprusside (2 µg/kg). The peak reductions in mean pulmonary arterial pressure 17±5 vs. 16±3% were similar, while the decrease in pulmonary vascular resistance tended to be greater with CK-165 (28±6 vs. 14±4%, $p=0.08$), accordingly, as was observed in the conscious pigs, there was a greater increase in peak pulmonary blood flow with CK-165 (15±3%) as compared to nitroprusside (1±2%) ($p<0.05$). Again the effects of CK-165 were more gradual in onset and longer lasting as compared with nitroprusside (Figure 4, Table 2).

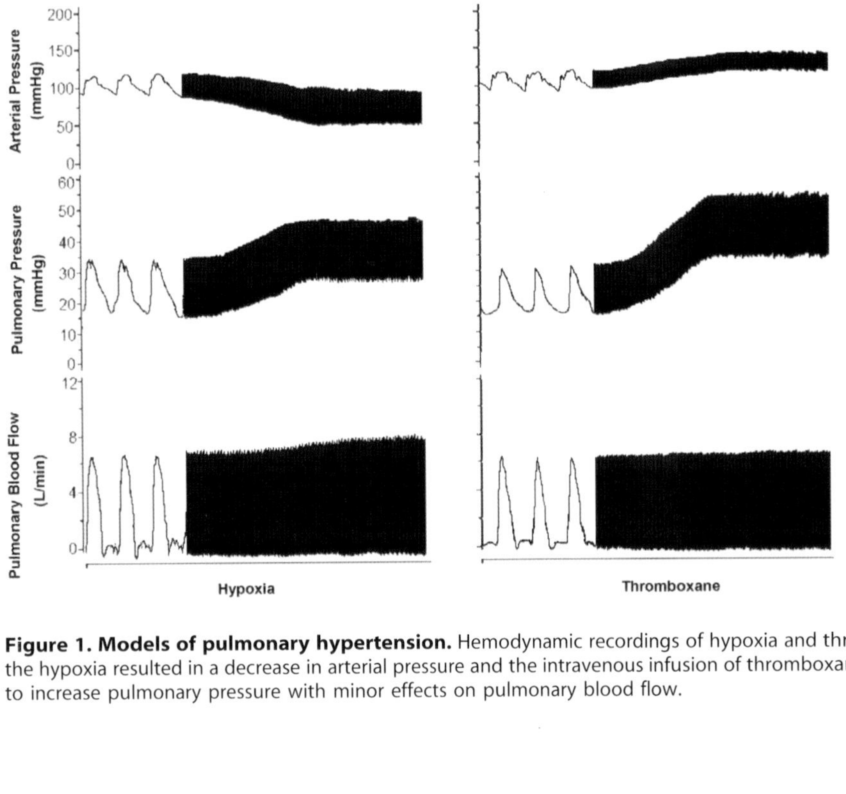

Figure 1. Models of pulmonary hypertension. Hemodynamic recordings of hypoxia and thromboxane pulmonary hypertension models. While the hypoxia resulted in a decrease in arterial pressure and the intravenous infusion of thromboxane resulted in an increase, both methods were able to increase pulmonary pressure with minor effects on pulmonary blood flow.

Table 1. Effects of Hypoxia and Subsequent CK-2019165 or Nitroprusside.

	Pre-Hypertension Baseline	Pulmonary Hypertension baseline	Hypoxia Model (CK-165) % change		Hypoxia Model (Nitroprusside) % change	
	(n = 6)	(n = 6)	Intravenous (n = 5)	Inhalation (n = 6)	Intravenous (n = 6)	Inhalation (n = 6)
Heart Rate (bpm)	125±7.7	146±9.4	8.7±1.0%‡	3.3±0.8%‡ ##	8.6±2.7%†	−0.4±0.8%
Mean Arterial Pressure (mmHg)	97±3.1	71±1.8**	−10.7±2.8%† ##	−0.6±1.0%	−25.9±2.5%‡	2.5±3.4%
Mean Pulmonary Artery Pressure (mmHg)	17.8±0.3	28.8±1.0**	−13.7±2.4%‡	−13.9±3.3%‡	−22.6±3.4%‡	−12.2±1.4%‡
Pulmonary Blood Flow (L/min)	2.6±0.1 (n = 5)	2.8±0.2 (n = 5)	9.4±1.1%‡ ##	1.5±1.3% (n = 5)	4.2±2.2% (n = 5)	1.5±1.0% (n = 5)
Pulmonary vascular resistance (mmHg/L/min)	4.0±0.3 (n = 5)	8.1±1.0** (n = 5)	−21.9±2.9%‡	−17.2±5.7%† (n = 5)	−14.7±4.7%† (n = 5)	−13.2±3.1%† (n = 5)

*p<0.05 Pulmonary Hypertension vs. Pre-Hypertension Baseline.
**p<0.01 Pulmonary Hypertension vs. Pre-Hypertension Baseline.
†p<0.05 Hypertension Baseline vs. Subsequent CK-2019165 or nitroprusside.
‡p<0.01 Hypertension Baseline vs. Subsequent CK-2019165 or nitroprusside.
#p<0.05 CK-2019165 vs. nitroprusside.
##p<0.01 CK-2019165 vs. nitroprusside.

In three conscious pigs, intravenous delivery of CK-165 compared with intravenous delivery of nitroprusside (2 μg/kg) reduced mean arterial pressure (10±2% vs. 8±2%) and mean pulmonary arterial pressure similarly (13±4 vs. 11±1%) while CK-165 decreased pulmonary vascular resistance somewhat more (17±1%) than nitroprusside (6±5%), resulting in a greater increase in peak pulmonary blood flow seen with CK-165 (11±3%) as compared to nitroprusside (1±3%) ($p<0.05$). Furthermore, the effects of CK-165 were more gradual in onset and longer lasting as compared to the rapid rise and fall seen with nitroprusside (Data not shown).

Rat Model of pulmonary artery hypertension against treprostinil and sildenafil

In anesthetized rats, pulmonary hypertension was induced by intravenous infusion of thromboxane (U-46619). Once the right ventricular systolic pressure (RVSP) and mean arterial pressure (MAP) were stable CK-165 was delivered via inhalation at 5 mg/kg (20.4±8.6%, $p<0.01$) and 30 mg/kg (58.2±6.9%, $p<0.01$), resulting in a significant reduction in RVSP compared with saline treated rats by the six minute time point (Figure 5). Furthermore, when compared against both the prostacyclin analog treprostinil and the phosphodiesterase 5 inhibitor sildenafil, a similar maximal reduction of RVSP was achieved with CK-165 (Figure 5).

Model of chronic pulmonary artery hypertension with monocrotaline in rats

Pulmonary artery hypertension was induced in rats via administration of a single dose of monocrotaline (60 mg/kg subcutaneously). After two weeks, animals were randomized to receive 100 mg/kg/day sildenafil or no sildenafil for 7 days and at the end of which the groups were randomized again to receive 30 mg/kg CK-165 or placebo. CK-165 was able to induce a similar reduction in RVSP with (20±4.5%, $p<0.01$) or without (18±3.8%, $p<0.05$) sildenafil compared with the monocrotaline only group (Figure 6).

Ex-vivo demonstration of vaso-relaxation via smooth muscle myosin inhibition

Pulmonary arteries were isolated from naïve rats as well as monocrotaline induced pulmonary artery hypertensive rats and

Table 2. Effects of Thromboxane and Subsequent CK-2019165 or Nitroprusside in Anesthetized Pigs.

	Pre-Hypertension Baseline	Pulmonary Hypertension baseline	Thromboxane Peak (CK-165) % Change	Thromboxane Peak (Nitroprusside) % Change
	(n = 5)	(n = 5)	(n = 4)	(n = 5)
Heart Rate (bpm)	128±4.3	130±6.9	6.7±2.7%	5.1±1.7%†
Mean Arterial Pressure (mmHg)	100±5.1	112±6.2	−24.5±2.5%‡ #	−13.6±3.6%‡
Mean Pulmonary Artery Pressure (mmHg)	18.5±0.9	34.7±1.4**	−17.4±5.4%†	−15.6±3.0%‡
Pulmonary Blood Flow (L/min)	3.2±0.4 (n = 4)	3.0±0.4 (n = 4)	14.85±3.4%† ##	1.42±1.8%
Pulmonary vascular resistance (mmHg/L/min)	4.5±0.9 (n = 4)	10.0±1.8* (n = 4)	−28.2±5.5%†	−14.3±4.2%†

*p<0.05 Pulmonary Hypertension vs. Pre-Hypertension Baseline.
**p<0.01 Pulmonary Hypertension vs. Pre-Hypertension Baseline.
†p<0.05 Hypertension Baseline vs. Subsequent CK-2019165 or nitroprusside.
‡p<0.01 Hypertension Baseline vs. Subsequent CK-2019165 or nitroprusside.
#p<0.05 CK-2019165 vs. nitroprusside.
##p<0.01 CK-2019165 vs. nitroprusside.

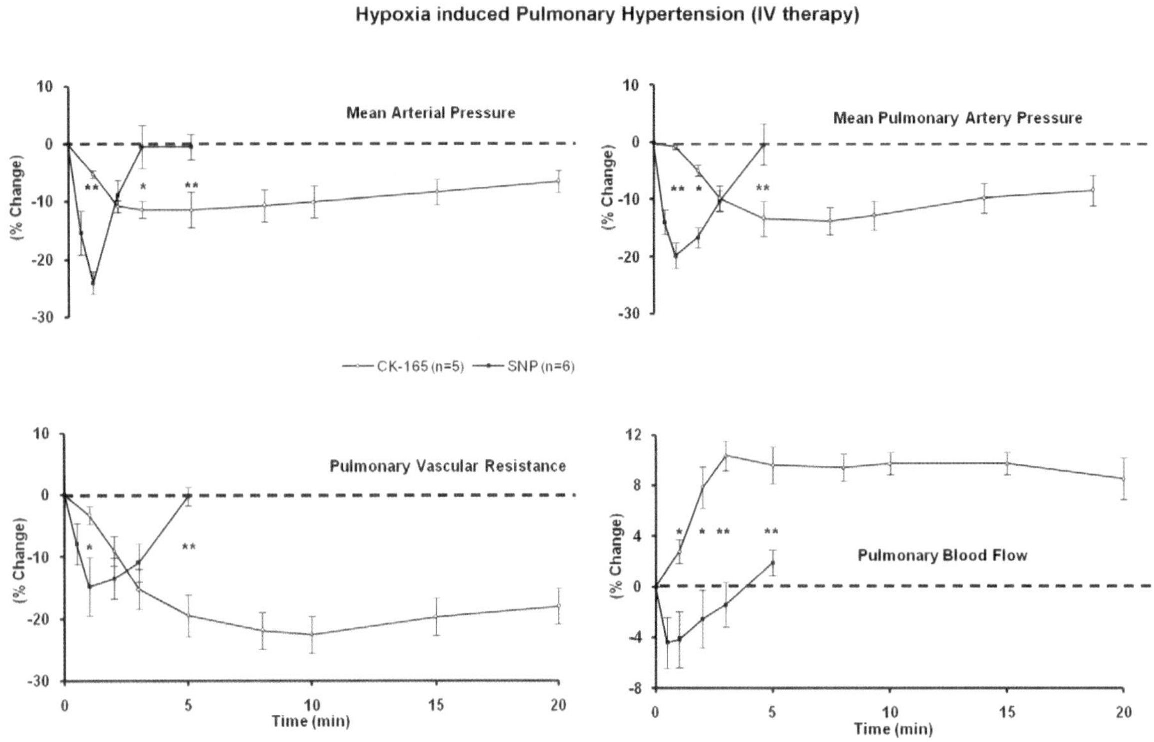

Figure 2. Effects of intravenous CK-165 on hypoxia induced pulmonary hypertension. The efficacy of intravenous CK-165 (4 mg/kg) and nitroprusside (2 μg/kg) were examined and compared in the porcine hypoxia model of pulmonary hypertension. All changes were plotted as percent change from baseline. The relatively longer half life, the more gradual and greater effects on mean pulmonary vascular resistance and blood flow were noted. (* $p<0.05$, ** $p<0.01$ CK-165 vs. nitroprusside).

contraction was stimulated via the addition of 1 μM phenylephrine. The addition of CK-2018571 (the parent of the more soluble pro-drug, CK-165) was able to relax phenylephrine induced contraction of pulmonary arterial rings from both naïve and monocrotaline induced pulmonary artery hypertensive rats with a similar EC_{50} of 6.08±0.03 μM and 6.08±0.10 μM, respectively (Figure 7).

Discussion

Since the final common effector of vascular constriction in pulmonary hypertension is smooth muscle myosin; it follows that an agent that relaxed smooth muscle at the level of smooth muscle myosin would be an effective approach to pulmonary vasodilation. Indeed, this mechanism appears effective in reducing arterial pressure in models of systemic hypertension [10]. The major finding of the current investigation is that the smooth muscle myosin inhibitors, CK-2019165, a soluble pro-drug of CK-2018571 were effective in reducing pulmonary vascular resistance in several models of pulmonary hypertension.

The effectiveness of smooth muscle myosin inhibition was demonstrated in two acute models of pulmonary hypertension (hypoxia and thromboxane) in chronically instrumented pigs with direct and continuous measurements of pulmonary and aortic arterial pressure, pulmonary blood flow and vascular resistance and compared to nitroprusside, a nitric oxide donor examined extensively in animal models of pulmonary hypertension [11–14]. Inhalation of nitric oxide is used in patients with pulmonary hypertension to establish the degree of acute reversibility and to reduce pulmonary artery pressure in the setting of adult respiratory distress syndrome without affecting systemic vascular tone [15]. The smooth muscle myosin inhibitor, CK-165, achieved similar efficacy to nitroprusside in these acute models of pulmonary hypertension.

Inhibition of smooth muscle myosin with CK-165 effectively reduced pulmonary artery pressure and pulmonary vascular resistance in both the hypoxia and thromboxane models of pulmonary hypertension regardless of whether the drug was delivered via the intravenous or inhalation route. When the drug was delivered intravenously, there was a fall in systemic arterial pressure suggesting the drug also affected systemic resistance vessels. However, when the drug was delivered through inhalation, this was not observed and the vasodilator effects were localized to the pulmonary vasculature.

A second goal of this study was to compare the effects of CK-165 in acute and chronic rat models of pulmonary hypertension. Smooth muscle myosin inhibition is capable of directly relaxing pulmonary artery vascular rings derived from rats with chronic pulmonary hypertension induced by monocrotaline to a similar degree and potency as those derived from naïve rats, consistent with a direct effect on the pulmonary vasculature. When delivered via nebulization in the thromboxane induced rat model of acute pulmonary hypertension, CK-165 reduced right ventricular systolic pressure (RVSP) consistent with a reduction in pulmonary artery pressure; further, CK-165 was able to reduce the RVSP to a similar extent (although not similar potency) as that seen with either treprostinil or sildenafil.

Finally, to address the question of efficacy in a setting where pulmonary vascular remodeling is present as is found in chronic pulmonary artery hypertension, we examined the efficacy of CK-165 in rats with monocrotaline induced chronic pulmonary artery hypertension. CK-165 reduced RVSP as an acute monotherapy to

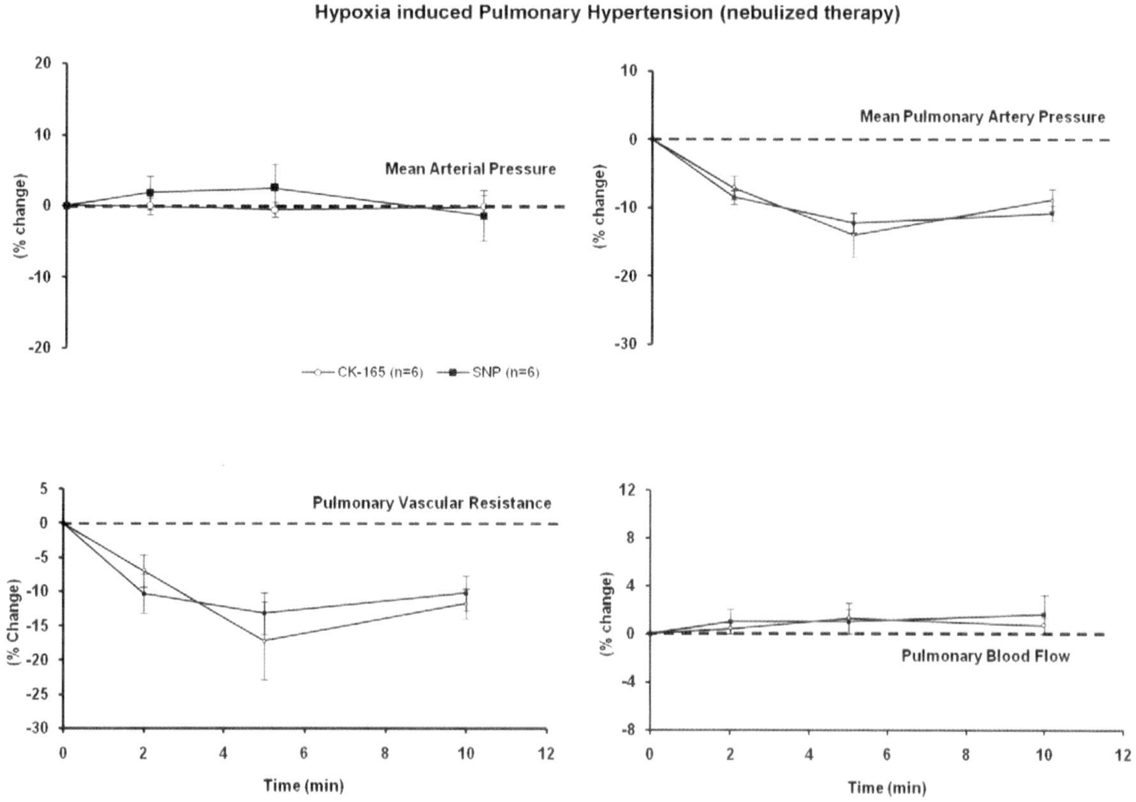

Figure 3. Effects of nebulized CK-165 on hypoxia induced pulmonary hypertension. The efficacy of nebulized CK-165 (4 mg/kg) and nitroprusside (2 μg/kg) were examined and compared in the porcine hypoxia model of pulmonary hypertension. All changes were plotted as percent change from baseline. When delivered continuously, similar effect profiles are observed between CK-165 and nitroprusside.

a similar extent as did 7 days of dosing with sildenafil; the level of reduction in RVSP was essentially the same when co-administrated with sildenafil, suggesting that a maximal effect on RSVP had been attained by each of these therapies.

In conclusion, inhibition of smooth muscle myosin is an effective means to reduce pulmonary vascular resistance and may be a potential therapeutic approach for pulmonary hypertension. Its effects compared with nitroprusside were more gradual and sustained when delivered intravenously, but quite similar when delivered by inhalation. Furthermore, it was able to produce similar effects when compared against both a prostacyclin analog as well as a phosphodiesterase 5 inhibitor in the case of acute pulmonary artery hypertension and against a phosphodiesterase 5 inhibitor in the setting of chronic pulmonary artery hypertension. Based on our results, inhibition of smooth muscle myosin appears to be efficacious in models of pulmonary hypertension. Although the duration of action of the current smooth muscle myosin inhibitor examined in this study may not be sufficient for chronic therapy in this disease, the current study provides proof of concept for this novel therapeutic target and its application to the treatment of pulmonary hypertension.

Materials and Methods

CK-2019165 and CK-2018571 were provided by Cytokinetics, Inc.

Animal Models

Animals used in this study were maintained in accordance with the *Guide for the Care and Use of Laboratory Animals of the National Health Institute (NIH, 2010)* and *New Jersey Medical School Institutional Animal Care and Use Committee or by the Institutional Animal Care and Use Committee at Cytokinetics, Inc.* This study has been approved by the *New Jersey Medical School Institutional Animal Care and Use Committee* protocol# 08088 and by the *Cytokinetics, Inc. Institutional Animal Care and Use Committee* under Protocol CK020-09.

Pig Models. Six domestic female pigs (15–20 kg) were anesthetized with thiopental (15 mg/kg i.v.) followed by endotracheal intubation and halothane (1.0–1.5 vol%) anesthesia. A left thoracotomy at the 5th intercostal space was performed, Tygon catheters were placed in the descending aorta, pulmonary artery and left atrium to measure their respective pressures. A Tygon catheter was also placed in the right atrium and used for drug administration. A transonic flow probe was placed around the main pulmonary artery to measure pulmonary blood flow. The chest was closed and post-operative analgesics were administered until the animals recovered fully from surgery. Female pigs were chosen over male pigs due to anatomical concerns for animal discomfort while in the sling during the extended experimental time period. All experiments in pigs were performed under anesthesia except for the experiments involving thromboxane induced pulmonary hypertension where experiments were performed in both conscious and anesthetized pigs.

Systemic hemodynamics in pigs were recorded using a Triton system (Triton, Inc.) and PowerLab data acquisition system (ADInstruments, Inc.). Aortic, pulmonary artery and atrial pressure were measured using strain gauge manometers that had been calibrated with a mercury manometer connected to the fluid-filled catheters. Pulmonary blood flow was measured with a

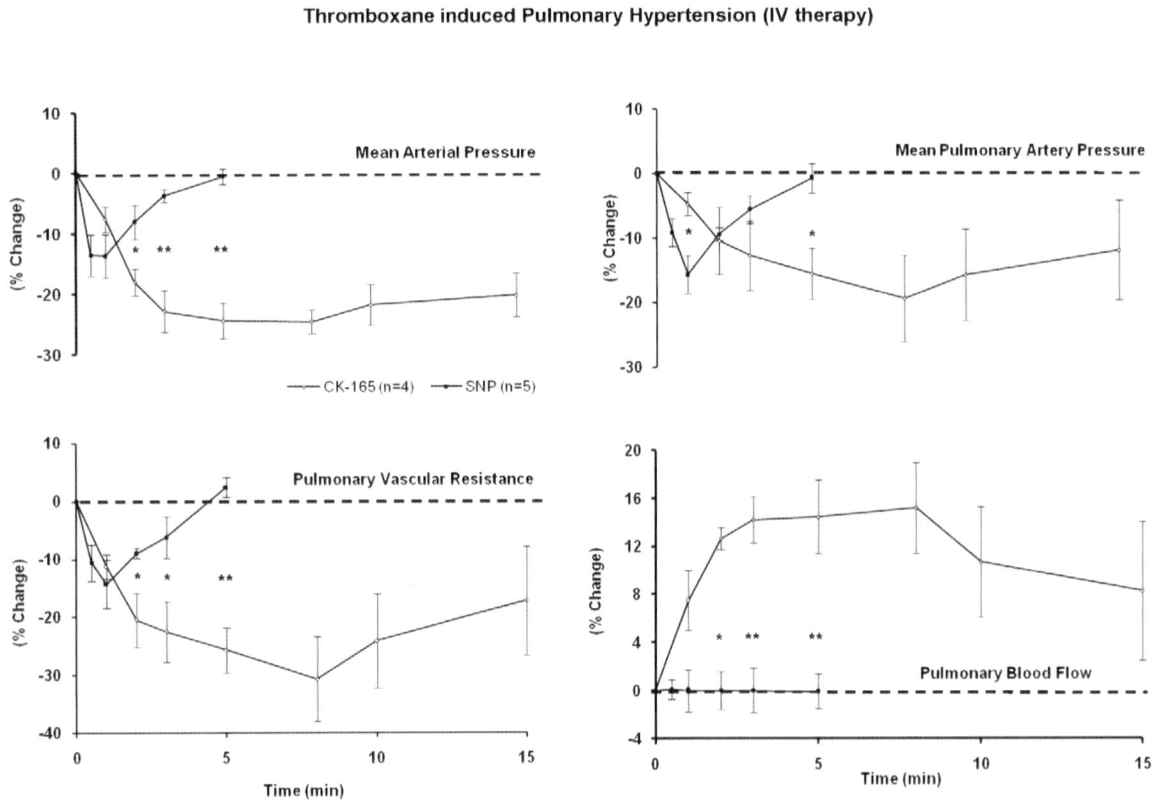

Figure 4. Effects of intravenous CK-165 on thromboxane induced pulmonary hypertension. The efficacy of intravenous CK-165 (4 mg/kg) and nitroprusside (2 μg/kg) were examined and compared in the porcine thromboxane model of pulmonary hypertension. All changes were plotted as percent change from baseline. The relatively longer half life, the more gradual and greater effects on mean arterial pressure, mean pulmonary vascular resistance and blood flow were noted. (* $p<0.05$, ** $p<0.01$ CK-165 vs. nitroprusside).

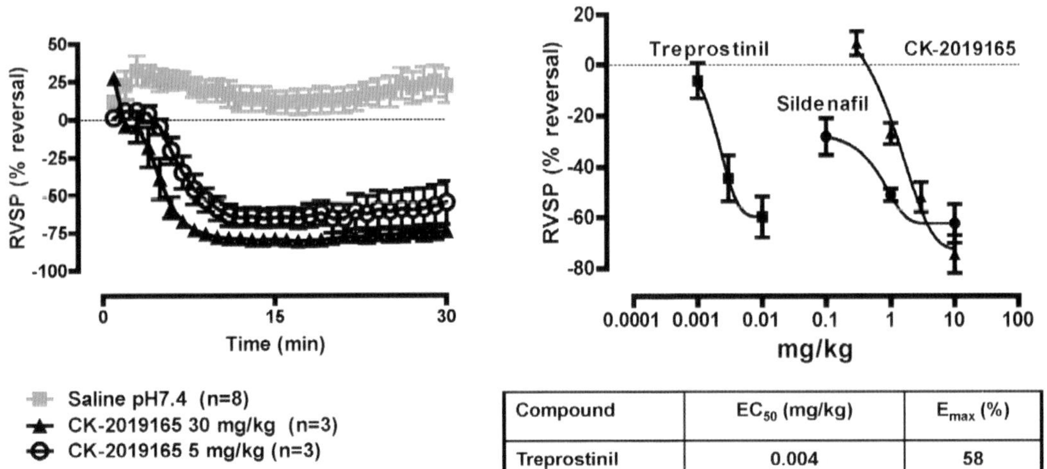

Compound	EC_{50} (mg/kg)	E_{max} (%)
Treprostinil	0.004	58
Sildenafil	0.92	61
CK-2019165	2.35	75

Figure 5. Dose response and pharmacodynamics of CK-165 in rats with U46619 induced pulmonary hypertension. CK-165 decreased RVSP rapidly after nebulization at both 5 mg/kg and 30 mg/kg by 20.4±8.6 and 58.2±6.9% at 6 minutes, respectively ($p<0.01$ compared with baseline). The maximum decrease in RVSP, E_{max}, observed with CK-165 (75±7.53%) is similar to that seen with the prostacyclin analog, treprostinil (58±8.09%) and the phosphodiesterase 5 inhibitor, sildenafil (61±7.65%).

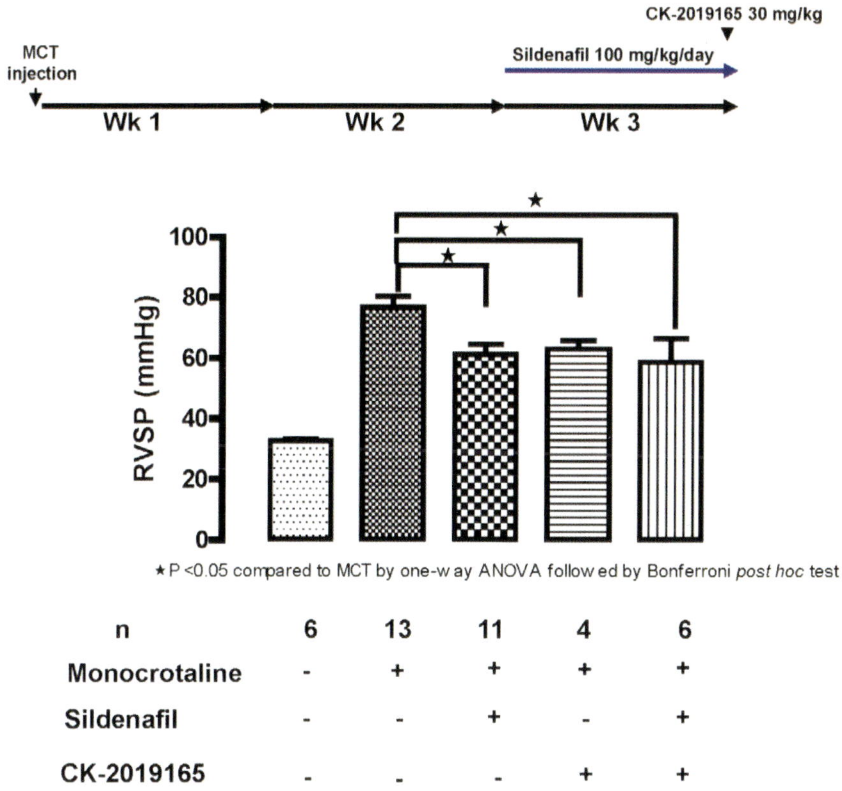

Figure 6. The effect of CK-165 and sildenafil in rats with monocrotaline-induced pulmonary hypertension. CK-165 decreased RSVP following intratracheal nebulization of 30 mg/kg in rats with monocrotaline induced pulmonary artery hypertension by 18.0±3.8% ($p<0.05$) when compared with vehicle treated group. The decrease is similar to that in monocrotaline rats treated with 100 mg/kg/day sildenafil (20.3±4.5%) for 7 days and treatment with CK-165 does not appear to have additive effects when co-administered with sildenafil.

Transonic flow meter (Transonic Systems Inc., T206). Pulmonary vascular resistance was calculated: (pulmonary arterial pressure - left atrial pressure)/pulmonary blood flow. Due to instrumentation failure not all hemodynamic variables were recorded for all experiments and animals.

Five to ten days after surgical instrumentation, pulmonary hypertension was induced with two different methods in the same animal at different times. 1) Hypoxic pig model: pigs were intubated, anesthetized with isoflurane, and ventilated at a reduced fraction of inspired O_2. Pulmonary hypertension resulted after the fraction of inspired O_2 was reduced to about 10% by adjusting the ratio of N_2/O_2 mixture in the inspiratory limb of the ventilator. Pulmonary hypertension was defined as a sustained elevation of mean pulmonary arterial pressure to ≥25 mmHg from an averaged baseline level of 18 mmHg. Arterial oxygen saturation was monitored continuously using a pulse oximeter

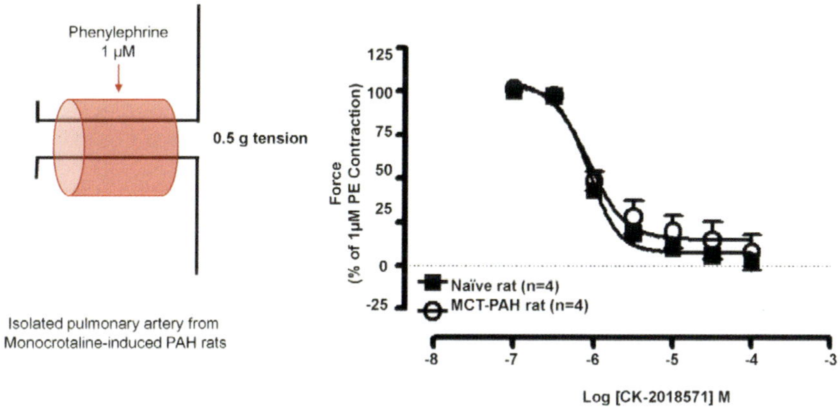

Figure 7. Determination of EC_{50} for CK-2018571 in pulmonary artery tissue rings. CK-2018571 inhibits phenylephrine-induced pulmonary artery contraction in isolated tissue rings from naïve and monocrotaline-treated rats. Pulmonary artery rings were pre-contracted with 1 μM phenylephrine and isometric tension was recorded in the presence of increasing concentrations of CK-2018571. CK-2018571 elicited relaxation in tissues from naïve rats with $pEC_{50}=6.08\pm0.03$, and in tissues from monocrotaline-treated rats with $pEC_{50}=6.08\pm0.10$.

during the entire experimental period. 2) Thromboxane model: pigs were placed in a sling and infused intravenously with the endoperoxide analog of thromboxane, U46619, at 0.1–0.5 μg/kg/min in the anesthetized state. These pigs were also studied with this procedure in the conscious state. Pulmonary hypertension was defined as a stable pulmonary artery pressure of greater than 30 mmHg. The animals were allowed to breathe spontaneously.

In the hypoxia pig model, once the pulmonary arterial pressure stabilized for 15 min, a volume of 2–3 ml of 10 mg/ml (CK-165) was nebulized over 4–5 min through the endotracheal tube using a Pari LC Plus compressed air nebulizer. The nebulizer was operated at 20 psi which results in an output of ~4.5 L/min. Sodium nitroprusside (4 mg/ml) was nebulized for the same duration as a control. After the drugs washed out, i.e., pulmonary artery pressure and mean arterial pressure returned to baseline levels and remained stable for 30 min, the smooth muscle myosin inhibitor CK-2019165 (4 mg/kg) was administered intravenously as was the positive control sodium nitroprusside (2 mg/kg). Without prior pharmacokinetic and pharmacodynamic data in the porcine model, the washout period for the animals was determined based on results of hemodynamic monitoring and was determined to be adequate after all hemodynamic variables returned to baseline and were stable for 30 min. In the thromboxane model, CK-165 and nitroprusside were administered intravenously in separate experiments under both the conscious and anesthetized states. In all models systemic and pulmonary vascular changes were monitored and compared.

Rat Models. Male Sprague-Dawley rats (Harlan, Indianapolis, IN) weighing between 180 and 210 g were housed in conventional conditions. Acute pulmonary artery hypertension was induced by continuous intravenous infusion of U-46619 (1 μg/kg/min). Chronic pulmonary artery hypertension was induced on day 0 by a single dose of monocrotaline (MCT) (60 mg/kg subcutaneously) (Sigma-Aldrich, St. Louis, MO). The rats were randomly assigned to five experimental groups: 1) Control; 2) MCT; 3) MCT+100 mg/kg/day Sildenafil for 7 days (days 15–21); 4) MCT+CK-2019165 30 mg/kg (on day 21), as a single nebulized dose; and 5) MCT+100 mg/kg Sildenafil (days 15–21)+CK-2019165 30 mg/kg (on day 21), as a single nebulized dose.

Hemodynamic measurements were made following anesthesia with a ketamine, xylazine and acepromazine cocktail at the dose of 80–100 mg/kg, 10 mg/kg and 1 mg/kg respectively, intramuscular. Rats were mechanically ventilated at 60–80 breaths/minute with a tidal volume of 2.0–3.0 ml/cycle using a Harvard rodent ventilator. The right ventricular pressure was recorded by advancing a 4.0 French pressure sensing catheter (Millar, Houston TX) into the right ventricle via right jugular vein. CK-2019165 was administrated via intra-tracheal nebulization at 30 mg/kg.

For preparation of pulmonary artery tissue rings for *in vitro* study, the main branch of pulmonary artery was isolated from naïve or monocrotaline (MCT)-treated rats and placed in oxygenated physiological salt solution. The pulmonary arteries were cleaned of adherent tissue and cut into rings (2 mm in length) and suspended in isolated tissue baths (volume 10 ml) containing oxygenated Krebs–Ringer bicarbonate buffer with the following composition (in mmol/l): NaCl (118), KCl (4.7), $CaCl_2$ (2.5), KH_2PO_4 (1.2), $MgSO_4$ (1.2), $NaHCO_3$ (25), dextrose (11.1) and disodium calcium edetate (0.026), maintained at 37°C and bubbled with 95% O_2 and 5% CO_2. A resting tension of 0.5 g was applied (determined by preliminary experiments to afford the optimum tension-length relationship). Following equilibration for 60 minutes, isometric dose response curves were recorded with increasing concentrations of CK-2018571 in rings pre-contracted with phenylephrine (1 μM). Results are mean ± SE, percent of maximum relaxation to CK-2018571 (E_{max}) and agonist sensitivity ($pEC_{50} = -logEC_{50}$; EC_{50} is concentration that evokes 50% relaxation). Values were determined using non-linear regression for both naïve and MCT-treated rat pulmonary arterial rings.

Statistical analysis

Data are expressed as mean±SE. Statistical significance was determined using a paired two tailed t-test when comparing CK-165 to baseline. An unpaired t-test was used to compare the peak responses of CK-165 to nitroprusside. In all experiments, the peak response time was chosen based on continuous monitoring and accordingly, in the CK-165 treated hypoxia model the peak response time was at 5 minutes. Due to a variation in peak times in the CK-165-treated thromboxane model, the average of 5 and 8 minute responses were used as peak for comparative analysis. For nitroprusside in the hypoxia model with inhalation delivery, the peak response time was 5 minutes, in all other pig models the peak response time was 1 minute. For chronic pulmonary artery hypertension studies, the statistical significance was determined by one-way ANOVA followed by Bonferroni's post-hoc test.

Acknowledgments

We would like to thank Serge Salganik for help in preparation of the manuscript.

Author Contributions

Conceived and designed the experiments: SFV DH YTS. Performed the experiments: DH LC YTS XZ ND MP. Analyzed the data: SFV DH LC YTS DEV ND MP. Contributed reagents/materials/analysis tools: FIM DJM ND MP. Wrote the paper: DH SVF DEV.

References

1. Galie N, Hoeper MM, Humbert M, Torbicki A, Vachiery JL, et al. (2009) Guidelines for the diagnosis and treatment of pulmonary hypertension: the Task Force for the Diagnosis and Treatment of Pulmonary Hypertension of the European Society of Cardiology (ESC) and the European Respiratory Society (ERS), endorsed by the International Society of Heart and Lung Transplantation (ISHLT). Eur Heart J 30: 2493–2537.
2. Badesch DB, Champion HC, Sanchez MA, Hoeper MM, Loyd JE, et al. (2009) Diagnosis and assessment of pulmonary arterial hypertension. J Am Coll Cardiol 54: S55–66.
3. Gomberg-Maitland M, Dufton C, Oudiz RJ, Benza RL (2011) Compelling evidence of long-term outcomes in pulmonary arterial hypertension? A clinical perspective. J Am Coll Cardiol 57: 1053–1061.
4. Badesch DB, Abman SH, Simonneau G, Rubin LJ, McLaughlin VV (2007) Medical therapy for pulmonary arterial hypertension: updated ACCP evidence-based clinical practice guidelines. Chest 131: 1917–1928.
5. Safdar Z (2011) Treatment of pulmonary arterial hypertension: the role of prostacyclin and prostaglandin analogs. Respir Med 105: 818–827.
6. Humbert M, Sitbon O, Yaici A, Montani D, O'Callaghan DS, et al. (2010) Survival in incident and prevalent cohorts of patients with pulmonary arterial hypertension. Eur Respir J 36: 549–555.
7. Morano S, Cipriani R, Gabriele A, Medici F, Pantellini F (2000) [Recurrent brown tumors as initial manifestation of primary hyperparathyroidism. An unusual presentation]. Minerva Med 91: 117–122.
8. Babu GJ, Loukianov E, Loukianova T, Pyne GJ, Huke S, et al. (2001) Loss of SM-B myosin affects muscle shortening velocity and maximal force development. Nat Cell Biol 3: 1025–1029.
9. Morano I, Chai GX, Baltas LG, Lamounier-Zepter V, Lutsch G, et al. (2000) Smooth-muscle contraction without smooth-muscle myosin. Nat Cell Biol 2: 371–375.
10. Zhao X, Ho D, Abarzua P, Dhar SK, Wang X, et al. (2011) Inhibition of smooth muscle myosin as a novel therapeutic target for hypertension. J Pharmacol Exp Ther 339: 307–312.
11. Adrie C, Ichinose F, Holzmann A, Keefer L, Hurford WE, et al. (1998) Pulmonary vasodilation by nitric oxide gas and prodrug aerosols in acute pulmonary hypertension. J Appl Physiol 84: 435–441.

12. Schutte H, Grimminger F, Otterbein J, Spriestersbach R, Mayer K, et al. (1997) Efficiency of aerosolized nitric oxide donor drugs to achieve sustained pulmonary vasodilation. J Pharmacol Exp Ther 282: 985–994.
13. Meadow W, Rudinsky B, Bell A, Hipps R (1998) Effects of nebulized nitroprusside on pulmonary and systemic hemodynamics during pulmonary hypertension in piglets. Pediatr Res 44: 181–186.
14. Yu XQ, Saugstad OD (1999) Nebulization of sodium nitroprusside in lung-lavaged newborn piglets. Pediatr Res 45: 255–259.
15. Rossaint R, Falke KJ, Lopez F, Slama K, Pison U, et al. (1993) Inhaled nitric oxide for the adult respiratory distress syndrome. N Engl J Med 328: 399–405.

Nicorandil Prevents Right Ventricular Remodeling by Inhibiting Apoptosis and Lowering Pressure Overload in Rats with Pulmonary Arterial Hypertension

Xiang-Rong Zuo[1,2]●, Qiang Wang[1]●, Quan Cao[2]●, Yan-Zhe Yu[1], Hui Wang[1], Li-Qing Bi[1], Wei-Ping Xie[1]*, Hong Wang[1]*

1 Department of Respiratory Medicine, The First Affiliated Hospital of Nanjing Medical University, Nanjing, Jiangsu, People's Republic of China, 2 Department of Critical Care Medicine, The First Affiliated Hospital of Nanjing Medical University, Nanjing, Jiangsu, People's Republic of China

Abstract

Background: Most of the deaths among patients with severe pulmonary arterial hypertension (PAH) are caused by progressive right ventricular (RV) pathological remodeling, dysfunction, and failure. Nicorandil can inhibit the development of PAH by reducing pulmonary artery pressure and RV hypertrophy. However, whether nicorandil can inhibit apoptosis in RV cardiomyocytes and prevent RV remodeling has been unclear.

Methodology/Principal Findings: RV remodeling was induced in rats by intraperitoneal injection of monocrotaline (MCT). RV systolic pressure (RVSP) was measured at the end of each week after MCT injection. Blood samples were drawn for brain natriuretic peptide (BNP) ELISA analysis. The hearts were excised for histopathological, ultrastructural, immunohistochemical, and Western blotting analyses. The MCT-injected rats exhibited greater mortality and less weight gain and showed significantly increased RVSP and RV hypertrophy during the second week. These worsened during the third week. MCT injection for three weeks caused pathological RV remodeling, characterized by hypertrophy, fibrosis, dysfunction, and RV mitochondrial impairment, as indicated by increased levels of apoptosis. Nicorandil improved survival, weight gain, and RV function, ameliorated RV pressure overload, and prevented maladaptive RV remodeling in PAH rats. Nicorandil also reduced the number of apoptotic cardiomyocytes, with a concomitant increase in Bcl-2/Bax ratio. 5-hydroxydecanoate (5-HD) reversed these beneficial effects of nicorandil in MCT-injected rats.

Conclusions/Significance: Nicorandil inhibits PAH-induced RV remodeling in rats not only by reducing RV pressure overload but also by inhibiting apoptosis in cardiomyocytes through the activation of mitochondrial ATP-sensitive K^+ (mitoK_{ATP}) channels. The use of a mitoK_{ATP} channel opener such as nicorandil for PAH-associated RV remodeling and dysfunction may represent a new therapeutic strategy for the amelioration of RV remodeling during the early stages of PAH.

Editor: Fadi N. Salloum, Virginia Commonwealth University Medical Center, United States of America

Funding: This work was partially supported by the National Natural Science Foundation of China (NSFC) (http://www.nsfc.gov.cn, No.30971319, HW), and by a research fund from the "Six Talent Peak" Project of Jiangsu Province (http://www.jshrss.gov.cn, No.08-B, WX). This work was also partially supported by the grant from Open Project Program of the key discipline of Public Health Department of Jiangsu Province (www.jswst.gov.cn, No.XK13_200902, XZ). No additional external funding received for this study. The funders had no role in study design, data collection and analysis, decision to publish, or preparation of the manuscript.

Competing Interests: The authors have declared that no competing interests exist.

* E-mail: wanghong.njmu@gmail.com (HW); xieweiping2002@yahoo.com (WX)

● These authors contributed equally to this work.

Introduction

Pulmonary arterial hypertension (PAH) is defined as a mean pulmonary artery pressure (mPAP) greater than 25 mmHg at rest with a pulmonary capillary wedge pressure, left atrial pressure, or left ventricular (LV) end-diastolic pressure less than or equal to 15 mmHg and a pulmonary vascular resistance (PVR) greater than 3 Wood units [1]. Severe PAH can cause death by progressively increasing PVR, which promotes right ventricular (RV) overload, pathological remodeling, dysfunction, and heart failure. The median survival time for patients with PAH is 2.8 years if left untreated. At present, prostanoids, endothelin-1 receptor antagonists, and phosphodiesterase-type 5 (PDE-5) inhibitors are used to improve the hemodynamics and the quality of life of patients with PAH [1]. However, these drugs produce only limited delays in the progress ion of PAH [2].

RV failure is the cause of at least 70% of deaths attributable to PAH [3]. The degree of RV remodeling is an independent prognostic indicator [4]. Many studies have confirmed that RV function is independently associated with prognosis of PAH [4,5,6,7,8]. Preventing and reversing RV remodeling and failure together with reducing pulmonary artery pressure (PAP) are therefore viable strategies for the treatment PAH [9,10].

Unlike that of LV remodeling, the pathophysiology of RV remodeling is not well understood, such that treatments successfully in the case of LV remodeling often have no beneficial effect on RV remodeling. Clinical and experimental evidence suggest that the mechanical stress created by elevated pressure on the pulmonary artery is not the only cause of PAH-induced RV remodeling and failure [11,12]. Some patients with severe PAH rapidly progress to RV failure but other patients do not [13]. RV myocardial function can also be impaired by factors such as sarcoidosis, scleroderma, and amyloidosis. These are potential contributing molecular mechanisms of RV remodeling independent of RV afterload [13]. For these reasons, the mechanisms underlying the development of RV hypertrophy (RVH) and remodeling merit further investigation.

Apoptosis plays an important role in the pathogenesis of LV remodeling. Inhibition of myocyte death is a viable therapeutic strategy [14]. In contrast, the development of PAH-induced RV remodeling and cardiomyocyte apoptosis is largely unknown. Recently, Maria et al. found that apoptosis plays a role in the progression of RV disease by using serial *in vivo* 99mTc-annexin scintigraphy [15]. This study may provide new insight into the course of cardiac cell apoptosis during RV remodeling and may aid in determining the optimal timing of antiapoptotic therapy to prevent or reverse RV remodeling.

Nicorandil, a mitochondrial ATP-dependent potassium (mitoK_{ATP}) channel opener, has been shown to be cardioprotective. Nicorandil can inhibit the development of monocrotaline (MCT)-induced PAH by reducing PAP and RVH [16]. These effects may be associated with up-regulation of lung eNOS protein, improvement in pulmonary vascular endothelial activation, and anti-inflammatory and anti-proliferative effects on lung tissue. Nicorandil can also inhibit cardiomyocyte apoptosis induced by oxidative stress and hypoxia [17,18,19], and prevent LV remodeling [20,21,22]. However, whether nicorandil can inhibit RV cardiomyocyte apoptosis and prevent RV remodeling is still unknown.

The purpose of this study is to investigate the influence of nicorandil on PAH-induced RV remodeling and the potential mechanisms. To determine whether the effects of nicorandil on RV remodeling are due to the activation of mitoK_{ATP} channels, these effects were also investigated in the presence of 5-hydroxydecanoate (5-HD), a mitoK_{ATP} channel blocker. MCT injection for three weeks caused pathological RV remodeling, characterized by hypertrophy, fibrosis, dysfunction, and RV mitochondrial impairment, as indicated by increased levels of apoptosis. Nicorandil improved RV function and prevented maladaptive RV remodeling in rats with MCT-induced severe PAH. The protective effects of nicorandil on PAH-induced RV remodeling were found to be mediated not only by reduction of RV systolic pressure (RVSP) but also by inhibition of apoptotic cell death through opening of mitoK_{ATP} channels.

Materials and Methods

Ethics Statement

All animal experiments were carried out according to the National Institutes of Health Guide for the Care and Use of Laboratory Animals (publication no. 85-23, revised 1996) and approved by the Animal Care and Use Committee of Nanjing Medical University (Approval ID 2010-SR-001).

In vivo model of PAH

Male Sprague-Dawley (SD) rats (200±20 g) were provided by the Sino-British SIPPR/BK Laboratory Animal Center (Shanghai, China). All animals were housed in groups of five per cage under standard laboratory conditions with free access to food and water at a constant room temperature of 22°C, 50–60%humidity, and a 12:12 day-night cycle. The rats were allowed to acclimate for 7 days before experimental procedures began.

Seventy-two rats received a single dose of 60 mg/kg of MCT injected intraperitoneally (ip). They were then randomly assigned to the following treatment groups: 0.9% saline (MCT-treated group), 7.5 $mg{\cdot}kg^{-1}{\cdot}d^{-1}$ nicorandil (nicorandil-treated group), and 5 $mg{\cdot}kg^{-1}{\cdot}d^{-1}$ 5-HD in combination with 7.5 $mg{\cdot}kg^{-1}{\cdot}d^{-1}$ of nicorandil (nicorandil and 5-HD-treated group). Treatments lasted 3 weeks. The age- and weight-matched control animals served as controls (control group) and received 0.9% saline. The doses of nicorandil and 5-HD used in this study were selected after review of previous studies [16,23]. MCT (Sigma-Aldrich, St. Louis, MO, U.S.) was dissolved in 1 N HCl neutralized with 1 N NaOH and diluted with 0.9% NaCl. Nicorandil (Tokyo Chemical Industry Co., Ltd, Tokyo, Japan) and 5-HD (Sigma) were dissolved in saline concentrations of 3 mg/ml and 2 mg/ml, respectively. All treatments were administered orally by gavage once daily for 3 weeks.

Body weight (BW) was measured twice a week to adjust the dose accordingly. At the end of each week of the study, 5–8 rats per group were randomly selected for a designated experimental protocol.

Hemodynamic Measurements

Twenty-one days after MCT/saline injection, all surviving rats were anesthetized with urethane (1.0 g/kg, ip) and measured for RVSP by right heart catheterization. Subcutaneous needle electrodes were inserted in the limbs for electrocardiogram (ECG) recording. The right jugular vein was isolated, and a small polyethylene catheter (PE10, Becton Dickinson, U.S.) was passed via a small transverse cut and then advanced into the RV under the guidance of the pressure tracing. After 20 minutes of stabilization, RVSP was recorded using a miniature pressure transducer (TSD104A,BIOPAC Systems, Inc., U.S.) digitized by a BIOPAC MP100 data acquisition system, and stored on a Dell PC. The femoral artery was cannulated with a small polyethylene catheter (PE 50, Becton Dickinson) for recording blood pressure (BP) with a transducer. The catheters were filled with heparinized saline (10 U/ml of heparin in 0.9% saline). ECG, RVSP and BP were simultaneously recorded on a polygraph. After hemodynamic measurements were completed, heparinized blood was collected for measurement of plasma brain natriuretic peptide (BNP). Whole lungs and hearts were also excised for Western blotting and histological analysis.

Assessment of Right Ventricular Hypertrophy

After the atria, pulmonary trunk and aorta were removed from the excised heart, the RV wall was separated from the LV wall and ventricular septum. Wet weights of the RV, free LV, and ventricular septum were determined. The ratio of RV weight to body weight (RV/BW) and the ratio of the RV weight to LV plus septum weight (RV/[LV+S]) were calculated for assessment of RVH [24].

Morphological Measurements

After being weighed, the RV was fixed with 10% neutral formalin (pH 7.40), embedded in paraffin, sectioned at a thickness of 4 μm, and stained with hematoxylin and eosin (HE) or Masson's Trichrome staining as needed. The cross-sectional area (CSA) of cardiomyocytes and the extents of interstitial and perivascular fibrosis were observed as described previously [9].

Ultrastructural Analysis

After being weighed, RV wall tissues (about 1 mm^3) were fixed in 2.5% cold glutaraldehyde solution (pH 7.40) for 3 hours, rinsed with 0.1 mol/l phosphate-buffered saline (PBS), and immersed in 1% osmium tetroxide for additional 2 hours at room temperature. Tissues were then dehydrated through a graded series of ethanol to propylene oxide solutions and embedded in epoxy resin. Ultrathin sections were cut and then visualized under transmission electron microscope (JEM-1010, JEOL, Japan).

TUNEL Assay

Detection of cardiomyocyte apoptosis was performed using a terminal transferase dUTP nick end labeling (TUNEL) assay kit (In Situ Cell Death Detection Kit, Fluorescein; Roche Diagnostics, Germany) to detect apoptotic cell nuclei. 4′, 6-diamidino-2-phenylindole (DAPI) (Sigma) was used to stain all cell nuclei. Briefly, sections were deparaffinized, digested with proteinase K (20 μg/ml) at room temperature for 15 minutes, and soaked in PBS for 5 minutes. Each section was then incubated with 50 μl of the TUNEL reaction mixture containing terminal deoxynucleotidyl transferase for 1 hour at 37°C in a dark, humidified chamber. Then slides were rinsed in water and counterstained with DAPI for cell nuclei. Sections incubated with PBS instead of TdT enzyme solution served as the negative controls. After two washes, the fluorescence images were observed and captured using a confocal microscope (Zeiss LSM510, Oberkochen, Germany) at the same magnification (×400). The rate of apoptosis is here expressed as a ratio of the number of TUNEL-positive myocytes to the total number of myocytes stained with DAPI from three different random fields per heart (n = 3). All of these assays were performed blind. Four rats from each group were evaluated.

Enzyme-linked Immunosorbent Assay (ELISA)

To determine the plasma level of rat BNP, blood samples from the RV were immediately centrifuged at 3000 rpm at 4°C for 15 minutes. Plasma samples were collected and stored at −80°C. These samples were analyzed using a commercial ELISA kit (Shanghai DoBio Biotech Co. Ltd., Shanghai, China) according to the manufacturer's instructions.

Western Blotting

All cardiac proteins were extracted and Western blot analysis was performed as described previously [25]. Frozen RV tissues taken from rats 1 week after MCT injection were weighed, homogenized in ice-cold lysis buffer, and quantified for protein levels using a commercial assay (KeyGen Biotech). One hundred milligrams of protein from each sample was loaded onto 15% SDS-PAGE gel and subjected to electrophoresis using a constant voltage. The proteins were transferred to polyvinylidence fluoride (PVDF) membrane (Millipore, Billerica, MA, U.S.). The membrane was incubated with rabbit anti-Bcl-2 monoclonal antibody, mouse anti-Bax monoclonal antibody (Cell Signaling Technology, Beverly, MA, U.S.), and glyceraldehyde-6-phosphate dehydrogenase (GAPDH, Santa Cruz Biotechnology, Santa Cruz, CA, U.S.) overnight at 4°C. After washing, the membranes were incubated for 1 hour with appropriate horseradish peroxidase-conjugated secondary antibodies. GAPDH was used as loading control. Then protein bands were detected by enhanced chemiluminescence (ECL, Cell Signaling Technology) and visualized using VersaDoc Imaging System (Bio-Rad, Hercules, CA, U.S.). The intensities of the bands were analyzed densitometrically using NIH Image 1.46 software.

Statistical Analysis

All data in tables and figures are shown in terms of the mean ± SD. Data were subjected to statistical analysis using SPSS 15.0 software (SPSS, Chicago, IL, U.S.). Comparisons between groups were made using one-way ANOVA and the least significant difference (LSD). P values of less than 0.05 were considered significant.

Results

Nicorandil Attenuated MCT-induced Growth Retardation and Mortality

There was no significant difference in BW among the experimental groups on days 0 and 7. However, the BW of MCT-treated rats were significantly lower than those of age-matched saline-treated control animals on days 14 and 21 (11.07% and 15.43%, $P<0.05$). Daily nicorandil treatment over the course of 3 weeks attenuated MCT-induced reductions in growth (BW values were 10.44% and 14.07% higher than those of rats treated with MCT at weeks 2 and 3, respectively) and this effect was abolished by 5-HD (Figure 1A). These results are in accordance with the literature [26,27,28].

Hongo et al. found that nicorandil improves survival in MCT-induced PAH rats [16]. During the 3-week treatment period and the following period of anesthesia, two rats from the MCT-treated group died, 4 from the Nico+5-HD-treated group died, and none from the control group or nicorandil-treated group died. Although our study was not designed to be a mortality study, these data also suggest that nicorandil reduced the death rate in the MCT-treated group. Consequently, at the end of week 2, hemodynamic measurements could be performed on only 7 rats from the Nico+5-HD-treated group. At week 3, there were only 6 in the MCT group and 5 in the Nico+5-HD-treated group.

Nicorandil Decreased MCT-induced Elevation of RVSP Levels

To determine the changes of hemodynamic parameters over the course of the development of MCT-induced PAH, we examined rats at the end of each week after injection with MCT and compared them to control animals. Mean blood pressure and heart rate did not differ significantly among the groups (data not shown). Compared to the controls, MCT-injected rats had higher RVSP. This appeared as early as the first week after injection, and showed a significant increase during the second week, which continued into the third week (MCT: 27.54±3.92 mmHg, 36.90±4.34 mmHg, 55.57±8.22 mmHg for weeks 1, 2, and 3 respectively vs. Control: 24.61±3.0 mmHg, 24.53±2.60 mmHg, 25.65±3.04 mmHg) (Figure 1B). Nicorandil decreased RVSP by 11.37%, 17.99%, and 38.29% in MCT-treated rats in weeks 1, 2, and 3, respectively. These effects of nicorandil were found to be blocked by 5-HD (Figure 1B).

Nicorandil Inhibited MCT-induced RVH

Chronic RV pressure overload secondary to PAH resulted in RVH, as indicated by RV/BW and RV/[LV+S] ratios in MCT rats. As shown in Figures 1C and 1D, RV/BW, and RV/[LV+S] were significantly higher in the MCT-treated group than in the control group on days 14 and 21. Nicorandil significantly decreased RV/BW (0.71±0.03 and 0.86±0.07 for the nicorandil group at weeks 2 and 3, respectively, vs. 0.90±0.03 and 1.19±0.06 for the MCT-treated group at the same times, $P<0.05$) and RV/[LV+S] (0.29±0.02 and 0.34±0.02 for the nicorandil group at weeks 2 and 3, respectively vs. 0.33±0.02 and

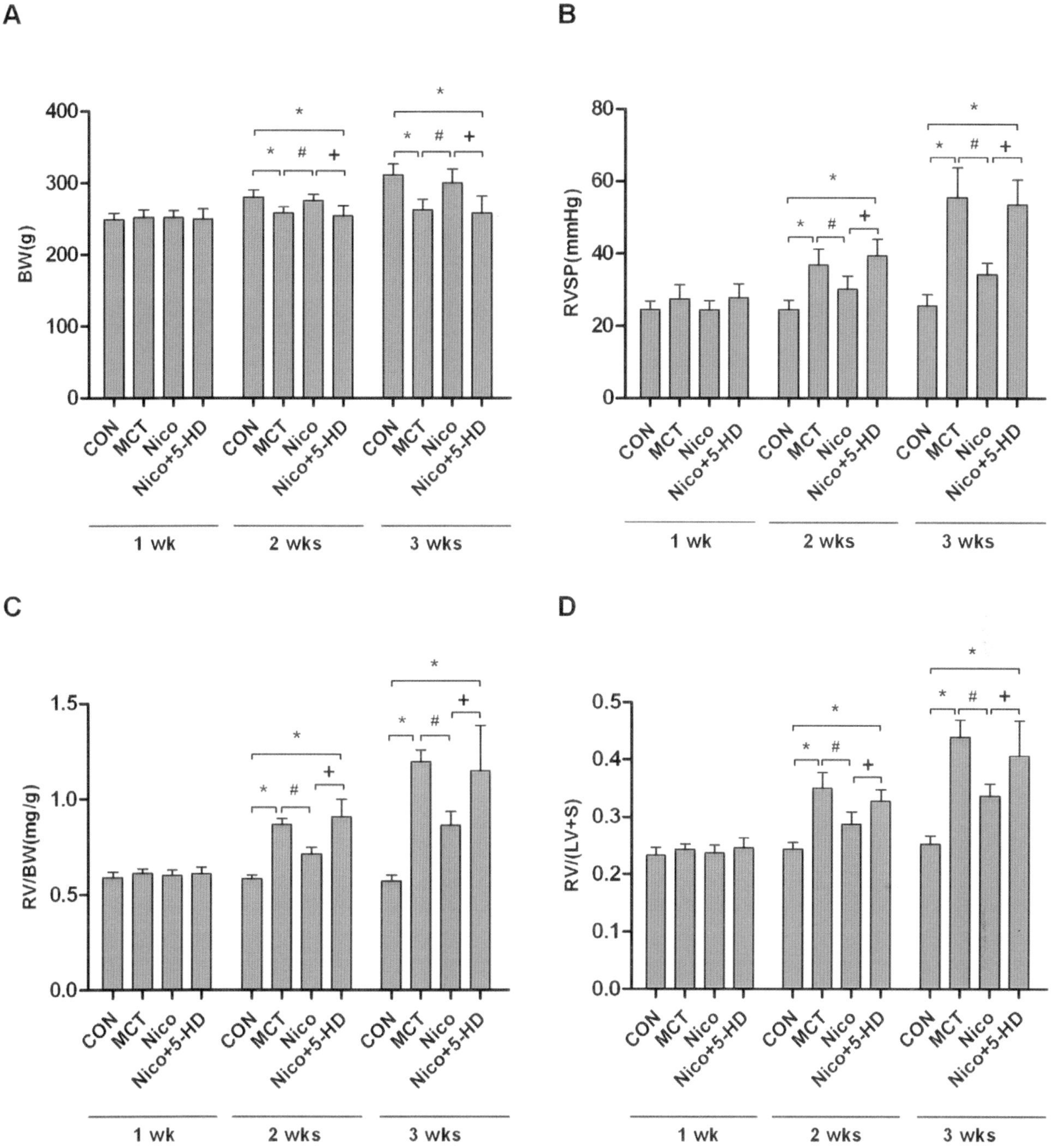

Figure 1. Effects of nicorandil on body weight, right ventricle systolic pressures and hypertrophy in rats on weeks 1–3 after monocrotaline administration. Measurements for the (A) BW, (B) RVSP, (C) RV/BW ratio, and (D) RV/(LV+S) ratio are presented as mean ± SD. BW, body weight; RVSP, right ventricle systolic pressures; MCT, monocrotaline. RV/BW represents the ratio of RV weight to BW, and RV/[LV+S] represents the ratio of the RV weight to left ventricular(LV) plus septum (S) weight. These are indicators of RV hypertrophy. Male SD rats were given a single dose (60 mg/kg) of MCT intraperitoneally and then fed 7.5 $mg \cdot kg^{-1} \cdot d^{-1}$ nicorandil (nicorandil-treated group), 5 $mg \cdot kg^{-1} \cdot d^{-1}$ 5-hydroxydecanoate (5-HD) combined with 7.5 $mg \cdot kg^{-1} \cdot d^{-1}$ nicorandil (nicorandil+5-HD-treated group), or saline (MCT-treated group) by oral gavage from day 1 to day 21. The age- and weight-matched control animals were injected with an equal volume of saline (control group) intraperitoneally, and then given saline for 21 d. CON represents the control group, MCT represents the MCT-treated group, Nico represents the nicorandil-treated group, Nico+5-HD group represents the nicorandil+5-HD-treated group. n = 8 for each group except for n = 7 in Nico+5-HD group at the second week, n = 6 in MCT group and n = 5 in Nico+5-HD group at third week after MCT injection. *$P<0.05$ compared with control group, #$P<0.05$ relative to the MCT-treated group. +$P<0.05$ relative to the nicorandil-treated group.

0.40±0.06 for the MCT-treated group). 5-HD inhibited the effect of nicorandil on RVH (Figures 1C and 1D), indicating that 5-HD inhibited the effect of nicorandil completely. RVH was determined by measuring the mean CSA of RV cardiomyocytes. HE staining of the RV tissues showed that the CSA of cardiomyocytes in the MCT group was significantly greater than in the control group at

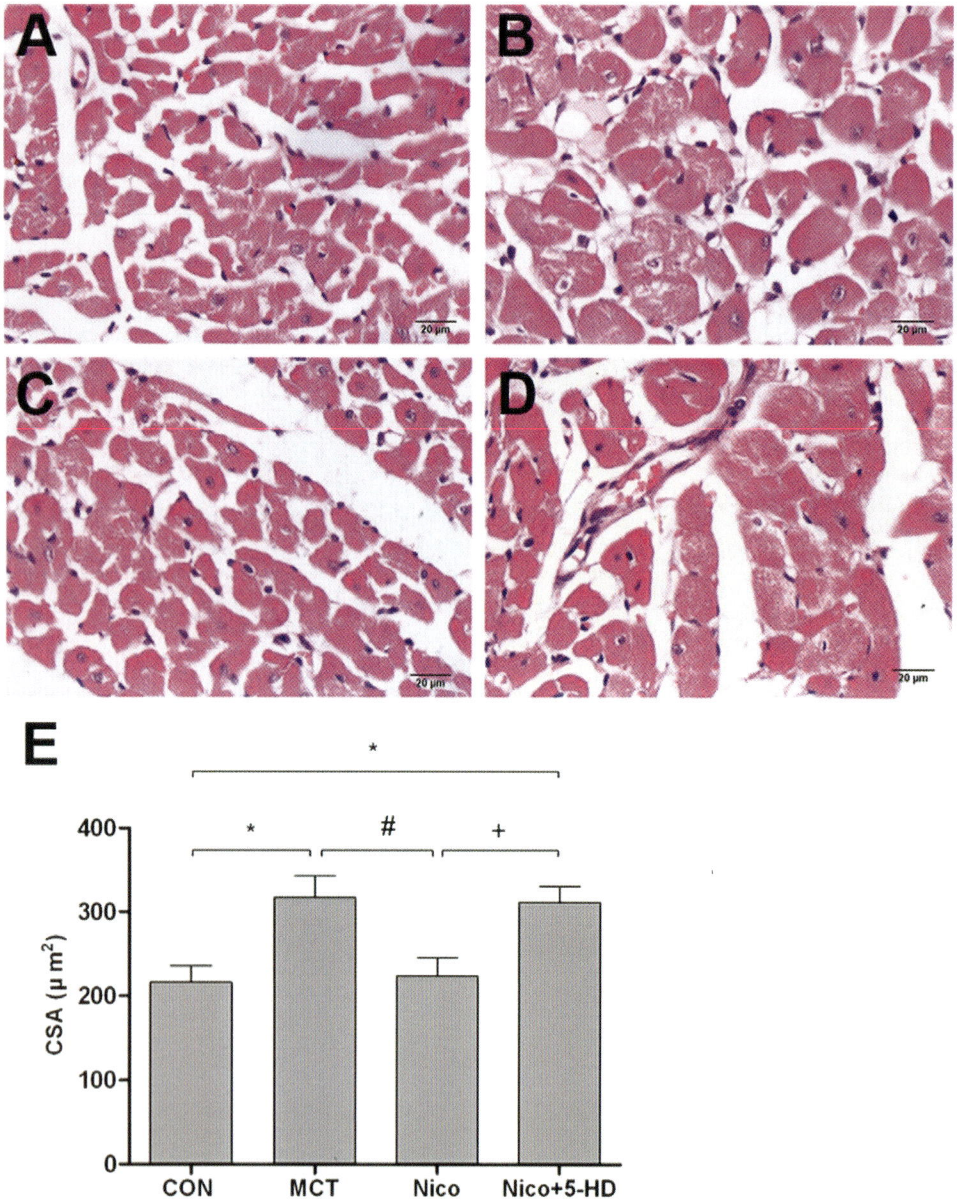

Figure 2. Effects of nicorandil on RV cardiomyocyte hypertrophy in rats with MCT-induced pulmonary arterial hypertension on day 21. Representative photomicrographs (HE stain) of cross-sections of RV myocytes from the following experimental groups: (A) Control group, (B) MCT-treated group, (C) nicorandil-treated group, and (D) nicorandil+5-HD-treated group. Abbreviations are the same as those given in Figure 1. Original magnification, ×400, scale bar = 20 μm. (E) Quantitative analysis of mean cross sectional area (CSA) of RV cardiomyocytes in rats. Abbreviations are the same as those used in Figure 1. Details of treatment groups are described in the legend of Figure 1. Data are presented as mean ± SD (n = 5). *$P<0.05$ relative to the control group, #$P<0.05$ relative to the MCT-treated group. +$P<0.05$ relative to the nicorandil-treated group.

day 21 (Figures 2A, 2B, and 2E $P<0.05$). Treatment with nicorandil at 7.5 mg/kg prevented the increase in the CSA of cardiomyocytes induced by MCT (Figure 2C). This change was inhibited by chronic administration of 5-HD as the values of the CSA of cardiomyocytes approached those of the MCT group (Figure 2D).

Nicorandil Diminished the Extent of Fibrosis Induced by MCT

RV remodeling is associated with both variations in the morphology of the cardiomyocytes and with increased interstitial fibrosis (increased myocardial collagen content). As demonstrated by Masson's Trichrome stain, significant interstitial and perivascular fibrosis was observed in the hypertrophic right-side hearts induced by MCT, while nicorandil treatment diminished the extent of fibrosis (Figure 3). However, the suppressive effects of nicorandil were reversed by 5-HD. These results suggest that 5-HD abolishes the inhibition of nicorandil in the case of interstitial fibrosis.

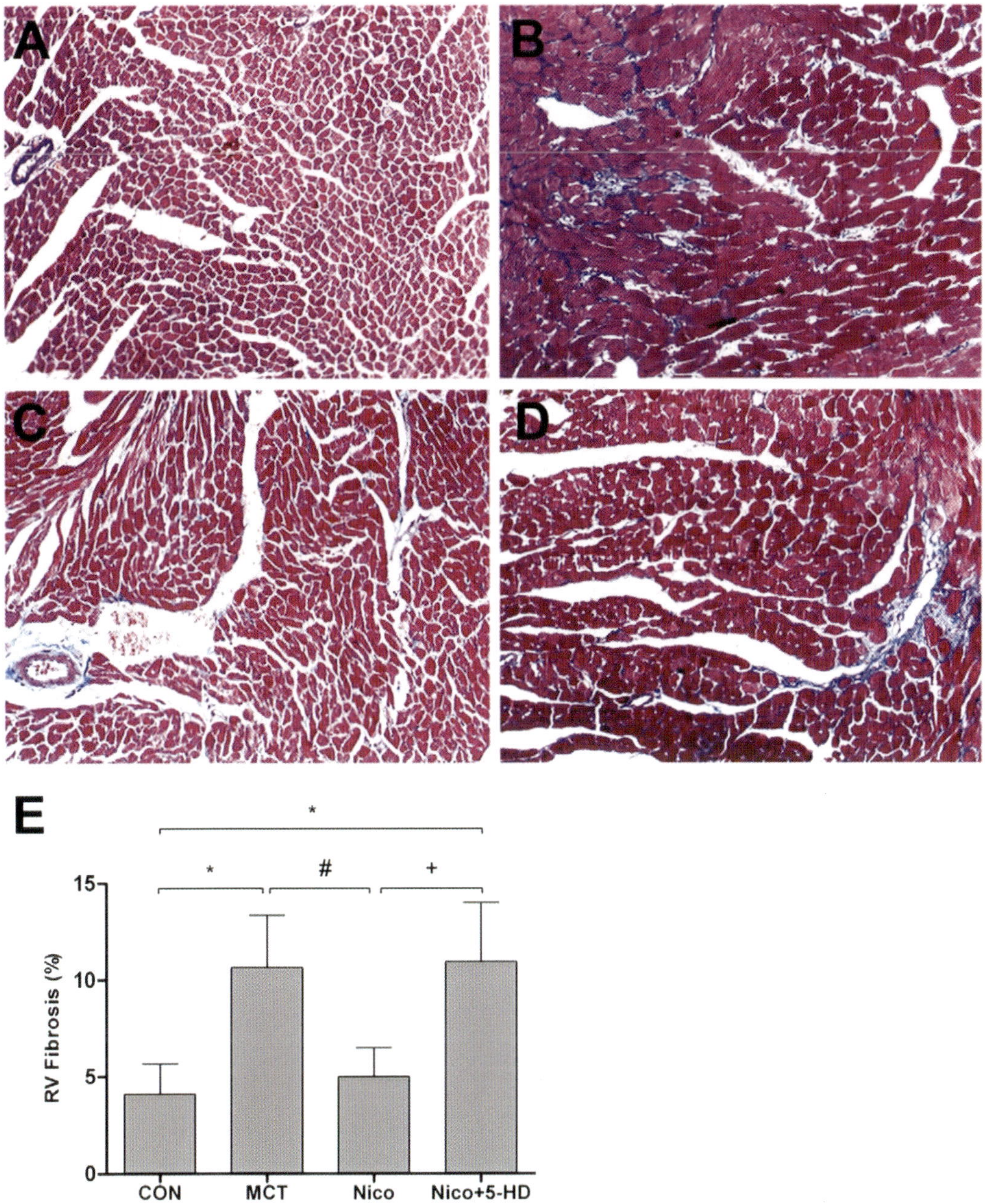

Figure 3. Effects of nicorandil on MCT-induced cardiomyocyte fibrosis in rat RV, 3 weeks after MCT injection. Representative Masson's Trichrome staining of cardiomyocyte sections showing the extent of interstitial and perivascular fibrosis in the RV-free walls for the following experimental groups: (A) Control group, (B) MCT-treated group, (C) nicorandil-treated group, and (D) nicorandil+5-HD-treated group. Original magnification, ×200. (E) Quantification of fibrosis in the stained cardiomyocyte sections (blue-stained areas expressed as percentage of total RV surface area) from CON, MCT, Nico, and Nico+5-HD groups. Abbreviations are the same as those used in Figure 1. Details of treatment groups are given in the legend of Figure 1. Data are presented as mean ± SD (n = 5). *$P<0.05$ relative to the control group, #$p<0.05$ relative to the MCT-treated group. +$P<0.05$ relative to the nicorandil-treated group.

Nicorandil Restored MCT-induced Ultrastructural Abnormalities in RV

Transmission electron microscopy of the RV cardiomyocytes revealed abnormalities in the MCT-treated group not visible in the control group. These included such as increased mitochondrial density, swelling, vacuolization, and medullary sheath-like degeneration, enlarged sarcoplasmic reticulum, dissolution of the myofilaments, broken Z-lines, and an irregular pattern of transverse striations (Figures 4A and 4B). Treatment with nicorandil prevented these abnormalities (Figure 4C), and treatment with the selective mitoK_{ATP} channel blocker 5-HD reversed the protective effects of nicorandil (Figure 4D).

Nicorandil Inhibited MCT-induced Cardiomyocyte Apoptosis in the RV

There were markedly more TUNEL-positive cardiomyocytes in the RV in the MCT-treated group than in the control group. This difference was observed as early as 1 week post MCT-injection

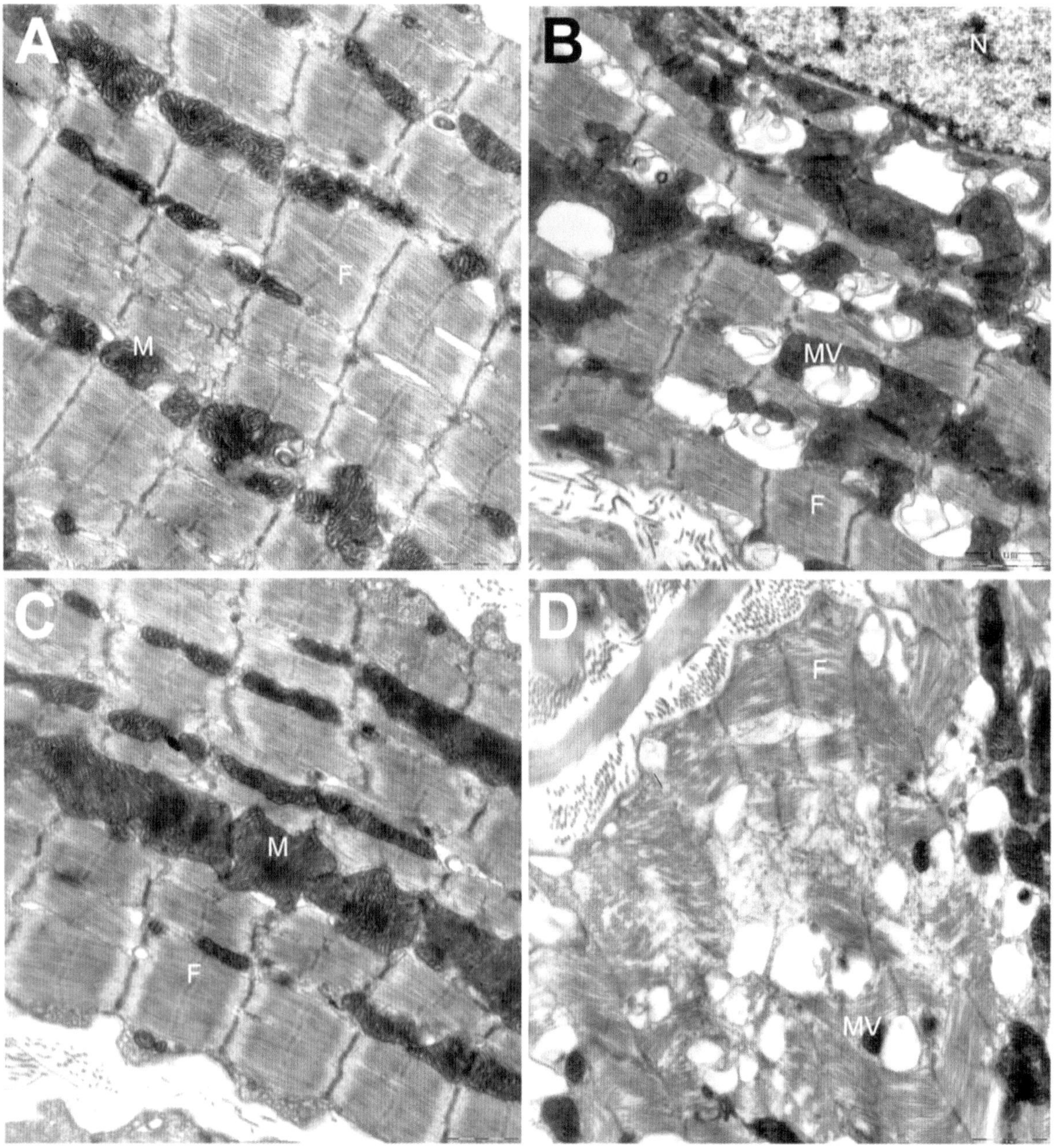

Figure 4. Effects of nicorandil on the ultrastructural changes in RV myocardial cells of MCT-induced pulmonary arterial hypertension rats. (A) The control group showed normal myocyte structure. (B) The MCT-treated group showed swelling and vacuolization of mitochondria, dilatation of the sarcoplasmic reticulum, dissolution of the myofilaments, and an irregular pattern of transverse striations not observed in the control group; (C) The nicorandil-treated group showed intact myocyte structure, suggesting that nicorandil ameliorates MCT-induced myocardial damage. (D) The nicorandil+5-HD-treated group showed disrupted myocyte ultrastructure similar to that observed in the MCT group, which suggests that 5-HD reversed the inhibitory effects of nicorandil. Details of treatment groups are given in legend of the Figure 1. M, mitochondria; N, nucleus; F, myofilaments; MV, mitochondrial vacuolization. Scale bar = 1 μm.

and continued into week 3 (Figures 5A and 5E). Photomicrographs of TUNEL-stained cells in RV in different groups during the second and third weeks after MCT injection are not shown. As shown in Figure 5C, nicorandil significantly inhibited cardiomyocyte apoptosis in the RV during the first week after MCT injection ($P<0.05$ vs MCT; Figures 5B and 5C). In contrast, treatment with 5-HD in combination with nicorandil resulted in TUNEL-positive cardiomyocytes in the RV, similar in number to time-matched MCT-treated rats. This demonstrates that 5-HD blocked the effect of nicorandil on apoptosis of cardiomyocytes induced by MCT (Figure 5D).

Nicorandil Suppressed the MCT-induced Increase in Plasma BNP

Plasma BNP is used for the diagnosis and staging of heart failure [29], because its levels become elevated in proportion to the degree of RV dysfunction and RV remodeling in PAH [30,31,32,33,34]. At 3 weeks, plasma BNP levels were markedly

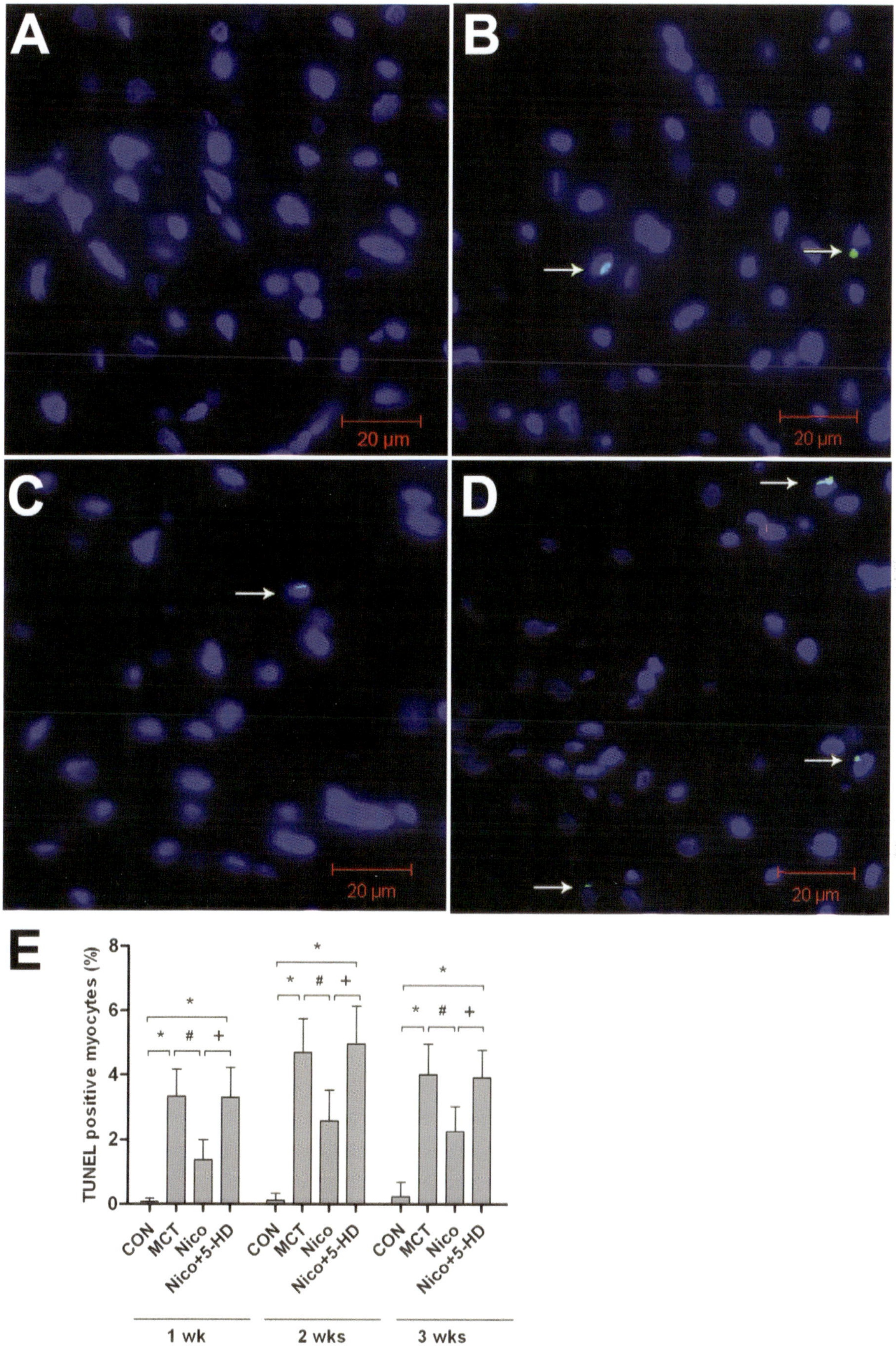
A
B
C
D
20 µm
20 µm
20 µm
20 µm
E
TUNEL positive myocytes (%)
8
6
4
2
0
CON
MCT
Nico
Nico+5-HD
1 wk
2 wks
3 wks

Figure 5. Effects of nicorandil on cardiac myocyte apoptosis in the RV myocardium. Apoptotic cardiomyocytes were detected by terminal deoxyribonucleotidyl transferase-mediated dUTP-digoxigenin nick end-labeling (TUNEL) staining in RV tissue from rats. Green fluorescence shows TUNEL-positive nuclei; blue fluorescence shows nuclei of total cardiomyocytes. (A–D) Representative photomicrographs of TUNEL-stained cells (white arrow) in RV at the first week after MCT injection. (E) Quantitative analysis of TUNEL-positive cardiomyocytes as the percentage of total cell number in right ventricles of the CON, MCT, Nico, and Nico+5-HD groups at 1–3 weeks post-MCT injection. Abbreviations are the same as those used in Figure 1. Representative photomicrographs of TUNEL-stained cells in RV in different groups at the second and third week after MCT injection are not shown. Details of treatment groups are given in the legend of Figure 1. Data are presented as mean ± SD (n = 4). *$P<0.05$ relative to the control group, #$P<0.05$ relative to the MCT-treated group. +$P<0.05$ relative to the nicorandil-treated group. Scale bars = 20 μm.

higher in MCT-injected animals than in age-matched control animals (59.16±4.96 pg/ml vs. 36.43±5.58 pg/ml). This increase was significantly suppressed by nicorandil. 5-HD also prevented the decrease in plasma BNP level induced by nicorandil (Figure 6).

Nicorandil Partially Reversed the MCT-induced Decrease in the Bcl-2/Bax Ratio

Western blotting was performed to examine the role of nicorandil on Bcl-2 and Bax in rat right heart tissue at week 1. As shown in Figure 7, the Bcl-2/Bax ratio was significantly lower in the MCT-injected animals than in controls at week 1 ($P<0.05$). Nicorandil partially reversed the decrease in the Bcl-2/Bax ratio at week 1 ($P<0.05$), whereas co-treatment with nicorandil and 5-HD decreased the ratio to the level observed in the MCT-injected rats (Figure 7).

Discussion

In this study, we successfully established an RV remodeling model *in vivo*. We induced PAH in rats using MCT for three weeks, and these rats displayed cardiac hypertrophy, fibrosis, and dysfunction consistent with previous studies [25,35,36]. We also demonstrated for the first time that nicorandil effectively attenuated the PAH-induced RV remodeling. This effect was probably associated not only with a reduction in RVSP but also inhibition of RV apoptosis.

In this study, injecting MCT (60 mg/kg, ip) into rats resulted in RV remodeling, as previously reported [25,35,36]. In MCT-injected rats, RVSP gradually increased from 24.61±3.0 mmHg at baseline to 36.90±4.34 mmHg at 2 weeks and 55.57±8.22 mmHg at 3 weeks. These results are consistent with the findings of previous studies in that MCT-induced PAH in rats is apparent by day 14 and worsens by day 21 (Figure 1B) [24,37,38]. The progression of RVH is indicated by the increased RV/BW and RV/[LV+S] ratios due to local pressure overload after 2 weeks [26,27,39]. The RV/BW ratio had a 108.77% increase and the RV/[LV+S] a 76.00% increase during the third week. This process was accompanied by increased CSA in RV cardiomyocytes (Figure 2B) and remarkable interstitial fibrosis in RV (Figure 3B). Plasma BNP levels increased by 62.39% in MCT-induced PAH rats. All of these observations strongly indicate that MCT can induce the formation of RV remodeling and dysfunction [25,35,36].

Nicorandil can ameliorate MCT-induced PAH in rats, possibly by significantly decreasing RV afterload and hypertrophy and by improving pulmonary artery remodeling [16,40]. Consistent with this, we found that nicorandil significantly decreased RVSP, RV/BW, RV/[LV+S], BNP, and interstitial fibrosis relative to the MCT group. In this way, we confirmed that nicorandil can improve RV remodeling and dysfunction induced by PAH.

Elevated PAP (RV afterload) is the main cause of PAH-induced RV maladaptive hypertrophy and failure. Recently, Bogaard et al. stated that an elevated PAP is not the only reason for PAH-associated RV remodeling and failure [12]. Apoptosis of the cardiomyocytes may also play a role in RV remodeling and in the subsequent development of heart failure [12,41,42,43]. Previous studies suggest that cardiomyocyte apoptosis is implicated in RV remodeling after acute left ventricular myocardial infarction [44] and pulmonary arterial banding [45,46]. However, the role of cardiomyocyte apoptosis in the development of PAH-induced RV remodeling and failure is still unknown. Maria et al. showed that apoptosis associated with fibrosis and capillary rarefaction is involved in RV hypertrophy, dilation, and failure in an angioproliferative pulmonary hypertension rat model, induced by combined exposure to the VEGF receptor blocker SU5416 and hypoxia [15]. Apoptosis is observed early and then declined when clinically manifest RV failure occurs. This may provide new insight into the time course of cardiac cell apoptosis in RV remodeling and aid in determining the optimal timing of antiapoptotic therapy to prevent or reverse RV remodeling. Theoretically, any drug capable of reducing both PAP and RV remodeling would be promising for the treatment of PAH. In the present study, our results show that in the MCT-induced cardiac remodeling rat model, there were significantly more apoptotic cardiomyocytes than in the control group. Apoptosis was observed as early as the first week after MCT treatment, even though there was no obvious elevation in RVSP. This indicated that early apoptosis might be involved in RV remodeling except for pressure overload. Nicorandil was found to reduce the number of apoptotic cardiomyocytes remarkably from the first week to the third week, in parallel to the reduction of RVH. This anti-apoptotic effect may contribute to the amelioration of MCT-induced RV remodeling.

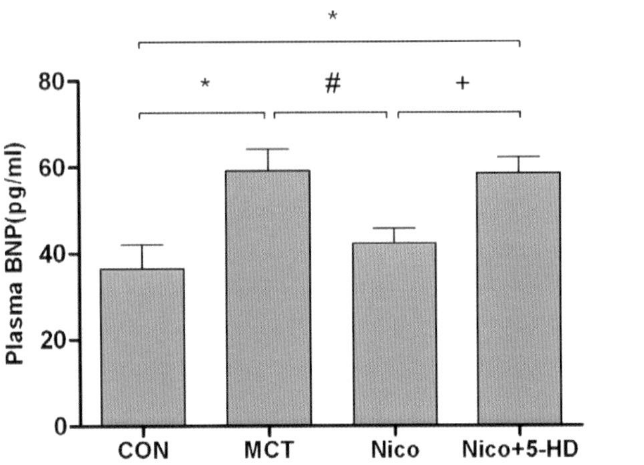

Figure 6. Effects of nicorandil on plasma levels of BNP in MCT-induced pulmonary arterial hypertension rats. Results of an enzyme-linked immunosorbent assay analysis of plasma BNP concentration from CON (n = 8), MCT (n = 6), Nico (n = 8), and Nico+5-HD (n = 5) groups. Abbreviations are the same as those used in Figure 1. Details of treatment groups are described in the legend of Figure 1. Data are presented as mean ± SD. *$P<0.05$ relative to the control group, #$P<0.05$ relative to the MCT-treated group. +$P<0.05$ relative to the nicorandil-treated group.

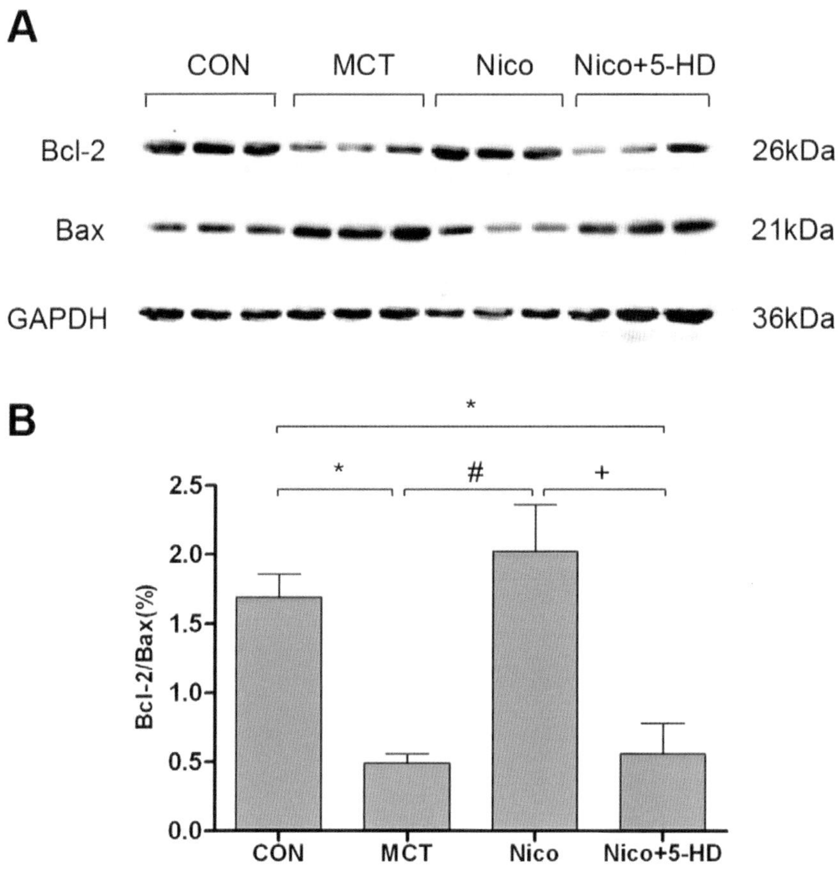

Figure 7. Effects of nicorandil on Bcl-2 and Bax protein expression in the RV, 1 week after MCT injection. The protein levels of Bcl-2 and Bax in the RV myocardium were determined by Western blot analysis. The levels of Bcl-2 and Bax protein were quantitatively analyzed with an image analyzer and expressed as the ratio of Bcl-2/Bax. Equal loading of protein was confirmed with anti-GAPDH antibody. (A) Representative Western blot results showing the expression of Bcl-2, Bax, and GAPDH protein in the right ventricle of rats from different experimental groups. (B) Bar graph showing the densitometric scanning of the ratio of Bcl-2/Bax. Abbreviations are the same as in the legend of Figure 1. Data are presented as mean ± SD (n = 3). *$P<0.05$ relative to the control group, #$P<0.05$ compared with MCT-treated group. +$P<0.05$ relative to the nicorandil-treated group.

Mitochondria are considered the central regulators of apoptosis [47], and play a vital role in cardiac remodeling and failure [48,49]. It is well established that the Bcl-2/Bax ratio determines cell apoptotic fate [50,51]. In our study, the Bcl-2/Bax ratio was reduced significantly ($P<0.05$) in the right myocardium 1 week after MCT injection compared with the control group (Figure 7). Apoptosis was detected by TUNEL assay as early as 1 week after MCT injection. This was consistent with the dramatic down-regulation of Bcl-2/Bax. This supports the hypothesis that apoptosis might be involved in a critical dysregulatory mechanism in the maladaptive cardiac response during the progression of pulmonary hypertension.

Many studies have demonstrated that mitoK_{ATP} channels are implicated in the mechanism of cell apoptosis [52]. Nicorandil, through its activation of mitoK_{ATP} channels, can inhibit apoptosis in cardiomyocytes by improving mitochondrial function, preventing calcium overload in the mitochondria, and preserving mitochondrial integrity [17,18,19,53]. In this study, nicorandil not only significantly reduced MCT-induced ultrastructural injuries to the mitochondria but also inhibited cardiomyocyte apoptosis in the RV as measured by the increase in the relative expression of Bcl-2/Bax in mitochondria. The anti-apoptotic effects of nicorandil may in part contribute to the amelioration of MCT-induced myocardial injuries and RV remodeling.

In conclusion, our results clearly show that nicorandil, a mitoK_{ATP} channel opener, can inhibit MCT-induced RV remodeling in rats. This effect is mediated not only by reduction of RVSP but also by inhibition of apoptotic cell death. Nicorandil can reduce mitochondrial impairment and inhibit the alteration of Bcl-2 and Bax in the mitochondria of cardiomyocytes in the MCT-treated rats. Its protective effect in PAH- induced RV remodeling may involve opening of the mitoK_{ATP} channel. For this reason, we believe that the use of a mitoK_{ATP} channel opener such as nicorandil may represent a new therapeutic strategy for ameliorating RV remodeling during the early stages of PAH.

Acknowledgments

The authors would like to thank Dr. Ji-Fu Wei (Clinical Experiment Center, The First Affiliated Hospital of Nanjing Medical University) for his helpful comments and valuable suggestions.

Author Contributions

Conceived and designed the experiments: XZ WX HW. Performed the experiments: XZ QW YY HW LB. Analyzed the data: XZ QW. Contributed reagents/materials/analysis tools: XZ QW QC. Wrote the paper: XZ QC.

References

1. McLaughlin VV, Archer SL, Badesch DB, Barst RJ, Farber HW, et al. (2009) ACCF/AHA 2009 expert consensus document on pulmonary hypertension a report of the American College of Cardiology Foundation Task Force on Expert Consensus Documents and the American Heart Association developed in collaboration with the American College of Chest Physicians; American Thoracic Society, Inc.; and the Pulmonary Hypertension Association. J Am Coll Cardiol 53: 1573–1619.
2. Rhodes CJ, Davidson A, Gibbs JS, Wharton J, Wilkins MR (2009) Therapeutic targets in pulmonary arterial hypertension. Pharmacol Ther 121: 69–88.
3. D'Alonzo GE, Barst RJ, Ayres SM, Bergofsky EH, Brundage BH, et al. (1991) Survival in patients with primary pulmonary hypertension. Results from a national prospective registry. Ann Intern Med 115: 343–349.
4. van Wolferen SA, Marcus JT, Boonstra A, Marques KM, Bronzwaer JG, et al. (2007) Prognostic value of right ventricular mass, volume, and function in idiopathic pulmonary arterial hypertension. Eur Heart J 28: 1250–1257.
5. Jing ZC, Xu XQ, Han ZY, Wu Y, Deng KW, et al. (2007) Registry and survival study in chinese patients with idiopathic and familial pulmonary arterial hypertension. Chest 132: 373–379.
6. Vonk Noordegraaf A, Naeije R (2008) Right ventricular function in scleroderma-related pulmonary hypertension. Rheumatology (Oxford) 47 Suppl 5: v42–43.
7. Humbert M, Sitbon O, Chaouat A, Bertocchi M, Habib G, et al. (2006) Pulmonary arterial hypertension in France: results from a national registry. Am J Respir Crit Care Med 173: 1023–1030.
8. Voelkel NF, Quaife RA, Leinwand LA, Barst RJ, McGoon MD, et al. (2006) Right Ventricular Function and Failure: Report of a National Heart, Lung, and Blood Institute Working Group on Cellular and Molecular Mechanisms of Right Heart Failure. Circulation 114: 1883–1891.
9. Bogaard HJ, Natarajan R, Mizuno S, Abbate A, Chang PJ, et al. (2010) Adrenergic receptor blockade reverses right heart remodeling and dysfunction in pulmonary hypertensive rats. Am J Respir Crit Care Med 182: 652–660.
10. Simon MA, Pinsky MR (2011) Right ventricular dysfunction and failure in chronic pressure overload. Cardiol Res Pract 2011: 568095.
11. Dore A, Houde C, Chan KL, Ducharme A, Khairy P, et al. (2005) Angiotensin receptor blockade and exercise capacity in adults with systemic right ventricles: a multicenter, randomized, placebo-controlled clinical trial. Circulation 112: 2411–2416.
12. Bogaard HJ, Natarajan R, Henderson SC, Long CS, Kraskauskas D, et al. (2009) Chronic Pulmonary Artery Pressure Elevation Is Insufficient to Explain Right Heart Failure. Circulation 120: 1951–1960.
13. Voelkel NF, Natarajan R, Drake JI, Bogaard HJ (2011) Right Ventricle in Pulmonary Hypertension. Comprehensive Physiology: John Wiley & Sons, Inc. p.525–540.
14. Dorn GW (2008) Apoptotic and non-apoptotic programmed cardiomyocyte death in ventricular remodelling. Cardiovascular Research 81: 465–473.
15. Campian ME, Verberne HJ, Hardziyenka M, de Bruin K, Selwaness M, et al. (2009) Serial Noninvasive Assessment of Apoptosis During Right Ventricular Disease Progression in Rats. Journal of Nuclear Medicine 50: 1371–1377.
16. Hongo M, Mawatari E, Sakai A, Ruan Z, Koizumi T, et al. (2005) Effects of nicorandil on monocrotaline-induced pulmonary arterial hypertension in rats. J Cardiovasc Pharmacol 46: 452–458.
17. Nagata K (2003) Nicorandil inhibits oxidative stress-induced apoptosis in cardiac myocytes through activation of mitochondrial ATP-sensitive potassium channels and a nitrate-like effect. Journal of Molecular and Cellular Cardiology 35: 1505–1512.
18. Nishikawa S, Tatsumi T, Shiraishi J, Matsunaga S, Takeda M, et al. (2006) Nicorandil regulates Bcl-2 family proteins and protects cardiac myocytes against hypoxia-induced apoptosis. Journal of Molecular and Cellular Cardiology 40: 510–519.
19. Akao M, Teshima Y, Marban E (2002) Antiapoptotic effect of nicorandil mediated by mitochondrial atp-sensitive potassium channels in cultured cardiac myocytes. J Am Coll Cardiol 40: 803–810.
20. Lee T-M, Lin M-S, Chang N-C (2008) Effect of ATP-Sensitive Potassium Channel Agonists on Ventricular Remodeling in Healed Rat Infarcts. Journal of the American College of Cardiology 51: 1309–1318.
21. Saeed M, Watzinger N, Krombach GA, Lund GK, Wendland MF, et al. (2002) Left ventricular remodeling after infarction: sequential MR imaging with oral nicorandil therapy in rat model. Radiology 224: 830–837.
22. Sanada S, Node K, Asanuma H, Ogita H, Takashima S, et al. (2002) Opening of the adenosine triphosphate-sensitive potassium channel attenuates cardiac remodeling induced by long-term inhibition of nitric oxide synthesis: role of 70-kDa S6 kinase and extracellular signal-regulated kinase. J Am Coll Cardiol 40: 991–997.
23. Eguchi Y, Takahari Y, Higashijima N, Ishizuka N, Tamura N, et al. (2009) Nicorandil attenuates FeCl(3)-induced thrombus formation through the inhibition of reactive oxygen species production. Circ J 73: 554–561.
24. Hardziyenka M, Campian ME, de Bruin-Bon HA, Michel MC, Tan HL (2006) Sequence of echocardiographic changes during development of right ventricular failure in rat. J Am Soc Echocardiogr 19: 1272–1279.
25. Okada M, Harada T, Kikuzuki R, Yamawaki H, Hara Y (2009) Effects of telmisartan on right ventricular remodeling induced by monocrotaline in rats. J Pharmacol Sci 111: 193–200.
26. Miyauchi T, Yorikane R, Sakai S, Sakurai T, Okada M, et al. (1993) Contribution of endogenous endothelin-1 to the progression of cardiopulmonary alterations in rats with monocrotaline-induced pulmonary hypertension. Circ Res 73: 887–897.
27. Buermans HP, Redout EM, Schiel AE, Musters RJ, Zuidwijk M, et al. (2005) Microarray analysis reveals pivotal divergent mRNA expression profiles early in the development of either compensated ventricular hypertrophy or heart failure. Physiol Genomics 21: 314–323.
28. Honda M, Yamada S, Goto Y, Ishikawa S, Yoshikane H, et al. (1992) Biochemical and structural remodeling of collagen in the right ventricular hypertrophy induced by monocrotaline. Jpn Circ J 56: 392–403.
29. de Lemos JA, McGuire DK, Drazner MH (2003) B-type natriuretic peptide in cardiovascular disease. Lancet 362: 316–322.
30. Nagaya N, Nishikimi T, Uematsu M, Satoh T, Kyotani S, et al. (2000) Plasma brain natriuretic peptide as a prognostic indicator in patients with primary pulmonary hypertension. Circulation 102: 865–870.
31. Nagaya N, Nishikimi T, Okano Y, Uematsu M, Satoh T, et al. (1998) Plasma brain natriuretic peptide levels increase in proportion to the extent of right ventricular dysfunction in pulmonary hypertension. J Am Coll Cardiol 31: 202–208.
32. Shiina Y, Funabashi N, Lee K, Daimon M, Sekine T, et al. (2009) Right atrium contractility and right ventricular diastolic function assessed by pulsed tissue Doppler imaging can predict brain natriuretic peptide in adults with acquired pulmonary hypertension. Int J Cardiol 135: 53–59.
33. Yap LB (2004) B-type natriuretic Peptide and the right heart. Heart Fail Rev 9: 99–105.
34. Reesink HJ, Tulevski, II, Marcus JT, Boomsma F, Kloek JJ, et al. (2007) Brain natriuretic peptide as noninvasive marker of the severity of right ventricular dysfunction in chronic thromboembolic pulmonary hypertension. Ann Thorac Surg 84: 537–543.
35. Hessel MH, Steendijk P, den Adel B, Schutte CI, van der Laarse A (2006) Characterization of right ventricular function after monocrotaline-induced pulmonary hypertension in the intact rat. Am J Physiol Heart Circ Physiol 291: H2424–2430.
36. Lourenco AP, Roncon-Albuquerque R, Jr., Bras-Silva C, Faria B, Wieland J, et al. (2006) Myocardial dysfunction and neurohumoral activation without remodeling in left ventricle of monocrotaline-induced pulmonary hypertensive rats. Am J Physiol Heart Circ Physiol 291: H1587–1594.
37. Henkens IR, Mouchaers KT, Vliegen HW, van der Laarse WJ, Swenne CA, et al. (2007) Early changes in rat hearts with developing pulmonary arterial hypertension can be detected with three-dimensional electrocardiography. Am J Physiol Heart Circ Physiol 293: H1300–1307.
38. Handoko ML, Schalij I, Kramer K, Sebkhi A, Postmus PE, et al. (2008) A refined radio-telemetry technique to monitor right ventricle or pulmonary artery pressures in rats: a useful tool in pulmonary hypertension research. Pflugers Arch 455: 951–959.
39. Lee JK, Nishiyama A, Kambe F, Seo H, Takeuchi S, et al. (1999) Downregulation of voltage-gated K(+) channels in rat heart with right ventricular hypertrophy. Am J Physiol 277: H1725–1731.
40. Sahara M, Sata M, Morita T, Hirata Y, Nagai R (2012) Nicorandil attenuates monocrotaline-induced vascular endothelial damage and pulmonary arterial hypertension. PLoS One 7: e33367.
41. Kret M, Arora R (2007) Pathophysiological basis of right ventricular remodeling. J Cardiovasc Pharmacol Ther 12: 5–14.
42. Haworth SG (2007) The cell and molecular biology of right ventricular dysfunction in pulmonary hypertension. European Heart Journal Supplements 9: H10–H16.
43. Bogaard HJ, Abe K, Vonk Noordegraaf A, Voelkel NF (2009) The Right Ventricle Under Pressure: Cellular and Molecular Mechanisms of Right-Heart Failure in Pulmonary Hypertension. Chest 135: 794–804.
44. Bussani R, Abbate A, Biondi-Zoccai GG, Dobrina A, Leone AM, et al. (2003) Right ventricular dilatation after left ventricular acute myocardial infarction is predictive of extremely high peri-infarctual apoptosis at postmortem examination in humans. J Clin Pathol 56: 672–676.
45. Ikeda S, Hamada M, Hiwada K (1999) Cardiomyocyte apoptosis with enhanced expression of P53 and Bax in right ventricle after pulmonary arterial banding. Life Sci 65: 925–933.
46. Braun M (2003) Right ventricular hypertrophy and apoptosis after pulmonary artery banding: regulation of PKC isozymes. Cardiovascular Research 59: 658–667.
47. Mignotte B, Vayssiere JL (1998) Mitochondria and apoptosis. Eur J Biochem 252: 1–15.
48. Tsutsui H, Kinugawa S, Matsushima S (2009) Mitochondrial oxidative stress and dysfunction in myocardial remodelling. Cardiovasc Res 81: 449–456.
49. Piao L, Marsboom G, Archer SL (2010) Mitochondrial metabolic adaptation in right ventricular hypertrophy and failure. J Mol Med 88: 1011–1020.
50. Gross A (2001) BCL-2 proteins: regulators of the mitochondrial apoptotic program. IUBMB Life 52: 231–236.

51. Adams JM, Cory S (1998) The Bcl-2 protein family: arbiters of cell survival. Science 281: 1322–1326.
52. Ardehali H, O'Rourke B (2005) Mitochondrial K(ATP) channels in cell survival and death. J Mol Cell Cardiol 39: 7–16.
53. Sanbe A, Marunouchi T, Yamauchi J, Tanonaka K, Nishigori H, et al. (2011) Cardioprotective effect of nicorandil, a mitochondrial ATP-sensitive potassium channel opener, prolongs survival in HSPB5 R120G transgenic mice. PLoS ONE 6: e18922.

6

Differentially Expressed Plasma MicroRNAs and the Potential Regulatory Function of Let-7b in Chronic Thromboembolic Pulmonary Hypertension

Lijuan Guo[1,2], Yuanhua Yang[1,2], Jie Liu[3], Lei Wang[1,2], Jifeng Li[1,2], Ying Wang[1], Yan Liu[4], Song Gu[4], Huili Gan[5,6], Jun Cai[4], Jason X.-J. Yuan[7], Jun Wang[1,3]*, Chen Wang[1,2,8]*

1 Beijing Key Laboratory of Respiratory and Pulmonary Circulation Disorders, Beijing Chao-Yang Hospital, Capital Medical University, Beijing, P.R. China, **2** Beijing Institute of Respiratory Medicine, Capital Medical University, Beijing, P.R. China, **3** Department of Physiology, Capital Medical University, Beijing, P.R. China, **4** Department of Cardiology, Beijing Chao-Yang Hospital, Capital Medical University, Beijing, P.R. China, **5** Department of Cardiac Surgery, Beijing Anzhen Hospital, Capital Medical University, Beijing, P.R. China, **6** Beijing Institute of Heart, Lung and Vessel Disease, Capital Medical University, Beijing, P.R. China, **7** Department of Medicine, University of Illinois at Chicago, Chicago, Illinois, United States of America, **8** Department of Beijing Hospital, Ministry of Health, Beijing, P.R. China

Abstract

Chronic thromboembolic pulmonary hypertension (CTEPH) is a progressive disease characterized by misguided thrombolysis and remodeling of pulmonary arteries. MicroRNAs are small non-coding RNAs involved in multiple cell processes and functions. During CTEPH, circulating microRNA profile endued with characteristics of diseased cells could be identified as a biomarker, and might help in recognition of pathogenesis. Thus, in this study, we compared the differentially expressed microRNAs in plasma of CTEPH patients and healthy controls and investigated their potential functions. Microarray was used to identify microRNA expression profile and qRT-PCR for validation. The targets of differentially expressed microRNAs were identified *in silico*, and the Gene Ontology database and Kyoto Encyclopedia of Genes and Genomes pathway database were used for functional investigation of target gene profile. Targets of let-7b were validated by fluorescence reporter assay. Protein expression of target genes was determined by ELISA or western blotting. Cell migration was evaluated by wound healing assay. The results showed that 1) thirty five microRNAs were differentially expressed in CTEPH patients, among which, a signature of 17 microRNAs, which was shown to be related to the disease pathogenesis by *in silico* analysis, gave diagnostic efficacy of both sensitivity and specificity >0.9. 2) Let-7b, one of the down-regulated anti-oncogenic microRNAs in the signature, was validated to decrease to about 0.25 fold in CTEPH patients. 3) ET-1 and TGFBR1 were direct targets of let-7b. Altering let-7b level influenced ET-1 and TGFBR1 expression in pulmonary arterial endothelial cells (PAECs) as well as the migration of PAECs and pulmonary arterial smooth muscle cells (PASMCs). These results suggested that CTEPH patients had aberrant microRNA signature which might provide some clue for pathogenesis study and biomarker screening. Reduced let-7b might be involved in the pathogenesis of CTEPH by affecting ET-1 expression and the function of PAECs and PASMCs.

Editor: Carol Feghali-Bostwick, Medical University of South Carolina, United States of America

Funding: This work was supported by the Fund of National Natural Science Foundation of China (81070041, 81070042, 81111130212, 81228001, 81370152, 81228001). URL:http://www.nsfc.gov.cn. The funders had no role in study design, data collection and analysis, decision to publish, or preparation of the manuscript.

Competing Interests: The authors have declared that no competing interests exist.

* Email: cyh-birm@263.net (CW); wang_jun@ccmu.edu.cn (JW)

Introduction

Chronic thromboembolic pulmonary hypertension (CTEPH) is characterized by continuously increased pulmonary vascular resistance due to unresolved emboli in major pulmonary arterials and/or pulmonary microvascular remodeling [1–3]. Recent epidemiology studies showed that the incidence of CTEPH in acute pulmonary thromboembolism survivors was about 2.7%–8.8% [4–6], and 2-year survival in untreated patients with a mean pulmonary artery pressure greater than 50 mmHg was as low as 10% [7]. However, recognition before CTEPH progression is difficult for the insidious onset and lack of effective biomarker of it.

MicroRNAs (miRNAs) are small endogenous non-coding RNAs that suppress gene expression post-transcriptionally by binding to the "seed sequences" in 3′ untranslated regions (UTRs) of target mRNAs. Dysregulation of miRNAs has been found in different diseases and biological processes [8]. Recent studies have shown that miRNAs were involved in pulmonary vascular remodeling and susceptibility of CTEPH [9,10], as well as pulmonary arterial smooth muscle cells (PASMCs) malproliferation of pulmonary arterial hypertension (PAH) [11–12].

Circulating miRNAs, known as stable cell-free miRNAs in serum or plasma, are passively and selectively released to blood by various cells, and may act as transmitter or messenger in cell communication [13,14]. During disease, aberrantly expressed miRNAs in the diseased cells are released into the circulation, and the circulating miRNA profile is endued with the disease properties [15]. Recently, circulating miRNAs have been extensively studied as potential blood-based biomarkers for disease diagnosis, especially in malignancies and cardiovascular diseases.

Plasma miR-134 has been shown to be a specific biomarker for acute pulmonary thromboembolism [16].

Multiple pathophysiologic processes have been reported to contribute to the progression of CTEPH [17–19], including imbalance of endothelin-1 (ET-1), nitric oxide and prostacyclin, dysfunction of pulmonary arterial endothelial cells (PAECs), and malproliferation of PASMCs. ET-1 is a key vasoconstrictor especially in pulmonary circulation, and can cause proliferation of many cells involved in vascular remodeling. ET-1 level was elevated in CTEPH patients [18], and endothelin receptor antagonists (ETAs) have been applied for CTEPH treatment [20]. Transforming growth factor (TGF)-β plays important regulatory roles in the balance of cell proliferation and apoptosis. The abnormal activation of TGF-β/transforming growth factor beta receptor 1 (TGFBR1) signaling was involved in development of idiopathic PAH [21,22]. Clarify the relationship between candidate miRNAs and these known mechanisms would intensify the recognition of disease pathogenesis.

Taking the complex pathophysiology of CTEPH and the extensive regulatory function of miRNAs into account, we hypothesized that circulating miRNA profile might reflect the miRNAs involved in the pathogenesis of CTEPH more comprehensively, thus could be used as candidate biomarker and shed light on the recognition of CTEPH pathogenesis. In this study, we identified a 17 miRNA signature in CTEPH plasma and investigated the potential functions of this signature *in silico*. Let-7b, one of the key miRNAs in it, was shown to influence ET-1 level and migration of PAECs and PASMCs.

Materials and Methods

Subjects

The study procedure was approved by the Medical Ethics Committee of Beijing Chao-Yang Hospital affiliated to Capital Medical University, and the written informed consent was obtained from each subject. The microarray cohort was composed of 10 CTEPH patients and 10 healthy control subjects. For further validation, another 40 pairs of subjects participated. The patients were recruited over approximate 4 years (from March, 2007 to November, 2010). Diagnosis of CTEPH was established based on standard protocol previously described [23]. Most of the CTEPH patients received the right heart catheterization. The exclusion criteria included malignancies, other cardiovascular diseases, and patients who had ever received any treatment for pulmonary hypertension except for anticoagulation.

Plasma Collection and RNA Extraction

Whole blood (2 mL) was drawn into Vacutainer (anti-coagulated with EDTA, BD, New Jersey, US), and plasma isolation was done within 2 hours by centrifugation at 1000 g for 10 minutes. Total RNA of plasma was harvested with the TRI Reagent (Sigma Aldrich, St. Louis, US). For real time PCR, an internal control of 5 fmol synthetic Syn-cel-miR-39 (Qiagen, Valencia, CA) was added to plasma after mixing with TRI Reagent, as previously described [24].

MiRNA Microarray and *In Silico* Analysis

The miRCURY LNA Array (version 14.0, Exiqon, Vedbaek, DK) was performed in microarray cohort. The dataset of microarray has been submitted to the repository of Gene Expression Omnibus, and the accession number is GSE56914. Random variance model (RVM) *t*-test was applied to filter the differentially expressed miRNAs. A greedy search, heuristic algorithm for making locally optimal choices at each stage with the hope of finding a global optimum, was taken to find different marker combinations, and during cross-validation of diagonal samples for each combination, seven diagnostic methods were applied [25]. More details can be found in File S1. TargetScan and miRDB were combined for target prediction. The Gene Ontology (GO) Database [26] and the KEGG PATHWAY Database [27] were used for functional investigation of target gene profile of differentially expressed miRNAs. The pathway analysis of let-7b alone was done using DIANA-miRPath [28].

Real-Time Quantitative Reverse-Transcription Polymerase Chain Reaction

A stem-loop real-time quantitative reverse transcription (qRT) polymerase chain reaction (PCR) was used to validate the data obtained by microarray in an enlarged independent cohort. TaqMan MicroRNA Assay, TaqMan MicroRNA Reverse Transcription Kit, and TaqMan Gene Expression Master Mix (Applied Biosystems, Foster, US) were used. The real-time PCR was performed on the ABI PRISM7500 system (Applied Biosystems, Foster, US).

Fluorescent Reporter Assay

The native 3′-UTR fragments of ET-1 and TGFBR1 containing the predicted hsa-let-7b binding sites were amplified from the human lung fibroblast cDNA of a health donor, and subcloned into pcDNA3.1/enhanced green fluorescent protein (EGFP) construct by *Not*I and *Xba*I (NEB, Ipswich, US) subsequently. The control constructs were generated by point mutation in the predicted "seed sequence" of hsa-let-7b using TaKaRa MutanB-EST Kit (TaKaRa, Dalian, CHN). The primer sets were shown in Table S1 in File S1.

Western Blotting and Enzyme-Linked Immunosorbent Assay

Expression of target genes TGFBR1 and ET-1 was detected by Western blotting and enzyme-linked immunosorbent assay (ELISA) respectively.

Wound Healing Assay

Migration of human PAECs and PASMCs (ScienCell, California, US) was evaluated by wound healing assay [29].

Statistical Analysis

Demographic and clinical characteristics of the subjects were described as mean ± SD, or median for abnormal distribution data. The Mann-Whitney *U* test, two-sample Kolmogorov-Smirnov test and χ^2 test were used to examine differences between two groups. Multiple comparison was done by two-way ANOVA with Student-Newman-Keuls method for Post Hoc Tests. Receiver-operating characteristic (ROC) curve analysis was also performed for candidate miRNA levels against CTEPH. Univariable linear and logistics regression analyses were conducted to evaluate the relationships between candidate miRNAs and clinically related indices. Age and sex were considered as controlled variables. SPSS 16.0 was used for all statistical analyses and $P<0.05$ (two-tailed) was considered statistically significant.

Additional details are available in File S1.

Results

Clinical Characteristics of Subjects

Ten CTEPH patients and 10 healthy controls matched in age and sex were involved in microarray cohort, and another 40 pairs in validation cohort. Baseline and clinical characteristics are shown in Table 1. In microarray cohort, all CTEPH patients received right heart catheterization, and acute vascular reaction test was positive in 1 out of 9 subjects (11.1%). The mean pulmonary artery pressure was 54.6 mmHg, and the pulmonary vascular resistance was 1071.2 dyn·s·cm^{-5}. In validation cohort, 36 CTEPH patients received right heart catheterization, and acute vascular reaction was positive in 6 subjects (16.7%). The mean pulmonary artery pressure was 51.5 mmHg, and pulmonary vascular resistance was 1079.4 dyn·s·cm^{-5}. There was no difference between CTEPH patients of the microarray and validation cohort in hemodynamic index, deep venous thrombosis, WHO functional class, 6-minute walk distance, acute vascular reaction and N-terminal pro-brain natriuretic peptide except C-reactive protein (Table S2 in File S1).

Aberrantly Expressed Circulating MiRNAs in CTEPH Patients

To determine the differential circulating miRNA profile of CTEPH, we employed the miRCURY LNA Array (version 14.0) system with plasma extracted RNA of 10 CTEPH patients and 10 healthy controls. As displayed in Table S3 in File S1, the circulating miRNA profiles differed significantly between CTEPH patients and healthy controls. Of 1700 probes on this array, we found 15 up-regulated and 20 down-regulated miRBase included miRNAs in CTEPH patients compared with healthy controls at $P<0.05$.

To further determine the molecular signature of CTEPH, the greedy search was applied. Based on the 35 differentially expressed miRNAs from the microarray, we identified a 17 miRNA combination showing the best diagnostic efficacy. The diagnostic models constructed with them gave diagnostic sensitivity and specificity of >0.9 for all the seven methods (Table S4 in File S1). Hierarchical cluster of miRNAs in the signature was shown in Figure 1. Among the included miRNAs, the top five of the six up-regulated miRNAs were miR-1260, miR-602, miR-129-5p, miR-1908 and miR-483-5p by foldchange, while the top five of eleven down-regulated miRNAs were miR-140-3p, miR-93, miR-22, miR-106b and let-7b.

Predictive Investigation of MiRNA Signature Functions

To illustrate the potential role of differentially expressed miRNAs in pathogenesis of the disease, pathway analysis and GO analysis were applied, and the significant pathways and the top 10% significant GO categories aligned by weight were shown in Figure S1 and Figure S2.

Taking the possible pathophysiology of CTEPH into account, we filtered these significant pathways and GO categories for the most important functions. As displayed in Table 2, the pathways associated with proliferation were the most important ones, and the pathways associated with immunity were up-regulated, while some cardiovascular related pathways were down-regulated. In the GO categories (Table 3), the cell function regulation categories were up-regulated, while the calcium transport regulation and negative regulation of cell proliferation categories were down-regulated.

Circulating Let-7b Significantly Decreased in CTEPH Patients

To confirm the findings obtained from the miRNA profile and attempt to find a candidate miRNA for further investigation on its role in the disease, after a detailed literature review (Table S5 in File S1), we selectively measured the expression of 3 miRNAs in an

Table 1. Clinical characteristics of the subjects.

Characteristics	miRNA microarray		qRT-PCR	
	Healthy control (n = 10)	CTEPH patient (n = 10)	Healthy control (n = 40)	CTEPH patient (n = 40)
Age (yr)*	49.7 (10.1)	49.8 (10.1)	49.6 (9.5)	51.9 (11.6)
Sex (Male/Total)	6/10	6/10	24/40	25/40
DVT (Positive/Total)	-	6/10	-	12/30
MBP (mmHg)*		91.2 (4.4)		93.3 (12.0)
sPAP (mmHg)*†	-	86.3 (13.5)	-	89.5 (19.7)
mPAP (mmHg)*†	-	54.6 (13.3)	-	51.5 (12.0)
PVR (dyn·s·cm^{-5})*†	-	1071.2 (243.9)	-	1079.4 (598.1)
CI (L·min^{-1}·m^{-2})*†	-	2.0 (0.6)	-	2.0 (0.6)
WHO functional class				
I	-	1/10	-	2/40
II	-	2/10	-	19/40
III	-	6/10	-	16/40
IV	-	1/10	-	3/40
6MWD (m)*‡	-	374.6 (27.0)	-	355.5 (109.0)
AVR (Positive/Total)	-	1/9	-	6/36
NTproBNP (pg/mL)*§	-	1436.6 (1577.1)	-	1456.2 (1433.5)
CRP (mg/L)*‖	-	6.0 (6.0)	-	4.7 (4.2)

Definition of abbreviations: DVT, deep venous thrombosis; MBP, mean blood pressure; sPAP, systolic pulmonary arterial pressure; mPAP, mean pulmonary arterial pressure; PVR, pulmonary vascular resistance; CI, cardiac index; 6MWD, 6-minute walk distance; AVR, acute vascular reaction; NTproBNP, N-terminal pro-brain natriuretic peptide; CRP, C-reactive protein. * Mean (SD); for microarray cohort, † n = 10, ‡ n = 7, § n = 8, ‖ n = 8; and for validation (qRT-PCR) cohort, † n = 36, ‡ n = 31, § n = 34, ‖ n = 29.

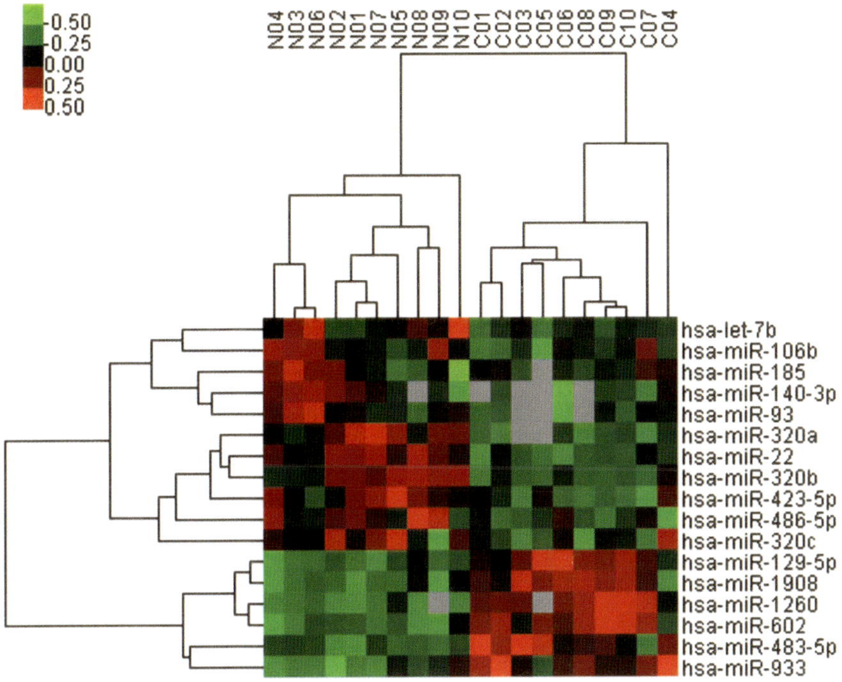

Figure 1. Circulating miRNAs signature in CTEPH patients and healthy controls. Heirarchical clustering and heatmap diagram of the optimum circulating miRNAs signature derived from the greedy search. RNA was isolated from EDTA-coagulated plasma from CTEPH patients (n = 10) and healthy controls (n = 10).

independent enlarged cohort of CTEPH patients (n = 40) and healthy controls (n = 40) using TaqMan qRT-PCR. Among the 3 included miRNAs, up-regulated miR-602 was oncogenic one, while down-regulated let-7b and miR-22 were anti-oncogenic ones involved in lung disease or cell migration and proliferation (Table S5 in File S1). As shown in Figure 2A, consistent with miRNA profile, let-7b and miR-22 levels were significantly reduced in CTEPH patient plasma ($P<0.001$). However, the up-regulation of miR-602 in the signature was not observed in the validation cohort. In CTEPH patients of validation cohort, the let-7b level

Table 2. Filtered pathways for potential pathogenesis of CTEPH.

Functions	KEGG pathway	Regulated	Weight (-lg*P*)
Associated with proliferation	MAPK signaling pathway	up/down	14.51/7.07
	ErbB signaling pathway	up/down	7.19/5.52
	TGF-β signaling pathway	up/down	6.67/4.67
	Wnt signaling pathway	up/down	2.32/2.90
	mTOR signaling pathway	up/down	5.43/4.03
	pathways in cancer	up/down	12.49/3.84
Associated with immunity	HTLV-1 infection	up	6.03
	T cell receptor signaling pathway	up	5.06
	Fc gamma R-mediated phagocytosis	up	4.47
	Bacterial invasion of epithelial cells	up	3.37
	Influenza A	up	2.48
	B cell receptor signaling pathway	up	2.43
Cardiovascular	Arrhythmogenic right ventricular cardiomyopathy	down	4.10
	Hypertrophic cardiomyopathy	down	3.77
	Vascular smooth muscle contraction	down	3.66
	Dilated cardiomyopathy	down	3.49
	Calcium signaling pathway	down	3.04
	Regulation of actin cytoskeleton	down	2.52

Table 3. Filtered GO categories for potential pathogenesis of CTEPH.

Function	GO category	Regulated	Weight (-lg*P*)
Cell functions	cell cycle	up	15.50
	cell differentiation	up	11.57
	cell adhesion	up	10.16
	cell division	up	8.86
	cell cycle arrest	up	6.69
	cell migration	up	6.51
Calcium signal and proliferation	regulation of calcium ion transport via voltage-gated calcium channel activity	down	5.22
	negative regulation of cell proliferation	down	4.94

was different between patients of positive and negative acute vascular reaction, while positively correlated with the level of plasminogen activator inhibitor 1 and D-Dimer, and inversely correlated with cardiac index (Table S6 in File S1 and Figure S3). ROC curve analysis revealed that let-7b and miR-22 had moderate value for CTEPH diagnosis with the area under the curve of 0.769 (95% CI: 0.664–0.874) and 0.751 (95% CI: 0.645–0.857) respectively (Figure 2B).

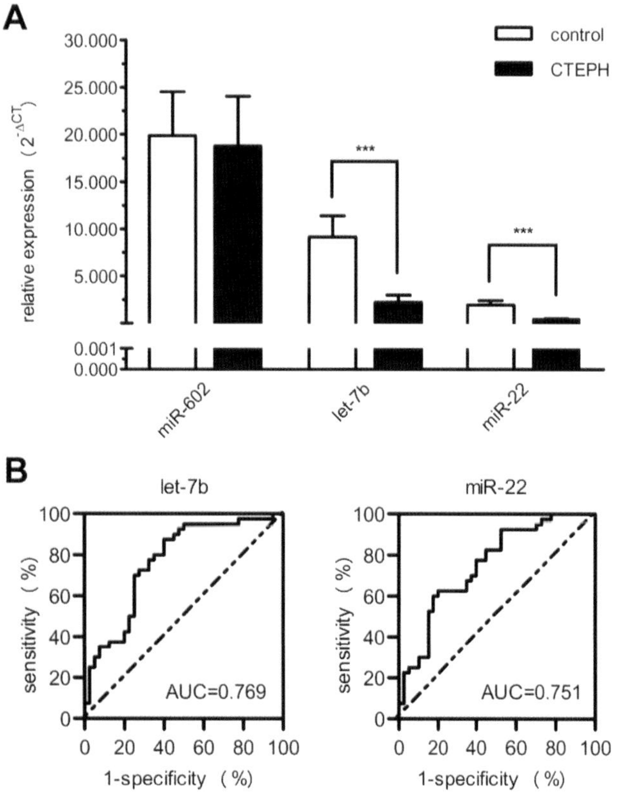

Figure 2. Independent validation of differentially expressed miRNAs. Three candidate miRNAs (miR-602, let-7b and miR-22) from the microarray were validated by qRT-PCR in an independent cohort of CTEPH patients (n = 40) and healthy controls (n = 40). (**A**) Relative expression ($2^{-\Delta CT}$) normalized to cel-miR-39 was shown as median with interquartile. *P* value was calculated by Mann-Whitney *U* test. ***$P<0.001$. (**B**) ROC curve analysis and AUC for 2 validated miRNAs (let-7b and miR-22) in the diagnosis of CTEPH.

ET-1 and TGFBR1 Were Direct Targets of Let-7b

In order to study the function of validated miRNAs in CTEPH, first we predicted their target genes by *in silico* analysis. The results showed that ET-1 and many important receptors in TGF-β and mitogen-activated protein kinase pathways contained let-7b binding sites in their 3′-UTRs, suggesting that they might be potential targets of let-7b. Thus we selected let-7b as the candidate miRNA in the following studies. The most highly targeted pathways and the potential targets of let-7b included in these pathways were displayed in Table S7 in File S1. Among the top 10 pathways, TGFBR1 was included in five of them, and this result suggested that TGFBR1 might be a core target of let-7b.

To determine whether let-7b directly targets ET-1 or TGFBR1 as predicted, we constructed an EGFP reporter carrying the putative let-7b binding sites in 3′-UTR of ET-1 or TGFBR1. Control constructs were generated from the wild ones by point mutation respectively (Figure 3A and 3B). Co-transfection of HEK293 cells with wild-type 3′-UTR TGFBR1 reporter constructs and 2′-OME modified let-7b mimics resulted in an approximately 45% reduction of EGFP fluorescence compared with control transfection (Figure 3C). The reduction was blunted when the seed binding site was mutated (Figure 3C). As predicted by Targetscan and RNAhybrid, there were two let-7b binding sites in the 3′-UTR of ET-1 (Figure 3B). Approximately 40% reduction of EGFP fluorescence with a construct containing a wild type 3′-UTR of ET-1 was detected compared to control transfection with all binding sites mutated construct(Figure 3D). The binding site, which was predicted by RNAhybrid (ET-1-mut2), seemed to be more powerful than the other one. These data suggested that TGFBR1 and ET-1 were direct targets of let-7b.

Let-7b Was Inversely Correlated with Plasma ET-1 Level in CTEPH Patients

As demonstrated above, ET-1 was one of the direct targets of let-7b. Literature showed that ET-1 was the key vasoconstrictor of pulmonary circulation, and has been indicated in the pathophysiology of pulmonary hypertension including CTEPH [18]. To further determine the association between ET-1 expression and let-7b, the plasma ET-1 level of the validation cohort was detected by ELISA. As shown in Figure 4A, the plasma ET-1 level was significantly elevated in CTEPH patients compared with healthy controls ($P<0.001$). This was consistent with previous report [18]. Furthermore, the ET-1 level was inversely related to the plasma let-7b level moderately ($r = -0.456$, $P<0.001$) (Figure 4B). These data suggested that the down-regulation of let-7b might be related to the elevated ET-1 level of CTEPH patients.

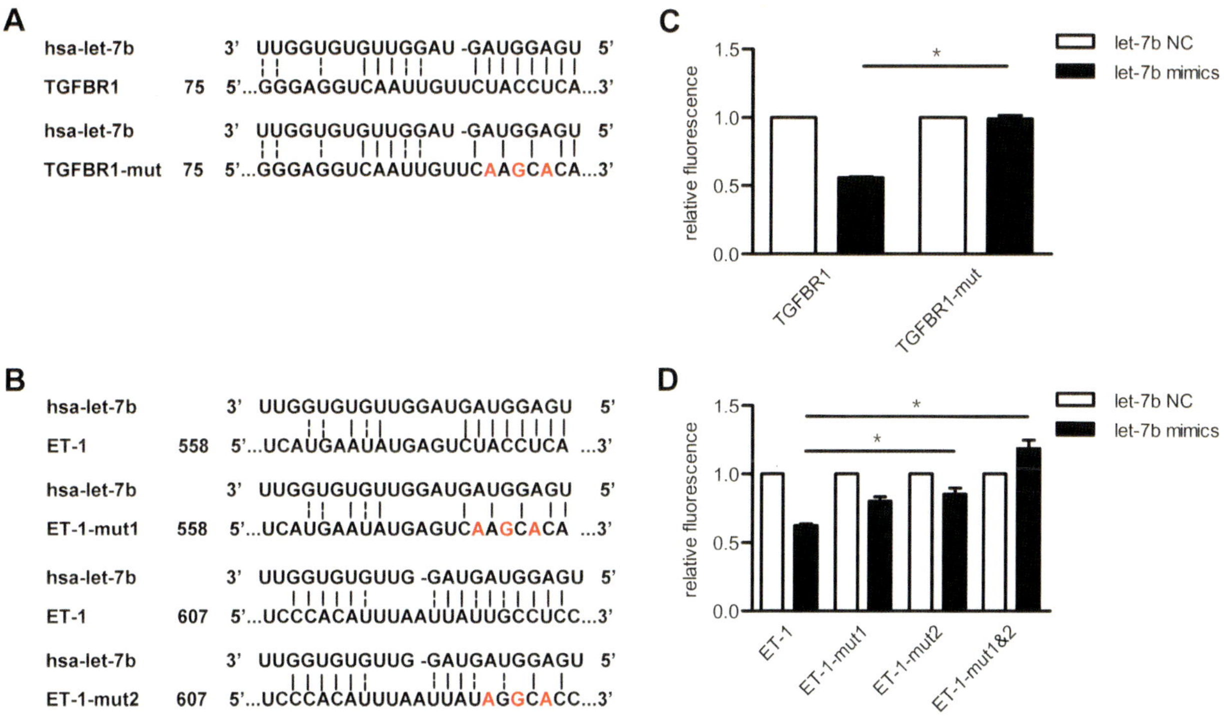

Figure 3. ET-1 and TGFBR1 were direct target genes of let-7b. EGFP reporter assay was applied for target validation in HEK 293 cells. Oligonucleotide mimics and negative control (NC) of let-7b were co-transfected with reporter plasmids and mutated controls, respectively. **(A)** & **(B)** Predicted duplex of let-7b and its target region of TGFBR1 and ET-1 with experimental mutation in seed sequences respectively. The number indicates the region position in its 3′-UTRs. The mutated nucleotide was shown in red, and the original nucleotide was its complementary one. **(C)** & **(D)** let-7b down-regulated EGFP expression through the predicted seed sequences in 3′-UTRs of ET-1 and TGFBR1. *P* value was calculated by two-sample Kolmogorov-Smirnov test. * $P<0.05$.

Altering Let-7b Regulated ET-1 and TGFBR1 Expression in PAECs

To further illustrate the function of let-7b, let-7b antagonist lentivirus or let-7b mimics were used to decrease or increase the let-7b expression in human PAECs. A multiplicity of infection of 20 achieved an infection rate of more than 90% for antagonist lentivirus and 80%–90% for let-7b mimics (data not shown), and the let-7b level was decreased approximately 45% and increased for 2 fold (Figure 5A). In the let-7b antagonized PAECs, TGFBR1 expression increased remarkably, and the reverse results were seen in let-7b over-expressed cells (Figure 5B). Similar results were also found for ET-1 level in the culture medium of PAECs (Figure 5C). ET-1 expression is a complex process regulated by multiple cytokines, including TGF-β. Previous studies showed that TGF-β stimulated expression of ET-1 preferentially through TGFBR1 [30]. As let-7b can also target TGFBR1, the effect of TGFBR1 on the let-7b regulation of ET-1 should be clarified. Thus, we silenced TGFBR1 in let-7b antagonized PAECs with siRNA. As shown in Figure 5D, the increased ET-1 level of let-7b antagonized PAECs was reversed to approximately normal level. These data indicated that TGFBR1 was involved in the let-7b regulation of ET-1, and this seemed to be over the effect of direct targeting.

Let-7b Regulated PAECs and PASMCs Migration through TGFBR1 and ET-1

Pulmonary vascular remodeling is the crucial pathological change in CTEPH, and activated migration of PAECs and/or PASMCs contributes to this process. We investigated the possible role of let-7b in migration of PAECs and PASMCs by wound healing assay after decreasing or increasing its expression using the antagonist lentivirus or let-7b mimics respectively as Figure 5. The PASMCs showed the similar efficiency as PAECs did, which was shown in Figure 5A. After Post Hoc Test, as shown in Figure 6A, migration of PAECs was slighted inhibited when let-7b was over-expressed, but antagonist showed no effect when PAECs were cultured in normal medium. For TGFBR1 and ET-1 have been identified as direct targets of let-7b, we supposed that they might participated in let-7b regulated cell migration. Then TGF-β (10 ng/mL) was added into the culture media. The results showed that TGF-β could induce the migration of let-7b NC PAECs, while when cultured in medium with TGF-β, migration of let-7b antagonized PAECs was further promoted. Similar results were observed for PASMCs except for induction of TGF-β on let-7b PASMCs (Figure 6B). The results above indicated the involvement of TGFBR1 in let-7b regulated migration of PASMCs and PAECs.

For ET-1, because there was no pro-migration effect observed by let-7b antagonist induced ET-1 increase (Figure 5C and Figure 6A), a selective endothelin A receptor antagonist (ETA, BQ-123, Sigma Aldrich, St. Louis, US) was used to observe the effect of derepression of ET-1 on migration of PAECs. As shown in Figure S4A, ETA (1 nM) could suppress normal PAECs migration, and the suppression effect was weakened by let-7b antagonist. For PASMCs, as they were not the chief cells for endogenous ET-1 expression, exogenous ET-1 was used to observe its effect on PASMCs migration. And we saw that ET-1 could promote the migration of both let-7b NC and let-7b antagonized PASMCs (Figure S4B). These results above indicated that although ET-1 was not the major mediator between let-7b and PAECs migration,

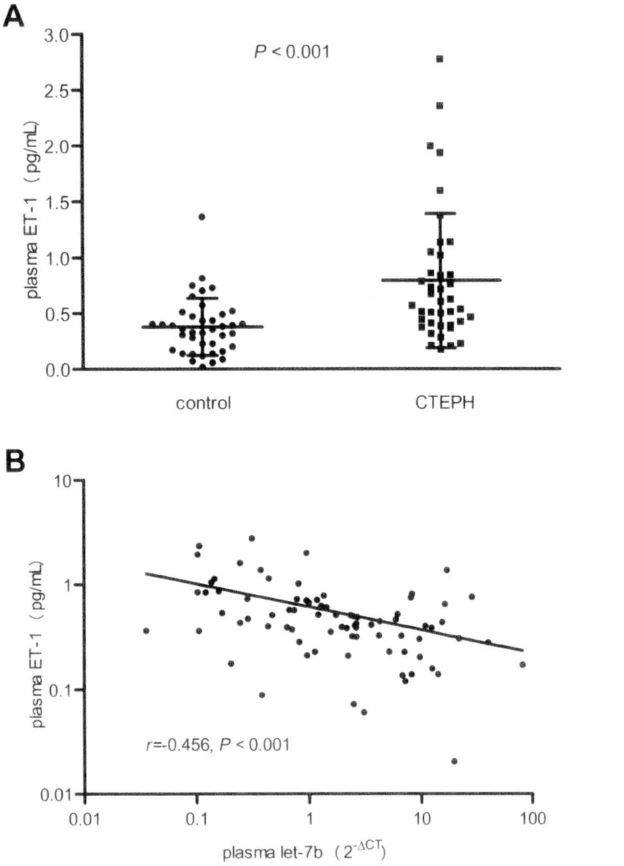

Figure 4. Elevated plasma ET-1 level in CTEPH patients and its correlation with let-7b. (**A**) Plasma endothelin-1 level of CTEPH patients (n = 40) and healthy controls (n = 40) measured by ELISA. *P* value was calculated by Mann-Whitney *U* test. $P<0.001$. (**B**) Spearman correlation and scatter plot of plasma endothelin-1 and let-7b (n = 80). The X- and Y-axis were log10 transformed. The correlation coefficient and *P* value were shown.

derepression of ET-1 by let-7b partially participated in the PAECs migration, and the elevated ET-1 also could induce PASMCs migration.

Discussion

In present study, we demonstrated that CTEPH patients had a differently expressed miRNA profile. And a signature of 17 miRNAs was shown to be related to the disease pathogenesis and gave the diagnostic efficacy of both sensitivity and specificity >0.9. Let-7b, one of the key miRNAs, might be involved in the pathogenesis of CTEPH by affecting ET-1 expression and the migration of PAECs and PASMCs.

Even though many studies have focused on the associated risk factors, genetic susceptibility, pathology, therapy, prognosis for CTEPH [2,7,10,31] in recent years, still there is much to be further recognized, especially for its pathogenesis. Early treatment before right heart insufficient by pulmonary endarterectomy or suitable medical treatment was crucial for prognosis improvement [32]. This highlighted the need to develop sensitive and reliable biomarkers for early diagnosis of CTEPH.

At present, possibly owing to the complex pathophysiology of CTEPH, the reported candidate molecular biomarkers for CTEPH, including asymmetric dimethylarginine [33], D-Dimer [34], heart-type fatty acid-binding protein [35] and brain natriuretic peptide [36] still were not sufficiently reliable for clinical application. Therefore, combination of some biomarkers representing different pathophysiological aspects of the disease might be the tendency for future biomarker screening. The emerging of microarray technology has made it possible to achieve tens of thousands of gene expression simutaneously as the base of screening. Biomarker signature have been studied in many diseases [37,38], including cancers, cardiovascular diseases. MiRNAs were recognized of limited amount to regulate most of protein-coding gene expression post-transcriptionally. Therefore, it seemed more practical to explore miRNAs as biomarkers for the diseases with complex etiology and pathophysiology. Studies on miRNA signature have increased steeply during recent few years [39,40]. These studies have shown that certain miRNA signature had satisfactory efficacy for disease diagnosis and evaluation.

As ideal diagnostic biomarker, miRNAs possess many sustaining properties. First, circulating miRNAs were remarkably stable even exposed to harsh environment [15,24] and this characteristics made detection reproducibly. Second, the pathognostic cell resource of miRNAs [14] determined the high specificity of circulating miRNAs for disease diagnosis. Third, miRNAs were small molecules that lacked post-processing modification. They could be detected by an extremely sensitive method at very low starting concentration [41]. Although large population verification of the results in our study is still needed, circulating miRNAs provide a promising prospect for CTEPH diagnosis. During verification, the signature can be further simplified for clinical application, and the efficacy and accuracy can be enhanced.

Since 2008, many studies have indicated that circulating miRNAs were functional molecules which might act in cell communication and suppress the translation of target genes in recipient cells. A recent study [15] showed that, in healthy subjects, circulating miRNA profile was similar to the profile of circulating blood cells, but this similarity was disturbed in diseased subjects, and the circulating miRNA profile was endued with characteristics of cells involved in the disease. In this study, we observed that the differentially expressed circulating miRNAs had important regulatory function in CTEPH pathogenesis, such as remodeling of pulmonary vascular, imbalance of vascular tone or inflammation. Many of these were regarded to be involved in CTEPH etiology. However, few of them have been thoroughly interpreted. Functions regulated by the aberrant miRNA signature were the cue for the comprehensive understanding of CTEPH pathogenesis. Based on these *in silico* results, we selectively focused on let-7b to study its cellular function relevant to the disease, because the predicted targets of it were likely to be involved in CTEPH pathogenesis. Let-7b has been reported to be an anti-oncogenic miRNA which is frequently lost in many tumors [13,42]. By the preliminary correlation analysis with clinical characteristics of CTEPH patients, we found that circulating let-7b levels were decreased in patients with negative AVR, which was generally regarded to be related with serious pulmonary vascular remodeling. This illuminating result indicated the possible role of let-7b in pulmonary vascular biology of CTEPH pathogenesis. In the further mechanism study, we found that let-7b could target ET-1 and TGFBR1, which have been reported to be closely related to the pathogenesis of CTEPH. Antagonizing let-7b could up-regulate ET-1 and TGFBR1 expression, which promoted PAECs and PASMCs migration. These effects would lead to persistent constriction or remodeling of pulmonary vascular bed and promote CTEPH development. Positive correlation was also found between let-7b and PAI-1 or D-Dimer, which were regarded to be elevated in thrombotic diseases. Therefore, the

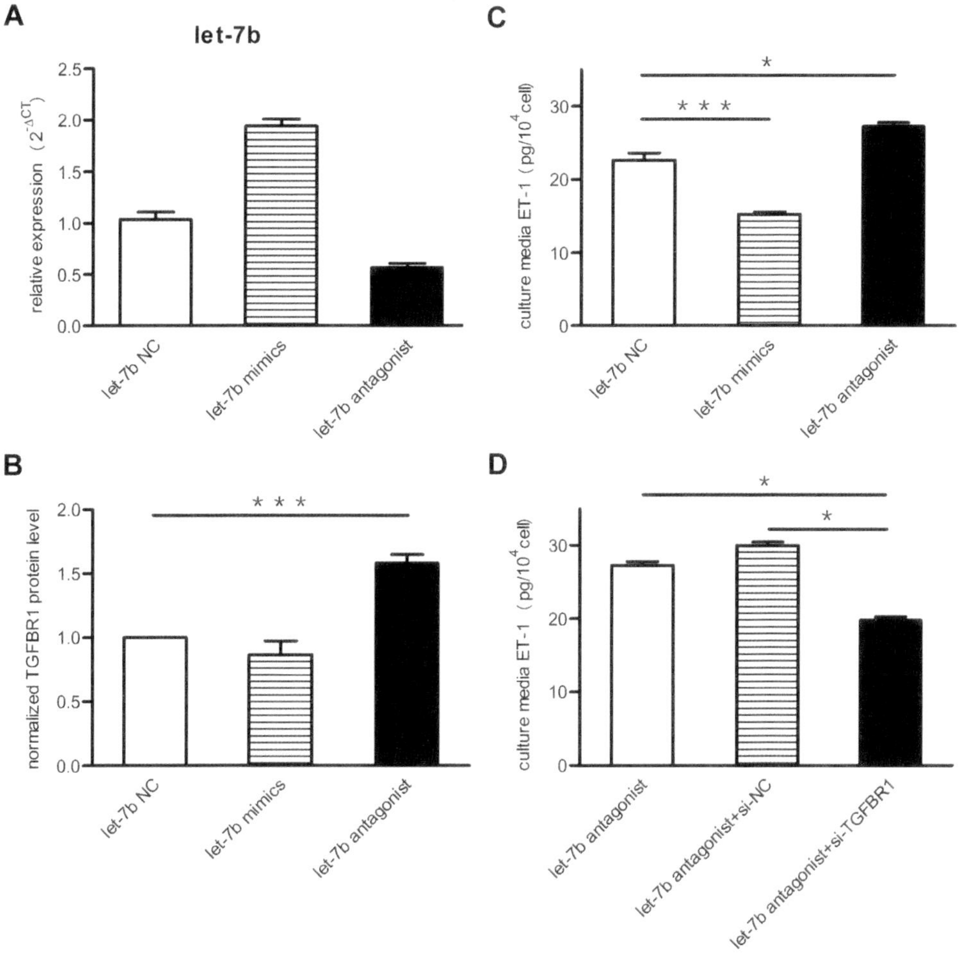

Figure 5. Altering let-7b regulated ET-1 and TGFBR1 expression in PAECs. Human pulmonary arterial endothelial cells (PAECs) were infected with a let-7b antagonist/\mimics lentivirus or empty control. (**A**) Endogenous let-7b was decreased to a level about 55% by antagonist lentivirus and was increased to about 2 fold by mimics. (**B**) After normalized by β-actin, TGFBR1 expression was increased about a half in let-7b antagonist infected PAECs and slightly decreased in let-7b over-expressed cells by western blotting. (**C**) Culture medium was collected after continuous culture for 48 h, and ET-1 levels were detected by ELISA. ET-1 level in culture medium of let-7b over-expressed PAECs was obviously decreased, and was increased in let-7b antagonized PAECs. (**D**) Let-7b antagonized cells were transfected with siRNA for TGFBR1 and control siRNA respectively. Silencing TGFBR1 with siRNA could reverse the increased ET-1 level causing by let-7b antagonist (n = 5). *P* value was calculated by two-sample Kolmogorov-Smirnov test. *** $P<0.001$. * $P<0.05$.

positive correlation gave no direct indication for the role of let-7b in coagulation process of CTEPH. The exact mechanism still needs further study.

ET-1 was a potent endothelium-derived vasoconstrictor [43]. It was mainly secreted by endothelial cells and mediate vascular constriction and PASMCs proliferation through endothelin A and B receptors [44,45]. In CTEPH patients, increases of ET-1 were significantly correlated with clinical characteristics [10]. In addition, elevated serum ET-1 was demonstrated to be a predictor of bad pulmonary endarterectomy outcome [46]. Endothelin receptor antagonists have emerged as cornerstone treatment for PAH for more than 10 years [47]. In CTEPH patients, especially inoperable ones, ETAs were also of benefit in hemodynamics [20]. ET-1 expression was a complex biological process. In the present study, we showed a new aspect of ET-1 expression regulation at the post-transcriptional level by a miRNA. The down-regulation of let-7b was correlated with elevation of plasma ET-1 level, and this might be accomplished through two ways. First, ET-1 was a direct target of let-7b, and it was derepressed when let-7b was down-regulated. Second, TGF-β was one of the most potent regulators of ET-1 expression [48]. It strongly increased ET-1 mRNA and protein expression in endothelial, and specifically, TGF-β induced ET-1 expression preferentially through the TGFBR1/Smad3 pathway [30,49]. Our results suggested that decreased let-7b up-regulated the expression of TGFBR1, which was in turn possibly involved in the elevation of ET-1 in CTEPH patients. In addition, ET-1 is a mitogenic growth factor especially in pulmonary circulation. By wound healing assay, we further illustrated that derepression of ET-1 by let-7b partially participated in the PAECs migration, and the elevated ET-1 could induce PASMCs migration. The aberrant migration of PAECs and PASMCs was further related to the pulmonary vascular remodeling of CTEPH patients.

Besides regulation of ET-1 expression, TGFBR1 and downstream signals played an important role in biology of pulmonary vessels. In monocrotaline induced pulmonary hypertension rat model, TGFBR1 was highly expressed in the lung [11]. And in isolated PASMCs of PAH patients, TGFBR1 was activated and implicated in pro-proliferative and anti-apoptotic phenotype of them [21]. In a study on TGF-β1 and related receptors of peripheral blood leucocytes, the TβRI/TβRII ratio was significant

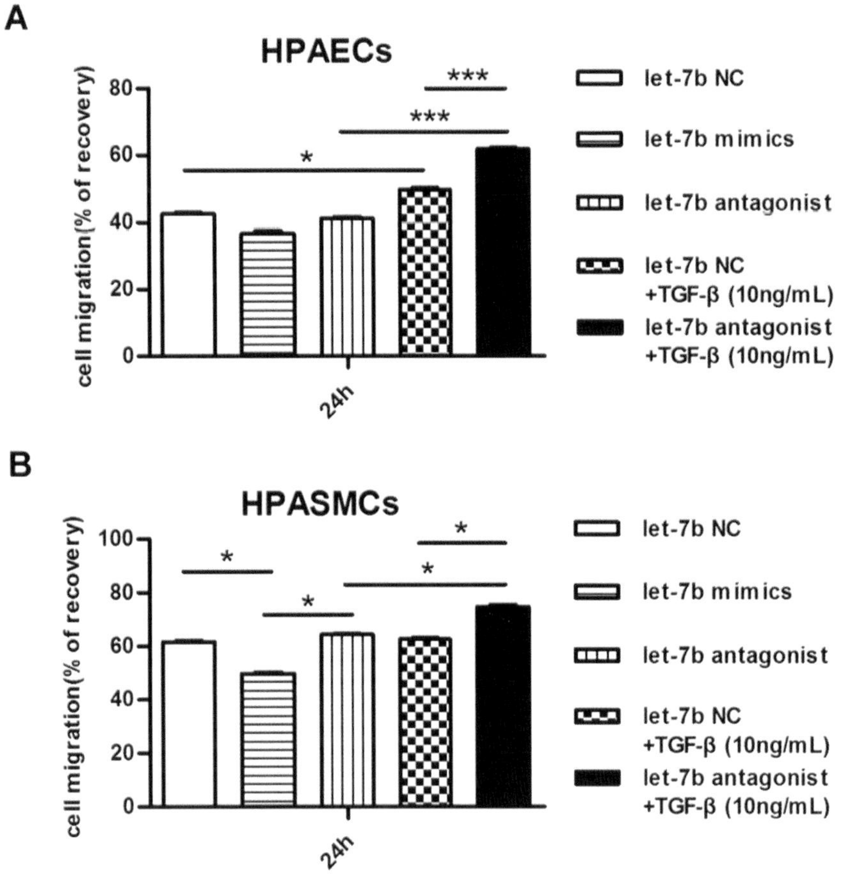

Figure 6. Let-7b regulated PAECs and PASMCs migration. Human PAECs or PASMCs were transfected with a let-7b antagonist lentivirus or let-7b mimics, and the migration was evaluated by wound healing assays. Pictures were taken at 0 h, 12 h, 24 h, and 48 h. The wounded area was expressed as the percentage of recovery. (**A**) Let-7b mimics suppressed PAECs migration, and its antagonist promoted TGF-β induced PAECs migration at 24 h (n = 5). (**B**).Let-7b mimics suppressed PASMCs migration, and its antagonist promoted TGF-β induced PASMCs migration at 24 h (n = 5). *P* value was calculated by two-way ANOVA, and Post Hoc Test was done by Student-Newman-Keuls method. *** $P<0.001$. * $P<0.05$.

increased in PAH [50]. These studies indicated an activated status of TGFBR1 during pulmonary hypertension, and in this study, we provide an indirect evidence for a potential role of TGFBR1 in CTEPH via let-7b. Up-regulation of TGFBR1 caused by let-7b, despite other receptors in TGF-β pathway, might lead to the proliferative vascular disease. During the experiment, we found a phenomenon that even with no effect on promoting PASMCs migration either by TGF-β or let-7b antagonist alone, the combinatorial treatment of them obviously promoted the migration of PASMCs. And we supposed the possible reason as follow: first, previous studies showed that TGF-β had dual role in vascular smooth muscle cell on phenotypic transformation [51,52]. It not only induced SMCs differentiation to the contractile phenotype, but also promoted SMCs dedifferentiation and induced the vascular remodeling. So we supposed that this phenomenon might just be a possible performance of normal PASMCs under TGF-β treatment. Second, TGFBR1 up-regulation has been reported to be related with pulmonary hypertension [11,21,50], and we have indentified that TGFBR1 was a direct target of let-7b. Thus we supposed that let-7b antagonist might be involved in cell migration by regulating TGFBR1 expression. As the target of let-7b was not TGF-β itself, let-7b antagonist alone did not induced PASMC migration without exogenous TGF-β. While under combinatorial treatment of let-7b antagonist and TGF-β, the derepressed TGFBR1 induced by let-7b antagonist was highlighted by its ligand TGF-β, and it led to the aberrant migration observed in let-7b antagonist PASMCs.

There are still some limitations in our study. First, these results were derived from relative small population, and the signature still needed to be validated and adjusted. Second, as miRNAs existing in plasma are in relative low concentration, some low abundance miRNAs might not be reliably detected in our microarray cohort. This might lead to some selection bias of miRNAs for pathogenesis study of CTEPH. However, as CTEPH is a multiple etiology disease, diverse sources of the circulating miRNA profile might be more advantageous for understanding the disease compared with relying on single profiles from single diseased tissue or cell. Third, regulation by miRNAs occurs at the network level. In this study, we selectively investigated the function of let-7b, but other miRNAs that contributed to the disease and their communication with let-7b, especially for the up-stream signal of let-7b and its role in CTEPH, still needed further study and evaluation. Fourth, our previous study of miRNA profile of PASMCs culture from pulmonary endarterectomy tissue also found let-7d, another member of let-7 family, was decreased and involved in the cell proliferation [9], which indicated the importance of let-7 family in pathogenesis of CTEPH. A hypothesis about the mechanism leading to the decrease of let-7 family is still needed to be set in our further study. We also should pay more attention to its possible effect in view of a future cure.

To our best knowledge, this is the first report of circulating miRNA profile of CTEPH. The results of this study provided us some clue and candidate for further pathogenesis investigation and clinical biomarker screening of this miscellaneous disease.

Supporting Information

Figure S1 The significant targeted pathways of miRNAs in the signature. Seventeen candidate miRNAs in the signature were included in target prediction and KEGG pathway analysis. The significance was defined with $P<0.05$, and the pathways were ranked by the weight (-lg$P$). (**A**) Significant targetgene related pathways of up-regulated miRNAs in CTEPH patients. (**B**) Significant targetgene related pathways of down-regulated miRNAs in CTEPH patients.

Figure S2 The top 10% significant targeted GO categories of miRNAs in the signature. Seventeen candidate miRNAs in the signature were included in target prediction and GO analysis. The significance was defined with $P<0.05$, and the top 10% significant GO categories were ranked by the weight (-lg$P$). (**A**) Top 10% significant targetgene related GO categories of up-regulated miRNAs in CTEPH patients. (**B**) Top 10% significant targetgene related pathways of down-regulated miRNAs in CTEPH patients.

Figure S3 Scatter plots of circulating miRNA concentrations of CTEPH patients against common clinical characteristics. The two validated candidate miRNAs were analyzed, and the index with statistical significance was displayed. (**A**) Plasma let-7b against CI (n = 35). (**B**) Plasma let-7b against PAI-I (n = 19). (**C**) Plasma let-7b against D-Dimer (n = 37). (**D**) Plasma miR-22 against total homocysteine (tHcy) (n = 28). (**E**) Plasma miR-22 against CI (n = 35). (**F**) Plasma miR-22 against PAI-I (n = 19). (**G**) Plasma miR-22 against D-Dimer (n = 37). (**H**) Plasma miR-22 against CRP (n = 29).

Figure S4 Let-7b regulated PASMCs/PAECs migration partially through ET-1. The two validated candidate miRNAs were analyzed, and the index with statistical significance was displayed. (**A**) Transfected PAECs was treated with endothelin A receptor antagonist (ETA, 1nM). ETA could inhibit control PAECs migration, and the inhibition role was weakened by let-7b antagonist (n = 5). (**B**) Normal and let-7b antagonized PASMCs were treated by ET-1 (1 nM). ET-1 could obviously promote migration of both cells, and no difference was observed between the promotion of both cells (n = 5). P-value was calculated by two-way ANOVA, and Post Hoc Test was done by Student-Newman-Keuls method. *** $P<0.001$. * $P<0.05$.

File S1 Supporting materials and methods and tables. Table S1, Sequences of the primers used in fluorescent reporter assay. Table S2, Differences in clinical characteristics between microarray cohort and validation cohort. Table S3, Properties of miRNAs of CTEPH patients and healthy controls differentially expressed in microarray. Table S4, Diagnostic efficacy of seven methods for the 17 miRNA signature. Table S5, Literature review for the functions of candidate miRNA in the signature. Table S6, Differences of circulating miRNA levels between different conditions of clinical characteristics. Table S7, Top ten powerfully target pathways of let-7b by DIANA-miRPath.

Acknowledgments

The authors thank professor Dian-hua Jiang of Duke University School of Medicine for his assistance with this manuscript preparation and technical support on this work.

Author Contributions

Conceived and designed the experiments: JW CW JC. Performed the experiments: LJG YHY JL LW JFL YW YL SG HLG. Analyzed the data: LJG. Wrote the paper: LJG JW CW. Major revision of the manuscript: JXJY.

References

1. Fedullo PF, Auger WR, Kerr KM, Rubin LJ (2001) Chronic thromboembolic pulmonary hypertension. N Engl J Med 345: 1465–1472.
2. Peacock A, Simonneau G, Rubin L (2006) Controversies, uncertainties and future research on the treatment of chronic thromboembolic pulmonary hypertension. Proc Am Thorac Soc 3: 608–614.
3. Lang I (2010) Advances in understanding the pathogenesis of chronic thromboembolic pulmonary hypertension. Br J Haematol 149: 478–483.
4. Pengo V, Lensing AW, Prins MH, Marchiori A, Davidson BL, et al. (2004) Incidence of chronic thromboembolic pulmonary hypertension after pulmonary embolism. N Engl J Med 350: 2257–2264.
5. Dentali F, Donadini M, Gianni M, Bertolini A, Squizzato A, et al. (2009) Incidence of chronic pulmonary hypertension in patients with previous pulmonary embolism. Thromb Res 124: 256–258.
6. Surie S, Gibson NS, Gerdes VE, Bouma BJ, van Eck-Smit BL, et al. (2010) Active search for chronic thromboembolic pulmonary hypertension does not appear indicated after acute pulmonary embolism. Thromb Res 125: e202–205.
7. Riedel M, Stanek V, Widimsky J, Prerovsky I (1982) Longterm follow-up of patients with pulmonary thromboembolism. Late prognosis and evolution of hemodynamic and respiratory data. Chest 81: 151–158.
8. Bartel DP (2004) MicroRNAs: genomics, biogenesis, mechanism, and function. Cell 116: 281–297.
9. Wang L, Guo LJ, Liu J, Wang W, Yuan JX, et al. (2013) MicroRNA expression profile of pulmonray artery smooth muscle cells and the effect of let-7d in chronic thromboembolic pulmonary hypertension. Pulm Circ 3: 654–664.
10. Chen Z, Nakajima T, Tanabe N, Hinohara K, Sakao S, et al. (2010) Susceptibility to chronic thromboembolic pulmonary hypertension may be conferred by miR-759 via its targeted interaction with polymorphic fibrinogen alpha gene. Hum Genet 128: 443–452.
11. Caruso P, MacLean MR, Khanin R, McClure J, Soon E, et al. (2010) Dynamic changes in lung microRNA profiles during the development of pulmonary hypertension due to chronic hypoxia and monocrotaline. Arterioscler Thromb Vasc Biol 30: 716–723.
12. Yang S, Banerjee S, De Freitas A, Cui H, Xie N, et al. (2012) miR-21 regulates chronic hypoxia induced pulmonary vascular remodeling. Am J Physiol Lung Cell Mol Physiol 302: 521–529.
13. Ohshima K, Inoue K, Fujiwara A, Hatakeyama K, Kanto K, et al. (2010) Let-7 microRNA family is selectively secreted into the extracellular environment via exosomes in a metastatic gastric cancer cell line. PLoS One 5: e13247.
14. Kosaka N, Iguchi H, Yoshioka Y, Takeshita F, Matsuki Y, et al. (2010) Secretory mechanisms and intercellular transfer of microRNAs in living cells. J Biol Chem 285: 17442–17452.
15. Chen X, Ba Y, Ma L, Cai X, Yin Y, et al. (2008) Characterization of microRNAs in serum: a novel class of biomarkers for diagnosis of cancer and other diseases. Cell Res 18: 997–1006.
16. Xiao J, Jing ZC, Ellinor PT, Liang D, Zhang H, et al. (2011) MicroRNA-134 as a potential plasma biomarker for the diagnosis of acute pulmonary embolism. J Transl Med 9: 159.
17. Sacks RS, Remillard CV, Agange N, Auger WR, Thistlethwaite PA, et al. (2006) Molecular biology of chronic thromboembolic pulmonary hypertension. Semin Thorac Cardiovasc Surg 18: 265–276.
18. Reesink HJ, Meijer RC, Lutter R, Boomsma F, Jansen HM, et al. (2006) Hemodynamic and clinical correlates of endothelin-1 in chronic thromboembolic pulmonary hypertension. Circ J 70: 1058–1063.
19. Ogawa A, Firth AL, Yao W, Madani MM, Kerr KM, et al. (2009) Inhibition of mTOR attenuates store-operated Ca2+ entry in cells from endarterectomized tissues of patients with chronic thromboembolic pulmonary hypertension. Am J Physiol Lung Cell Mol Physiol 297: L666–676.
20. Confalonieri M, Kodric M, Longo C, Vassallo FG (2009) Bosentan for chronic thromboembolic pulmonary hypertension. Expert Rev Cardiovasc Ther 7: 1503–1512.

21. Thomas M, Docx C, Holmes AM, Beach S, Duggan N, et al. (2009) Activin-like kinase 5 (ALK5) mediates abnormal proliferation of vascular smooth muscle cells from patients with familial pulmonary arterial hypertension and is involved in the progression of experimental pulmonary arterial hypertension induced by monocrotaline. Am J Pathol 174: 380–389.
22. Long L, Crosby A, Yang X, Southwood M, Upton PD, et al. (2009) Altered bone morphogenetic protein and transforming growth factor-beta signaling in rat models of pulmonary hypertension: potential for activin receptor-like kinase-5 inhibition in prevention and progression of disease. Circulation 119: 566–576.
23. Barst RJ, McGoon M, Torbicki A, Sitbon O, Krowka MJ, et al. (2004) Diagnosis and differential assessment of pulmonary arterial hypertension. J Am Coll Cardiol 43: 40S–47S.
24. Mitchell PS, Parkin RK, Kroh EM, Fritz BR, Wyman SK, et al. (2008) Circulating microRNAs as stable blood-based markers for cancer detection. Proc Natl Acad Sci U S A 105: 10513–10518.
25. Man TK, Chintagumpala M, Visvanathan J, Shen J, Perlaky L, et al. (2005) Expression profiles of osteosarcoma that can predict response to chemotherapy. Cancer Res 65: 8142–8150.
26. Ashburner M, Ball CA, Blake JA, Botstein D, Butler H, et al. (2000) Gene ontology: tool for the unification of biology. The Gene Ontology Consortium. Nat Genet 25: 25–29.
27. Kanehisa M, Goto S, Kawashima S, Okuno Y, Hattori M (2004) The KEGG resource for deciphering the genome. Nucleic Acids Res 32: D277–280.
28. Papadopoulos GL, Alexiou P, Maragkakis M, Reczko M, Hatzigeorgiou AG (2009) DIANA-mirPath: Integrating human and mouse microRNAs in pathways. Bioinformatics 25: 1991–1993.
29. Lauder H, Frost EE, Hiley CR, Fan TP (1998) Quantification of the repair process involved in the repair of a cell monolayer using an in vitro model of mechanical injury. Angiogenesis 2: 67–80.
30. Castanares C, Redondo-Horcajo M, Magan-Marchal N, Lamas S, Rodriguez-Pascual F (2006) Transforming growth factor-beta receptor requirements for the induction of the endothelin-1 gene. Exp Biol Med (Maywood) 231: 700–703.
31. Bonderman D, Wilkens H, Wakounig S, Schafers HJ, Jansa P, et al. (2009) Risk factors for chronic thromboembolic pulmonary hypertension. Eur Respir J 33: 325–331.
32. Condliffe R, Kiely DG, Gibbs JS, Corris PA, Peacock AJ, et al. (2008) Improved outcomes in medically and surgically treated chronic thromboembolic pulmonary hypertension. Am J Respir Crit Care Med 177: 1122–1127.
33. Skoro-Sajer N, Mittermayer F, Panzenboeck A, Bonderman D, Sadushi R, et al. (2007) Asymmetric dimethylarginine is increased in chronic thromboembolic pulmonary hypertension. Am J Respir Crit Care Med 176: 1154–1160.
34. Arunthari V, Burger CD (2009) Utility of d-dimer in the diagnosis of patients with chronic thromboembolic pulmonary hypertension. Open Respir Med J 3: 85–89.
35. Lankeit M, Dellas C, Panzenbock A, Skoro-Sajer N, Bonderman D, et al. (2008) Heart-type fatty acid-binding protein for risk assessment of chronic thromboembolic pulmonary hypertension. Eur Respir J 31: 1024–1029.
36. Reesink HJ, Tulevski, II, Marcus JT, Boomsma F, Kloek JJ, et al. (2007) Brain natriuretic peptide as noninvasive marker of the severity of right ventricular dysfunction in chronic thromboembolic pulmonary hypertension. Ann Thorac Surg 84: 537–543.
37. Aldea M, Clofent J, Nunez de Arenas C, Chamorro M, Velasco M, et al. (2011) Reverse phase protein microarrays quantify and validate the bioenergetic signature as biomarker in colorectal cancer. Cancer Lett 311: 210–218.
38. Kittleson MM, Hare JM (2005) Molecular signature analysis: using the myocardial transcriptome as a biomarker in cardiovascular disease. Trends Cardiovasc Med 15: 130–138.
39. Youssef YM, White NM, Grigull J, Krizova A, Samy C, et al. (2011) Accurate molecular classification of kidney cancer subtypes using microRNA signature. Eur Urol 59: 721–730.
40. Liu N, Chen NY, Cui RX, Li WF, Li Y, et al. (2012) Prognostic value of a microRNA signature in nasopharyngeal carcinoma: a microRNA expression analysis. Lancet Oncol 13: 633–641.
41. Kroh EM, Parkin RK, Mitchell PS, Tewari M (2010) Analysis of circulating microRNA biomarkers in plasma and serum using quantitative reverse transcription-PCR (qRT-PCR). Methods 50: 298–301.
42. Schultz J, Lorenz P, Gross G, Ibrahim S, Kunz M (2008) MicroRNA let-7b targets important cell cycle molecules in malignant melanoma cells and interferes with anchorage-independent growth. Cell Res 18: 549–557.
43. Yanagisawa M, Kurihara H, Kimura S, Tomobe Y, Kobayashi M, et al. (1988) A novel potent vasoconstrictor peptide produced by vascular endothelial cells. Nature 332: 411–415.
44. Rodriguez-Pascual F, Busnadiego O, Lagares D, Lamas S (2011) Role of endothelin in the cardiovascular system. Pharmacol Res 63: 463–472.
45. Wang C, Wang J, Zhao L, Wang Y, Liu J, et al. (2008) Sildenafil inhibits human pulmonary artery smooth muscle cell proliferation by decreasing capacitative Ca2+ entry. J Pharmacol Sci 108: 71–78.
46. Langer F, Bauer M, Tscholl D, Schramm R, Kunihara T, et al. (2005) Circulating big endothelin-1: an active role in pulmonary thromboendarterectomy? J Thorac Cardiovasc Surg 130: 1342–1347.
47. Dupuis J, Hoeper MM (2008) Endothelin receptor antagonists in pulmonary arterial hypertension. Eur Respir J 31: 407–415.
48. Kurihara H, Yoshizumi M, Sugiyama T, Takaku F, Yanagisawa M, et al. (1989) Transforming growth factor-beta stimulates the expression of endothelin mRNA by vascular endothelial cells. Biochem Biophys Res Commun 159: 1435–1440.
49. Castanares C, Redondo-Horcajo M, Magan-Marchal N, ten Dijke P, Lamas S, et al. (2007) Signaling by ALK5 mediates TGF-beta-induced ET-1 expression in endothelial cells: a role for migration and proliferation. J Cell Sci 120: 1256–1266.
50. Jachec W, Foremny A, Domal-Kwiatkowska D, Smolik S, Tomasik A, et al. (2008) Expression of TGF-beta1 and its receptor genes (TbetaR I, TbetaR II, and TbetaR III-betaglycan) in peripheral blood leucocytes in patients with idiopathic pulmonary arterial hypertension and Eisenmenger's syndrome. Int J Mol Med 21: 99–107.
51. Tsai S, Hollenbeck ST, Ryer EJ, Edlin R, Yamanouchi D, et al. (2009) TGF-beta through Smad3 signaling stimulates vascular smooth muscle cell proliferation and neointimal formation. Am J Physiol Heart Circ Physiol 297: H540–549.
52. Shi X, Direnzo D, Guo LW, Franco SR, Wang B, et al. (2014) TGF-beta/Smad3 Stimulates Stem Cell/Developmental Gene Expression and Vascular Smooth Muscle Cell De-Differentiation. PLoS One 9: e93995.

7

Modification of Hemodynamic and Immune Responses to Exposure with a Weak Antigen by the Expression of a Hypomorphic BMPR2 Gene

Sung-Hyun Park[1], Wen-Chi Chen[1], Carol Hoffman[1], Leigh M. Marsh[2], James West[3], Gabriele Grunig[1,4]*

1 Department of Environmental Medicine, New York University School of Medicine, Tuxedo, New York, United States of America, **2** Ludwig Boltzmann Institute for Lung Vascular Research, Graz, Austria, **3** Division of Allergy, Pulmonary, and Critical Care Medicine, Department of Medicine, Vanderbilt University Medical Center, Nashville, Tennessee, United States of America, **4** Division of Pulmonary Medicine, Department of Medicine, New York University School of Medicine, New York, New York, United States of America

Abstract

Background: Hypomorphic mutations in the bone morphogenic protein receptor (BMPR2) confer a much greater risk for developing pulmonary arterial hypertension (PAH). However, not all carriers of a mutation in the BMPR2 gene suffer from PAH. We have previously shown that prolonged T helper 2 (Th2) responses in the lungs to a mild antigen delivered via the airways induce severe pulmonary arterial remodeling, but no pulmonary hypertension. The current studies were designed to test the idea that Th2 responses to a mild antigen together with the expression of a hypomorphic BMPR2 gene would trigger pulmonary hypertension.

Methodology/Principal Findings: Mice that expressed a hypomorphic BMPR2 transgene (transgene-positive) and transgene-negative mice were either exposed to saline, or primed and exposed to a mild antigen (Ovalbumin) over a prolonged period of time. Only transgene-positive but not transgene-negative mice exposed to antigen developed significantly increased right ventricular systolic pressures, while both groups showed pulmonary artery remodeling with severe muscularization and airway inflammation to a similar degree. Antigen exposure resulted in a smaller increase in the percentage of Interleukin (IL)-13 positive T cells in the lymph nodes, and in a smaller increase in resistin-like-molecule (RELM)α expression and a decreased ratio of expression of IL-33 relative to its receptor (IL-1-receptor-like 1, IL1RL1-ST2) in the right ventricles of transgene-positive mice compared to transgene-negative animals. Furthermore, only antigen-challenged transgene-positive mice showed a significant increase in Interferon (IFN)γ positive T cells over saline-exposed controls.

Conclusions/Significance: Our study suggests that exposure with a mild Th2 antigen can trigger pulmonary hypertension on the background of the expression of a hypomorphic BMPR2 gene and that conversely, the expression of the hypomorphic BMPR2 gene can alter the immune response to a mild, inhaled antigen.

Editor: Marco Idzko, University Hospital Freiburg, Germany

Funding: The work was funded in part by the National Institutes of Health 1R21HL092370-01 (G.G.), 1R01 HL095764-01 (GG); R01HL082694 (J.W.); American Heart Association, Founders affiliate (0855943D, G.G.); Stony Wold – Herbert Fund, New York; (S.H.P.). The NIEHS Center Grant 5P30ES00260-47 and the Cancer Center Support Grant (C.C.S.G.) 5P30CA016087-31 provided Core Facility support. These funders had no role in study design, data collection and analysis, decision to publish, or preparation of the manuscript.

* E-mail: ggrunig1@earthlink.net

Introduction

Pulmonary arterial hypertension (PAH) is characterized by increased right ventricular systolic pressures and severe thickening of arteries due to smooth muscle cell hypertrophy and impaired ability to terminate repair responses [1,2]. Our group has reported that severe pulmonary arterial remodeling can be caused by a T helper 2 (Th2) immune response to inhaled antigen [3].

Bone morphogenic protein receptor (BMPR) 2 is a member of the transforming growth factor (TGF) β superfamily of transmembrane serine/threonine kinases which binds bone morphogenetic proteins (BMP) [4]. BMPR2 signaling controls many developmental processes through multiple downstream pathways [5–7]. TGFβ and BMP regulate endothelial and smooth muscle cell proliferation and apoptosis with opposite and antagonistic effects [6,8]. In humans, mutations in BMPR2 and the dysfunction of BMPR2 are a cause of hereditary PAH [9–12]. Reduced BMPR2 signaling disturbs the balance between BMPR2 and TGFβ signaling resulting in enhanced TGFβ signaling, and contributes to abnormal growth responses to BMPs and TGFβ [6,8,13]. Increased TGFβ signaling induces smooth muscle cell proliferation [9].

However, even though patients who are BMPR2 mutation carriers have a much greater chance of developing PAH, not all of them do [14,15]. The variability in penetrance is thought to depend on genetic and environmental modifiers, including female gender [13,16,17]. Inflammatory responses are also thought to exacerbate the consequences of mutations in the BMPR2 gene [8,18–21]. However, the exact mechanism by which inflammatory processes would initiate or exacerbate the PAH phenotype in BMPR2 mutation carriers remains to be elucidated.

Many mutations occur in the BMPR2 tail domain [15]. One such mutation is an arginine to nonsense mutation at amino acid 899 (R899X) found in family US33 [22]. Dr. West's group created transgenic mice that express the BMPR2 R899X mutation ($BMPR2^{R899X}$) under the control of specific promoters to express the transgene in smooth muscle cells, or in all cells when induced by doxycycline [22–24]. Upon the expression of the hypomorphic BMPR2 transgene for several weeks, the mice developed elevated right ventricular systolic pressure and muscularization of pulmonary vessels. Using the $BMPR2^{R899X}$ mouse, we tested the idea that the Th2 immune response to inhaled antigen would exacerbate the pulmonary hypertension phenotype in mice that express the hypomorphic BMPR2 transgene.

Results

Groups of animals studied

When housed in our mouse facility at the Department of Environmental Medicine, New York University, Tuxedo, NY, all $BMPR2^{R899X}$ mice expressed the $BMPR2^{R899X}$ transgene in the hearts (Fig. 1A) and lungs (data not shown). The expression of the $BMPR2^{R899X}$ transgene was detected from the first day of birth and persisted at similar levels through the life of the animals (Fig. 1A). Expression levels in the heart were similar in the hearts of saline and antigen exposed animals (Fig. 1A) and independent of doxycycline administration in the food (data not shown). Four groups of animal were studied: mice that expressed the $BMPR2^{R899X}$ transgene or were transgene-negative that were either given saline intranasally, or intraperitoneally primed and intranasally challenged with antigen (Fig. 1B, C).

Right ventricular systolic pressure was increased in transgene-positive mice exposed to antigen

Transgene-positive animals that were primed and challenged with antigen had significantly increased right ventricular systolic pressures compared to saline exposed transgene-positive or transgene-negative groups of mice (Fig. 2). In contrast, antigen-exposed transgene-negative animals showed a trend to increased right ventricular systolic pressures that failed to reach statistical significance (Fig. 2). The significant increase in right ventricular systolic pressures in antigen-exposed transgene-positive but not in antigen-exposed transgene-negative mice (when compared to the respective saline exposed controls) was seen using two different analysis methods: comparison of the means (Fig. 2A), or analysis of the frequency of animals being below or above a threshold cutoff value for right ventricular systolic pressures that was set using the data from the saline-exposed animals (Fig. 2B). Of note, in our mouse facility, transgene-positive animals given saline did not show an increase in right ventricular systolic pressures when compared to the transgene-negative saline exposed group (Fig. 2).

Muscularization of small pulmonary blood vessels

Muscularization of pulmonary blood vessels was studied using a very sensitive, automated technique that is based on the detection of smooth muscle actin staining [25,26]. Antigen exposure induced severe muscularization in small (50–100 μm in diameter) and very small (less than 50 μm in diameter) blood vessels (Fig. 3A, B). The percent of fully muscularized small and very small blood vessels was significantly correlated with right ventricular pressures (Fig. 3C, D). As previously reported by Dr. West's group [22], among the saline exposed groups of mice, transgene-positive mice had a higher percentage of fully muscularized very small blood vessels when compared to transgene-negative animals (Fig. 3A). There was no difference between groups of antigen exposed transgene-negative or transgene positive animals with respect to the degree of muscularization or the relative smooth muscle actin positive area of the pulmonary blood vessels (Fig. 3A, B).

Histological changes in the lungs of antigen challenged animals

Lung histology was analyzed by scoring using previously published techniques [3,27–30] from each of the animals included in this study (Fig. 4). Antigen-exposed transgene-positive or transgene–negative animals developed pulmonary arterial remodeling (Fig. 4A), perivascular inflammation (Fig. 4B), alveolar inflammation (Fig. 4C), and an increase in mucus producing goblet cells (Fig. 4D) to a moderate to severe degree as shown in representative digital scans of lung sections (Fig. 4E–H). While pulmonary arterial remodeling, perivascular inflammation, and alveolar inflammation had similar severity scores in the antigen-exposed mice that were transgene-positive or transgene–negative (Fig. 4A–C), the goblet cell score was increased to a significantly lower level in the antigen-exposed transgene-positive mice when compared to the transgene-negative animals (Fig. 4D). Saline exposed groups of transgene-negative or transgene-positive mice showed normal lung histology (Fig. 4A–F).

Effects of antigen challenge on body and heart weights

The next analyses were performed to study growth adaptation to antigen exposure, and right heart hypertrophy responses to increased right ventricular systolic pressures (Fig. 5A, B). The antigen exposure protocol slowed growth and this effect was significant in transgene-positive but not transgene-negative mice (Fig. 5A). Consequently, body weight was significantly negatively correlated with right ventricular pressures (Fig. 5C). As expected from previous findings in Dr. West's laboratory with the $BMPR2^{R899X}$ strain [22], right ventricular weights (corrected for the weight of the left ventricle and septum, Fig. 5B, or for body weight) did not increase with antigen exposure, and were not positively correlated with right ventricular systolic pressures (Fig. 5D, E). Surprisingly, the weights of the left ventricle and septum showed a weak positive correlation with right ventricular systolic pressures (Fig. 5F), perhaps reflecting changes in the systemic circulation of antigen-exposed mice.

Airway inflammation and cellular changes in lung draining lymph nodes

Antigen exposure induced a large influx of neutrophils, eosinophils, and lymphocytes into the airways as measured by analysis of bronchoalveolar lavage (Fig. 6A–C). In addition, bronchoalveolar lavage CD11c+ cells expressed much higher major histocompatibility complex type II (MHCII) levels in antigen-exposed animals when compared to saline exposed (Fig. 6D). Finally, antigen-exposure induced an increase in the numbers of CD4+ T cell in the lung draining lymph nodes, combined with a decrease in the percentage of lymph node CD4+ T cells expressing Helios (Fig. 7A–B). The transcription factor Helios can be expressed by a subtype of T regulatory cells that counterbalance pro-inflammatory effector T cells [31,32], and in CD4+ T cells differentiating to Th2 or follicular helper cells [33].

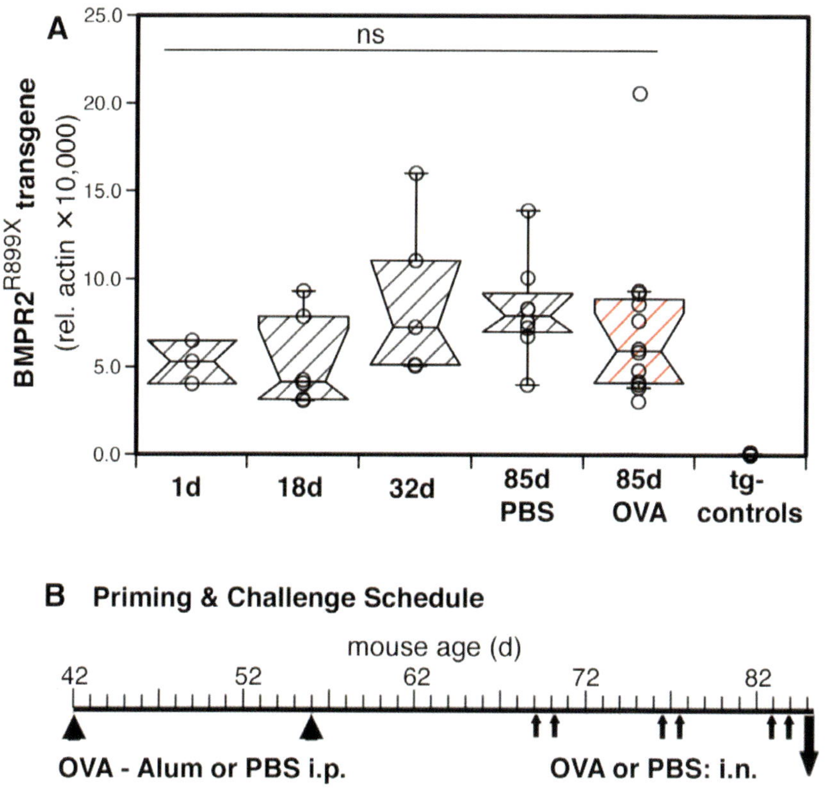

C Groups

	tg- PBS	tg+ PBS	tg- OVA	tg+ OVA
BMPR2^{R899X} expression	no	yes	no	yes
Antigen priming & challenge	no	no	yes	yes

Figure 1. Expression of BMPR2^{R899X} transgene, experimental schedule and groups of animals studied. (**A**) Notched box and whisker plots extending to the 10th and 90th percentiles showing expression of mRNA for transgenic BMPR2^{R899X} (relative to β-actin; ×10,000) in heart tissues from animals aged 1 to 85 days old and transgene-negative (tg−) controls (n = 3–12). Data of individual mice are represented as dots. At 85 days old, mice were from the saline (PBS) or antigen (OVA) exposed groups as indicated. There were no statistically significant differences between pairs of groups (Mann Whitney U test, $p>0.05$). (**B**) Schematic representation of the experimental schedule for antigen (Ovalbumin, OVA) priming by intraperitoneal (i.p.) injections of OVA-Alum followed by intranasal (i.n.) challenge with soluble OVA. Control animals were given saline (PBS). (**C**) Study groups of animals as defined by BMPR2^{R899X} transgene expression and exposure to antigen or saline.

The inflammatory responses to antigen exposure were similar in transgene-positive and -negative animals (Fig. 6A–D, 7A–B). In contrast, saline exposed transgene-positive mice had mild inflammation as shown by a significant increase in the numbers of eosinophils in the bronchoalveolar lavage (Fig. 6B), significantly increased numbers of CD4+ T cells (Fig. 7A) and a significantly decreased percentage of Helios+ CD4+ T cells (Fig. 7B) in the lung draining lymph nodes. The inflammatory phenotype in the saline exposed transgene-positive mice was expected based on previous reports from Dr. West's group [22].

Unique immune phenotype in antigen-exposed BMPR2^{R899X} mice in lung draining lymph nodes

Exposure to antigen induced a significantly increased percentage of CD4+ or CD8+ T cells capable of making IL-13 in both transgen-positive and transgene-negative animals, albeit to a significantly lower level in trangene-positive animals (Fig. 7C, D). In addition, only antigen exposed transgene-positive, but not antigen exposed transgene-negative animals had a significant increase in T cells capable of producing IFNγ that was most noticeable in the CD8+ T cell compartment (Fig. 7E, F). In contrast, the percentage of CD4+ T cells capable of producing IL-17A/F was increased to a similar significant degree in antigen exposed transgene-negative or transgene–positive mice (Fig. 7G).

Unique cytokine and extracellular matrix protein expression in the right ventricles of transgene-positive mice

Next, we tested the idea that an immune response in the lungs combined with severe pulmonary vascular remodeling could be reflected in the right ventricle by changes in the expression of cytokines, their receptors and extracellular matrix proteins. The data show that antigen exposure significantly increased the expression of RELMα in the right ventricle in both transgene-

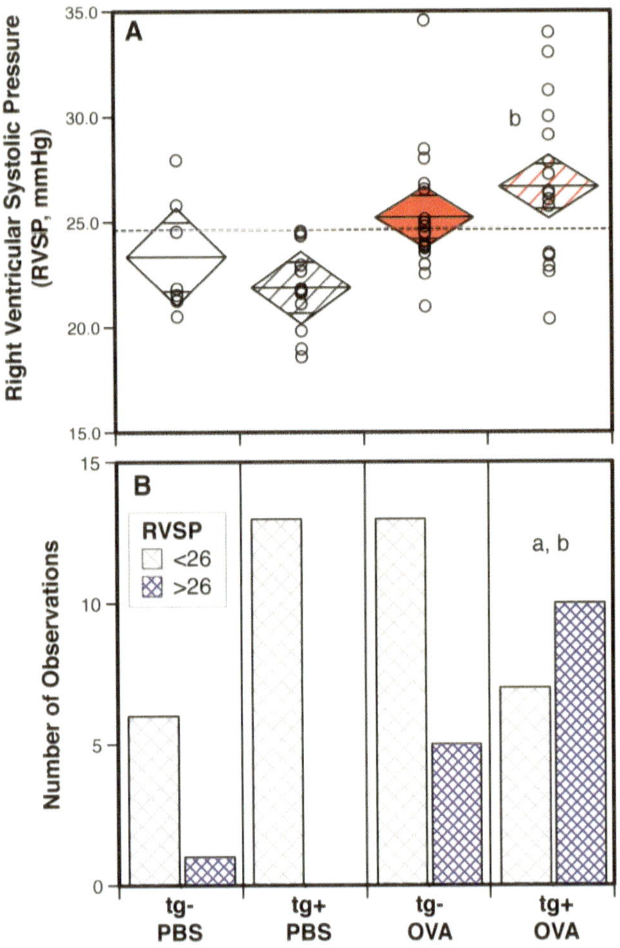

Figure 2. Increased right ventricular systolic pressures in mice that express the hypomorphic BMPR2 transgene and are exposed to antigen. (**A**) Diamond mean comparison plots show group means, upper and lower 95% confidence limits, overlap marks, for right ventricular systolic pressures (RVSP, mmHg) of saline (PBS) versus antigen (OVA) exposed mice stratified by transgene-negative (tg−) versus -positive (tg+). The dashed line represents the overall mean. Dots represent data from individual mice. Data were pooled from three independent experiments (n = 7 to 18). Pair-wise comparisons between groups were calculated with the Mann-Whitney U test ($p<0.05$; b: transgene-positive saline vs. antigen). (**B**) Bar graphs show the frequency of RVSP measurements that were lower or higher than 26 mmHg for each of the groups of animals. Chi-Square analysis of the data distribution between all groups was $p=0.0039$; pair-wise comparisons calculated $p<0.05$ for a: transgene-positive antigen (OVA) vs. transgene negative saline (PBS); b: transgene-positive antigen vs. transgene-positive saline).

negative and -positive mice, albeit to a significantly smaller degree in antigen-exposed transgene-positive animals (Fig. 8A). The expression of RELMγ followed similar trends, but there was no significant difference between groups (Fig. 8B). Transgene-negative antigen-exposed mice showed a non-significant trend towards increase in the expression of IL-33 and decrease of ST2-IL1RL1, an IL-33 receptor, resulting in a significant increase in the ratio of IL-33 to ST2-IL1RL1 when compared to saline controls (Fig. 8 C–E). In contrast, antigen-exposed transgene-positive animals showed no changes in IL-33 or ST2-IL1RL1 expression or in the ratio of IL-33 to ST2-IL1RL1 relative to saline controls (Fig. 8C–E). Furthermore, comparison of the two antigen-exposed groups showed a significantly lower ratio of IL-33 to ST2-IL1RL1 in transgene-positive animals (Fig. 8E). Comparison of the two saline exposed groups revealed significant differences between transgene-negative and transgene-positive mice in the ratio of IL-33 to ST2-IL1RL1 (Fig. 8E) and in the expression of biglycan (Fig. 8F).

Discussion

Inflammation is now considered to be a critical pathogenetic component in PAH [19,34–39]. Furthermore, recent reports indicate that mutations in the BMPR2 gene and inflammatory responses are linked, together contributing to the pulmonary hypertension phenotype: Dr. Morrell and colleagues, examining smooth muscle cells isolated from patients who carry a BMPR2 mutation found an abnormal inflammatory phenotype in these cells that contributed to the abnormal responses to TGFβ [8]. Dr. Zhang and colleagues showed that monocrotaline induced inflammation was one of the requisite secondary triggers of pulmonary hypertension in mice that have a heterozygous BMPR2 deletion [21].

Our study tested the hypothesis that a Th2 immune response in the lungs induced in response to a mild antigen would trigger or exacerbate the pulmonary hypertension phenotype in mice carrying a BMPR2 transgene [22] that models a hypomorphic mutation found in a family of patients affected with PAH [22,24]. In our animal facility at New York University, saline exposed $BMPR2^{R899X}$ mice expressing the hypomorphic transgene had mild inflammation and vascular remodeling in the lungs but normal right ventricular systolic pressures relative to transgene-negative littermates. In contrast, antigen-exposed mice that expressed the hypomorphic BMPR2 transgene showed significantly increased right ventricular systolic pressures.

A recent publication by Dr. Le Cras and colleagues [18] tested the same idea using BMPR2 hypomorphic mice that carry one normal BMPR2 allele and one BMPR2 allele that has a deletion of exon 2. The authors found that chronic exposure with house dust mite antigen extract induced the pulmonary hypertension phenotype in wild type and BMPR2 hypomorphic mice to a similar degree, while airway hyperreactivity, a cardinal sign of asthma, was induced to a more severe degree in the BMPR2 hypomorphic animals [18]. The major difference to our experimental system was that exposure to antigen in wild type mice was sufficient to induce the pulmonary hypertension phenotype in the study by Dr. Le Cras and colleagues [18] but not in ours. Compared to house dust mite antigen that primes for Th2 responses when given via the intranasal route [18], the antigen used in our studies, Ovalbumin, is much milder and therefore the mice in our study were primed by the intraperitoneal route with antigen and adjuvants. Ovalbumin is so mild that when given only via the intranasal route to unprimed, naïve animals a tolerance response is induced [28]. In addition, the mouse strains used in our study (FVB) was different from the mouse strain (BALB/c) used by Dr. Le Cras and colleagues [18]. The combined differences in the experimental protocols are likely the reason why antigen-exposure did not induce the pulmonary hypertension phenotype in transgene-negative, wild type animals in our current study, supporting our previously published data [3].

The mechanism that led to the increase in right ventricular systolic pressure in antigen-challenged transgene-positive animals remains unclear. Our data indicate that the severity of pulmonary arterial remodeling or the degree of vessel muscularization in the lungs in response to exposure with the mild antigen were not associated with the increased right ventricular systolic pressures.

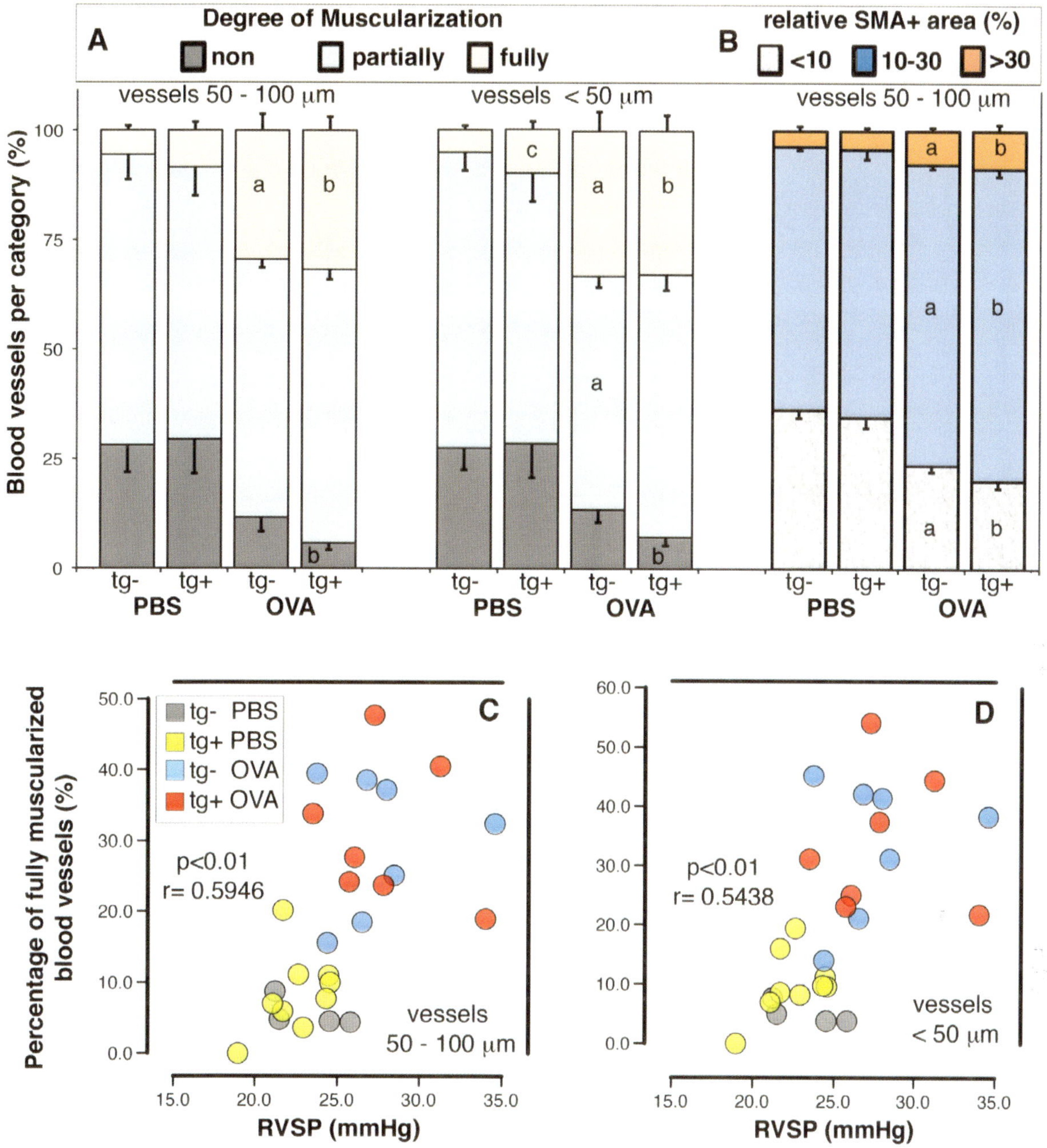

Figure 3. Muscularization of small blood vessels in the lungs: effects of the hypomorphic BMPR2 transgene and antigen exposure. **A**) Stacked bar graphs represent the percentage of non-muscularized, partially muscularized, and fully muscularized blood vessels that are 50–100, or <50 μm in diameter. **B**) Stacked bar graphs represent the percentage of bloods vessels (50–100 μm in diameter) for which the smooth muscle actin positive area was <10%, 10–30%, or >30% relative to the area of the total vessel. Data were pooled from two independent experiments (n = 4–9 per group with 60–1000, mean 400 vessels analyzed per mouse). Pair-wise comparisons were calculated with the t test with Welch's correction (p<0.05; a: transgene-negative saline (PBS) vs. antigen (OVA); b: transgene-positive saline vs. antigen; c: saline exposed transgene negative vs. transgene-positive). (**C, D**) Individual data points from two independent experiments (n = 4–7 per group) are shown. Each data point plots the percentage of fully muscularized blood vessels sized 50–100 μm (**C**) or <50 μm (**D**) in diameter against the right systolic ventricular pressure (RVSP, mmHg). Combined data from saline or antigen exposed groups of transgene-negative or trangene-positive mice (indicated by color code) were analyzed with the Spearman's Rank Order Correlation Coefficient test (p- and r- values are indicated).

An alternative explanation, that needs to be addressed in future experiments, would be that the increased right ventricular pressures in the transgene-positive animals reflect a significant difference in the composition of the extracellular matrix of the lungs or heart when compared to the transgene-negative mice, mediated by a skewed balance in BMPR2 and TGFβ receptor signaling in response to injury induced by antigen exposure. The idea that mutations in BMPR2 confer a phenotype of maladaption to injury is supported by studies in human patients, which demonstrate a more severe clinical phenotype of PAH in carriers of a mutated BMPR2 allele [40–44].

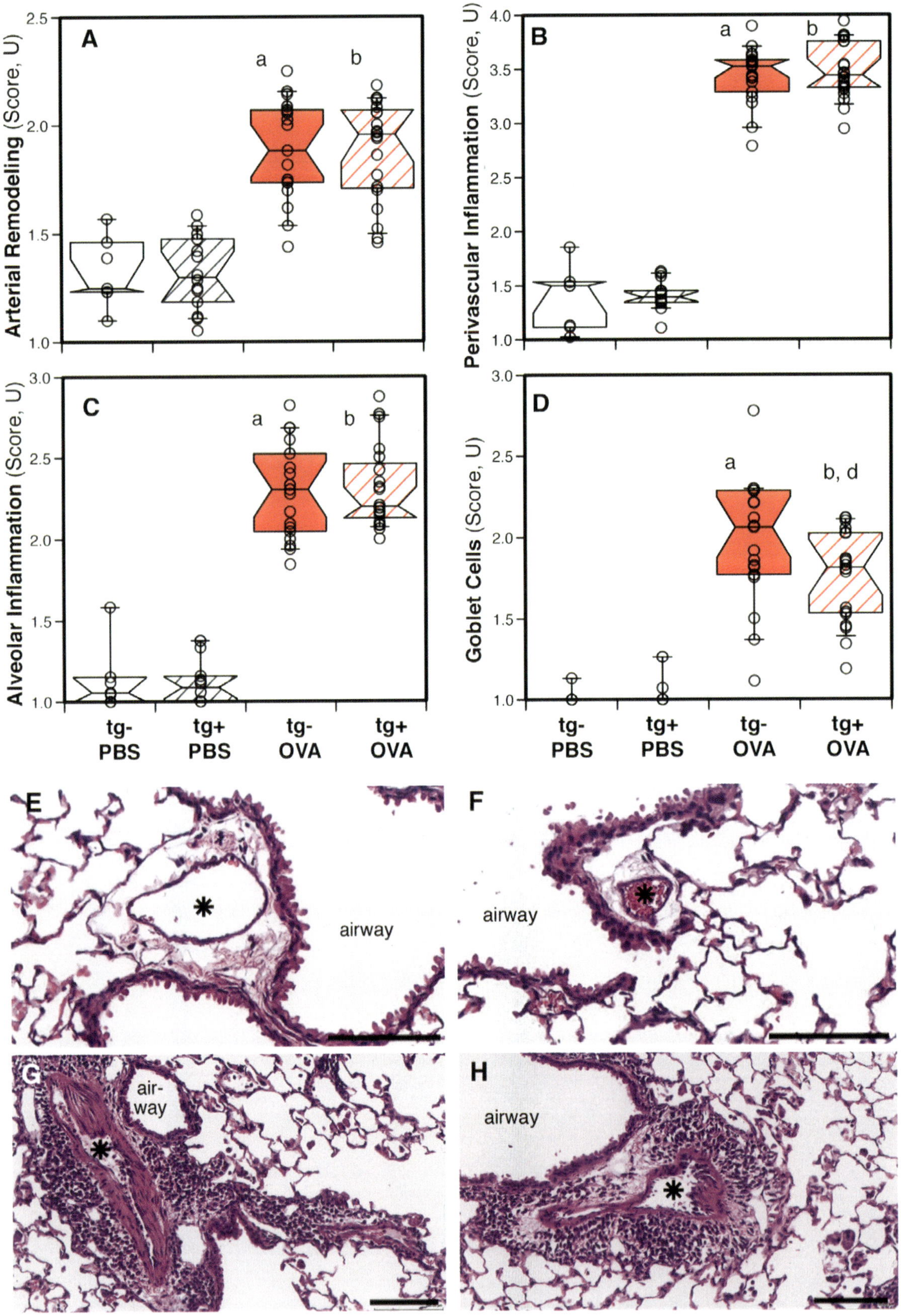

Figure 4. Histological changes in the lungs: effects of the hypomorphic BMPR2 transgene and antigen exposure. (**A–D**) Notched box and whisker plots extending to the 10th and 90th percentiles showing scores (1-normal to 4-severe change) for (**A**) pulmonary arterial remodeling, (**B**) perivascular inflammation, (**C**) alveolar inflammation, and (**D**) goblet cells. Data of individual mice are represented as dots. Data were pooled from

three independent experiments (n = 7 to 20 per group). Pair-wise comparisons between groups were calculated with the Mann-Whitney U test ($p<0.05$; a: transgene-negative saline (PBS) vs. antigen (OVA); b: transgene-positive saline vs. antigen; d: antigen exposed transgene-negative vs. transgene-positive). (**E–H**) Scanned representative images show sections of lungs from saline, transgene-negative (**E**), saline, transgene-positive (**F**), antigen, transgene-negative (**G**), or antigen, transgene-positive (**H**) mice. The images of the antigen exposed mice show pulmonary arterial remodeling, perivascular inflammation and alveolar inflammation. For reference the airways (airway) and pulmonary arteries (*) are indicated; the scale bar represents 100 µm. Sections were stained with hematoxylin and eosin.

Surprisingly, we report for the first time that the immune response phenotype in the lungs and lung draining lymph nodes corresponded with changes in the right heart based on the measurement of the Th2 response associated genes [45–49], RELMα and IL-33, but not the Th2-independent molecules, RELMγ and biglycan. A Th2 inflammatory phenotype in the lungs was reflected by an increase in the ratio of IL-33 expression relative to its receptor ST2-IL1RL1 in the right ventricles and an increase in RELMα expression. This observation was made in two groups of mice: A) Saline-exposed transgene-positive animals that had a mild Th2 type inflammation (mild increase in BAL eosinophils but not neutrophils, mild increase in lung lymph node cellularity). B) Antigen-exposed transgene-negative mice that demonstrated a polarized Th2 response with significantly increased IL-13 but not IFNγ. In a similar pattern, in the right ventricle of antigen-exposed transgene-positive animals the increase in RELMα was less pronounced when compared to antigen-exposed transgene-negative mice and there was no upregulation of the IL-33 to ST2-IL1RL1 expression ratio when compared to saline exposed groups of mice. This may be a reflection of the decreased Th2 polarization in the lymph nodes of these transgene-positive, antigen-exposed mice (significantly less IL-13, increased IFNγ). The decreased Th2 polarization may also explain the development of significantly less pronounced mucus cell hyperplasia in the airways (a sensitive sign of IL-13 dependent Th2 inflammation [30,50]) of these transgene-positive antigen-

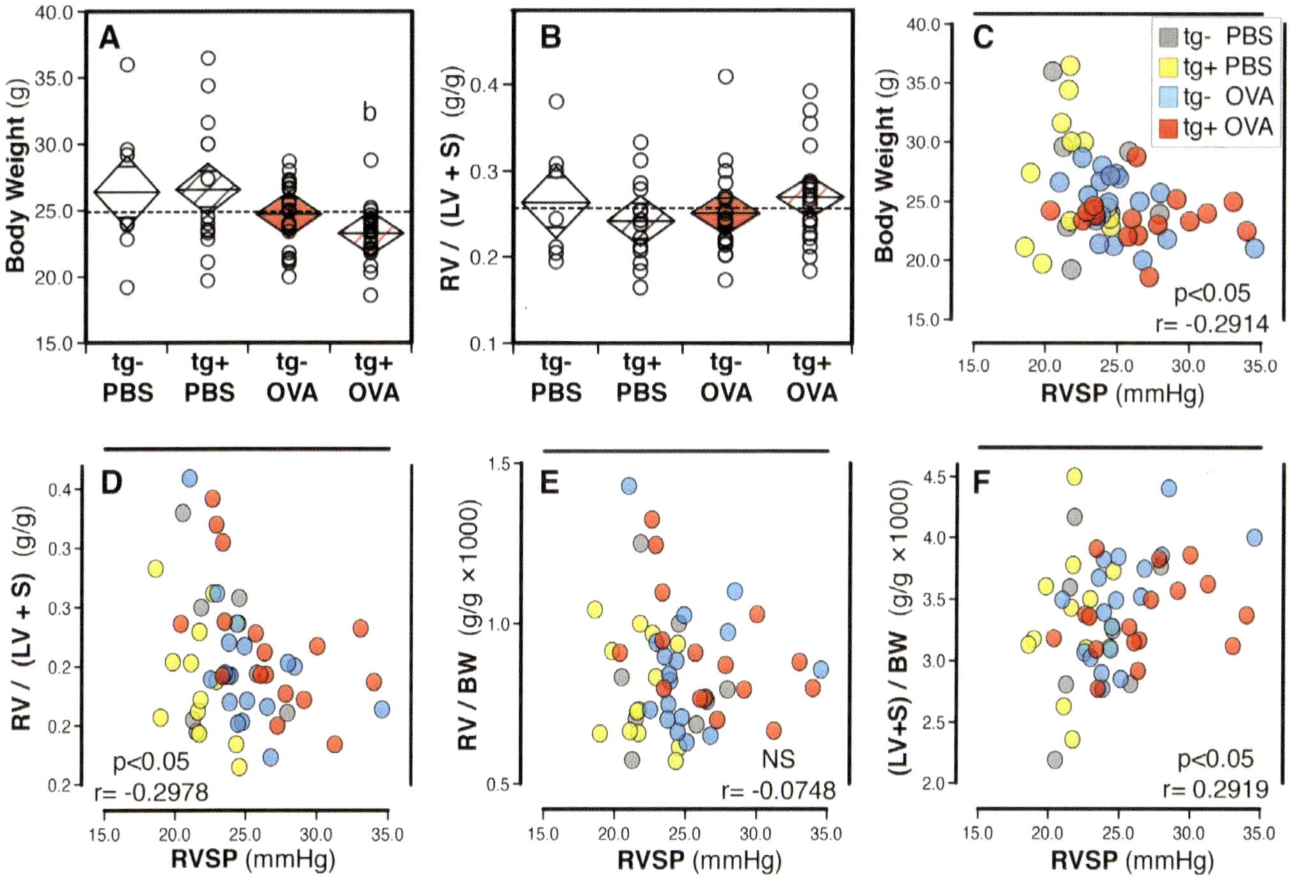

Figure 5. Body and heart weights: effects of the hypomorphic BMPR2 transgene and antigen exposure. (**A, B**) Diamond mean comparison plots show group means, upper and lower 95% confidence limits, overlap marks, for body weight (**A**) and right ventricular weight relative to the weight of the left ventricle and septum, RV/LV+S (**B**). Data are shown for groups of saline (PBS) versus antigen (OVA) exposed mice stratified by transgene-negative (tg−) versus -positive (tg+). The dashed line represents the overall mean. Dots represent data from individual mice. Data were pooled from three independent experiments (n = 7 to 19). Pair-wise comparisons were performed with the Mann-Whitney U test (b: transgene-positive saline vs. antigen, $p<0.05$). (**C–F**) Dot plots show individual data points for right ventricular systolic pressure (RVSP, mmHg) plotted against body weight (**C**), right ventricular weight relative to the weight of the left ventricle and septum (**D**), right ventricular weight relative to body weight (**E**), and weight of left ventricle and septum relative to body weight (**F**). Data were pooled from three independent experiments (n = 7 to 18 per group). Combined data from saline (PBS) or antigen (OVA) exposed groups of transgene-negative or trangene-positive mice (indicated by color code) were analyzed with the Spearman's Rank Order Correlation Coefficient test (p- and r- values are indicated).

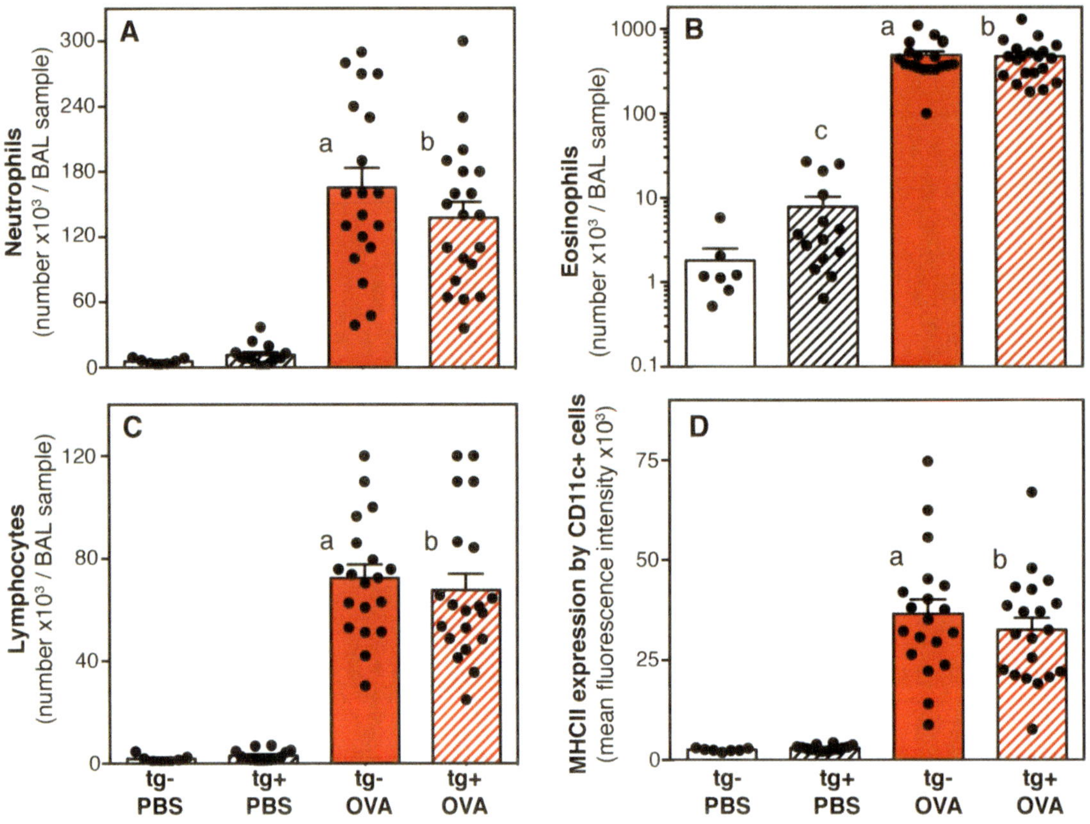

Figure 6. Inflammatory cell responses in the airways: effects of the hypomorphic BMPR2 transgene and antigen exposure. Bar graphs show means and standard error of the means (SEM) for cellular analysis of bronchoalveolar lavage (BAL): numbers per sample of (**A**) neutrophils, (**B**) eosinophils, (**C**) lymphocytes (sum of CD4+ and CD8+ cells) and (**D**) MHCII expression by CD11c+ cells (mean fluorescence intensity, MFI). Data of individual mice are represented as dots. Data were pooled from three independent experiments (n = 7 to 20 per group). Pair-wise comparisons between groups were calculated with the Mann-Whitney U test ($p<0.05$; a: transgene-negative saline (PBS) vs. antigen (OVA); b: transgene-positive saline vs. antigen; c: saline exposed transgene-negative vs. transgene-positive).

challenged animals when compared to transgene-negative antigen-challenged mice. While future studies will need to be designed to elucidate the molecular regulation and functional role of the expression changes of these cytokines in the right heart, our study furthers the emerging topic of the role of inflammation in chronic heart disease [51,52].

The Th2 response associated cytokines expressed in the right heart could have protective or detrimental effects. For example, IL-33 has been reported to enhance the asthma phenotype induced by exposure to a Th2 antigen [45–47], however, by signaling through its receptor, ST2-IL1RL1, IL-33 has been shown to have significant protective function in the left heart [53,54]. Similarly, RELMα has been shown to enhance hypoxia induced pulmonary hypertension [55], while on the other hand anti-inflammatory effects of this cytokine have been reported [56,57].

It is tempting to speculate that the changes in the immune response to antigen exposure in mice expressing the hypomorphic BMPR2 transgene were caused by an imbalance of BMPR2 and TGFβ signaling controlling T cell function. T cells are known to express TGFβ receptors and integration of signals from this receptor determines the activity of these cells [58,59], controlling for example the function of regulatory T cells, the cytokine production profile of effector T cells, and Th17 responses. In addition, signals through BMPR2 have been reported to be important for the development of T cells from thymocytes [60].

In conclusion, our study suggests the possibility that exposure via the airways with mild antigens could exacerbate or trigger the pulmonary hypertension phenotype in patients carrying a BMPR2 mutation, causing an unusual immune response phenotype, and potentially mal-adaptive responses in the right ventricle. Our findings support the idea that there is a molecular connection between a hypomorphic BMPR2, asthma-like responses and pulmonary hypertension as previously suggested by studies performed in pediatric pulmonary hypertension patients [61]. These intriguing findings require further in-depth mechanistic analysis.

Materials and Methods

Ethics Statement

All animal experiments were performed according to guidelines outlined by the United States Department of Agriculture and the American Association of Laboratory Animal Care under the supervision and specific approval of the Institutional Animal Care and Use Committees at New York University (IACUC numbers 081114, 111107, most recent approval date: 11/9/2011) (New York, NY). The named IACUC committee specifically approved this study.

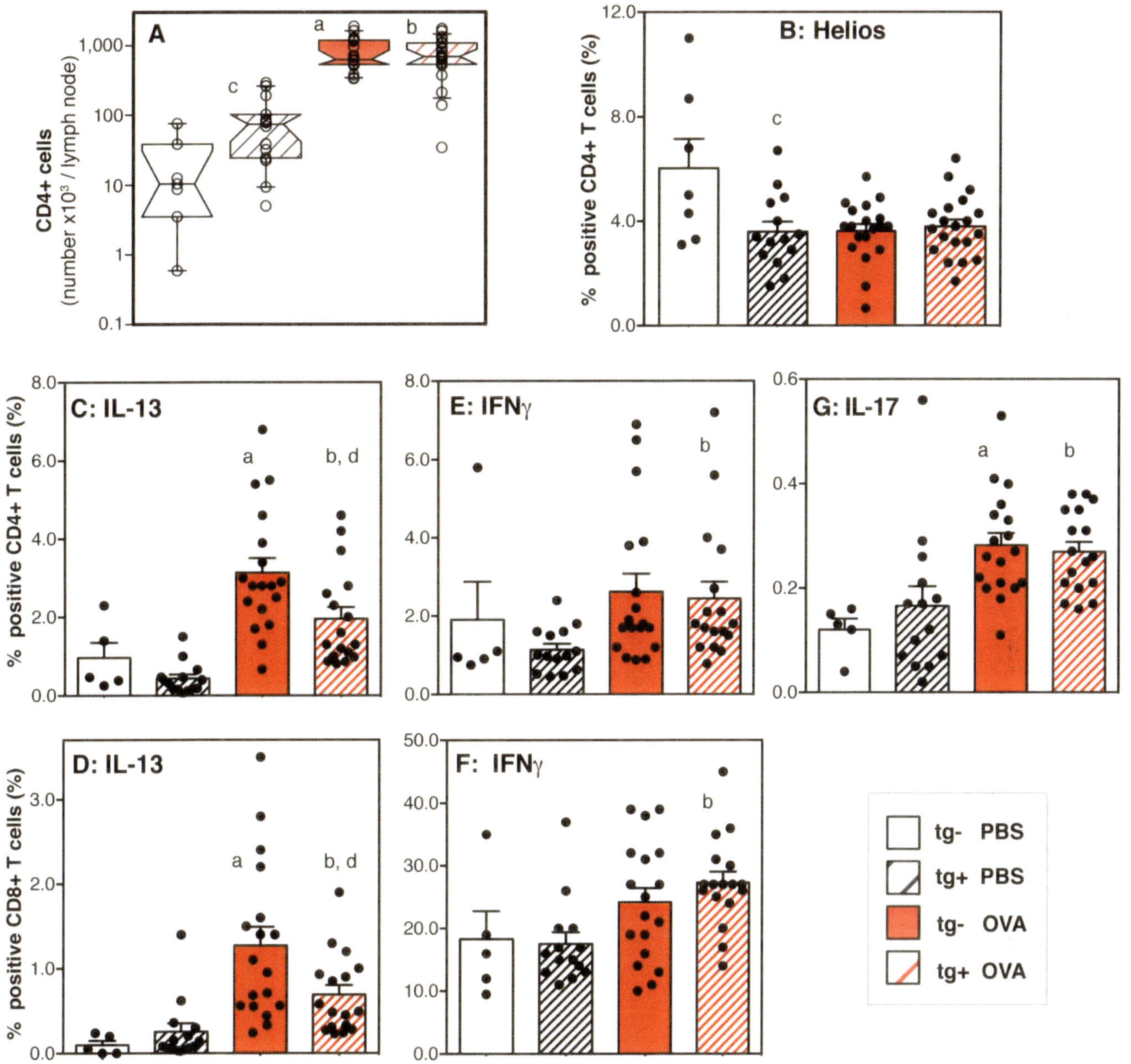

Figure 7. Responses in the lung draining lymph nodes: effects of the hypomorphic BMPR2 transgene and antigen exposure. (**A**) Notched box and whisker plot extending to the 10th and 90th percentiles shows the numbers of CD4+ T cells per lymph node. (**B**) Bar graph shows means and standard error of the means (SEM) of the percentage of CD4+ T cells that were positive for intracellular Helios. (**C–G**) Bar graphs show means and SEM of the percentage of CD4+ or CD8+ T cells that were positive for intracellular cytokines IL-13 (**C, D**), IFNγ (**E, F**), or IL-17A/F (**G**). Data of individual mice are represented as dots. Data were pooled from three independent experiments (n = 6 to 20 per group). Pair-wise comparisons between groups were calculated with the Mann-Whitney U test ($p<0.05$; a: transgene-negative saline (PBS) vs. antigen (OVA); b: transgene-positive saline vs. antigen; c: saline exposed transgene-negative vs. transgene–positive; d: antigen exposed transgene-negative vs. transgene-positive).

Mice

BMPR2 hypomorphic mice (BMPR2^{R899X}) on the FVB background were from Dr. West's laboratory at Vanderbilt University [22–24]. This mouse strain was crossed to ROSA promoter transgenic mice, resulting in ROSA26rtTAXTetO(7)-tet-BMPR2(R899X) mice that can express the hypomorphic BMPR2 transgene in every cell type [23,24]. The BMPR2 transgene has an arginine to nonsense mutation at amino acid 899, modeling a mutation found in a family of patients affected with PAH [22]. Cross-breeding of mice positive or negative for the BMPR2 transgene was performed to generate littermates for the experiments. Only female mice were used for the study being 5–7 weeks of age at the start of the experiment. For each experiment, littermate mice were randomized into cages holding up to 4 mice each. The mice tested negative for mouse pathogens and were housed in filter-top cages under specific pathogen free conditions at Sterling Forest, Tuxedo, NY.

All experiments were performed according to guidelines outlined by the United States Department of Agriculture and the American Association of Laboratory Animal Care under the supervision of the Institutional Animal Care and Use Committee at New York University (New York, NY).

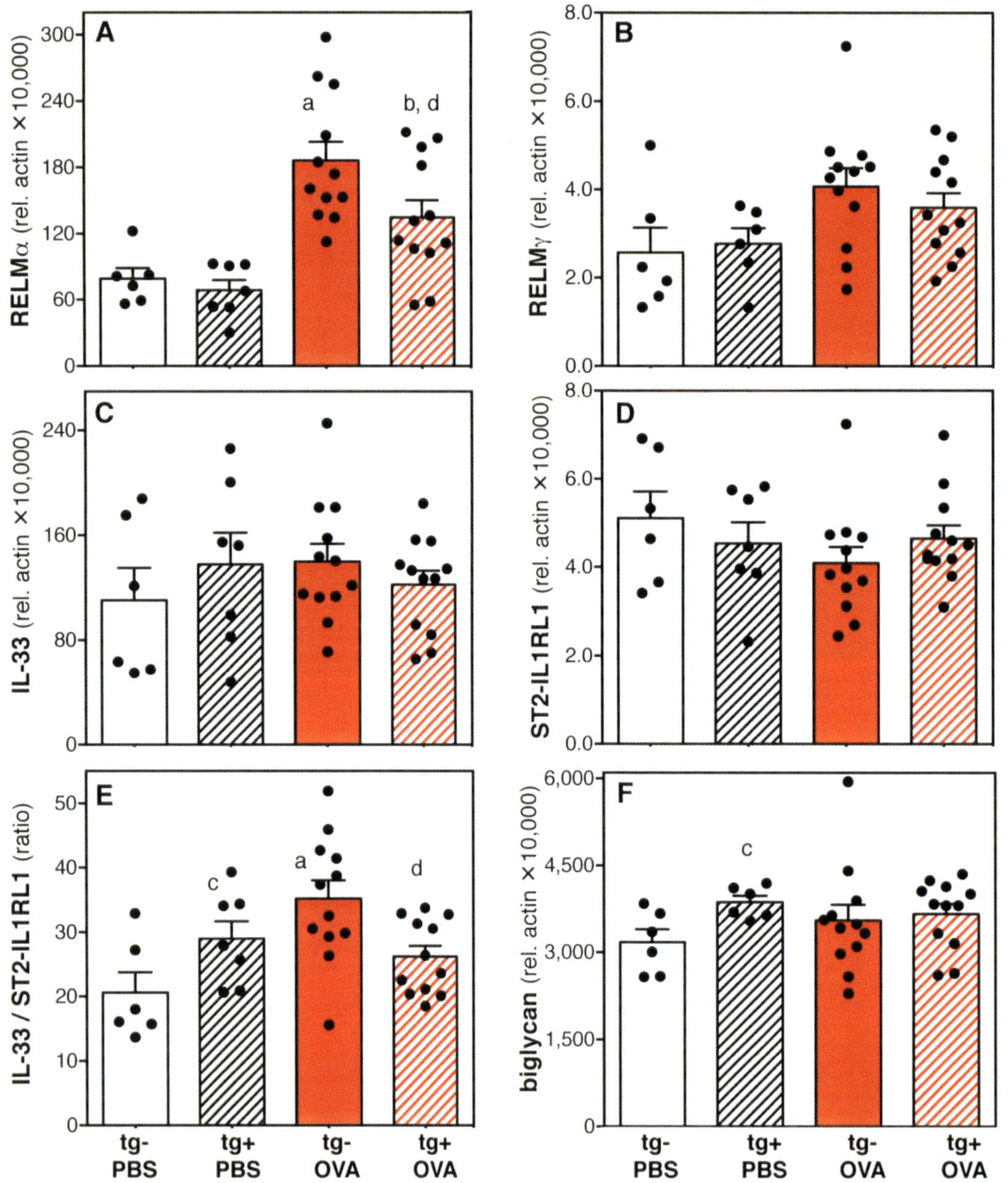

Figure 8. Expression of cytokines and extracellular matrix proteins in the right ventricle: effects of the hypomorphic BMPR2 transgene and antigen exposure. Bar graphs show means and standard error of the means (SEM) of mRNA expression in right ventricles relative (rel.) to β-actin (×10,000) or ratio of expression of cytokine to cytokine receptor. Data are shown for the cytokines RELMα (**A**), RELMγ (**B**), and IL-33 (**C**); the IL-33 receptor ST2-IL1RL1 (**D**); the ratio of IL-33 to ST2-IL1RL1 expression (**E**); and the extracellular matrix protein biglycan (**F**). Data of individual mice are represented as dots. Data were pooled from two independent experiments (n = 6 to 12 per group). Pair-wise comparisons between groups were calculated with the Mann-Whitney U test ($p<0.05$; a: transgene-negative saline (PBS) vs. antigen (OVA); b: transgene-positive saline vs. antigen; c: saline exposed transgene-negative vs. transgene–positive; d: antigen exposed transgene-negative vs. transgene-positive).

Antigen priming and challenge

Animals were primed and challenged with antigen as previously published [3]. Briefly, mice were injected intraperitoneally with Ovalbumin (OVA) (grade V; Sigma-Aldrich, St. Louis, MO; 50 µg/dose) adsorbed to Alum (Imject Alum; Thermo Fisher Scientific, Rockford, IL; 2 mg/dose) to prime the immune response at a two-week interval. Two weeks later, the mice were intranasally challenged with OVA (100 µg/dose) for two times each week, for a total of 6 doses given over a three week period. Control mice were given saline (phosphate buffered saline, PBS) intranasally. The experimental conditions are outlined in Figure 1.

Right Ventricular Systolic Pressure

The analysis was performed without prior knowledge of group designation of the mice [62] using a protocol developed in Dr. West's laboratory [22]. Mice were anaesthetized by intraperitoneal injection of Avertin (tribromoethanol, Sigma-Aldrich, up to 500 mg/kg). Once the pain reflex ceased, mice were shaved with shaving lotion, placed on a surgical table, and fixed with tape. The surgical area was exposed using scissors and surgical forceps. The thyroid grand was dissected upward to expose the right jugular vein. Two sutures were placed under the clearly exposed jugular vein. The cranial suture was tightly tied and the caudal suture was loosely tied. A hole was made between two sutures using small surgical microdissecting scissors. A pressure catheter (F1.4, Millar Instruments, Inc. Houston, Texas) was inserted and advanced into the right ventricle. The pressure signal was monitored to determine the position of the catheter. Once in the correct position, right ventricular pressures were recorded for two minutes. The right ventricular pressure data were analyzed using the LabChart 7 program (ADInstruments, Colorado Springs, CO). Without knowledge of group designation, more than 20 curves were selected randomly for each animal. The difference between maximum and minimum pressure for each curve was measured and averaged to derive the right ventricular systolic pressure for each mouse. Once the catheter was removed, the second suture was tied off tightly. Mice were euthanized with an overdose of sodium pentobarbital.

Bronchoalveolar lavage and tissue harvest

Bronchoalveolar lavage and tissue harvest was performed as described [3,27–30,62]. Briefly, a tracheal catheter was inserted and bronchoalveolar lavage (BAL) was performed by gently washing with three 1 ml aliquot of Hanks Balanced Salt solutions. Following BAL, lungs, lung draining lymph nodes and ventricles were recovered. The right lung lobe was snap frozen in liquid nitrogen, the remainder of the lungs was inflated with buffered formaldehyde and removed into formaldehyde for histology. The lung draining lymph nodes were removed for preparation of single cell suspensions. In our laboratory, the BAL does not wash out all inflammatory cells from the lungs, and is performed gently to minimize the potential for mechanical damage of the tissue. This consecutive protocol allows us to reduce the number of animals used for each study.

Right Ventricular Hypertrophy

The right ventricle, and left ventricle plus septum were removed and weighed. The body weight was also determined. Weight determinations were performed without prior knowledge of group designation of the mice. The data were used to calculate a) the right ventricular weight relative to the combined weight of the left ventricle and septum and b) ventricular weights relative to body weight.

Quantification of pulmonary vascular muscularization

The degree of muscularization was quantified in sections that were stained by dual-immunohistochemistry with a rabbit anti-von Willebrand factor antibody (Dako, Glostrup, Danemark) recognizing endothelial cells and goat anti-smooth muscle actin antibody (Everest Biotech, Upper Heyford, UK) to detect muscularization as described [25,26]. Slides were scanned using an Aperio slide scanner and the images analyzed with the VisiomorphDP^{TM} software (Visiopharm, Hoersholm, Denmark). From each slide 60–1000, mean 400, vessels were identified and analyzed for muscularization by calculating a) the length of smooth muscle actin staining relative to the length of the vessel circumference for vessels less than 50 μm, or 50–100 μm in diameter, b) the area of smooth muscle positivity relative to the total area for vessels 50–100 μm in diameter. For each parameter, the vessels were categorized in 3 groups. The categories for the relative length of smooth muscle actin staining were non-muscularized (<0.2); partially (0.2–0.8); fully (>0.8) muscularized. The categories for the percentage of the smooth muscle actin positive area were <10%; 10–30%; >30%.

Scoring of histological changes

Lung tissue was recovered after taking BAL. The lung was placed into formaldehyde for fixation and preparation of histological slides. Lungs were stained with H&E (hematoxylin and eosin) and PAS (periodic acid schiff). Lung sections were coded and randomized to obscure the group identity. Sections were examined with a light microscope at 200× or 400× magnification. Scores were determined without prior knowledge of group designation of the sections as described [3,27–30]. Random, consecutive view fields were scored. Fifteen to thirty fields per lung were scored, and the mean score was calculated for each parameter. Digital images were taken from slides scanned using the Leica Biosystems SlidePath Gateway and the Leica SCN400 slide scanner (Leica Microsystems Inc., Buffalo Grove, IL).

Pulmonary arterial remodeling was scored on small- to medium-sized arteries that are located close to the airways and could be examined under the view field given with 400× magnification as follows [3]: (1) normal; (2) thickened vascular wall with intact lumen and circular media (all cells follow the form given by the endothelium); (3) the wall is thickened and lined with disorganized layers of cells (cells in the blood vessel wall assume a pattern that differs from the lumen); or (4) thickening is more pronounced as for score '3' and lumen is nearly closed.

Perivascular inflammation was scored as follows [3,27–30]: (1) normal with very few inflammatory cells; (2) scattered inflammatory cells up to two rings in depth; (3) cuffs of inflammatory cells measuring three rings or more in depth; or (4) dense ring of inflammatory cells.

Alveolar inflammation was scored as [3,27–29]: (1) normal; (2) alveolar walls normal, few macrophages in alveoli; (3) mild thickening of alveolar walls and increased alveolar macrophages and eosinophils; or (4) marked thickening of alveolar walls and alveolar multinucleated giant cells, and inflammatory cells (eosinophils, neutrophils, macrophages, lymphocytes) in 30–50% of the field.

Goblet cell hyperplasia [3,27–30]: Medium-sized airways were scored in sections stained with periodic acid Schiff as: (1) less than 5% goblet cells; (2) 5–25%; (3) 25–50%; or (4) more than 50% goblet cells.

mRNA expression

RNA isolation, cDNA conversion, qPCR and analysis of the data was performed without prior knowledge of group designation of the samples. Total RNA from right heart tissue was isolated with the RNeasy Mini Kit (QIAGEN Inc, Valencia CA) and reverse transcribed using the High-Capacity cDNA Reverse Transcription kit (Applied Biosystems, Foster City, CA). Real time PCR was performed in triplicate with 20 ng of cDNA using the 7900HT Fast Real-Time PCR system (Applied Biosystems). The qPCR for the detection of the expression of the BMPR2 transgene, IL-33, ST2-IL1RL1, biglycan, and β-actin was performed with SYBR Green (Invitrogen, Grand Island, NY). For the specific detection of RELMα and RELMγ, we used the TaqMan Gene expression Assay (Applied Biosystems) based on a FAM labeled probe and the corresponding TaqMan gene expression assay for β-actin. The sequences for the primers or probes, respectively, are indicated in Table 1. The following conditions were used: 95°C for 10 min, followed by 40 cycles of 95°C for 15 s and 60°C for 1 min, followed by a hold at 4°C. Raw data was then analyzed with SDS Relative Quantification Software version 2.3 (Applied Biosystems) to determine cycle threshold (Ct). Mean values were determined and standardized for β-actin. Within each experiment, the β-actin Ct values were tightly

Table 1. Sequences of Primers and Probes.

Name	Sequence
BMPR2-transgene-F[1]	GACGAGAGCAACAGGCTGG
BMPR2-transgene-R	CCCTGAAGTTCTCAGCTCTAGATCATTTATC
IL-33-F	ACTGCATGAGACTCCGTTCTG
IL-33-R	CCTAGAATCCCGTGGATAGGC
IL1RL1-ST2-F	TGACTGTCTGGCCCTGAACCT
IL1RL1-ST2-R	TCTCTCCAGAACAGAGCAACCTCAA
Biglycan-F	TGAACCAGGAGCCTTTGATGGC
Biglycan-R	GTCCTCCAACTCAATAGCCTGG
β-actin-F	GGCTGTATTCCCCTCCATCG
β-actin-R	CCAGTTGGTAACAATGCCATGT
RELMα(TaqMan Gene expression assay)	CTTGCCAATCCAGCTAACTATCCCT
RELMγ(TaqMan Gene expression assay)	AAACCTGGCTCATATCCCATTGATG
Actin, β(TaqMan Gene expression assay)	ACTGAGCTGCGTTTTACACCCTTTC

[1]Abbreviations: F- forward, R-reverse.

clustered with standard deviations of less than 2% of the mean demonstrating the consistent quality of the RNA from each sample (data not shown).

Immune responses

BAL cells and lung lymph node cells were analyzed by flow cytometry as described [3,27,28] using a MACS Quant (Miltenyi Biotec, Auburn, CA) instrument and FloJo (TreeStar Inc, Ashland, OR) software. Cell counts were performed using the feature provided by the MACS Quant flow cytometer. All cell analysis was performed without prior knowledge of the group designation of the samples.

BAL samples

BAL samples were analyzed as described [27] for the presence of eosinophils ($CD11b^{high}$, $CCR3^{high}$, $GR1^{low}$, $CD11c^{low\text{-}intermediate}$, $MHCII^{low\text{-}intermediate}$), neutrophils ($CD11b^{high}$, $GR1^{high}$, $CD11c^{low\text{-}intermediate}$, $MHCII^{low\text{-}intermediate}$), lymphocytes (cells expressing CD4 or CD8 and falling into the lymphocyte gate by forward and side scatter profile), and CD11c+ cells that co-express CD205. The mean fluorescence intensity of CD11c+CD205+ cells stained with anti MHCII antibody was determined as a measure of the capacity of these cells to present antigen [27,28].

Single cell suspensions from lung draining lymph nodes were analyzed as described [3,27,28,63] following brief fixation with 2% PBS buffered formaldehyde (20–30 minutes at room temperature). The cell suspensions were analyzed for cellularity (cell count per sample) and numbers of T cells (CD3 positive, B220 negative cells that are also positive for CD4 or CD8). CD4+ T cells were intracellularly stained using a published protocol [3,63] following permeabilization with saponin-containing buffer with anti-Helios antibody and the frequency of this subpopulation was determined.

Intracellular cytokine staining was performed on cell suspensions prepared from the lung draining lymph nodes, as previously described [3,27–29,63]. The cells were cultured in the presence of phorbol-myristate-acetate (PMA) and ionomycin for 4 h, with the addition of Brefeldin A for the last 2 h of culture. The cells were harvested, fixed in 2% buffered formaldehyde, permeabilized, and stained with anti-cytokine (anti-IL-13, anti–IFN-γ, and anti- IL-17A/F monoclonal antibodies). The cells were surface stained with anti-CD3 combined with anti-CD8α and anti-CD4 labeled monoclonal antibodies. The cells were examined on a MACS-Quant cytometer. Electronic gates were set using the forward and side scatter profiles in combination with the surface labels to capture CD3+ T cells that were either CD4+ or CD8+. Intracellular isotype control monoclonal antibodies were used to set the quadrants that demarcated cytokine-positive cells.

The cell populations were analyzed using monoclonal antibodies tagged with Pacific Blue, AlexaFluor, fluorescein (FITC), phycoerythrin (PE), peridinin-chlorophyll (PerCP), Allophycocyanin (APC), or cyanine (Cy) tandem dyes that were purchased from BD Bioscience (San Jose, California), Ebioscience (San Diego, California) or Biolegend (San Diego, California). BAL cells were stained with anti-CD11c-PacificBlue (clone N418); anti-CD11b-PE (clone M1/70); anti-MHCII-FITC (I-A/I-E, clone M5/114.15.2); anti-Ly-6G/Ly-6C-APC-Cy7 (clone GR1); PerCp-anti-CD4 (clone GK1.5) and PerCP-anti-CD8α (clone 53-6.7); anti-CCR3-AlexaFluor 647 (clone TG14, Biolegend, or clone 83103, BD Bioscience); anti-CD205-PE-Cy7 (clone Dec205 Biolegend). Lung lymph node cells were stained with anti-CD45R/B220-PacificBlue (clone RA3-6B2, Biolegend); anti-CD3-FITC (clone 17A2, ebioscience), anti-CD8α-PE-Cy7 (clone 53-6.7, Biolegend), anti-CD4-APC-Cy7 or -PerCp (clone GK1.5, Biolegend), anti-Helios-APC (clone 22F6, Biolegend). Intracellular staining was performed with anti-IL-13-PE (clone eBio13A, Ebioscience), anti-IFNγ –AlexaFluor 645 (clone XMG1.2, Biolegend), and anti-IL-17A/F-PE-Cy7 (clone TC11-18H10.1, Biolegend), on cells that were surface stained with anti-CD3-FITC, anti-CD8α-PerCP, and anti-CD4-APC-Cy7. IgG1-isotype control antibodies were from ebioscience or biolegend.

Statistical analysis

Statistical analysis and graphs were generated using the Aable 3 software (Gigawiz) or Prism 5 (Graphpad). Data from multiple groups were analyzed for significant differences using the Kruskal Wallis test (tie corrected). Pair-wise comparisons were conducted with the unpaired, two-tailed Mann-Whitney U test, or the unpaired, two-tailed t test with Welch's correction for unequal variances. Categorical data were analyzed with the chi-square test. Analysis for correlation was performed with the Spearman's Rank Order Correlation Coefficient test (two-tailed). A p value <0.05 was considered to mean statistical significance.

Acknowledgments

The authors gratefully acknowledge the help of Linda R. Robinson, Dr. West laboratory, Department of Medicine, Vanderbilt University Medical Center, Nashville, Tennessee, USA, for helping us to set up hemodynamics measurements in the Grunig laboratory.

Author Contributions

Edited the manuscript: GG SHP LM JW. Conceived and designed the experiments: GG SHP. Performed the experiments: SHP WCC CH LM GG. Analyzed the data: GG SHP LM. Contributed reagents/materials/analysis tools: LM JW GG. Wrote the paper: GG SHP.

References

1. Zaiman A, Fijalkowska I, Hassoun PM, Tuder RM (2005) One hundred years of research in the pathogenesis of pulmonary hypertension. Am J Respir Cell Mol Biol 33: 425–431.
2. West J (2010) Cross talk between Smad, MAPK, and actin in the etiology of pulmonary arterial hypertension. Adv Exp Med Biol 661: 265–278.
3. Daley E, Emson C, Guignabert C, de Waal Malefyt R, Louten J, et al. (2008) Pulmonary arterial remodeling induced by a Th2 immune response. J Exp Med 205: 361–372.
4. Gilboa L, Nohe A, Geissendorfer T, Sebald W, Henis YI, et al. (2000) Bone morphogenetic protein receptor complexes on the surface of live cells: a new oligomerization mode for serine/threonine kinase receptors. Mol Biol Cell 11: 1023–1035.
5. Phillips JA 3rd, Poling JS, Phillips CA, Stanton KC, Austin ED, et al. (2008) Synergistic heterozygosity for TGFbeta1 SNPs and BMPR2 mutations modulates the age at diagnosis and penetrance of familial pulmonary arterial hypertension. Genet Med 10: 359–365.
6. Eickelberg O, Morty RE (2007) Transforming growth factor beta/bone morphogenic protein signaling in pulmonary arterial hypertension: remodeling revisited. Trends Cardiovasc Med 17: 263–269.
7. Upton PD, Morrell NW (2009) TGF-beta and BMPR-II pharmacology implications for pulmonary vascular diseases. Curr Opin Pharmacol 9: 274–280.
8. Davies RJ, Holmes AM, Deighton J, Long L, Yang X, et al. (2012) BMP type II receptor deficiency confers resistance to growth inhibition by TGF-beta in pulmonary artery smooth muscle cells: role of proinflammatory cytokines. Am J Physiol Lung Cell Mol Physiol 302: L604–615.
9. Morrell NW, Yang X, Upton PD, Jourdan KB, Morgan N, et al. (2001) Altered growth responses of pulmonary artery smooth muscle cells from patients with primary pulmonary hypertension to transforming growth factor-beta(1) and bone morphogenetic proteins. Circulation 104: 790–795.
10. Deng Z, Morse JH, Slager SL, Cuervo N, Moore KJ, et al. (2000) Familial primary pulmonary hypertension (gene PPH1) is caused by mutations in the bone morphogenetic protein receptor-II gene. Am J Hum Genet 67: 737–744.
11. Newman JH, Wheeler L, Lane KB, Loyd E, Gaddipati R, et al. (2001) Mutation in the gene for bone morphogenetic protein receptor II as a cause of primary pulmonary hypertension in a large kindred. N Engl J Med 345: 319–324.
12. Lane KB, Machado RD, Pauciulo MW, Thomson JR, Phillips JA 3rd, et al. (2000) Heterozygous germline mutations in BMPR2, encoding a TGF-beta receptor, cause familial primary pulmonary hypertension. The International PPH Consortium. Nat Genet 26: 81–84.
13. Machado RD, Pauciulo MW, Thomson JR, Lane KB, Morgan NV, et al. (2001) BMPR2 haploinsufficiency as the inherited molecular mechanism for primary pulmonary hypertension. Am J Hum Genet 68: 92–102.
14. Newman JH, Trembath RC, Morse JA, Grunig E, Loyd JE, et al. (2004) Genetic basis of pulmonary arterial hypertension: current understanding and future directions. J Am Coll Cardiol 43: 33S–39S.
15. Rabinovitch M (2008) Molecular pathogenesis of pulmonary arterial hypertension. J Clin Invest 118: 2372–2379.
16. Austin ED, Hamid R, Hemnes AR, Loyd JE, Blackwell T, et al. (2012) BMPR2 expression is suppressed by signaling through the estrogen receptor. Biol Sex Differ 3: 6.
17. West J, Cogan J, Geraci M, Robinson L, Newman J, et al. (2008) Gene expression in BMPR2 mutation carriers with and without evidence of Pulmonary Arterial Hypertension suggests pathways relevant to disease penetrance. BMC Med Genomics 1: 45.
18. Mushaben EM, Hershey GK, Pauciulo MW, Nichols WC, Le Cras TD (2012) Chronic allergic inflammation causes vascular remodeling and pulmonary hypertension in BMPR2 hypomorph and wild-type mice. PLoS One 7: e32468.
19. Price LC, Wort SJ, Perros F, Dorfmuller P, Huertas A, et al. (2012) Inflammation in pulmonary arterial hypertension. Chest 141: 210–221.
20. Perros F, Dorfmuller P, Humbert M (2005) Current insights on the pathogenesis of pulmonary arterial hypertension. Semin Respir Crit Care Med 26: 355–364.
21. Song Y, Coleman L, Shi J, Beppu H, Sato K, et al. (2008) Inflammation, endothelial injury, and persistent pulmonary hypertension in heterozygous BMPR2-mutant mice. Am J Physiol Heart Circ Physiol 295: H677–690.
22. West J, Harral J, Lane K, Deng Y, Ickes B, et al. (2008) Mice expressing BMPR2R899X transgene in smooth muscle develop pulmonary vascular lesions. Am J Physiol Lung Cell Mol Physiol 295: L744–755.
23. Talati M, West J, Blackwell TR, Loyd JE, Meyrick B (2010) BMPR2 mutation alters the lung macrophage endothelin-1 cascade in a mouse model and patients with heritable pulmonary artery hypertension. Am J Physiol Lung Cell Mol Physiol 299: L363–373.
24. Johnson JA, Hemnes AR, Perrien DS, Schuster M, Robinson LJ, et al. (2012) Cytoskeletal defects in Bmpr2-associated pulmonary arterial hypertension. Am J Physiol Lung Cell Mol Physiol 302: L474–484.
25. Schermuly RT, Dony E, Ghofrani HA, Pullamsetti S, Savai R, et al. (2005) Reversal of experimental pulmonary hypertension by PDGF inhibition. J Clin Invest 115: 2811–2821.
26. Crnkovic S, Hrzenjak A, Marsh LM, Olschewski A, Kwapiszewska G (2011) Origin of neomuscularized vessels in mice exposed to chronic hypoxia. Respir Physiol Neurobiol 179: 342–345.
27. Hoffman C, Park SH, Daley E, Emson C, Louten J, et al. (2011) Interleukin-19: a constituent of the regulome that controls antigen presenting cells in the lungs and airway responses to microbial products. PLoS One 6: e27629.
28. Padilla J, Daley E, Chow A, Robinson K, Parthasarathi K, et al. (2005) IL-13 Regulates the Immune Response to Inhaled Antigens. J Immunol 174: 8097–8105.
29. Ford JG, Rennick D, Donaldson DD, Venkayya R, McArthur C, et al. (2001) IL-13 and IFN-gamma: interactions in lung inflammation. J Immunol 167: 1769–1777.
30. Grunig G, Warnock M, Wakil AE, Venkayya R, Brombacher F, et al. (1998) Requirement for IL-13 Independently of IL-4 in Experimental Asthma. Science 282: 2261–2263.
31. Gottschalk RA, Corse E, Allison JP (2012) Expression of Helios in peripherally induced Foxp3+ regulatory T cells. J Immunol 188: 976–980.
32. Thornton AM, Korty PE, Tran DQ, Wohlfert EA, Murray PE, et al. (2010) Expression of Helios, an Ikaros transcription factor family member, differentiates thymic-derived from peripherally induced Foxp3+ T regulatory cells. J Immunol 184: 3433–3441.
33. Serre K, Benezech C, Desanti G, Bobat S, Toellner KM, et al. (2011) Helios is associated with CD4 T cells differentiating to T helper 2 and follicular helper T cells in vivo independently of Foxp3 expression. PLoS One 6: e20731.
34. Hassoun PM, Mouthon L, Barbera JA, Eddahibi S, Flores SC, et al. (2009) Inflammation, growth factors, and pulmonary vascular remodeling. J Am Coll Cardiol 54: S10–19.
35. Perros F, Dorfmuller P, Montani D, Hammad H, Waelput W, et al. (2012) Pulmonary lymphoid neogenesis in idiopathic pulmonary arterial hypertension. Am J Respir Crit Care Med 185: 311–321.
36. Said SI, Hamidi SA, Gonzalez Bosc L (2010) Asthma and pulmonary arterial hypertension: do they share a key mechanism of pathogenesis? Eur Respir J 35: 730–734.
37. Soon E, Holmes AM, Treacy CM, Doughty NJ, Southgate L, et al. (2010) Elevated levels of inflammatory cytokines predict survival in idiopathic and familial pulmonary arterial hypertension. Circulation 122: 920–927.
38. Tamosiuniene R, Tian W, Dhillon G, Wang L, Sung YK, et al. (2011) Regulatory T cells limit vascular endothelial injury and prevent pulmonary hypertension. Circ Res 109: 867–879.
39. Hoffmann J, Yin J, Kukucka M, Yin N, Saarikko I, et al. (2011) Mast cells promote lung vascular remodelling in pulmonary hypertension. Eur Respir J 37: 1400–1410.
40. Liu D, Liu QQ, Eyries M, Wu WH, Yuan P, et al. (2012) Molecular genetics and clinical features of Chinese idiopathic and heritable pulmonary arterial hypertension patients. Eur Respir J 39: 597–603.
41. Girerd B, Montani D, Eyries M, Yaici A, Sztrymf B, et al. (2010) Absence of influence of gender and BMPR2 mutation type on clinical phenotypes of pulmonary arterial hypertension. Respir Res 11: 73.
42. Sztrymf B, Coulet F, Girerd B, Yaici A, Jais X, et al. (2008) Clinical outcomes of pulmonary arterial hypertension in carriers of BMPR2 mutation. Am J Respir Crit Care Med 177: 1377–1383.
43. Pfarr N, Szamalek-Hoegel J, Fischer C, Hinderhofer K, Nagel C, et al. (2011) Hemodynamic and clinical onset in patients with hereditary pulmonary arterial hypertension and BMPR2 mutations. Respir Res 12: 99.
44. Rosenzweig EB, Morse JH, Knowles JA, Chada KK, Khan AM, et al. (2008) Clinical implications of determining BMPR2 mutation status in a large cohort of children and adults with pulmonary arterial hypertension. J Heart Lung Transplant 27: 668–674.
45. Louten J, Rankin AL, Li Y, Murphy EE, Beaumont M, et al. (2011) Endogenous IL-33 enhances Th2 cytokine production and T-cell responses during allergic airway inflammation. Int Immunol 23: 307–315.
46. Kurowska-Stolarska M, Kewin P, Murphy G, Russo RC, Stolarski B, et al. (2008) IL-33 induces antigen-specific IL-5+ T cells and promotes allergic-induced airway inflammation independent of IL-4. J Immunol 181: 4780–4790.
47. Schmitz J, Owyang A, Oldham E, Song Y, Murphy E, et al. (2005) IL-33, an interleukin-1-like cytokine that signals via the IL-1 receptor-related protein ST2 and induces T helper type 2-associated cytokines. Immunity 23: 479–490.
48. Munitz A, Cole ET, Karo-Atar D, Finkelman FD, Rothenberg ME (2012) Resistin-like molecule-alpha regulates IL-13-induced chemokine production but not allergen-induced airway responses. Am J Respir Cell Mol Biol 46: 703–713.
49. Munitz A, Waddell A, Seidu L, Cole ET, Ahrens R, et al. (2008) Resistin-like molecule alpha enhances myeloid cell activation and promotes colitis. J Allergy Clin Immunol 122: 1200–1207 e1201.
50. Wills-Karp M, Luyimbazi J, Xu X, Schofield B, Neben TY, et al. (1998) Interleukin-13: central mediator of allergic asthma. Science 282: 2258–2261.
51. Baum JR, Long B, Cabo C, Duffy HS (2012) Myofibroblasts cause heterogeneous Cx43 reduction and are unlikely to be coupled to myocytes in the healing canine infarct. Am J Physiol Heart Circ Physiol 302: H790–800.
52. Ma F, Li Y, Jia L, Han Y, Cheng J, et al. (2012) Macrophage-stimulated cardiac fibroblast production of IL-6 is essential for TGF beta/Smad activation and cardiac fibrosis induced by angiotensin II. PLoS One 7: e35144.
53. Kakkar R, Lee RT (2008) The IL-33/ST2 pathway: therapeutic target and novel biomarker. Nat Rev Drug Discov 7: 827–840.

54. Sanada S, Hakuno D, Higgins LJ, Schreiter ER, McKenzie AN, et al. (2007) IL-33 and ST2 comprise a critical biomechanically induced and cardioprotective signaling system. J Clin Invest 117: 1538–1549.
55. Angelini DJ, Su Q, Yamaji-Kegan K, Fan C, Skinner JT, et al. (2009) Hypoxia-induced mitogenic factor (HIMF/FIZZ1/RELMalpha) induces the vascular and hemodynamic changes of pulmonary hypertension. Am J Physiol Lung Cell Mol Physiol 296: L582–593.
56. Nair MG, Du Y, Perrigoue JG, Zaph C, Taylor JJ, et al. (2009) Alternatively activated macrophage-derived RELM-{alpha} is a negative regulator of type 2 inflammation in the lung. J Exp Med 206: 937–952.
57. Pesce JT, Ramalingam TR, Wilson MS, Mentink-Kane MM, Thompson RW, et al. (2009) Retnla (relmalpha/fizz1) suppresses helminth-induced th2-type immunity. PLoS Pathog 5: e1000393.
58. Li MO, Wan YY, Sanjabi S, Robertson AKL, Flavell RA (2006) Transforming growth factor-beta regulation of immune responses. Annual Review of Immunology 24: 99–146.
59. Reynolds LA, Maizels RM (2012) Cutting Edge: In the Absence of TGF-beta Signaling in T Cells, Fewer CD103(+) Regulatory T Cells Develop, but Exuberant IFN-gamma Production Renders Mice More Susceptible to Helminth Infection. Journal of Immunology 189: 1113–1117.
60. Hager-Theodorides AL, Outram SV, Shah DK, Sacedon R, Shrimpton RE, et al. (2002) Bone morphogenetic protein 2/4 signaling regulates early thymocyte differentiation. J Immunol 169: 5496–5504.
61. Rastogi D, Ngai P, Barst RJ, Koumbourlis AC (2004) Lower airway obstruction, bronchial hyperresponsiveness, and primary pulmonary hypertension in children. Pediatr Pulmonol 37: 50–55.
62. Chen WC, Park SH, Hoffman C, Philip C, Robinson L, et al. (2012) Right ventricular systolic pressure measurements in combination with harvest of lung and immune tissue samples in mice. J Visualized Experiments in press.
63. Grunig G, Corry DB, Leach MW, Seymour BW, Kurup VP, et al. (1997) Interleukin-10 is a natural suppressor of cytokine production and inflammation in a murine model of allergic bronchopulmonary aspergillosis. J Exp Med 185: 1089–1099.

8

Diagnostic Value of Echocardiography in the Diagnosis of Pulmonary Hypertension

Christoph Hammerstingl [¶], Robert Schueler* [¶], Lisa Bors, Diana Momcilovic, Stefan Pabst, Georg Nickenig, Dirk Skowasch

Department of Internal Medicine II, Cardiology/Pneumology, University of Bonn, Bonn, Germany

Abstract

Aims: To determine the value of echocardiography including tissue Doppler imaging (TDI) and right ventricular (RV) speckle tracking analysis for the diagnosis of pulmonary hypertension (PH) and discrimination between pre- and postcapillary PH.

Methods and Results: 155 consecutive patients (mean age 70.5±13.0 years, 81 [52%] male gender, BMI 27.2±6.1 kg/m^2) with PH undergoing right heart catheterization (RHC) and transthoracic echocardiography (TTE) with TDI between January 2008 and December 2009 were retrospectively evaluated including offline speckle tracking analysis of RV contractility. After RHC 23.2% of patients (36) were diagnosed with precapillary PH. Invasive results from RHC were significantly correlated to TTE measurements (E/é, postcapillary wedge pressure [PCWP], r = 0.61, P<0.001; mean, systolic pulmonary arterial pressure [mPAP, sPAP], r = 0.43, P<0.001). Single echocardiographic parameters were of good predictive value for final PH-diagnosis (sPAP, area under the curve [AUC] 0.63, P = 0.025; lateral apical RV longitudinal strain [RVaSl)], AUC 0.76, P = 0.001; E/é, AUC 0.84, P<0.001) which could be increased by combining most predictive parameters after receiver operating curves (ROC) cut off analysis (sPAP>69 mmHg, E/é<12, RVaSl ≥−8.4%). TTE had a sensitivity of 33.33% and a specificity of 100% to identify patients with precapillary PH, and a negative predictive value of 84.72% to rule out precapilary PH.

Conclusion: Echocardiography allows feasible and reliable estimation of PH and seems helpful to distinguish between pre- and postcapillary PH. Further prospective studies on patients with different manifestations of PH must validate the predictive value of echocardiography in this clinical setting.

Editor: Fikret Er, University of Cologne, Germany

Funding: This study has been supported by an unrestricted grand of Actelion Pharmaceuticals Deutschland GmbH. The funders had no role in study design, data collection and analysis, decision to publish, or preparation of the manuscript.

Competing Interests: The authors have received an unrestricted grant from Actelion Pharmaceuticals Germany.

* E-mail: robert.schueler@ukb.uni-bonn.de

¶ These authors contributed equally to this work.

Introduction

Precapillary pulmonary arterial hypertension (PAH) is a severe and life threatening disease, leading to death if untreated within 2–3 years after diagnosis [1]. Definite diagnosis of PAH is often delayed with a median of 3 years from onset of first symptoms to start of effective therapy [2]. Therefore, current guidelines emphasize the importance of early diagnosis of precapillary PAH and differentiation from other entities of pulmonary hypertension (PH) [3]. Up to now definite diagnosis of PAH can only be confirmed by invasive right heart catheterization (RHC) which is not widely available, puts the patients at risk for rare but serious complications, and which is inconvenient for frequent follow up evaluations [4]. Furthermore, PAH is a rare disease and invasive RHC confirms postcapillary PH in most cases with elevated pulmonary pressure. TTE is a non-invasive method which is widely available, cost effective, and has been established as non-invasive screening technique for the detection of PH. Furthermore, echocardiographic studies are recommended at regular intervals during the follow up of patients with proven PAH under specific therapy [5]. It would be of great interest to identify a simple, non-invasive diagnostic algorithm which allows for (a) adequate PH diagnosis with a sufficient high reliability, and (b) discriminates between pre-and postcapillary PH.

Therefore, we sought to determine the value of an echocardiographic algorithm for the diagnosis of PH in patients with typical clinical symptoms which were transferred to our hospital for further evaluation.

Results

155 consecutive patients with PH undergoing standardized two dimensional TTE before RHC between January 2008 and December 2009 were analysed. Baseline characteristics as well as results from RHC and TTE are presented in ***table 1***. After RHC 36 (23.2%) patients were diagnosed with precapillary PH; in 119 (76.8%) patients PH was found to be postcapillary.

Echocardiographically determined sPAP was >30 mmHg in all patients leading to a sensitivity of this parameter of 100% for the

Table 1. Baseline data, groups divided with regard to findings from right heart catheterization.

	All patients (n = 155)	Precapillary PH (n = 36)	Postcapillary PH (n = 119)	*p-value*
Age (years)	70.5±13.0	65.9±16.8	71.3±11.4	**0.002**
BMI (kg/m^2)	27.2±6.1	26.2±6.0	27.6±6.4	0.37
Male gender (n, %)	81 (52%)	13 (36%)	68 (57%)	**0.03**
Hypertension (n, %)	91 (59%)	12 (36%)	78 (65%)	**0.002**
Diabetes mellitus (n, %)	33 (21%)	7 (19%)	26 (22%)	0.82
Smokers (n, %)	29 (19%)	7 (19%)	22 (18%)	1.0
Stroke (n, %)	3 (2%)	0 (0%)	3 (2%)	1.0
Lipid disorder (n, %)	45 (29%)	5 (14%)	40 (33%)	**0.02**
CAD (n, %)	80 (51%)	14 (39%)	66 (55%)	0.09
NYHA FC II (n, %)	28 (18%)	4 (11%)	24 (20%)	0.25
NYHA FC III (n, %)	93 (60%)	27 (75%)	66 (55%)	0.47
NYHA FC IV (n, %)	34 (22%)	5 (14%)	29 (24%)	0.31
Medication				
Aspirin (n, %)	89 (57%)	17 (47%)	72 (60%)	0.18
ß-blocker (n, %)	115 (74%)	16 (44%)	99 (83%)	**<0.0001**
ARB/ACEI (n, %)	24 (15%)	3 (8%)	21 (18%)	0.29
Diuretics (n, %)	128 (83%)	23 (64%)	105 (88%)	**0.002**
Statin (n, %)	86 (55%)	14 (39%)	72 (60%)	**0.03**
CCB (n, %)	30 (19%)	8 (21%)	23 (19%)	1.0
OAC (n, %)	64 (41%)	12 (33%)	52 (44%)	0.33
Right heart catheterization				
mPAP [mmHg]	38.7±10.7	39.3±13.3	38.5±9.8	0.70
sPAP [mmHg]	55.0±17.6	60.3±17.4	53.5±17.4	**0.04**
CO [l/min]	3.6±3.8	3.2±2.3	3.4±4.2	0.42
PCWP [mmHg]	22.9±9.3	11.2±2.6	26.6±7.3	**<0.0001**
RV systolic pressure [mmHg]	54.2±20.1	58.1±18.8	53.1±20.5	0.18
RV diastolic pressure [mmHg]	5.3±5.8	4.3±5.8	5.6±5.8	0.24
RV mean pressure [mmHg]	9.4±8.6	11.9±12.1	8.6±7.1	**0.04**
RA mean pressure [mmHg]	13.5±13.1	12.7±5.4	13.8±14.7	0.69
Echocardiography				
sPAP [mmHg]	51.8±17.1	58.3±23.6	49.9±14.2	**0.009**
LVEF [%]	53.2±18.1	61.8±13.9	50.6±18.5	**0.001**
LAV [ml]	84.0±52.7	79.9±64.9	85.2±48.7	0.6
RVDs [cm]	2.4±1.1	2.4±1.2	2.4±1.1	0.8
RVDd [cm]	3.3±1.4	3.4±1.6	3.3±1.3	0.88
E/é	16.5±7.9	9.9±2.9	18.5±7.9	**<0.0001**
MV E [m/s]	1.1±0.7	0.9±0.5	1.2±0.8	0.18
MV A [m/s]	0.6±0.5	0.6±0.5	0.6±0.5	0.77
MV é [m/s]	0.07±0.06	0.07±0.04	0.07±0.07	0.79
MV A [m/s]	0.07±0.04	0.07±0.04	0.07±0.05	0.80
é/A	1.3±0.8	1.5±0.9	1.2±0.7	0.07
E/A	1.5±1.2	1.1±0.9	1.7±1.2	**0.01**
IVSd [cm]	1.2±0.6	1.1±0.3	1.3±0.6	0.08
2D RV longitudinal lateral apical strain [%]	−8.0±4.6	5.7±3.4	−10.4±4.5	**0.003**

BMI, body mass index; CAD, coronary artery disease; NYHA FC, NYHA functional class; CCB, calcium channel blocker; ARB/ACEI, angiotensin receptor blockers/ angiotensin converting enzyme inhibitor; mPAP, mean pulmonary arterial pressure; sPAP, systolic pulmonary arterial pressure; PCWP, pulmonary capillary wedge pressure; RV, right ventricle; RA, right atrium; LVEF, left ventricular ejection fraction; E, early; A, atrial; MV, mitral velocity; RVDs/d, systolic/diastolic right ventricular diameter; LAV, left atrial volume; IVSd, diastolic interventricular septum thickness.

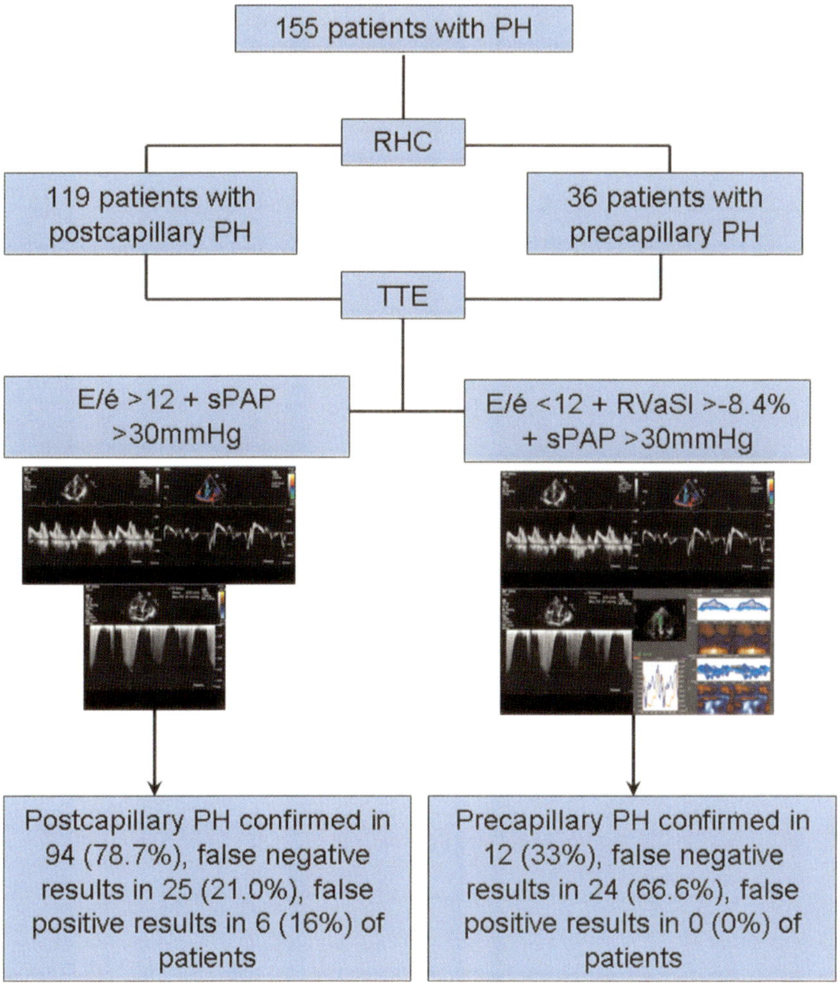

Figure 1. Incremental diagnostic value of apical strain and E/é in addition to echocardiographically determined sPAP for identification of patients with precapillary PH. *AUC, area under the curve; CI, confidence interval; sPAP, systolic pulmonary arterial pressure; RVSl, right ventricular longitudinal strain.*

identification of patients with PH; however, sPAP alone can not discriminate pre-from postcapillary PH; its specificity was 0%.

When compared with results from RHC, non-invasive determined sPAP was significantly correlated with invasively measured mPAP ($r = 0.43$; $P<0.0001$), but not with invasive sPAP ($r = 0.15$, $P = 0.06$). PCWP values from RHC were significantly correlated with TTE derived E/é values ($r = 0.61$, $P<0.0001$).

When comparing patient groups based on final PH diagnosis several echocardiographic parameters and demographic parameters showed significant differences (***table 1***). Patients with precapillary PH tended to have a lower LV EF, lower E/é values, higher sPAP and higher RVaSl values. Mean values of invasively measured sPAP (60.3±17.4 mmHg vs. 53.5±17.4 mmHg, $P = 0.04$) and sPAP derived from echocardiography (58.3±23.6 mmHg vs. 49.9±14.2 mmHg, $P = 0.009$) were significantly different in patients with precapillary and postcapillary PH. Interestingly, only in patients with precapillary PH, there was a significant correlation between invasive and non-invasive measurements of sPAP-values (TTE: 58.3±23.6 mmHg, RHC: 60.3±17.4, mmHg; $P = 0.008$; $r = 0.37$), whereas in patients with postcapillary PH this correlation was not found to be significant (TTE: 49.9±14.2 mmHg, RHC: 53.5±17.4 mmHg; $P = 0.07$; $r = 0.15$).

Echocardiographic Parameters Identifying Subjects with Postcapillary PH.

When comparing groups with regard to invasive findings from RHC only in patients with postcapillary PH a significant correlation was found between PCWP and E/e ($r = 0.44$, $P<0.001$ vs. $r = 0.07$, $P = 0.67$), with increasing E/e values in patients with postcapillary PH. ROC curve analysis confirmed the predictive value of this parameter to identify patients with postcapillary PH (AUC, 0.84, $P<0.001$) with an optimal cut off value of >12. This parameter alone had a sensitivity of 78.69% and specificity of 81.82%, a positive predictive value of 94.12%, and a negative predictive value of 50.94% to identify patients with postcapillary PH.

Echocardiographic Parameters Identifying Subjects with Precapillary PH

Logistic stepwise backwards regression analysis of most predictive variables after univariate regression analysis (LV EF, E/A, sPAP, E/é and RVaSl) identified only E/é ($P = 0.003$) and RVaSl ($P = 0.004$) to be independently associated with the presence of precapillary PH.

This finding was confirmed by ROC analsis of RVaSl, (AUC 0.76, P = 0.001; cut off value, >−8.4%) with a sensitivity of 33.33% and a specificity of 95.08% of this parameter for the identification of patients with precapillary PH.

When combining sPAP with RVaSl, TTE showed a sensitivity of 88.24%, and specificity of 68.75% to identify patients with precapillary PH. Finally, when adding sPAP to RVaSl and E/é the diagnostic value of echocardiography for the diagnosis of precapillary PH showed a sensitivity of 33.33% and a specificity of 100%, a positive predictive value of 100% and a negative predictive value of 84.72% (***figure 1***).

Discussion

In our study we aimed to evaluate the diagnostic value of echocardiography as non invasive screening method in patients with suspected PH by using a simple algorithm which was evaluated in a large cohort of symptomatic patients undergoing non-invasive and invasive testing. The most important findings of our study are that (a) estimation of PCWP with echocardiography is feasible and of high value to identify subjects with postcapillary PH and (b) echocardiography in combination with 2D speckle tracking analysis of RV deformation capability has a high predictive value to identify patients with precapillary PH.

Echocardiographic Parameters Predicting Postcapillary PH

Hadano could show a relevant correlation of E/é ratio with PCWP and LVEDP, respectively in patients with heart failure undergoing RHC which correlates with the results from our study. However, this group did not investigate the diagnostic value of this parameter in patients with suspected PH but without known structural heart disease. [6,7].

More recently, Ruan and colleagues found normal or reduced E/é ratios in 70 patients with primary PH and increasing E/é values in patients with PH due to cardiac aetiology were similarly to the findings in our study group [8].

In contrast to this study group who suggested the use of lateral mitral annulus systolic velocities [8] we used the average of septal and lateral mitral annulus velocities as recommended by the American and European society of echocardiography [9,10]. Additionally, we were able to show the high discriminative value of E/é to distinguish pre-from postcapillary PH in a considerably larger patient group.

Echocardiographic Assessment of Patients with Precapillary PH

Transthoracic echocardiography provides several different variables which correlate well with right heart hemodynamics and function, and therefore should always be performed in the case of suspected PH [2]. However, up to now echocardiography alone is considered inaccurate for the determination of pulmonary arterial pressure in symptomatic subjects due to its limited sensitivity and specificity [11] and, moreover, TTE is supposed unable to differentiate between pre-and postcapillary PH, as suggested in a recently published study by Bonderman et al. [12]. This group evaluated a non-invasive algorithm to exclude precapillary pulmonary hypertension (PH) in 372 (251 retrospective, 121 prospective subjects) symptomatic patients with PH combining echocardiography, ECG and laboratory testing (NT-proBNP). In this study on highly selected patients the non-invasive diagnostic algorithm including TTE had a good sensitivity of 100% and a low specificity of 19.3% for the detection of precapillary PH [12].

In our study TTE derived sPAP did not correlate well with sPAP from RHC. This finding may partly be explained by to the fact that all patients underwent TTE ≥1 day before invasive measurements and were fasting for at least 12 hours before undergoing RHC leading to volume depletion and a decrease in sPAP values. Importantly, invasive and non-invasive sPAP were not significantly different in patients with precapillary PH (60.3±17.4 mmHg, 58.3±23.6 mmHg, P = 0.64), but in patient with postcapillary PH after RHC (53.5±17.4 mmHg, 49.8±14.2 mmHg, P = 0.04), indicating on a stronger volume-load dependency of PAP in patients with postcapillary PH. These finding supports current PH guidelines [2] suggesting a systemic volume challenge in patients with suspected postcapillary PH when invasive results are not decisive.

RV Strain Analysis in Patients with Pulmonary Hypertension

Studies on 2D RV speckle tracking in patients with PH are scarce. Ahmad et al. showed in 63 patients with different aetiologies of RV impairment that 2D ST derived RV strain correlated well with global RV function as determined with cardiac magnetic resonance imaging (cMRI) [13].

In another study Fukuda and colleagues examined 45 patients with precapillary PH and found RV free wall longitudinal strain values to be of high diagnostic value of for the determination of RV function before and after pharmacological treatment. Interestingly, in this study RV free wall longitudinal strain values was highly significant correlated with changes in 6 minute walking distance [14].

This is the first study to evaluate the value the combination of non-invasive measurements for the estimation of PCWP, PAP, and RVaSl to diagnose precapillary PH in symptomatic patients with suspected PH. We found echocardiography to be of good sensitivity and specificity for the detection of precapillary PH and to be of reasonable good value to rule out precapillary PH which is of great importance in this patient cohort.

Limitations

Our study cohort consisted of patients with invasively proven PH. We did not follow a control group and our study design was retrospective. However, our results indicate on a high reliability of echocardiographic diagnostic in the setting of PH and suggest a high reliability of this non invasive strategy for the differentiation of pre-and postcapillary PH.

We did not evaluate the underlying aetiology of PAH or postcapillary PH in this study. Sensitivity and specificity of this test might not be the same in different patient groups with rare aetiologies of PH. Therefore, further prospective studies on different patients populations are required to confirm our findings.

Clinical Impact

RHC is often delayed in symptomatic patients with suspected PH. Echocardiography provides reliable estimation of pulmonary pressure and left ventricular filling pressures and is therefore a valuable tool for the assessment of PH in clinical symptomatic patients. Since the combination of sPAP, RVaSl and E/é was of high specificity to identify patients with precapillary PH, this non invasive approach including RV speckle tracking analysis might be an appropriate tool during the diagnostic work up of patients with suspected PH.

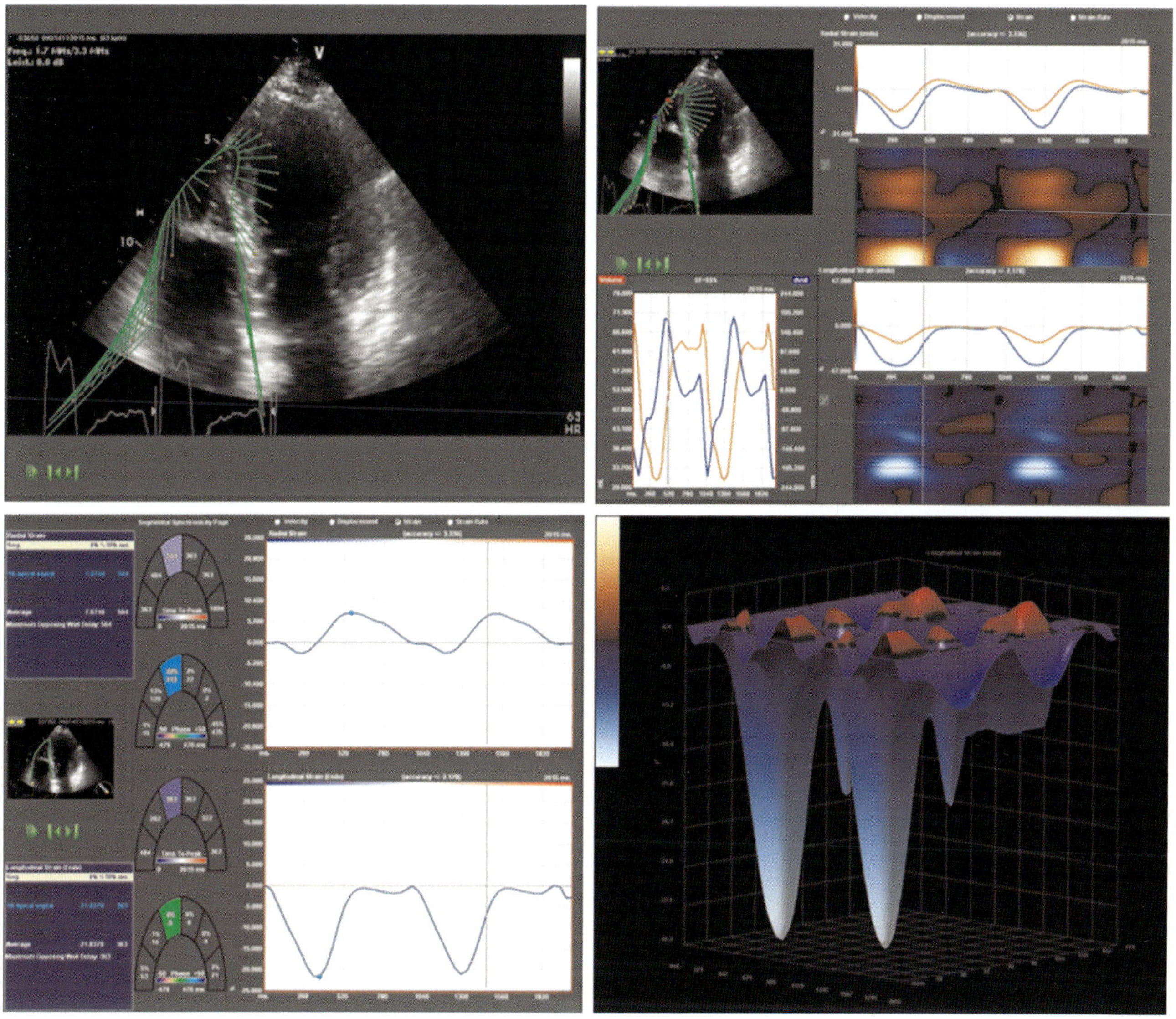

Figure 2. Patient distribution according to results of right heart catheterization; flow chart of the study design. *PH, postcapillary pulmonary hypertension; RHC, right heart catheterization; TTE, transthoracic echocardiography; sPAP, systolic pulmonary arterial pressure; RVaSl, apical right ventricular longitudinal strain.*

Conclusion

Echocardiography allows feasible and reliable estimation of PH and seems helpful to distinguish between pre-and postcapillary PH. Further prospective studies on patients with different manifestations of PH must validate the predictive value of echocardiography in this clinical setting.

Methods

Ethics Statement

The study has been approved by the ethics committee of the University of Bonn. Informed consent was obtained by all patients before study inclusion. Furthermore all the data were analyzed anonymously. This study has been conducted according to the principles expressed in the Declaration of Helsinki.

Study Concept

Figure 2 shows a flow chart of our study concept. Consecutive patients with suspected PH undergoing standardized two dimensional TTE ≤7 days before RHC were retrospectively analysed. Based on the invasive hemodynamic evaluation during RHC, precapillary or postcapillary PH was diagnosed according to current guidelines [3]. Patients with significant valvular heart disease and cardiomyopathies of any aetiology were excluded from the analysis. Precapillary PH was defined as mean pulmonary arterial pressure (mPAP) ≥25 mmHg and pulmonary capillary wedge pressure (PCWP) of ≤15 mmHg; patients with an Mpap ≥25 mmHg and a PCWP >15 mmHg were defined as suffering from postcapillary PH.

The following echocardiographic parameters were used to evaluate the presence of PH and the concomitant finding of an elevated PCWP which mainly distinguishes postcapillary PH from precapillary PH.

Systolic pulmonary artery pressure (sPAP) was estimated with continuous wave Doppler of systolic tricuspid regurgitant velocity and considered elevated when reaching values >30 mmHg. *PCWP* was assumed to be elevated (>15 mmHg) in cases with E/é ratio >12, a echocardiographic parameter which reflects on left ventricular filling pressure and is defined as the ration of peak mitral inflow velocities and peak mitral annulus velocity. Subjects with sPAP>30 mmHg and E/é <12 were assumed to have precapillary PAH, whereas in patients with sPAP>30 mmHg and E/é >12 PH was considered postcapillary. Furthermore, offline speckle tracking (ST) analysis of right ventricular (RV) contractility was performed in all subjects and compared with the results from RHC aiming to determine the diagnostic value of this new imaging technique in this clinical setting.

Transthoracic Echocardiography

Each patient underwent standardized two-dimensional transthoracic echocardiography for the determination of left and right ventricular functional parameters and dimensions according to the recommendations of the American Society of Echocardiography [15,16] using commercially available ultrasound scanner (Vivid 7, General Electric Medical Health, Waukesha, Wisconsin, USA; iE 33, Philips Medical Systems, Koninklijke N.V.) with a 2.5-MHz phased-array transducer. Echocardiographic views, including apical four-and two-chamber views (4CV,2CV) and parasternal (long-and short-axis views), with the patient in the left lateral decubitus position, were obtained in two-dimensional, three-dimensional and colour tissue Doppler imaging (TDI) modes. 2D ejection fraction (EF) was calculated by Simpsons rule from 4 CV. Mitral inflow velocities were recorded by standard pulsed-wave Doppler at the tips of the mitral valve leaflets in an apical 4CV. E/é ratio was determined by measuring TDI derived systolic and diastolic velocities of the septal and lateral mitral valve annulus and averaging the values and conventional measurement of mitral valve inflow velocities according to recommendations of the American Society of Echocardiography [9]. During echo sPAP was estimated by measuring the peak systolic tricuspid regurgitant velocity flow at continuous wave Doppler if applicable.

2D Speckle Tracking Analysis of Right Ventricular Deformation Capabilities

Figure 3 shows an example of RV ST analysis of RV deformation capabilities. Two cine loops from apical four chamber view were digitized and stored on an echocardiographic imaging server (XCELERA, Philips Medical Systems, Koninklijke N.V.). Offline 2D ST analyses of the gray scale images obtained by 2D echocardiography were done by using commercially available software (TomTec Imaging Systems GmbH, Unterschleissheim, Germany). The endocardium of the free RV wall was manually traced starting from the lateral tricuspidal annulus to RV apex, and was tracked by the 2D strain software along the border throughout two cardiac cycles. Accuracy of border tracking was manually verified and adjusted if needed. The free right ventricular wall was segmented visually in a basal, midventricular and apical segment. For the determination of regional RV impairment we followed the approach of Dambrauskaite [17] and Lopez-Candalez [18]. Therefore only longitudinal lateral apical RV Sl (RVaSl) entered further analysis. Of note, RV speckle tracking analysis of free RV wall was applicable in all patients.

Statistical Analysis

Exploratory data analysis was performed and no adjustment was made for multiple tests.

Normal distribution of continuous variables was examined using the Kolmogorov – Smirnov test. Continuous data was expressed as mean values±standard deviation. Two-tailed P-values were calculated and considered to be significant if ranging below

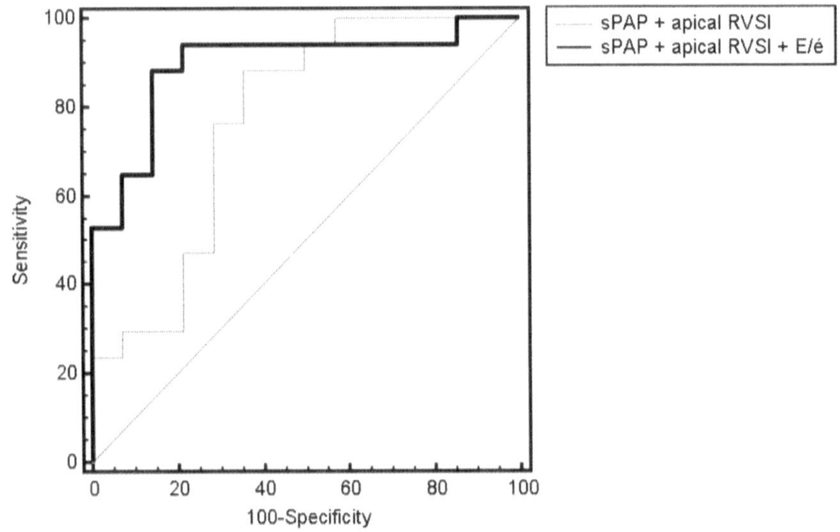

	AUC	95% CI	P
sPAP + apical RV SI	0.787	0.61 - 0.91	0.0003
sPAP + apical RV SI +E/é	0.89	0.73 - 0.97	<0.0001

Figure 3. Right ventricular speckle tracking and 3 dimensional visualisation of longitudinal right ventricular strain values. *Right ventricular; 3D, three dimensional; RVSI, right ventricular longitudinal strain.*

0.05. Comparisons between two groups were performed with using students t test for paired samples or pair wise comparisons with Wilcoxon signed rank test for paired continuous variables. For categorical data Fisher's exact test were calculated. Statistics were performed using SPSS for Windows (PASW statistic., Version 17.0.2, SPSS Inc., Chicago, Illinois, USA) and MedCalc statistical software (MedCalc Software, Version 11.4.1.0, Mariakerke, Belgium).

To assess the predictive ability of the echocardiographic parameters logistic regression was performed. Associated receiver operating characteristic (ROC) curves for predicted probabilities were drawn for a diagnostic model including sPAP, 2D RVaSl and E/é. The corresponding areas under the curve along with their 95% CIs were calculated. Furthermore, we aimed to determine the diagnostic value of single parameters, as well as the combination of most predictive parameters for PH diagnosis by calculating the sensitivity, specificity, negative and positive predictive values for each parameter and its combination.

Author Contributions

Conceived and designed the experiments: CH DS GN. Performed the experiments: RS LB SP DM. Analyzed the data: RS DS CH. Contributed reagents/materials/analysis tools: DM LB SP RS. Wrote the paper: RS CH.

References

1. Simonneau G, Robbins IM, Beghetti M, Channick RN, Delcroix M, et al. (2009) Updated clinical classification of pulmonary hypertension. J Am Coll Cardiol 54: S43–S54.
2. Galie N, Hoeper MM, Humbert M, Torbicki A, Vachiery JL, et al. (2009) Guidelines for the diagnosis and treatment of pulmonary hypertension: the Task Force for the Diagnosis and Treatment of Pulmonary Hypertension of the European Society of Cardiology (ESC) and the European Respiratory Society (ERS), endorsed by the International Society of Heart and Lung Transplantation (ISHLT). Eur Heart J 30: 2493–2537.
3. Proceedings of the 4th World Symposium on Pulmonary Hypertension (2009) February 2008, Dana Point, California, USA. J Am Coll Cardiol 54: S1–117.
4. Hoeper MM, Lee SH, Voswinckel R, Palazzini M, Jais X, et al. (2006) Complications of right heart catheterization procedures in patients with pulmonary hypertension in experienced centers. J Am Coll Cardiol 48: 2546–2552.
5. Lang IM, Plank C, Sadushi-Kolici R, Jakowitsch J, Klepetko W, et al. (2010) Imaging in pulmonary hypertension. JACC Cardiovasc Imaging 3: 1287–1295.
6. Paulus WJ, Tschope C, Sanderson JE, Rusconi C, Flachskampf FA, et al. (2007) How to diagnose diastolic heart failure: a consensus statement on the diagnosis of heart failure with normal left ventricular ejection fraction by the Heart Failure and Echocardiography Associations of the European Society of Cardiology. Eur Heart J 28: 2539–2550.
7. Hadano Y, Murata K, Liu J, Oyama R, Harada N, et al. (2005) Can transthoracic Doppler echocardiography predict the discrepancy between left ventricular end-diastolic pressure and mean pulmonary capillary wedge pressure in patients with heart failure? Circ J 69: 432–438.
8. Ruan Q, Nagueh SF (2007) Clinical application of tissue Doppler imaging in patients with idiopathic pulmonary hypertension. Chest 131: 395–401.
9. Nagueh SF, Appleton CP, Gillebert TC, Marino PN, Oh JK, et al. (2009) Recommendations for the evaluation of left ventricular diastolic function by echocardiography. J Am Soc Echocardiogr 22: 107–133.
10. Nagueh SF, Appleton CP, Gillebert TC, Marino PN, Oh JK, et al. (2009) Recommendations for the evaluation of left ventricular diastolic function by echocardiography. Eur J Echocardiogr 10: 165–193.
11. Fisher MR, Forfia PR, Chamera E, Housten-Harris T, Champion HC, et al. (2009) Accuracy of Doppler echocardiography in the hemodynamic assessment of pulmonary hypertension. Am J Respir Crit Care Med 179: 615–621.
12. Bonderman D, Wexberg P, Martischnig AM, Heinzl H, Lang MB, et al. (2011) A noninvasive algorithm to exclude pre-capillary pulmonary hypertension. Eur Respir J 37: 1096–1103.
13. Ahmad H, Mor-Avi V, Lang RM, Nesser HJ, Weinert L, et al. (2011) Assessment of Right Ventricular Function Using Echocardiographic Speckle Tracking of the Tricuspid Annular Motion: Comparison with Cardiac Magnetic Resonance. Echocardiography. In press.
14. Fukuda Y, Tanaka H, Sugiyama D, Ryo K, Onishi T, et al. (2011) Utility of right ventricular free wall speckle-tracking strain for evaluation of right ventricular performance in patients with pulmonary hypertension. J Am Soc Echocardiogr 24: 1101–1108.
15. Douglas PS, Garcia MJ, Haines DE, Lai WW, Manning WJ, et al. (2011) ACCF/ASE/AHA/ASNC/HFSA/HRS/SCAI/SCCM/SCCT/SCMR 2011 Appropriate Use Criteria for Echocardiography. J Am Soc Echocardiogr 24: 229–267.
16. Gottdiener JS, Bednarz J, Devereux R, Gardin J, Klein A, et al. (2004) American Society of Echocardiography recommendations for use of echocardiography in clinical trials. J Am Soc Echocardiogr 17: 1086–1119.
17. Dambrauskaite V, Delcroix M, Claus P, Herbots L, D'hooge J, et al. (2007) Regional right ventricular dysfunction in chronic pulmonary hypertension. J Am Soc Echocardiogr 20: 1172–1180.
18. Lopez-Candales A, Rajagopalan N, Gulyasy B, Edelman K, Bazaz R (2009) Differential strain and velocity generation along the right ventricular free wall in pulmonary hypertension. Can J Cardiol 25: e73–e77.

Homocysteine Level and Risk of Abdominal Aortic Aneurysm

Hui Cao, Xinhua Hu*, Qiang Zhang, Jun Li, Junpeng Wang, Yang Shao, Bing Liu, Shijie Xin

Department of Vascular and Thyriod Surgery, the First Affiliated Hospital of China Medical University, Shenyang, China

Abstract

Objectives: Previous studies have reported inconsistent findings regarding the association between elevated plasma homocysteine (Hcy) levels and abdominal aortic aneurysm (AAA). We investigated this association between Hcy levels in patients with AAA and unaffected controls by conducting a meta-analysis and systematic review.

Methods: We conducted a systematic literature search (up to August 2013) of the PubMed database and Embase. We selected observational studies that evaluated Hcy levels in subjects with AAA compared to unaffected controls. Criteria for inclusion were the assessment of baseline Hcy and risk of AAA as an outcome. The results were presented as odd ratio (OR) and corresponding 95% confidence intervals (CI) comparing AAA patients to the control subjects.

Results: 7 studies with 6,445 participants were identified and analyzed. Overall, elevated plasma Hcy was associated with an increased risk of AAA (3.29; 95% CI 1.66–6.51). The pooled adjusted OR from a random effect model of only men participants in the AAA compared with the control group was 2.36 (95% CI 0.63–8.82).

Conclusion: This meta-analysis and systematic review suggested that Hcy significantly increased the risk of AAA.

Editor: Utpal Sen, University of Louisville, United States of America

Funding: This work was supported by National Nature Science Foundation of China (81070254, 30872527 and 30672048). URL: http://www.nsfc.gov.cn/Portal0/default152.htm. The funders had no role in study design, data collection and analysis, decision to publish, or preparation of the manuscript.

Competing Interests: The authors have declared that no competing interests exist.

* E-mail: xhhu@mail.cmu.edu.cn

Introduction

Abdominal aortic aneurysm (AAA) is an abnormal dilatation of the abdominal aorta, exceeding the normal aortic diameter by at least 50%. Aortic aneurysms do not tend to cause any symptoms and are often diagnosed incidentally on physical examination or imaging investigations for other unrelated conditions [1,2]. Screening demonstrates that disease prevalence ranges from 1.3% (45–54 years of age) to 12.5% in men (75–84 years of age), and in women from 0% in the youngest to 5.2% in the oldest age groups [3]. Currently there are no recognized treatments to diminish aneurysm progression at an early stage and a pharmacological treatment that targeted the processes underlying aortic dilatation [4].

Homocysteine (Hcy) is a branch-point intermediate of methionine metabolism, which can be further metabolised via two alternative pathways: degraded irreversibly through the transsulfuration pathway or remethylated to methionine by the remethylation pathway [5,6]. Vitamin B and folate are major determinants of Hcy metabolism and supplementation with vitamin B and folic acid has been shown to be effective in normalizing Hcy levels [7–10]. Elevated total plasma level of Hcy has been shown to correlate strongly with coronary artery disease [11,12], stroke [13,14], fracture [9,15], venous thrombosis [13], and may increase the risk of retinal artery [16] and vein occlusion [17] and nonarteritic anterior ischemic optic neuropathy [18]. Several studies reported that the elevated Hcy concentrations were identified as a potentially modifiable risk factor for abdominal aortic aneurysms [5,6,19-23]. Based on the previously published clinical evidence, a clinical review demonstrated there is evidence for an association between Hcy and AAA [24]. However, it is not strong enough to conclude that it plays a causal role in the pathogenesis of AAA. In the current study, we performed a meta-analysis to assess the relationship between Hcy and AAA in the literature. The aim of the current meta-analysis and systematic review was to quantitatively evaluate findings from observational studies on the plasma level of Hcy and the incidence of AAA.

Methods

This study was conducted in accordance with the 'preferred reporting items for systematic reviews and meta-analyses' (PRISMA) guidelines. No protocol exists for this meta-analysis.

Search strategy

We conducted a PubMed database and Embase search (up to August 2013) for studies assessing the association between AAA and Hcy. Papers could be published in English and Chinese. Potentially relevant studies were identified by various combinations of the following search terms: abdominal aortic aneurysm, hyperhomocysteinemia, homocysteine, folate, folic acid, vitamin B_6, and pyridoxine. In addition, we also manually searched the reference lists to detect additional eligible studies.

Study selection

Studies satisfying the following criteria were included in the observational meta-analysis: 1) providing raw data dealing with AAA and Hcy level and the risk of AAA; 2) AAA was defined as computed tomography (CT) and ultrasonographically proven infrarenal aortic diameter ≥30 mm); 3) Hcy level was measured at baseline using a technique standardized in each study; 4) providing adjusted odd ratio (OR) and the 95% confidence interval (CI) comparing the Hcy level of AAA to the control group. Exclusion criteria were: reviews, letters, case-reports, animal studies or the participants in a highly selected disease.

Data extraction and quality assessment

Two reviewers (Xinhua Hu and Qiang Zhang) independently extracted the data according to predefined criteria using a "AAA associated with Hcy extraction form" developed specifically for the review. The OR and 95% CI were extracted. When both crude and adjusted OR were provided, we used the most fully adjusted OR for all the included studies. We also extracted the following items from each individual study: author; year of publication; the country of study; the sample size; gender; and the mean age or age range of participants; Hcy level; case and control number. Where discrepancies were identified, reviewers resolved these by discussion.

Quality assessment that was performed with consideration of the following aspects followed the Newcastle-Ottawa Scale [25]: 1) Selection (4 scores): is the case definition, representativeness of the cases, selection of controls, and definition of controls. 2) Comparability (2 scores): select the most important factor, the criteria could be modified to indicate specific control for as second important factor. 3) Exposure (3 scores): ascertainment of exposure, same method of ascertainment for cases and controls, and non-response rate.

Statistical analysis

The OR was used as the common measure across studies. Data analysis used multivariate-adjusted OR and 95% CI. If the publications reported separately OR for smoker, we chose the separate OR estimates for the different items comparing AAA to the control from individual study. Before pooling the data, adjusted OR from each study was converted to their logOR to stabilize the variances and to normalize the distributions. The standard errors (SEs) for logOR were calculated from reported 95% CI. Homogeneity of OR across studies was assessed by using the Cochrane Q statistic ($p<0.10$ was considered indicative of statistically significant heterogeneity) and I^2 statistic (values of less than 40% as "heterogeneity might not be important " and of more than 75% as "considerable heterogeneity", based on the suggestion of the Cochrane Handbook for Systematic Review of Interventions) [26]. The pooled OR was computed using either fixed-effects models or, in the presence of heterogeneity, random-effects models [27].

We constructed a funnel plot with logOR and their SEs of logOR using AAA by visual inspection to assess the potential publication bias. Potential publication bias was also assessed by both Begg' rank correlation test [28] and Egger linear regression test at the $p<0.10$ level of significance [29]. Finally, sensitivity analysis was used to investigate the influence of a single study on the overall risk estimate, and was carried out by sequentially omitting one study at each turn with the metaninf algorithm in STATA. All analysis was performed using STATA version 12.0 statistical software (Stata Corp LP, College Station). A p value < 0.05 was considered as statistically significant.

Results

Literature search

After the application of search strategy, a total of 85 potentially relevant citations were identified in our initial literature search. After reviewing the full-texts, only 7 studies met the inclusion criteria [5,6,19–23]. Analysis was carried out on 1410 patients with an AAA (infrarenal aortic diameter ≥30 mm) and 5035 age and sex matched controls. A flow chart showing the study selection is presented in Fig 1. No additional studies were identified through our hand search of references from published studies.

Baseline characteristics and quality assessment

Characteristics of the included studies were listed in Table 1. The qualities of the included studies were listed in Table 2.

Association of plasma Hcy with all AAA

7 studies [5,6,19–23] reported AAA and Hcy. The total number of participants included in this meta-analysis was 6445 with 1410 total AAA patients. As shown in Fig 2, the pooled adjusted OR from a random effect model for all studies combined for the Hcy levels that was associated from a random effect model of participants with AAA was 3.29 (95% CI 1.66–6.51), with evidence of significant heterogeneity ($I^2 = 92.9\%$; $p = 0.000$). The pooled OR from a fixed-effect model was 1.21 (95% CI, 1.11–1.31).

Of the 7 included studies 3 actually had more than 100 subjects within each cohort [5,6,20], and the pooled adjusted OR from a random effect model for the 3 studies combined for the Hcy levels that was associated from a random effect model of participants with AAA was 2.20 (95% CI 1.01–4.80), with evidence of significant heterogeneity ($I^2 = 96.3\%$; $p = 0.000$) (Fig 3). 4 studies had less than 100 subjects [19,21–23], and the pooled adjusted OR from a random effect model for the 4 studies combined for the Hcy levels that was associated from a random effect model of participants with AAA was 5.43 (95% CI 1.47–20.01), with evidence of significant heterogeneity ($I^2 = 69.8\%$; $p = 0.019$) (Fig 4).

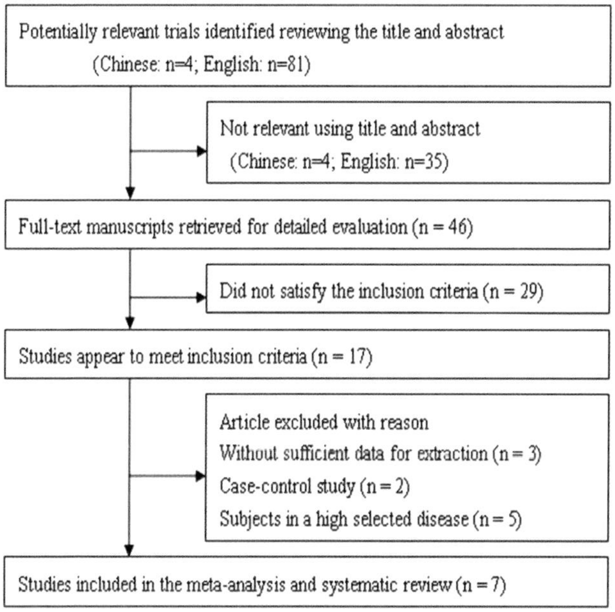

Figure 1. Flow chart of study selection process for meta-analysis.

Table 1. Summary of clinical studies included in meta-analysis.

Study/year	Country	Design	Subjects	Age/range Mean(SD)	Male	Hcy levels (Mean±SD), μmol/L		OR (95% CI)	Adjustment for covariates
			cases/controls	cases/controls	cases/controls	AAA patients	controls		
Wong YYE (2013)	Australia	case-control study	318/3930	77.7±4.1/76.5±3.6	318/3930	15.1±6.1	13.2±5.1	1.45(1.10–1.91)	Age, sex,smoking, hypertension, BMI, aortic diameter, dyslipidemia, diabetes, Cardiovascular disease, hsCRP
Giusti B (2008)	Italy	case-control study	423/423	73.5(40–94)/72(41–94)	376/366	15.3(6.7–144.3)	14.1(6.1–94.9)	1.1(1.01–1.20)	Age, sex,smoking, hypertension, dyslipidemia, diabetes mellitus, and COPD
Peeters AC (2007)	Netherlands	case-control study	88/88	69(45–85)/67(44–83)	81/81	quartil 9.33,11.8,15.1	N	0.78(01.7–3.62)	Age, sex,smoking, hypertension, dyslipidemia, concentration of creatinine, vitamin B_6, B_{12}, and folate
Sofi F(2005)	Italy	case-control study	438/438	74(40–94)/73.4(48–84)	397/391	16.2(7.3–93.6)	11(6–24.6)	7.8(4.60–13.20)	Age, sex,smoking, hypertension, aortic diameter, dyslipidemia
Warsi AA (2004)	UK	case-control study	38/36	70(53–79)/66(48–79)	35/21	19.4	10.9	9.75(2.17–43.77)	Age, sex,smoking, hypertension, aortic diameter, dyslipidemia, diabetes, cardiac disease, stroke
Spark JI (2003)	Australia	case-control study	47/60	N	N	17.9(14.8–20.8)	8.5(7.0–11.8)	15.9(4.96–51.00)	Age, sex,smoking, hypertension, aortic diameter, dyslipidemia,diabetes, cholesterol
Brunelli T (2000)	Italy	case-control study	58/60	69.3±6.7/67.6±7.0	58/60	15.7±6.5	9.6±3.9	6(1.23–29.6)	Age, smoking, hypertension, aortic diameter, diabetes mellitus, Hypercholesterolemia, Hypertriglyceridemia

Abbreviations: Body mass index, BMI; odd ratio, OR; not provide, N; chronic obstructive pulmonary disease, COPD; high-sensitivity C-reactive protein, hsCRP.

Table 2. The Newcastle-Ottawa Quality Assessment Scale for case–control studies.

Study	Selection	Comparability	Outcome	Summary
Wong YYE (2013)	4	2	2	8
Giusti B (2008)	4	2	2	8
Peeters AC (2007)	4	2	3	9
Sofi F (2005)	4	2	3	9
Warsi AA (2004)	4	2	3	9
Spark JI (2003)	4	2	2	8
Brunelli T (2000)	4	2	3	8

As shown in Fig 5, the pooled adjusted OR in two studies [5,23] from a random effect model of participants with AAA in the high Hcy group compared with the normal Hcy concentrations group only men was 2.36 (95% CI 0.63–8.82), with evidence of significant heterogeneity ($I^2 = 66.4\%$; $p = 0.085$).

Sensitive analysis on AAA

As shown in Fig 6, in the metainf analysis, there was little change in the quantitative summary measure of OR or 95% CI.

Assessment of publication bias

Evidence of publication bias for studies reporting adjusted OR of AAA was noted in asymmetrical funnel plot on visual inspection, and Egger' s linear regression test ($p = 0.049$), but not in the Begg's rank correlation test ($p = 1.000$). There was no evidence of publication bias for studies reporting adjusted OR of abdominal aortic diameter, this was further confirmed by Begg's rank correlation test ($p = 0.806$) and Egger's linear regression test ($p = 0.136$).

Discussion

The findings of the current meta-analysis provided evidence that Hcy was a predictor of increased AAA risk. Subjects with elevated Hcy increased risk of AAA (OR 3.29; 95% CI 1.66–6.51).

The major environmental exposures associated with AAA development include sex, advancing age, cigarette smoking, dyslipidaemia, and hypertension [30]. In the current meta-analysis, male was not associated with a markedly increase AAA risk (OR 2.36; 95% CI 0.63–8.28). However, due to the limited included study number and low proportion (376 of 1410) of AAA, the apparent lack of association with AAA and gender might be not convincing.

Pathological characterization of AAA includes intimal atheroma, infiltration of inflammatory cells, such as macrophages, T lymphocytes, neutrophils and dendritic cells and activated platelets into the aortic wall. These early events are followed by extracellular matrix (ECM) destruction and remodelling, vascular smooth muscle cell (VSMC) depletion and dysfunction [31].

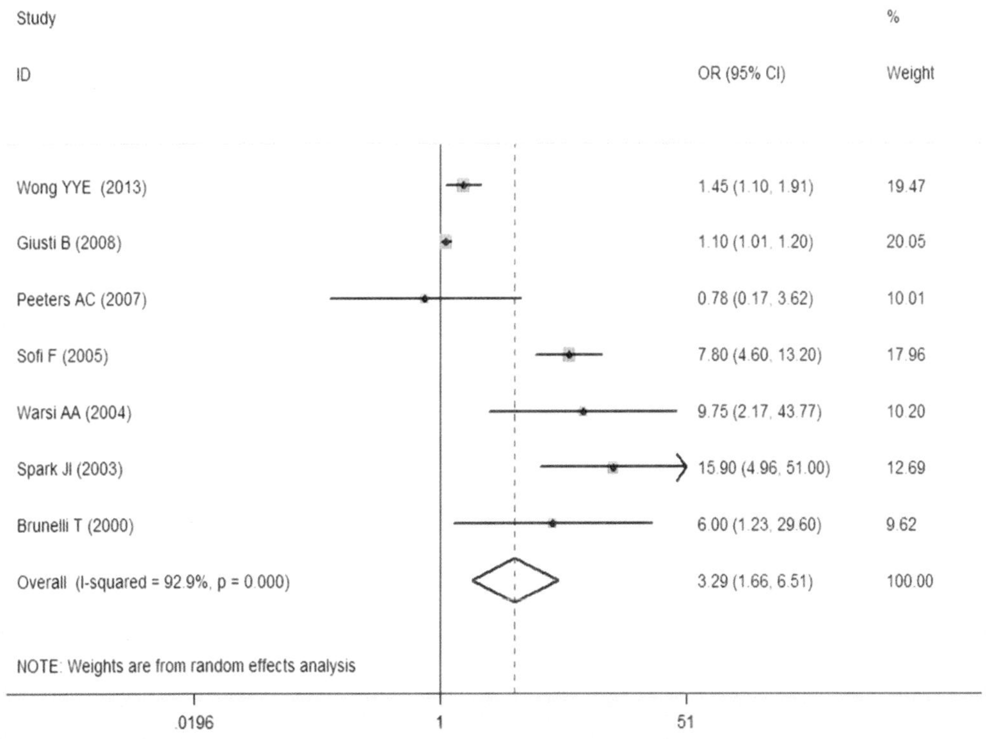

Figure 2. OR and 95% CI from the included studies of plasma Hcy level and AAA.

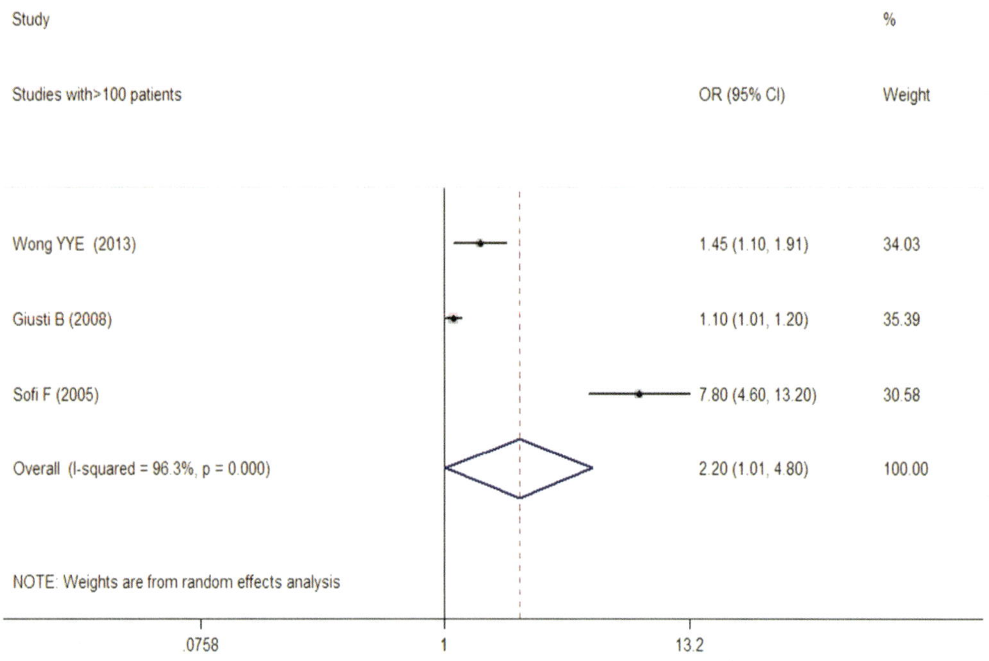

Figure 3. OR and 95% CI from the studies with >100 patients of plasma Hcy level and AAA.

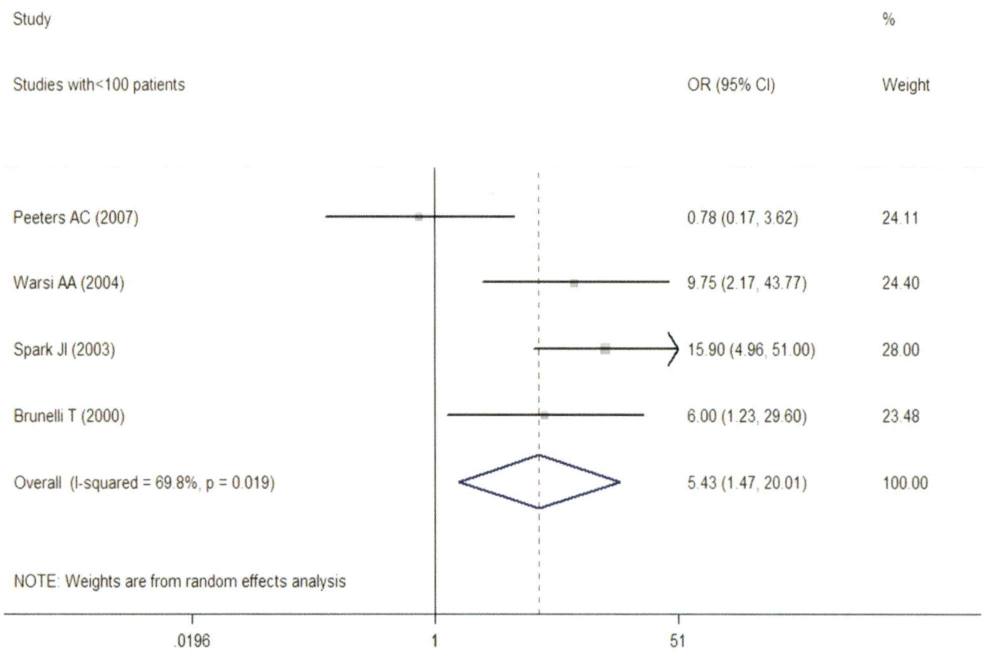

Figure 4. OR and 95% CI from the studies with <100 patients of plasma Hcy level and AAA.

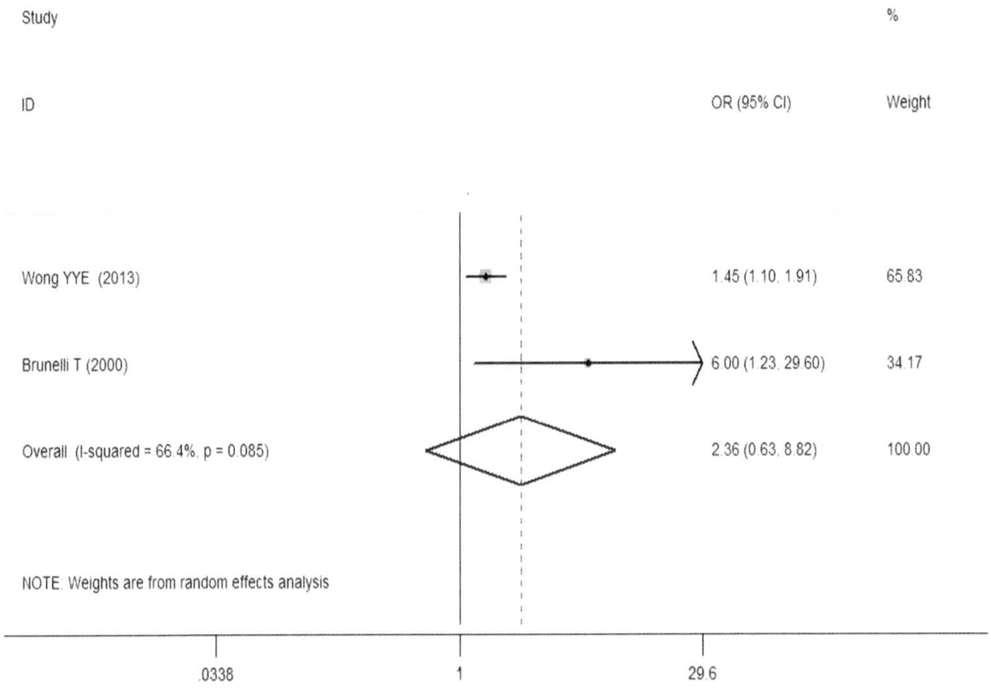

Figure 5. OR and 95% CI from the included studies of plasma Hcy level and AAA by men.

Experiments had demonstrated that Hcy stimulates chemokine and cytokine secretion from cultured human monocytes and has been implicated in suppressing regulatory T-cell function [32]. A recent interesting study by Liu Z et al., within an angiotensin II induced AAA mouse model suggests that hyper-Hcy exaggerates

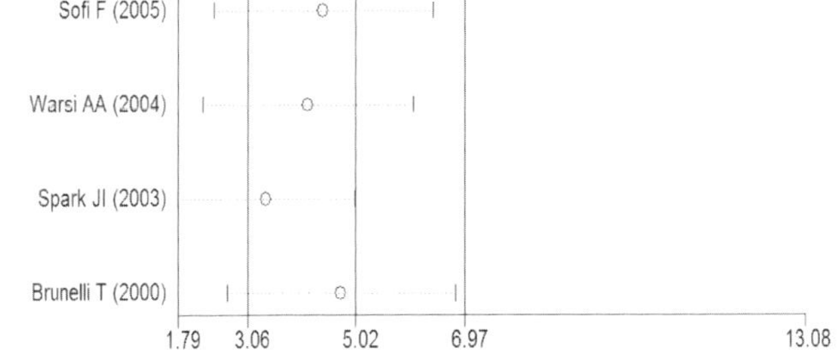

Figure 6. OR and 95% CI by omitting each study from the included studies of plasma Hcy and AAA.

adventitial inflammation, promoting AAA [33]. Hcy induces the synthesis of serine elastase in arterial smooth muscle cells, causing elastolysis by degradation of the extracellular matrix and release of reactive oxygen species, which are implicated in AAA pathogenesis [34,35]. Whether Hcy plays a role in aneurysm formation and/or in aneurysm expansion or Hcy is simply a marker of the condition need to be investigated.

Plasma Hcy levels are also influenced by several factors such as genetic factors [36,37], plasma folate and vitamin B_{12} concentrations. Selhub and colleagues have suggested that inadequate plasma concentrations of one or more B vitamins are contributing factors in approximately two thirds of all cases of hyperhomocysteinaemia and that vitamin supplementation can normalise high homocysteine concentrations [7]. As lack of well-designed RCTs, we were unable to perform a meta-analysis of the clinical effects of Hcy-lowering therapy among the limited studies because of the in consistent outcomes. Hcy-lowering therapy by folic acid, vitamins B_6 and B_{12} supplement will help to reduce rates of AAA or not, the answer maybe urgent in the development of interventions to prevent AAA. More well-design RCTs are needed to test the effects of Hcy-lowering therapy on the AAA incident.

Although we only included the case-control studies in the analysis, there are still several potential limitations. First, because of the cross-sectional design, the studies are unable to determine if the altered parameters are causally related to the presence of AAA. Second, we only included the study in English and Chinese, and some relevant studies might be not included in the review. There was a low risk of publication bias in studies of Hcy concentrations in relation to all AAA, as suggested by asymmetrical funnel plot on visual inspection and Egger's linear regression test ($p = 0.049$). Third, there was significant heterogeneity ($I^2 = 92.9\%$ in all AAA) among the included studies. Another potential source of heterogeneity was the lack of uniform definition of subjects. Forth, a major limitation was the possibility of uncontrolled confounding, and the individual studies did not adjust for potential risk factors in a consistent way. A wide spectrum of diseases was associated with elevated plasma Hcy concentrations, such as cardiovascular disease, stroke and cognitive impairment. These diseases were also associated with AAA; some residual confounding factors still affected the results. None of the analyzed studies seems to have adjusted Hcy levels for its most important covariate, glomerular filtration rate (GFR), and this is a major problem for the outcome. The lack of adjustment for these confounding factors might have resulted in a slight over estimation of the OR. Finally, the studies of Wong YYE and the Brunelli T contained only men, and that may make the findings have only limited relevance to AAA in women [5,23].

Conclusions

In conclusion, this meta-analysis and systematic review provided evidence that Hcy was associated with AAA. Whether this link is causal remained to be clarified further by future studies. More well-design RCTs on the effect of Hcy-lowering therapy on the prevention or treatment of AAA would be helpful to clarify this question.

Author Contributions

Conceived and designed the experiments: HC XHH. Performed the experiments: HC JL. Analyzed the data: XHH QZ. Contributed reagents/materials/analysis tools: JPW YS BL SJX. Wrote the paper: HC XHH QZ.

References

1. Cosford PA, Leng GC (2007) Screening for abdominal aortic aneurysm. Cochrane Database Syst Rev 2:CD002945.
2. Maegdefessel L, Spin JM, Adam M, Raaz U, Toh R, et al. (2013)Microman-Micromanaging abdominal aortic aneurysms. Int J Mol Sci 14:14374–14394.
3. Go AS, Mozaffarian D, Roger VL, Benjamin EJ, Berry JD, et al. (2013) Executive summary: Heart disease and stroke statistics 2013 update: A report from the american heart association. Circulation 127:143–152.
4. Harrison SC, Smith AJ, Jones GT, Swerdlow DI, Rampuri R, et al. (2012) Interleukin-6 receptor pathways in abdominal aortic aneurysm. Eur Heart J. doi: 10.1093/eurheartj/ehs354.
5. Wong YY, Golledge J, Flicker L, McCaul KA, Hankey GJ, et al. (2013) Plasma total homocysteine is associated with abdominal aortic aneurysm and aortic diameter in older men. J Vasc Surg 58:364–370.
6. Giusti B, Saracini C, Bolli P, Magi A, Sestini I, et al. (2008) Genetic analysis of 56 polymorphisms in 17 genes involved in methionine metabolism in patients with abdominal aortic aneurysm. J Med Genet 45:721–730.
7. Selhub J, Jacques PF, Wilson PW, Rush D, Rosenberg IH (1993) Vitamin status and intake as primary determinants of homocysteinemia in an elderly population. JAMA 270:2693–2698.
8. Homocysteine lowering trialists' collaboration (1998) Lowering blood homocysteine with folic acid based supplements: Meta-analysis of randomised trials. BMJ 316:894–898.
9. van Wijngaarden JP, Doets EL, Szczecinska A, Souverein OW, Duffy ME, et al. (2013) Vitamin B12, folate, homocysteine, and bone health in adults and elderly people: A systematic review with meta-analyses. J Nutr Metab 2013:486186.
10. Berti C, Fekete K, Dullemeijer C, Trovato M, Souverein OW, et al (2012) Folate intake and markers of folate status in women of reproductive age, pregnant and lactating women: A meta-analysis. J Nutr Metab 2012:470656.
11. Humphrey LL, Fu R, Rogers K, Freeman M, Helfand M (2008) Homocysteine level and coronary heart disease incidence: A systematic review and meta-analysis. Mayo Clin Proc 83:1203–1212.
12. Marti-Carvajal AJ, Sola I, Lathyris D, Karakitsiou DE, Simancas-Racines D (2013) Homocysteine-lowering interventions for preventing cardiovascular events. Cochrane Database Syst Rev 1:CD006612.
13. Wald DS, Law M, Morris JK (2002) Homocysteine and cardiovascular disease: Evidence on causality from a meta-analysis. BMJ 325:1202.
14. Casas JP, Bautista LE, Smeeth L, Sharma P, Hingorani AD (2005) Homocysteine and stroke: Evidence on a causal link from mendelian randomisation. Lancet 365:224–232.
15. Yang J, Hu X, Zhang Q, Cao H, Wang J, et al (2012) Homocysteine level and risk of fracture: A meta-analysis and systematic review. Bone 51:376–382.
16. Cahill MT, Stinnett SS, Fekrat S (2003) Meta-analysis of plasma homocysteine, serum folate, serum vitamin B(12), and thermolabile MTHFR genotype as risk factors for retinal vascular occlusive disease. Am J Ophthalmol 136:1136–1150.
17. McGimpsey SJ, Woodside JV, Cardwell C, Cahill M, Chakravarthy U (2009) Homocysteine, methylenetetrahydrofolate reductase C677T polymorphism, and risk of retinal vein occlusion: A meta-analysis. Ophthalmology 116:1778–1787.
18. Pianka P, Almog Y, Man O, Goldstein M, Sela BA, et al. (2000) Hyperhomocystinemia in patients with nonarteritic anterior ischemic optic neuropathy, central retinal artery occlusion, and central retinal vein occlusion. Ophthalmology 107:1588–1592.
19. Peeters AC, van Landeghem BA, Graafsma SJ, Kranendonk SE, Hermus AR, et al. (2007) Low vitamin B6, and not plasma homocysteine concentration, as risk factor for abdominal aortic aneurysm: A retrospective case-control study. J Vasc Surg 45:701–705.
20. Sofi F, Marcucci R, Giusti B, Pratesi G, Lari B, et al. (2005) High levels of homocysteine, lipoprotein (a) and plasminogen activator inhibitor-1 are present in patients with abdominal aortic aneurysm. Thromb Haemost 94:1094–1098.
21. Warsi AA, Davies B, Morris-Stiff G, Hullin D, Lewis MH (2004) Abdominal aortic aneurysm and its correlation to plasma homocysteine, and vitamins. Eur J Vasc Endovasc Surg 27:75–79.
22. Spark JI, Laws P, Fitridge R (2003) The incidence of hyperhomocysteinaemia in vascular patients. Eur J Vasc Endovasc Surg 26:558–561.
23. Brunelli T, Prisco D, Fedi S, Rogolino A, Farsi A, et al. (2000) High prevalence of mild hyperhomocysteinemia in patients with abdominal aortic aneurysm. J Vasc Surg 32:531–536.
24. Moroz P, Le MT, Norman PE (2007) Homocysteine and abdominal aortic aneurysms. ANZ J Surg 77:329–332.
25. Wells GA, Shea B, O'Connell D, Peterson J, Welch V, et al. (2013) The Newcastle-Ottawa Scale (NOS) for assessing the quality if nonrand omized studies in meta-analyses. http://www.ohri. ca/programs/clinical_epidem iology/oxford.asp. [last accessed 30/3/2013].
26. Higgins JP, Thompson SG, Deeks JJ, Altman DG (2003) Measuring inconsistency in meta-analyses. BMJ 327:557–560.
27. DerSimonian R, Laird N (1986) Meta-analysis in clinical trials. Control Clin Trials 7:177–188.
28. Begg CB, Mazumdar M (1994) Operating characteristics of a rank correlation test for publication bias. Biometrics 50:1088–1101.
29. Egger M, Davey Smith G, Schneider M, Minder C (1997) Bias in meta-analysis detected by a simple, graphical test. BMJ 315:629–634.
30. Forsdahl SH, Singh K, Solberg S, Jacobsen BK (2009) Risk factors for abdominal aortic aneurysms: A 7-year prospective study: The tromso study, 1994–2001. Circulation 119:2202–2208.
31. Krishna SM, Dear A, Craig JM, Norman PE, Golledge J (2013) The potential role of homocysteine mediated DNA methylation and associated epigenetic changes in abdominal aortic aneurysm formation. Atherosclerosis 228:295–305.
32. Feng J, Zhang Z, Kong W, Liu B, Xu Q, et al. (2009) Regulatory T cells ameliorate hyperhomocysteinaemia-accelerated atherosclerosis in apoE-/- mice. Cardiovasc Res 84:155–163.
33. Liu Z, Luo H, Zhang L, Huang Y, Liu B, et al. (2012) Hyperhomocysteinemia exaggerates adventitial inflammation and angiotensin II-induced abdominal aortic aneurysm in mice. Circ Res 111:1261–1273.
34. Jourdheuil-Rahmani D, Rolland PH, Rosset E, Branchereau A, Garcon D (1997) Homocysteine induces synthesis of a serine elastase in arterial smooth muscle cells from multi-organ donors. Cardiovasc Res 34:597–602.
35. Ke XD, Foucault-Bertaud A, Genovesio C, Dignat-George F, Lamy E, et al. (2010) Homocysteine modulates the proteolytic potential of human arterial smooth muscle cells through a reactive oxygen species dependant mechanism. Mol Cell Biochem 335:203–210.
36. den Heijer M, Graafsma S, Lee SY, van Landeghem B, Kluijtmans L, et al. (2005) Homocysteine levels before and after methionine loading in 51 Dutch families. Eur J Hum Genet 13:753–762.
37. Jee SH, Song KS, Shim WH, Kim HK, Suh I, et al. (2002) Major gene evidence after MTHFR-segregation analysis of serum homocysteine in families of patients undergoing coronary arteriography. Hum Genet 111:128–135.

10

ANG-1 TIE-2 and BMPR Signalling Defects Are Not Seen in the Nitrofen Model of Pulmonary Hypertension and Congenital Diaphragmatic Hernia

Harriet Jane Corbett[1,2]*, Marilyn Gwen Connell[1], David Garth Fernig[3], Paul Damion Losty[1,2]¶, Edwin Chitran Jesudason[1,2]¶

1 Division of Child Health, Institute of Translational Medicine, The University of Liverpool, Liverpool, United Kingdom, 2 Department of Paediatric Surgery, Alder Hey Children's National Health Service (NHS) Foundation Trust, Liverpool, United Kingdom, 3 Department of Chemical and Structural Biology, Institute of Integrative Biology, The University of Liverpool, Liverpool, United Kingdom

Abstract

Background: Pulmonary hypertension (PH) is a lethal disease that is associated with characteristic histological abnormalities of the lung vasculature and defects of angiopoetin-1 (ANG-1), TIE-2 and bone morphogenetic protein receptor (BMPR)-related signalling. We hypothesized that if these signalling defects cause PH generically, they will be readily identifiable perinatally in congenital diaphragmatic hernia (CDH), where the typical pulmonary vascular changes are present before birth and are accompanied by PH after birth.

Methods: CDH (predominantly left-sided, LCDH) was created in Sprague-Dawley rat pups by e9.5 maternal nitrofen administration. Left lungs from normal and LCDH pups were compared at fetal and postnatal time points for ANG-1, TIE-2, phosphorylated-TIE-2, phosphorylated-SMAD1/5/8 and phosphorylated-ERK1/2 by immunoprecipitation and Western blotting of lung protein extracts and by immunohistochemistry on lung sections.

Results: In normal lung, pulmonary ANG-1 protein levels fall between fetal and postnatal life, while TIE-2 levels increase. Over the corresponding time period, LCDH lung retained normal expression of ANG-1, TIE-2, phosphorylated-TIE-2 and, downstream of BMPR, phosphorylated-SMAD1/5/8 and phosphorylated-p44/42.

Conclusion: In PH and CDH defects of ANG-1/TIE-2/BMPR-related signalling are not essential for the lethal vasculopathy.

Editor: James West, Vanderbilt University Medical Center, United States of America

Funding: HJC was supported by a Clinical Training Fellowship awarded by the Royal College of Surgeons of England, and Medical Research Council (Medical Research Council grant number G84/6485). ECJ is supported by a Medical Research Council New Investigator Award. DGF is funded by Cancer and Polio Research Fund Laboratories and North West Cancer Research Fund. MGC was the Senior Experimental Officer, Funded by The University of Liverpool. PDL is Professor of Paediatric Surgery, funded by the University of Liverpool. The funders had no role in study design, data collection and analysis, decision to publish, or preparation of the manuscript.

Competing Interests: The authors have declared that no competing interests exist.

* E-mail: harriet.corbett@alderhey.nhs.uk

¶ These authors contributed equally to this work.

Introduction

Pulmonary arterial hypertension (PH) remains a lethal disease: understanding its pathogenesis is a key priority in the search for effective therapies. Receptors for the TGF-beta super-family appear to play pivotal roles since mutations in the genes for bone morphogenetic protein receptor 2 (*bmpr2*) and anaplastic lymphoma kinase-1 (ALK-1) are implicated in familial PAH [1–3]. Even in non-familial PAH, altered BMPR-2 signalling may result from reduced pulmonary expression of BMPR-1A (with which BMPR-2 normally heterodimerizes for function) [4]. Reduced BMPR-1A expression is induced in vitro by vascular growth factor, angiopoetin-1 (ANG-1) signalling through TIE-2; elevations in both of these are strongly correlated with disease severity in non-familial PAH lung [4]. Increased ANG-1/TIE-2 signalling is therefore proposed to interfere indirectly with BMPR-2 activity to cause non-familial PH. Conversely, however, the ANG-1 and TIE-2 changes are argued by others to result from, rather than cause, PH [5–7].

Given these contrasting views, we sought to test if dysregulated ANG-1/TIE-2/BMPR-related signalling is required for PH. Human newborns with congenital diaphragmatic hernia (CDH) frequently die due to refractory PH despite inhaled nitric oxide (iNO) and extracorporeal membrane oxygenation (ECMO) [8,9]. We sought to test ANG-1/TIE-2/BMPR-related signalling in an experimental rodent model of CDH induced by maternal administration of nitrofen [10]. Resulting CDH fetuses and newborns have hypoplastic lungs featuring diminished airway and vascular branching, reduced cell proliferation, abnormal growth factor responses and heparan sulphate co-factor expression, altered smooth muscle contractility and Ca2+ signalling, as well as striking histological features of PH in the vasculature [10–

21]. Therefore, if dysregulated ANG-1/TIE-2/BMPR-related signalling really is a significant driver of PH, we hypothesize that such dysfunction should be apparent prenatally in the nitrofen CDH model.

Materials and Methods

Animal Model: Creation of CDH and Lung Harvest

All experiments were approved under the Animals - UK Scientific Procedures Act 1986, project licence number PPL 40/2293 and personal licence number PIL 40/8001. All efforts were made to minimize suffering and all surgery was performed under general anaesthesia. Time-mated Sprague-Dawley rats were used to create CDH. Day 0 of gestation was taken as the day of discovery of a vaginal plug (term = day 22). To induce left CDH (LCDH), 100 mg of nitrofen was dissolved in 2 mL of olive oil and gavage fed to dams on day 9.5 of gestation [10]. Untreated animals served as controls [22,23]. Fetal lungs were harvested on days 17.5, 18.5, 20.5 and 21.5 of gestation (Figure 1). Control and nitrofen exposed dams were given a lethal dose of intraperitoneal sodium pentobarbital (100 mg/Kg) and fetuses delivered by caesarean section. Since the vasculopathy is more severe in ipsilateral CDH lung, left lungs were harvested from control and LCDH fetuses [24]. Postnatal lung tissue was also harvested from rat pups after a short period of air-breathing. These pups were delivered by caesarean section with the dam under general anaesthesia. Pups were rubbed dry to stimulate them and encourage the onset of spontaneous breathing, placed in a warm incubator at 30°C in ambient air and observed for respiratory effort, movement and colour. Pups from both nitrofen treated and control dams were sacrificed after fixed time periods (between 5 min and 1 h) by cervical dislocation. Control lung tissue from older animals was harvested after cervical dislocation (12 h old pups) or a lethal dose of intraperitoneal sodium pentobarbital (1 week old and adult rats). Lung tissue for Western blotting and immunoprecipitation was snap-frozen in liquid nitrogen and stored at −80°C. Lung tissue for immunohistochemistry was fixed in 4% (w/v) paraformaldehyde in phosphate-buffered saline pH 7.4 (PBS) for 4 h, washed in PBS and then cryoprotected by immersion in 20% (w/v) sucrose overnight. The tissue was then either embedded in gelatine (7.5% (w/v) gelatine in 15% (w/v) sucrose in PBS) and coated with embedding medium or directly coated with embedding medium before freezing by immersion in pre-chilled isopentone at −40°C. Frozen fixed tissue was stored at −35°C until use.

Western blotting and immunoprecipitation

Western blotting of samples from e17.5 and e18.5 lungs comprised 2–3 pooled left lungs. A single left lung was used as an independent sample in older age groups with the exception of 1 week old and adult rats where a left lung fragment of equivalent volume to an e21.5 left lung was used. Tissue was manually homogenized in 0.5–1 mL of ice-cold modified radio-immuno-precipitation assay (RIPA) buffer (50 mM Tris-HCl pH 7.4, 1% (v/v) NP-40, 0.25% (w/v) Na-deoxycholate, 150 mM NaCl, 1 mM EDTA, 1 mM PMSF, 1 mM activated Na3VO4, 1 mM NaF and 1× complete mini protease tablet/10 mL buffer). The homogenate was left on ice for 10 min then centrifuged at 14,000 rpm for 10 min at 4°C. The insoluble material in the pellet was discarded. Total protein content of the supernatant was determined using a bicinchoninic acid kit based on the method described by Smith et al. (1985) and total protein concentration of the supernatant was adjusted to between 0.75 and 1.25 μg/mL with RIPA buffer. Electrophoresis sample buffer (5×, 250 mM Tris-HCl pH 6.8, 10% (w/v) SDS, 5% (v/v) beta mercaptoethanol, 10% (v/v) glycerol, 0.01% (w/v) bromophenol blue) was added to give a final 1× concentration of buffer and the sample was boiled for 5 min.

Samples containing approximately 24 μg of total lung protein were separated in 8, 10 and 12% (w/v) polyacrylamide gels by SDS-PAGE. A C6 BMP4-stimulated cell lysate was used as a positive control for phosphorylated SMAD1/5/8 (p-SMAD1/5/8) and phosphorylated ERK1/2 (p-ERK1/2). Separated polypeptides were electro-transferred onto nitrocellulose membrane. Membranes were blocked by incubating in 5% (w/v) non-fat milk solution/TRIS- or phosphate-buffered saline (TBS/PBS)/0.1% (v/v) Tween-20 for 1 h at room temperature. Membranes were then incubated with primary antibody at 4°C. Antibodies against p-SMAD1/5/8 and p-ERK1/2 were used at 1:1000 dilution in TBS/0.1% (v/v) Tween-20 with 2.5% (w/v) bovine serum albumin (p-SMAD1/5/8) or 5% (w/v) non-fat milk (p-ERK1/2). Antibodies against ANG-1 and TIE-2 were used at 1:1000 dilution in PBS/0.1% (v/v) Tween-20 with 5% (w/v) non-fat milk.

Following overnight incubation with primary antibody, membranes were washed five times in TBS/0.1% (v/v) Tween-20 (TBS/T) over 25 min, then incubated with horse-radish peroxidase (HRP) labelled anti-goat (ANG-1, TIE-2), anti-rabbit (p-SMAD1/5/8) or anti mouse (p-ERK1/2) antibodies for 1 h at room temperature. After a further wash cycle, membranes were incubated with chemiluminescence reagent and immunoreactive bands were imaged with the ChemiDoc XRS System using Quantity-One software. After imaging, membranes probed for p-ERK1/2 were incubated with stripping buffer (40 mM Tris-HCl pH 6.8, 0.67% (w/v) SDS, 0.3% beta mercaptoethanol) for 30 min at room temperature, washed in TBS/T and re-incubated overnight with antibodies against ERK1/2 or actin. Membranes were re-washed and incubated with appropriate secondary antibodies. All other membranes were simply washed, re-incubated with anti-actin followed by the appropriate secondary antibody. After a final wash cycle membranes were incubated with chemiluminescence reagent and imaged, as described above.

Immunoprecipitation

Lung protein extracts from e20.5 and e21.5 (800–900 μg protein) were made up to 400 μL with RIPA buffer. The protein extract was incubated overnight with 40 μL of anti-phosphorylated tyrosine cross-linked to protein-A agarose beads (clone 4G10) on a rotating wheel at 4°C. The samples were then centrifuged (14,000 rpm, 10 min, 4°C), the supernatant discarded and the agarose bead slurry washed with ice-cold RIPA buffer, then ice-cold PBS to reduce detergent levels. The beads were re-suspended in electrophoresis sample buffer to give a final 1× concentration of buffer and the mixture boiled for 5 minutes. Equal volumes of supernatant were subjected to SDS-PAGE and Western blotting with TIE-2 antibody.

Immunohistochemistry

Tissue sections 7 μM thick were cut using a cryostat and thaw-mounted onto slides, dried at room temperature and re-frozen until use. Slides for incubation with p-SMAD1/5/8 antibody were incubated in antigen retrieval buffer (10 mM sodium citrate, pH 6.0) at just below 100°C for 10 min, cooled in the buffer for 30 min then washed. Sections were incubated with blocking buffer (PBS, 20% (v/v) goat serum) for 30 min then incubated overnight at 4°C with p-SMAD1/5/8 antibody in buffer (PBS, 0.1% (v/v) Tween-20, 5% (v/v) goat serum). Slides for incubation with TIE-2 antibody were incubated directly with blocking buffer (PBS, 20% (v/v) rabbit serum) for 30 min then incubated overnight at 4°C

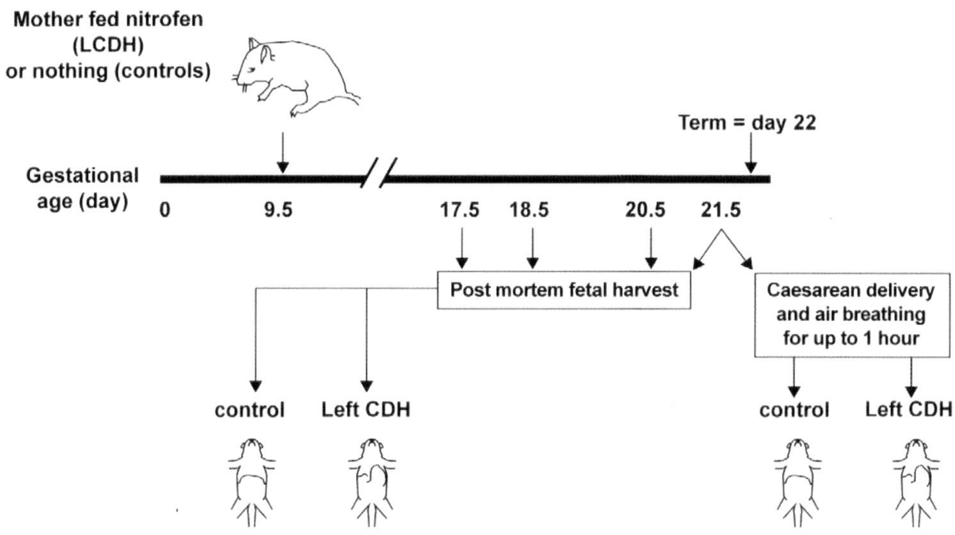

Figure 1. The experimental model. Outline of the experimental model.

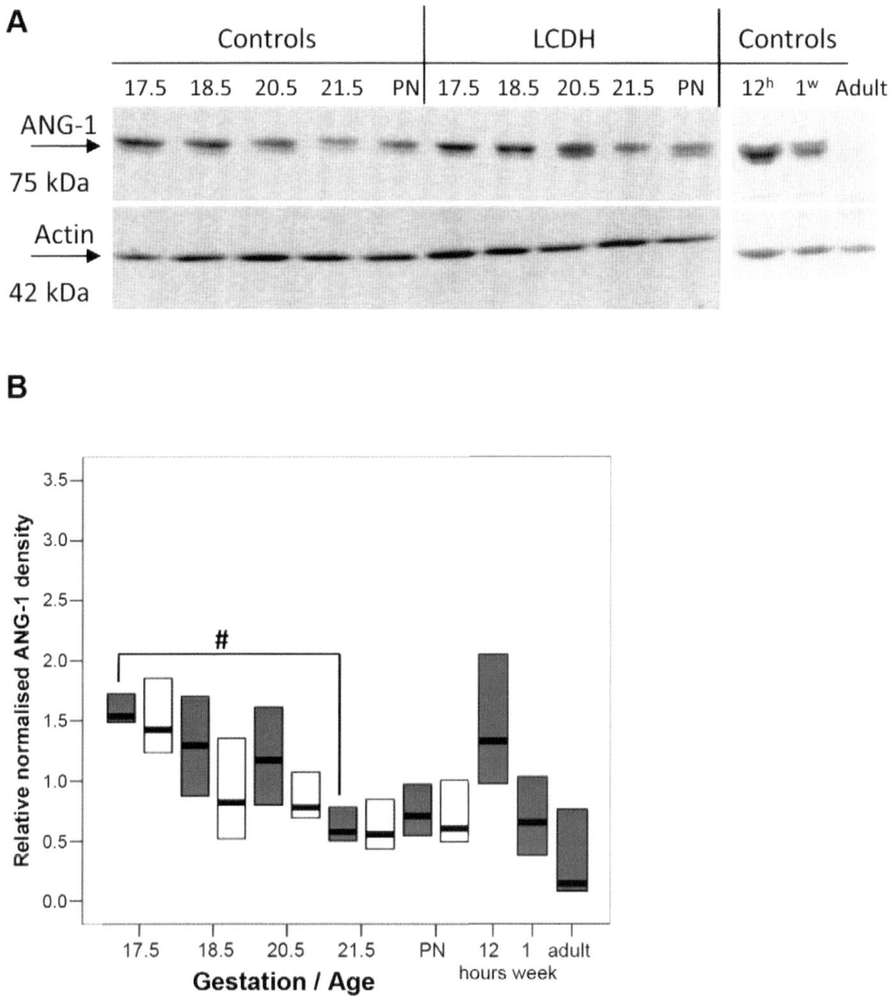

Figure 2. Western blots and graphs showing ANG-1 and actin immunoreactivity. Western blots showing ANG-1 and actin immunoreactivity in control and LCDH lung (**a**). ANG-1 immunoreactivity in control (grey) and LCDH lung (white boxes) expressed as median (bar) and inter-quartile ranges (box) (**b**). Statistical analysis found a significant linear trend (#) in the fall in ANG-1.

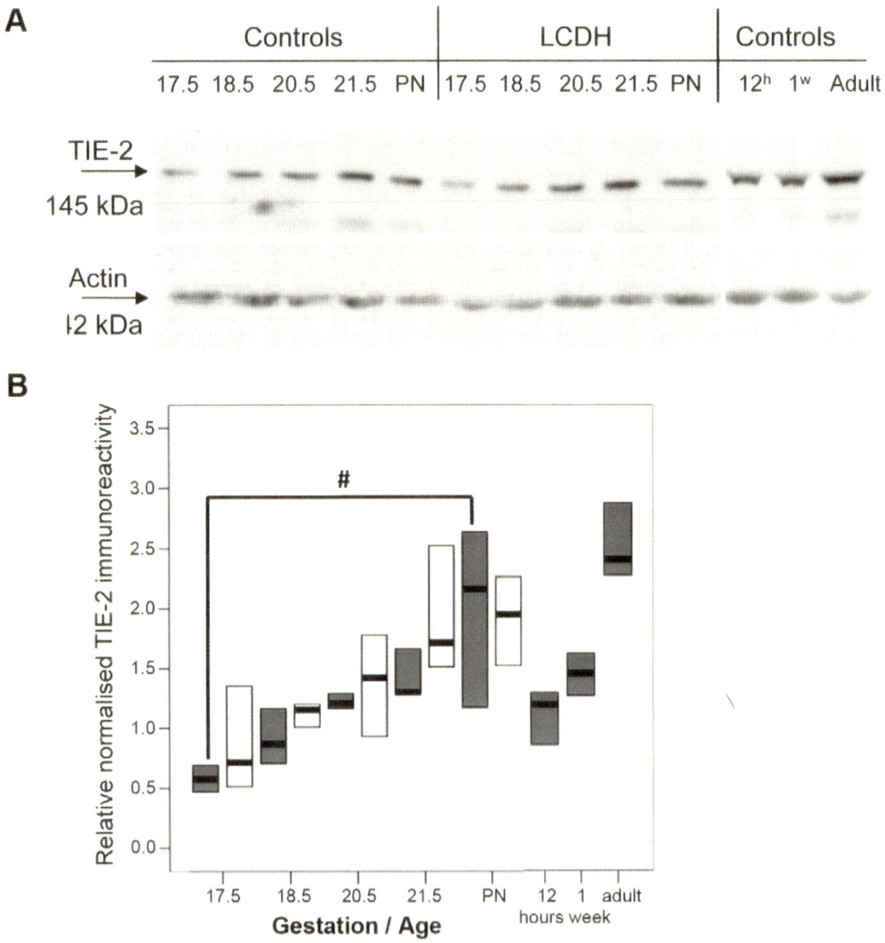

Figure 3. Western blots and graphs showing TIE-2 and actin immunoreactivity. Western blots showing TIE-2 and actin immunoreactivity in control and LCDH lung (**a**). TIE-2 immunoreactivity in control (grey) and LCDH lung (white boxes) expressed as median (bar) and inter-quartile ranges (box) (**b**). Statistical analysis found a significant linear trend (#) in the rise in TIE-2.

with TIE-2 antibodies in buffer (PBS, 0.1% (v/v) Tween-20, 5% (v/v) rabbit serum). Slides were then washed in PBS and sections incubated with fluoroscein isothiocyanate conjugated (FITC) anti-goat antibodies (TIE-2) or anti-rabbit antibodies (p-SMAD1/5/8) in PBS for 2 h. Following further washes the slides were mounted in fluorescent mounting medium and visualized using fluorescence and the appropriate filter. Control sections were treated as above except the primary antibody was omitted.

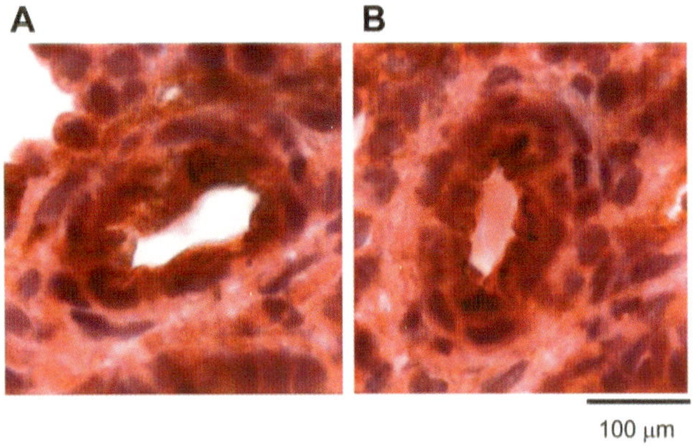

Figure 4. Photomicrographs showing TIE-2 immunoreactivity. Photomicrographs showing similar TIE-2 immunoreactivity (brown DAB staining) in the endothelium of rat pulmonary vasculature at gestation e20.5 in (**A**) control lung (manification ×100) and (**B**) LCDH lung (×100).

For diaminobenzidine (DAB) staining, after incubation in blocking buffer (TBS, 20% (v/v) serum) slides were incubated in 0.3% (v/v) hydrogen peroxide in TBS for 15 minutes to block endogenous peroxide activity, then rinsed in TBS. Sections were incubated overnight at 4°C with TIE-2 or p-SMAD1/5/8 antibody in buffer (TBS, 0.1% (v/v) Tween-20, 5% (v/v) serum). The following morning slides were washed in TBS then sections were incubated with biotin conjugated anti-goat or anti-rabbit antibodies in TBS for 45 min, washed and then incubated with a streptavidin-biotinylated peroxidase mixture for a further 45 min. Slides were washed again before incubating with DAB (Fast 3,3′-diaminobenzidine tablet set) for 3–5 min and then thoroughly rinsed with running water. Slides were lightly stained with Mayer's haemalum and 1% aqueous eosin before mounting with DPX mounting medium and visualisation with light microscopy. Control sections were treated as above except the primary antibody was omitted.

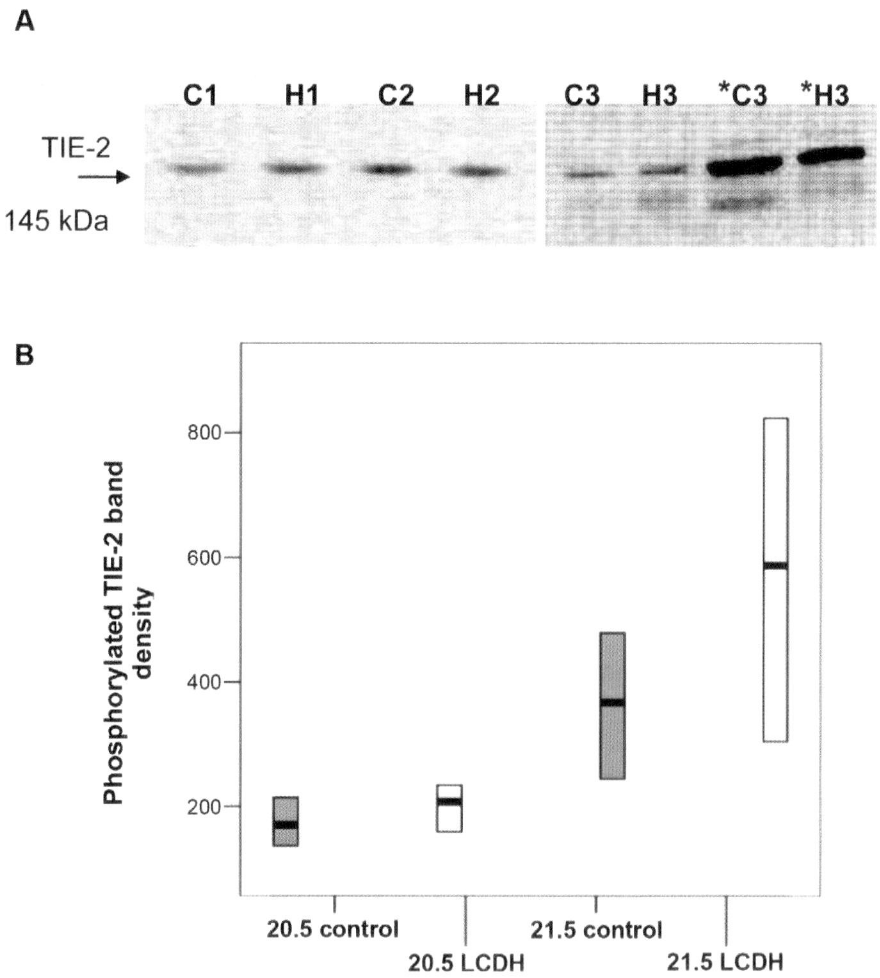

Figure 5. Western blot and graph showing phosphorylated (p) TIE-2 immunoreactivity. Western blot showing p-TIE-2 immunoreactivity in e20.5 lung in three contempraneously prepared sample pairs, 1,2 and 3 (C = control, H = LCDH). Total TIE-2 expression in sample pair 3 is shown (*C3 & *H3) as a positive control (**a**). Normalised p-TIE-2 immunoreactivity in control (grey) and LCDH lung (white boxes) expressed as median and inter-quartile ranges (**b**).

Materials

Rats were purchased from Charles River Ltd., UK. Nitrofen was purchased from Zheijang Chemicals, China. Embedding medium (Cryo-M-bed) was purchased from Bright Instrument Company, Huntingdon, UK. Complete mini protease tablets were purchased from Roche, Switzerland. The bicinchoninic acid Kit, Tween-20, anti-actin antibody, FITC-conjugated anti-goat and anti-rabbit antibodies and the Fast 3,3′-diaminobenzidine tablet set were purchased from Sigma-Aldrich, UK. Antibodies against p-SMAD1/5/8, p-ERK1/2 and ERK1/2 were purchased from Cell Signaling Technology, USA. The C6 BMP4-stimulated cell lysate was donated by Cell Signaling Technology. Antibodies against ANG-1 and TIE-2 were purchased from R & D Systems, UK. The nitrocellulose membrane (Hi-bond) was purchased from Amersham Biosciences, GE Healthcare UK Ltd. SuperSignal West Dura Substrate chemiluminescence reagent was purchased from Pierce, UK. The anti-phosphorylated tyrosine antibody cross-linked to protein-A agarose beads (clone 4G10) was purchased from Upstate, Millipore Corporation, USA. Biotin conjugated anti-goat and anti-rabbit antibodies, and the strepta-vidin-biotinylated peroxidase mixture was purchased from Dako, Denmark.

Data analysis

Photon output originating from individual bands of immunoreactivity was recorded as intensity per mm2 (INT/mm2) and only measurements that were not saturated, as determined by the ChemiDoc imager, were used. Background intensity for each membrane was measured and subtracted from the intensity measurements recorded from immunoreactive bands to give normalised density. Protein level per immunoreactive band was calculated relative to actin level to give normalised relative protein levels. Each experiment was repeated between 4 and 7 times and normalised relative band densities reported as medians and inter-quartile ranges (IQR). Statistical differences between median band density for the groups (control and LCDH) at and between each gestational time-point were determined by Mann-Whitney U test using SPSS version 13. Analysis of the trends seen according to gestational age was done by Oneway ANOVA with polynomial contrasts (SPSS version 13). A p-value of <0.05 was considered significant.

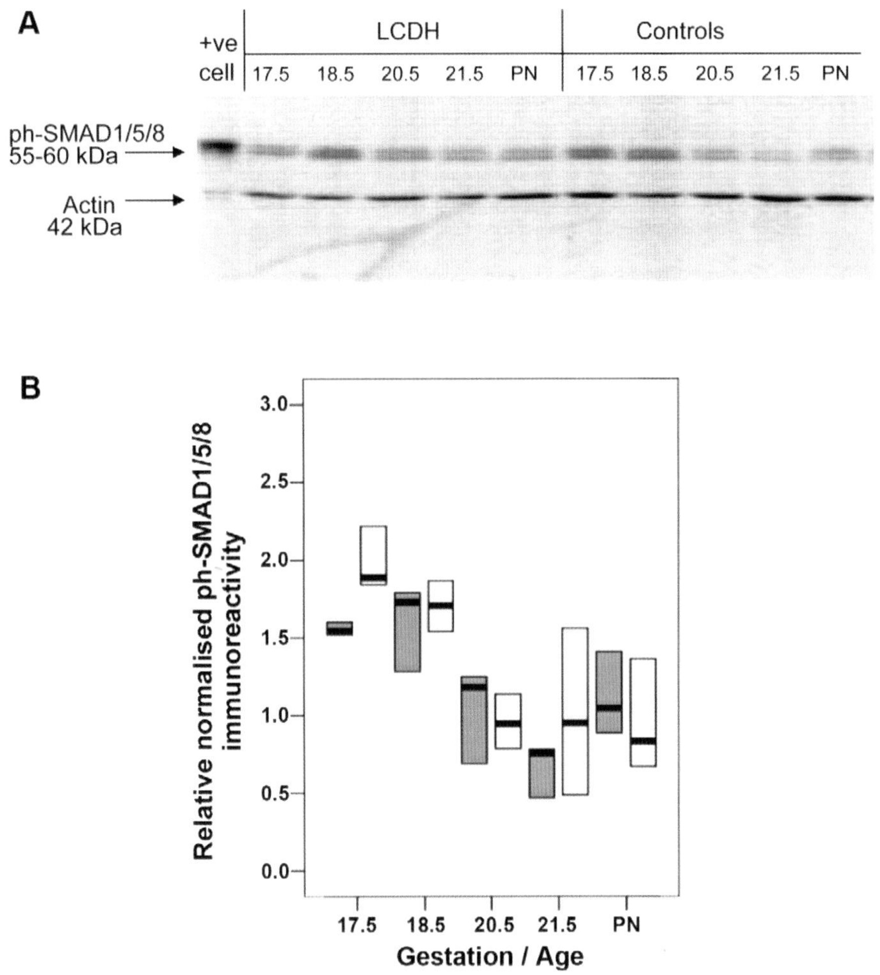

Figure 6. Western blot and graph showing p-SMAD1/5/8 and actin immunoreactivity. Western blot showing p-SMAD1/5/8 and actin immunoreactivity (+ve cell = positive control cell lysate, BMP stimulated C6 cells) (**a**). p-SMAD1/5/8 immunoreactivity in control (grey) and LCDH lung (white boxes) expressed as median (bar) and inter-quartile ranges (box) (**b**).

Results

ANG-1 and TIE-2 are developmentally regulated but unaltered in perinatal CDH lung

To test if increased ANG-1/TIE-2 activity suppresses BMPR signalling to generate PH as postulated in human adult studies, we first tested if ANG-1/TIE-2 activity was abnormally increased in the perinatal CDH lung with its established pulmonary vascular changes typical of PH. Immunoblotting with the antibody to ANG-1 revealed a single band of immunoreactivity corresponding to 75 kDa (Figure 2a). There was a significant change in ANG-1 protein level with the developmental stage of the lung (Figure 2b & c). ANG-1 protein levels in control lung fall significantly from e17.5 and e18.5 to a low level at e21.5. From the low level at e21.5 there is a marked rise by 12 h after birth. The ANG-1 level detected in adult lung was significantly lower than in e17.5, e18.5 and e20.5 fetal lung, as well as being significantly lower than the level recorded in 12 h old lung (Figure 2c). Statistical analysis of the fall in ANG-1 between e17.5 and postnatal by Oneway ANOVA found an unweighted linear trend F value of 6.87 with a p value of 0.015, suggesting a significant linear trend. There was no significant difference between the level of ANG-1 protein between control and LCDH lung (Figure 2b). The decline of ANG-1 protein levels in control lung between the early (e17.5) and late fetal period (e21.5) was also mirrored in LCDH lung with a significant linear trend (F value 12.38, $p = 0.002$). Later postnatal time-points could not be examined in LCDH lung, since survival for nitrofen-exposed pups is usually less than 30 min.

Immunoblotting with an antibody to TIE-2 revealed a dominant band of immunoreactivity corresponding to a size of 145 kDa (Figure 3a). There was a significant change in the level of TIE-2 and the stage of development of the lung (Figure 3b & c). TIE-2 levels in control lung rise significantly from low levels at e17.5 to a high level in PN lung. From the high level in PN lung there is a fall by 12 h of age and then TIE-2 levels rise to a maximum in adult lung (Figure 3c). Statistical analysis of the rise in TIE-2 between e17.5 and PN by Oneway ANOVA found an unweighted linear trend F value of 21.16 with a p value of <0.0001 suggesting a significant linear trend. There was no significant difference between the level of TIE-2 protein between control and LCDH lung (Figure 3b). Again, the same trend of a rise in TIE-2 protein level was observed in LCDH lung between the early fetal period (e17.5) and postnatal. Analysis of this trend in LCDH lung also showed a significant linear trend (F value 13.17, $p = 0.001$).

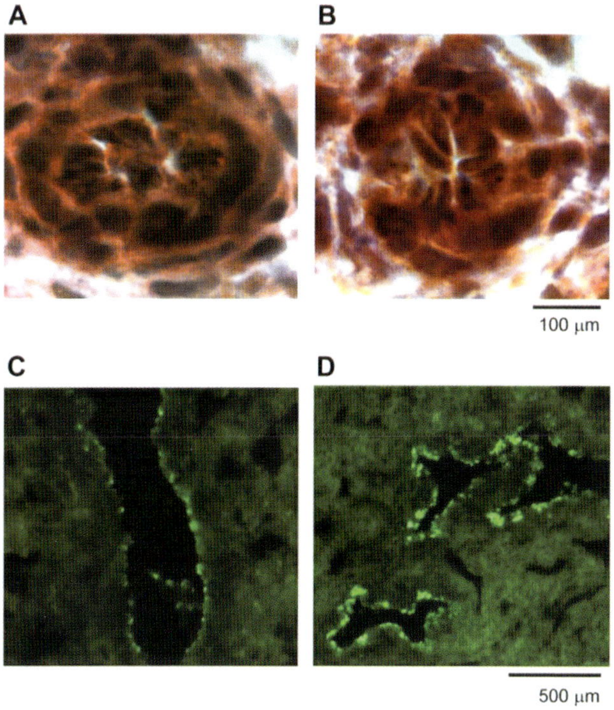

Figure 7. Photomicrographs showing p-SMAD1/5/8 immunoreactivity. Photomicrographs showing similar p-SMAD1/5/8 immunoreactivity (brown DAB staining) in the endothelium of rat pulmonary vasculature in (**A**) control lung at gestation e19.5 (manification ×100) and (**B**) LCDH lung, at gestation e19.5 (×100). p-SMAD1/5/8 immunoreactivity in the airway epithelium in (**C**) control lung at gestation e21.5 (manification ×25) and (**D**) LCDH lung, at gestation e21.5 (×25).

Furthermore, TIE-2 immunoreactivity and activation appeared comparable between normal and CDH lung: TIE-2 localised to the endothelium in fetal (e20.5) and adult pulmonary arteries (Figure 4) with no gross differences in immunohistochemical staining intensity; phosphorylated (activated) TIE-2 protein levels determined by Western blotting were not significantly different between control and LCDH lung at e20.5 and e21.5 (Figures 5a & b).

Signalling downstream of BMPR appears normal in perinatal CDH lung

In the absence of pathological changes in ANG-1/TIE-2 signalling, we next tested if BMPR signalling was being dysregulated by another pathway by comparing normal and perinatal CDH lung for the pulmonary SMAD and ERK1/2 elements of downstream BMPR signalling. Immunoblotting with antibody to p-SMAD1/5/8 revealed a dual band of immunoreactivity corresponding to a size of 55–60 kDa in control and LCDH lung extracts, and the positive control cell lysate (Figure 6a). There was no significant difference between the level of p-SMAD1/5/8 protein between control and LCDH lung at any gestation time studied (Figure 6b). p-SMAD1/5/8 immunoreactivity was localised to the vascular endothelium and the airway epithelium in fetal rat lung (Figure 7). High power images acquired using diaminobenzidine staining (Figures 7 A & B) revealed staining of the cytoplasm and nuclei of the endothelial cells of the pulmonary vasculature. Low power images acquired using FITC staining (Figures 7 C & D) revealed airway epithelial p-SMAD1/5/8 staining, but vascular endothelial staining was not detected by this method. There were no gross differences in localisation or intensity of p-SMAD1/5/8 staining between control and LCDH lung at e19.5 and e21.5.

Immunoblotting with antibody to p-ERK1/2 revealed two bands of immunoreactivity corresponding to sizes of 42 and 44 kDa in control and LCDH lung extract (Figure 8a). Using actin to calculate relative protein expression, there was no significant difference between the level of p-ERK1/2 protein between control and LCDH lung at the gestation times studied (Figure 8b). Using a total ERK1/2 antibody to calculate the protein activity relative to the total amount of ERK1/2 (Figure 8c), it was confirmed that there was no significant difference between the level of p-ERK1/2 protein between control and LCDH lung.

Discussion

Pulmonary hypertension is associated with high mortality in newborns, children and adults. Uncovering the signalling abnormalities that underpin PH remains a key component in the search for new and effective therapies. TGF-beta super family signalling appears critical as familial PH is associated with not only *bmpr2* mutations but also alterations in other related pathways such as ALK [1,2,3]. Signalling downstream of the TGF-beta super family receptors includes SMADs and, in certain cell types, mitogen-activated protein kinases (MAPKs) such as ERK1/2, with some context-dependent variation [25,26]. Experimental PH and *bmpr2* insufficiency models appear to reduce SMAD signalling with similar findings observed in humans with familial PH [27–33]. It is noteworthy that upregulation of MAPKs in experimental PH varies throughout the course of disease. Intriguingly, *bmpr2* gene therapy attenuates experimental PH even in the absence of *bmpr2* mutations [34].

A unifying model of BMPR dysfunction to explain both familial and non-familial PH has emerged from human data showing enhanced ANG-1/TIE-2 signalling suppresses BMPR1A, and hence BMPR2 activity in non-familial PH [4]. To evaluate this further, it is critical to determine whether the signalling defects observed in PH in this and other studies represent causal changes, mere correlation or even a protective response to PH [5,6]. Given the insidious onset of adult PH, it is not currently feasible to test this in human subjects. Similarly debate persists about the characteristic pathological changes observed in the pulmonary vasculature and whether they are the cause of PH, or conversely, a consequence of it.

Newborns with CDH frequently die as a result of refractory PH [35,36]. Unlike those developing persistent pulmonary hypertension of the newborn (PPHN) from other causes (notably meconium aspiration syndrome), infants with CDH do not respond consistently well to inhaled nitric oxide (iNO) [8,37]. While this may indicate the inherent heterogeneity of PH, the refractory nature of PH in CDH suggests it may have more in common with adult PH. Taking these concepts, it is striking to note that the pulmonary vascular changes that are so characteristic of adult PH are also present in prenatal CDH lung. This supports the view that such vascular abnormalities precede and are perhaps causative of PH. In view of these shared pathological defects, we sought to determine if the signalling aberrations identified in adult humans with PH could also be observed in prenatal and newborn CDH lung. We sought to also explore whether such signalling defects were responsible for PH.

To access prenatal and neonatal CDH lung, we utilised the leading CDH experimental model which closely phenocopies human CDH possessing both the characteristic pulmonary vascular changes of PH and some abnormalities of endothelial

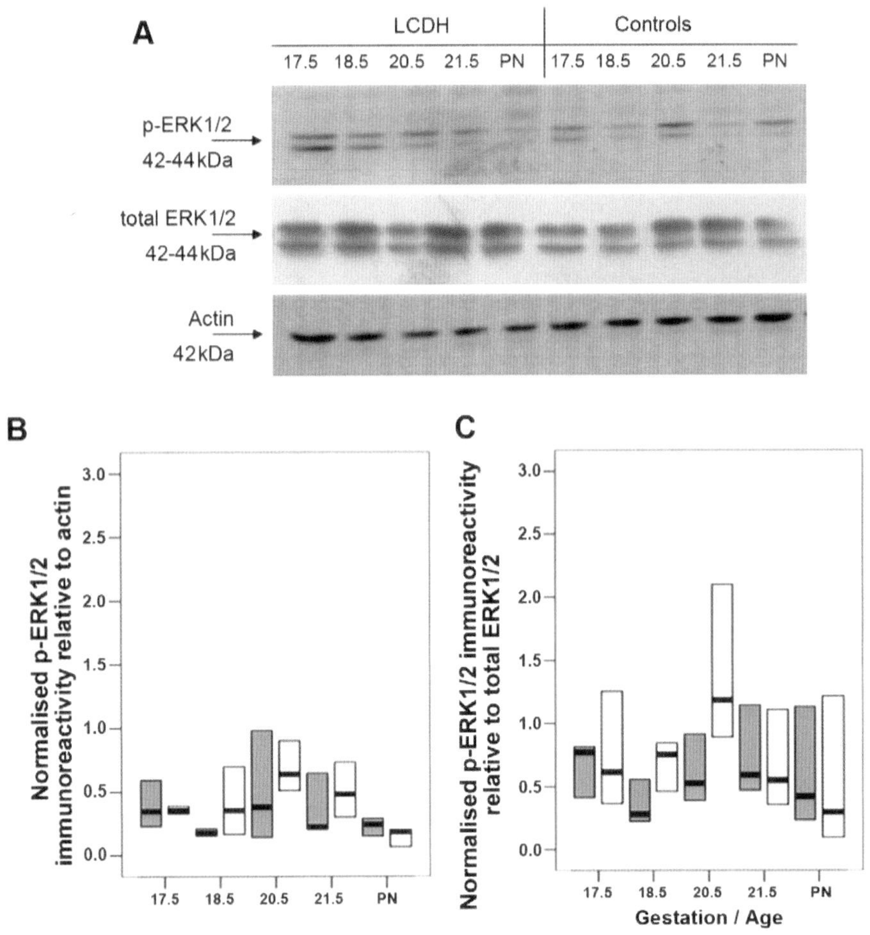

Figure 8. Western blots and graphs showing p-ERK1/2, total ERK1/2 and actin immunoreactivity. Western blot showing p-ERK1/2, total ERK1/2 and actin immunoreactivity (**a**). p-ERK1/2 immunoreactivity relative to actin (**b**) and total ERK1/2 (**c**) in control lung (grey boxes) and LCDH lung (white boxes) expressed as median (bar) and inter-quartile ranges (box).

nitric oxide synthase (eNOS) signalling too [23,38,39]. In this model, we have shown that the ANG-1/TIE-2/BMPR-related signalling defects observed in adult PH patients are not present prenatally or even in the newborn period despite the presence of the shared pulmonary vasculopathy. We also demonstrated that both pulmonary levels of ANG-1 and TIE-2 are developmentally regulated with significant changes noted during the critical transition of the pulmonary vasculature from prenatal to postnatal life. Hence, while our data indicate that ANG-1/TIE-2 signalling is not dysregulated as a cause of PH in CDH, this pathway may still be crucially important in adaptations of the lung vasculature at birth.

There are a number of important caveats to these findings. Firstly, different species may intrinsically regulate ANG-1 and TIE-2 differently through development [40]: hypoplastic human fetal lung associated with a range of conditions including CDH showed minimal gestational change in ANG-1 but a fall in TIE-2 [41]; in baboon lung both ANG-1 and TIE-2 mRNA levels have been reported to rise during gestation [42]; in a murine CDH model, raised ANG-1 protein levels were transiently observed in late gestation lung but, in keeping with our observations, normal levels returned after birth [26]. Secondly, we found striking p-SMAD1/5/8 staining with FITC in large airway epithelium at the time points studied. Vascular endothelial staining was only detected with DAB stained tissue using high powered magnification. Predominant airway staining has been described previously and it is possible that most SMAD1/5/8 activity on Western blotting was of airway rather than vascular origin [43,44]. Hence, relevant changes in vascular SMAD1/5/8 activity may have been masked by larger and invariant airway expression. Third, unlike studies that have reported respectively either increased total lung ERK1/2 activity or reduced ERK1/2 activity, we identified no differences in ERK1/2 activation between normal and LCDH lung [23,45]. Different experimental protocols and species differences may underlie some of this variation, but our data indicate that altered pulmonary ERK1/2 activity is not causative in PH associated with CDH. A further observation herein reported relates to the expression of activated protein levels relative to total actin or total ERK1/2. Takahashi *et al.* reported activated protein as a ratio of the total amount of ERK1/2 and concluded that changes in MAPK activity were not due to induction of total protein [28]. Further, our findings show that when levels of activated ERK1/2 protein were measured relative to both actin and total ERK1/2, we still detected no significant differences.

In summary, ANG-1 and TIE-2 are developmentally regulated in perinatal lung and may participate in pulmonary adaptation to extrauterine life. However, ANG-1/TIE-2/BMPR-related signalling defects are not essential for the pulmonary vasculopathy characteristic of PH in CDH. Therefore, therapies to reduce elevated levels of ANG-1/TIE-2 signalling in adult humans with

PH must be interpreted with caution since these signalling changes may be either epiphenomena or even protective responses. Interestingly, ANG-1 is currently being tested therapeutically in a range of conditions including myocardial infarction and sepsis [46,47]. Even if such strategies to modulate ANG-1/TIE-2 signalling prove effective for adult PH, our findings indicate they are likely to be ineffective in CDH and that the pathogenesis of CDH related PH is sufficiently different from adult diseases to warrant dedicated research endeavors for this unsolved problem.

Author Contributions

Conceived and designed the experiments: HJC MGC DGF PDL ECJ. Performed the experiments: HJC MGC. Analyzed the data: HJC. Contributed reagents/materials/analysis tools: HJC MGC DGF. Wrote the paper: HJC DGF PDL ECJ.

References

1. International PPH Consortium, Lane KB, Machado RD, Pauciulo MW, Thomson JR, et al. (2000) Heterozygous germline mutations in BMPR2, encoding a TGF-beta receptor, cause familial primary pulmonary hypertension. Nat Genet 26: 81–84.
2. Machado RD, Pauciulo MW, Thomson JR, Lane KB, Morgan NV, et al. (2001) BMPR2 haploinsufficiency as the inherited molecular mechanism for primary pulmonary hypertension. Am J Hum Genet 68: 92–102.
3. Harrison RE, Flanagan JA, Sankelo M, Abdalla SA, Rowell J, et al. (2003) Molecular and functional analysis identifies ALK-1 as the predominant cause of pulmonary hypertension related to hereditary haemorrhagic telangiectasia. J Med Genet 40: 865–871.
4. Du L, Sullivan CC, Chu D, Cho AJ, Kido M, et al. (2003) Signaling molecules in nonfamilial pulmonary hypertension. N Engl J Med 348: 500–509.
5. Zhao YD, Campbell AI, Robb M, Ng D, Stewart DJ (2003) Protective role of angiopoietin-1 in experimental pulmonary hypertension. Circ Res 92: 984–991.
6. Brindle NP, Saharinen P, Alitalo K (2006) Signaling and functions of angiopoietin-1 in vascular protection. Circ Res 98: 1014–1023.
7. Kugathasan L, Ray JB, Deng Y, Rezaei E, Dumont DJ, et al. (2009) The angiopietin-1-Tie2 pathway prevents rather than promotes pulmonary arterial hypertension in transgenic mice. J Exp Med 206: 2221–2234.
8. Finer NN, Barrington KJ (2006) Nitric oxide for respiratory failure in infants born at or near term. Cochrane Database Syst Rev Oct 18(4): CD000399.
9. Mugford M, Elbourne D, Field D (2008) Extracorporeal membrane oxygenation for severe respiratory failure in newborn infants. Cochrane Database Syst Rev Jul 16(3): CD001340.
10. Kluth D, Kangah R, Reich P, Tenbrinck R, Tibboel D, et al. (1990) Nitrofen-induced diaphragmatic hernias in rats: an animal model. J Pediatr Surg 25: 850–854.
11. Tenbrinck R, Gaillard JL, Tibboel D, Kluth D, Lachmann B, et al. (1992) Pulmonary vascular abnormalities in experimentally induced congenital diaphragmatic hernia in rats. J Pediatr Surg 27: 862–865.
12. Coleman C, Zhao J, Gupta M, Buckley S, Tefft JD, et al. (1998) Inhibition of vascular and epithelial differentiation in murine nitrofen-induced diaphragmatic hernia. Am J Physiol 274: L636–646.
13. Okoye BO, Losty PD, Lloyd DA, Gosney JR (1998) Effect of prenatal glucocorticoids on pulmonary vascular muscularisation in nitrofen-induced congenital diaphragmatic hernia. J Pediatr Surg 33: 76–80.
14. Kanai M, Kitano Y, von Allmen D, Davies P, Adzick NS, et al. (2001) Fetal tracheal occlusion in the rat model of nitrofen-induced congenital diaphragmatic hernia: tracheal occlusion reverses the arterial structural abnormality. J Pediatr Surg 36: 839–845.
15. Taira Y, Yamataka T, Miyazaki E, Puri P (1998) Comparison of the pulmonary vasculature in newborns and stillborns with congenital diaphragmatic hernia. Pediatr Surg Int 14: 30–35.
16. Jesudason EC, Connell MG, Fernig DG, Lloyd DA, Losty PD (2000) Heparin and in-vitro experimental lung hypoplasia. Pediatr Surg Int 16: 247–251.
17. Jesudason EC, Connell MG, Fernig DG, Lloyd DA, Losty PD (2000) In vitro effects of growth factors on lung hypoplasia in a model of congenital diaphragmatic hernia. J Pediatr Surg 35: 914–922.
18. Jesudason EC, Connell MG, Fernig DG, Lloyd DA, Losty PD (2000) Cell proliferation and apoptosis in experimental lung hypoplasia. J Pediatr Surg 35: 129–133.
19. Jesudason EC, Connell MG, Fernig DG, Lloyd DA, Losty PD (2000) Early lung malformations in congenital diaphragmatic hernia. J Pediatr Surg 35: 124–127.
20. Thompson SM, Connell MG, van Kuppevelt TH, Xu R, Turnbull JE, et al. (2011) Structure and epitope distribution of heparan sulfate is disrupted in experimental lung hypoplasia: a glycobiological epigenetic cause for malformation? BMC Dev Biol 11: 38. Available: http://www.biomedcentral.com/1471-213X/11/38.
21. Featherstone NC, Connell MG, Fernig DG, Wray S, Burdyga TV, et al. (2006) Airway smooth muscle dysfunction precedes teratogenic congenital diaphragmatic hernia and may contribute to hypoplastic lung morphogenesis. Am J Respir Cell Mol Biol 35: 571–578.
22. Cilley RE, Zgleszewski SE, Krummel TM, Chinoy MR (1997) Nitrofen dose-dependent gestational day-specific murine lung hypoplasia and left-sided diaphragmatic hernia. Am J Physiol 272: L362–371.
23. Chinoy MR, Graybill MM, Miller SA, Lang CM, Kauffman GL (2002) Angiopoietin-1 and VEGF in vascular development and angiogenesis in hypoplastic lungs. Am J Physiol Lung Cell Mol Physiol 283: L60–66.
24. Geggel RL, Murphy JD, Langleben D, Crone RK, Vacanti JP, et al. (1985) Congenital diaphragmatic hernia: arterial structural changes and persistent pulmonary hypertension after surgical repair. J Pediatr 107: 457–464.
25. Morrell NW, Adnot S, Archer SL, Dupuis J, Jones PL, et al. (2009) Cellular and molecular basis of pulmonary arterial hypertension. J Am Coll Cardiol 54: S20–31.
26. Nohe A, Keating E, Knaus P, Petersen NO (2004) Signal transduction of bone morphogenetic protein receptors. Cell Signal 16: 291–299.
27. Frank DB, Lowery J, Anderson L, Brink M, Reese J, et al. (2008) Increased susceptibility to hypoxic pulmonary hypertension in Bmpr2 mutant mice is associated with endothelial dysfunction in the pulmonary vasculature. Am J Physiol Lung Cell Mol Physiol 294: L98–109.
28. Takahashi H, Goto N, Kojima Y, Tsuda Y, Morio Y, et al. (2006) Downregulation of type II bone morphogenetic protein receptor in hypoxic pulmonary hypertension. Am J Physiol Lung Cell Mol Physiol 290: L450–458.
29. Long L, MacLean MR, Jeffery TK, Morecroft I, Yang X, et al. (2006) Serotonin increases susceptibility to pulmonary hypertension in BMPR2-deficient mice. Circ Res 98: 818–827.
30. West J, Tada Y, Fagan KA, Steudel W, Fouty BW, et al. (2005) Suppression of type II bone morphogenic protein receptor in vascular smooth muscle induces pulmonary arterial hypertension in transgenic mice. Chest 128: 553S.
31. Yu PB, Beppu H, Kawai N, Li E, Bloch KD (2005) Bone morphogenetic protein (BMP) type II receptor deletion reveals BMP ligand-specific gain of signaling in pulmonary artery smooth muscle cells. J Biol Chem 280: 24443–24450.
32. Yang X, Long L, Southwood M, Rudarakanchana N, Upton PD, et al. (2005) Dysfunctional Smad signaling contributes to Abnormal smooth muscle cell proliferation in familial pulmonary arterial hypertension. Circ Res 96: 1053–1063.
33. Ihida-Stansbury K, McKean DM, Lane KB, Loyd JE, Wheeler LA, et al. (2006) Tenascin-C is induced by mutated BMP type II receptors in familial forms of pulmonary arterial hypertension. Am J Physiol Lung Cell Mol Physiol 291: L694–702.
34. Reynolds AM, Holmes MD, Danilov SM, Reynolds PN (2012) Targeted gene delivery of BMPR-2 attenuates pulmonary hypertension. Eur Respir J 39: 329–343.
35. Rocha GM, Bianchi RF, Severo M, Rodrigues MM, Baptista MJ, et al. (2008) Congenital diaphragmatic hernia - the neonatal period (part I). Eur J Pediatr Surg 18: 219–223.
36. Gallot D, Boda C, Ughetto S, Perthus I, Robert-Gnansia E, et al. (2007) Prenatal detection and outcome of congenital diaphragmatic hernia: a French registry-based study. Ultrasound Obstet Gynecol 29: 276–283.
37. Thérèse P (2006) Persistent pulmonary hypertension of the newborn. Paediatr Respir Rev 7: S175–176.
38. Solari V, Piotrowska AP, Puri P (2003) Expression of heme oxygenase-1 and endothelial nitric oxide synthase in the lung of newborns with congenital diaphragmatic hernia and persistent pulmonary hypertension. J Pediatr Surg 38: 808–813.
39. Okoye BO, Losty PD, Fisher MJ, Wilmott I, Lloyd DA (1998) Effect of dexamethasone on endothelial nitric oxide synthase in experimental congenital diaphragmatic hernia. Arch Dis Child Fetal Neonatal Ed 78: F204–208.
40. Stewart DJ (2005) Bone morphogenetic protein receptor-2 and pulmonary arterial hypertension: unraveling a riddle inside an enigma? Circ Res 96: 1033–1035.
41. Boucherat O, Franco-Montoya ML, Delacourt C, Martinovic J, Masse V, et al. (2010) Defective angiogenesis in hypoplastic human fetal lungs correlates with nitric oxide synthase deficiency that occurs despite enhanced angiopoietin-2 and VEGF. Am J Physiol Lung Cell Mol Physiol 298: L849–856.
42. Maniscalco WM, Watkins RH, Pryhuber GS, Bhatt A, Shea C, et al. (2002) Angiogenic factors and alveolar vasculature: development and alterations by injury in very premature baboons. Am J Physiol Lung Cell Mol Physiol 282: L811–823.
43. Richter A, Yeager ME, Zaiman A, Cool CD, Voelkel NF, et al. (2004) Impaired transforming growth factor-beta signaling in idiopathic pulmonary arterial hypertension. Am J Respir Crit Care Med 170: 1340–1348.
44. Chen C, Chen H, Sun J, Bringas P, Jr., Chen Y, et al. (2005) Smad1 expression and function during mouse embryonic lung branching morphogenesis. Am J Physiol Lung Cell Mol Physiol 288: L1033–1039.

45. Kling DE, Narra V, Islam S, Kinane TB, Alessandrini A, et al. (2001) Decreased mitogen activated protein kinase activities in congenital diaphragmatic hernia-associated pulmonary hypoplasia. J Pediatr Surg 36: 1490–1496.
46. Thurston G, Rudge JS, Ioffe E, Zhou H, Ross L, et al. (2000) Angiopoietin-1 protects the adult vasculature against plasma leakage. Nat Med 6: 460–463.
47. Sun L, Cui M, Wang Z, Feng X, Mao J, et al. (2007) Mesenchymal stem cells modified with angiopoietin-1 improve remodeling in a rat model of acute myocardial infarction. Biochem Biophys Res Commun 357: 779–784.

11

Key Role of the Endothelial TGF-β/ALK1/Endoglin Signaling Pathway in Humans and Rodents Pulmonary Hypertension

Benoît Gore[1], Mohamed Izikki[1], Olaf Mercier[3], Laurence Dewachter[2], Elie Fadel[3], Marc Humbert[1], Philippe Dartevelle[3], Gerald Simonneau[1], Robert Naeije[2], Franck Lebrin[4], Saadia Eddahibi[1,3]*

1 INSERM U999, Le Plessis-Robinson, France, **2** Laboratory of Physiology, Faculty of Medicine, Free University of Brussels, Brussels, Belgium, **3** Centre Chirurgical Marie Lannelongue, Le Plessis-Robinson, France, **4** INSERM U833, Collège de France, Paris, France

Abstract

Mutations affecting transforming growth factor-beta (TGF-β) superfamily receptors, activin receptor-like kinase (ALK)-1, and endoglin (ENG) occur in patients with pulmonary arterial hypertension (PAH). To determine whether the TGF-β/ALK1/ENG pathway was involved in PAH, we investigated pulmonary TGF-β, ALK1, ALK5, and ENG expressions in human lung tissue and cultured pulmonary-artery smooth-muscle-cells (PA-SMCs) and pulmonary endothelial cells (PECs) from 14 patients with idiopathic PAH (iPAH) and 15 controls. Seeing that ENG was highly expressed in PEC, we assessed the effects of TGF-β on Smad1/5/8 and Smad2/3 activation and on growth factor production by the cells. Finally, we studied the consequence of ENG deficiency on the chronic hypoxic-PH development by measuring right ventricular (RV) systolic pressure (RVSP), RV hypertrophy, and pulmonary arteriolar remodeling in ENG-deficient ($Eng^{+/-}$) and wild-type ($Eng^{+/+}$) mice. We also evaluated the pulmonary blood vessel density, macrophage infiltration, and cytokine expression in the lungs of the animals. Compared to controls, iPAH patients had higher serum and pulmonary TGF-β levels and increased ALK1 and ENG expressions in lung tissue, predominantly in PECs. Incubation of the cells with TGF-β led to Smad1/5/8 phosphorylation and to a production of FGF2, PDGFb and endothelin-inducing PA-SMC growth. Endoglin deficiency protected mice from hypoxic PH. As compared to wild-type, $Eng^{+/-}$ mice had a lower pulmonary vessel density, and no change in macrophage infiltration after exposure to chronic hypoxia despite the higher pulmonary expressions of interleukin-6 and monocyte chemoattractant protein-1. The TGF-β/ALK1/ENG signaling pathway plays a key role in iPAH and experimental hypoxic PH via a direct effect on PECs leading to production of growth factors and inflammatory cytokines involved in the pathogenesis of PAH.

Editor: Rory Edward Morty, University of Giessen Lung Center, Germany

Funding: This study was supported by grants from the INSERM, and the Agence National de la Recherche (ANR-08-GENOPAT-004 to S.E., A.L-V and M.H.). This article reflects only the authors' views and under no circumstances is the European Community liable for any use that may be made of the information it contains. The funders had no role in study design, data collection and analysis, decision to publish, or preparation of the manuscript.

Competing Interests: The authors have declared that no competing interests exist.

* Email: saadia.eddahibi@inserm.fr

Introduction

Pulmonary arterial hypertension (PAH) is an uncommon but potentially life-threatening disease. Incompletely understood pathogenic mechanisms cause a progressive increase in pulmonary vascular resistance that ultimately leads to right ventricular (RV) failure [1]. Among patients with heritable forms of PAH, many have germline mutations in genes encoding receptors of the transforming growth factor-beta (TGF-β) receptor superfamily, usually the bone morphogenetic protein (BMP) receptor type 2 gene (*BMPR2*) and less often the *ACVRL1* or *ENG* gene encoding activin receptor-like kinase 1 (ALK1) and endoglin (ENG), respectively. These germline mutations have also been linked to hereditary hemorrhagic telangiectasia (HHT), an autosomal dominant vascular disorder characterized by telangiectasia and arteriovenous malformations [2].

TGF-β is a multifunctional cytokine whose signals are mediated by specific type I and II serine/threonine kinase receptors. Upon binding of active TGF-β to the constitutively activated type II receptor (TβRII), a specific type I receptor (TβRI) is recruited. Activation of this second receptor via phosphorylation initiates intracellular signaling through the phosphorylation of a set of receptor-regulated Smads (R-Smad), which subsequently form a complex with co-Smad (Smad4). The R-Smad/co-Smad complex enters the nucleus, where it modulates the transcription of target genes. In most cells, the TGF-β signaling pathway involves the TβRII/ALK5 complex, which induces Smad2/3 phosphorylation. However, in endothelial cells, TGF-β activates two distinct type I receptors, ALK5 and ALK1, which transmit signals via the ALK5/Smad2/3 and ALK1/Smad1/5 pathways, respectively [3]. ALK5/Smad2/3 inhibits and ALK1/Smad1/5 stimulates endothelial-cell proliferation and migration. ENG, which is a transmembrane accessory receptor for TGF-β signaling, plays a pivotal role in the balance of ALK1 and ALK5 signaling that regulates endothelial cell proliferation. ENG is predominantly expressed on proliferating endothelial cells *in vitro* and on angiogenic blood vessels *in vivo* [4].The TGF-β/ALK1/ENG signaling pathway plays a key role in vessel formation and maintenance [4]. However, its contribution to the pathogenesis of PAH is poorly understood [4]. In the present study, we evaluated the susceptibility of ENG-deficient mice ($Eng^{+/-}$) to PAH induced by 3 weeks of chronic hypoxia. We also evaluated pulmonary vascular remodeling and inflammation in these mice comparatively with wild-type mice exposed to chronic hypoxia. We investigated the expression pattern of the TGF-β/ALK1/ENG signaling pathway in lung tissue and in pulmonary-artery smooth-muscle-cells (PA-SMCs) and pulmonary endothelial cells (PECs) from patients with iPAH comparatively with controls. In a recent study, we found that serum-free medium of quiescent human PECs elicited marked PA-SMC proliferation [5]. We therefore evaluated whether TGF-β exposure of cultured PECs from controls increased the growth-promoting activity of the PEC culture medium and modified the expression of growth-promoting factors implicated in PAH development.

Methods

Ethics Statement

This study was approved by the institutional review board and the local ethics committee (Comité de Protection des Personnes, Ile-de-France VII, Le Kremlin-Bicêtre, France). Written, informed consent was given by all the patients prior to their contribution to the study.

Experiments were conducted according to the European Union regulations (Directive 86/609 EEC) for animal experiments and complied with our institution's guidelines for animal care and handling. The animal facility is licensed by the French Ministry of Agriculture (agreement N° B92-019-01). This study was approved by the Committee on the Ethics of Animal Experiments CEEA26 CAPSud. All animal experiments were supervised by Dr. Olaf Mercier (agreement delivered by the French Ministry of Agriculture for animal experiment N° A92–396). All efforts were made to minimize animal suffering.

Studies of human lung tissue samples

Tissue sampling. Lung tissue and pulmonary arteries were collected during lung transplantation in 14 patients (8 men and 6 women) with idiopathic pulmonary hypertension (iPAH) and during lobectomy or pneumonectomy for localized cancer in 15 controls (9 men and 6 women). All iPAH patients had New York Heart Association class III or IV heart failure and were treated with intravenous epoprostenol. In the controls, preoperative transthoracic echocardiography showed no evidence of PAH and the study samples were taken at a distance from tumor sites. Neither the iPAH patients nor the controls had *BMPR2*, *ACVRL1*, or *ENG* mutations or polymorphisms.

In the patients with iPAH, mean pulmonary artery pressure was 61±4 mm Hg (range, 28 to 90 mm Hg), mean pulmonary vascular resistance was 12.53±1.30 mm Hg $\cdot L^{-1}\cdot min^{-1}\cdot m^{-2}$ (range, 5.67 to 22.40 mm Hg$\cdot L^{-1}\cdot min^{-1}\cdot m^{-2}$), and mean cardiac index was 2.42± 0.2 $L\cdot min^{-1}\cdot m^{-2}$ (range, 1.2 to 3.4 $L\cdot min^{-1}\cdot m^{-2}$).

Isolation and culture of human PA-SMCs and PECs. Human PA-SMCs were cultured from pulmonary artery explants, as previously described [6]. To characterize the PA-SMC phenotype, we assessed the expression of muscle-specific contractile and cytoskeletal proteins including smooth-muscle-cell α-actin, desmin, and vinculin [6]. PA-SMCs were used between passages 3 and 6.

Human PECs were obtained by exposing lung tissue fragments to Dispase I digestion (Roche Diagnostics, Penzbeg, Germany) at 37°C overnight, as previously described [5]. The suspension was filtered, plated onto 0.1% gelatin-coated wells, and grown in MCDB131 medium (Invitrogen, Cergy-Pontoise, France) supplemented with 10% fetal calf serum (FCS), 50 U/mL penicillin/streptomycin, 4 mmol/L L-glutamine, 25 mmol/L HEPES, 10 U/mL heparin, 1 μg/mL human endothelial cell growth supplement, and 10 ng/mL vascular endothelial growth factor (Promocell, Heidelberg, Germany). PECs were purified using the immunomagnetic technique with anti-PECAM-1 (CD31) monoclonal antibody-labeled DynaBeads14 (Dynal, Biotech, Compiègne, France). For endothelial-cell phenotype characterization, the cells were labeled with acetylated low-density lipoprotein (LDL) coupled to a fluorescent carbocyanine dye (Dil-Ac-LDL, Tebu, Le Perray en Yvelines, France) and stained with antibodies against the endothelial cell-specific lectin *Ulex europaeus* agglutinin-1 (UEA-1, Sigma, Lyon, France). Experiments were also performed using monoclonal antibodies against desmin and vimentin (Dako, Trappes, France). Cells positive for Dil-Ac-LDL and UEA-1 and negative for desmin and vimentin were classified as endothelial cells and constituted >95% of our PEC cultures. Cells were used for the study at passage 6 [5].

Protein extraction and Western blotting. Lung samples were homogenized, and PECs and PA-SMCs were sonicated in lysis CHAPS Buffer (150 mM NaCl, 10 mM Tris HCl pH = 7.5, 1 mM EDTA, 1 mM EGTA, 1 mM Leupeptin, 1 mM PMSF, and 1% CHAPS). Protein concentrations were measured using the Bradford technique, and 30 μg of protein per sample was used for Western blotting (10% acrylamide), as previously described [5]. Proteins were electrophoretically transferred to a nitrocellulose membrane (Sigma-Aldrich, Ayrshire, UK), which was then saturated in 5% bovine serum albumin (BSA) in Tris-buffered saline Tween 20 (TBS-T). TGF-β receptor protein expression was evaluated using goat anti-human ALK1, ALK5, and ENG antibodies (R&D System, Lille), diluted 1:1000 in BSA with 1% TBS-T. Detection was with an anti-goat antibody coupled to horseradish peroxidase (HRP) (Dakocytomation, Trappes, France) diluted 1:2000 in BSA, 1% TBS-T, and ECL kit substrate (GE Healthcare, Vélizy, France). A polyclonal antibody against β-actin (diluted 1:3000; Sigma Aldrich) served as the internal control. Densitometric quantification of the immunoblot bands was performed using Bio-Rad Quantity One software.

Enzyme-linked immunosorbent assay (ELISA). TGF-β protein levels were evaluated in lung samples and serum from patients with iPAH and controls using an ELISA (R&D systems, Lille, France). ENG protein concentrations were determined in the same serum samples and in supernatants from PECs isolated from patients with iPAH and controls using ELISA kits, according to the manufacturer's instructions (R&D Systems, Lille).

Effect of TGF-β on Smad phosphorylation. PECs (300 000 cells per well, 6-well plates coated with 0.1% gelatin) were plated in 10% FCS/MCB131 medium for 24 hours then starved for 24 hours in serum-free medium. PECs were then treated with TGF-β (0, 5, or 50 ng/mL) for 30 min. The protein was harvested by scraping in a cell lysis buffer containing an anti-phosphatase mixture (Cell Signaling, Saint-Quentin, France) then sonicated. Protein concentrations were measured using the Bradford technique, and 10 μg samples were then used for Western blotting as previously described [5]. Immunoblotting assays were performed as described above with rabbit anti-human phospho-Smad1/5/8 (Cell Signaling, Saint-Quentin, France) and rabbit anti-human Smad 1/5/8 (Santa Cruz Biotechnology, Le Perray en Yvelines, France) diluted 1:1000 to determine the ratio of phospho-Smad1/5/8 over Smad1/5/8. Detection was performed with anti-rabbit antibody coupled to HRP (Dakocytomation, Trappes, France).

RNA extraction. Total RNA was extracted from lung tissue, PECs, and PA-SMCs using RNeasy Mini kit (Qiagen SA, Courtaboeuf, France), according to the manufacturer's instructions. RNA integrity was evaluated by visual inspection of ethidium bromide-stained agarose gels and the RNA concentration was determined from optical density measurements.

Preparation of cDNA and quantitative real-time polymerase chain reaction (QRT-PCR). First-strand cDNA synthesis was with the SuperScript II RT reverse transcriptase system (Invitrogen, Cergy Pontoise). A mix containing 1 μg of total RNA, 100 ng of random primers, and 1 μL of dNTP (10 mM) in a total of 12 μL was incubated for 5 min at 65°C and chilled on ice. After addition of a second mixture of 4 μL of first-strand buffer, 2 μL of dithiothreitol (0.1 M), and 40 U of RNase inhibitor (RNaseOUT; Invitrogen, Cergy Pontoise), the samples were left at 25°C for 2 min. Finally, after addition of 1 μL of SuperScript II RT (200 units/μL), the reaction was incubated for 10 min at 25°C, 50 min at 42°C, and 15 min at 70°C. The cDNA was diluted 1:20 for use in a quantitative real-time-polymerase chain reaction (QRT-PCR).

The primers were designed using Primer Express Software (Applied Biosystems, Courtabœuf, France) for human *TGF-β*, *ALK1*, *ALK5*, and *ENG* and for both human and mouse preproendothelin-1 (preproET-1), platelet-derived growth factor (PDGF)-A and -B, fibroblast growth factor (FGF)-2, epidermal growth factor (EGF), interleukin (IL)-6, and monocyte chemoattractant protein (MCP)-1. Specific QRT-PCR primer sequences for all genes were listed in Table S1. To avoid inappropriate amplification of residual genomic DNA, intron-spanning primers were selected and internal control 18S rRNA primers were used. For each sample, the amplification reaction was performed in duplicate using Syber Green mix and specific primers. Signals were detected and results analyzed using ABI-Prism 7000 sequence detection software (Applied Biosystems). The expression level of the genes of interest was computed relative to the mRNA expression level of the internal standard r18S as follows: relative mRNA = $1/2^{(\text{Ctgene of interest-Ctr 18S})}$.

PA-SMC growth assays. PA-SMCs from controls were seeded at a density of $5 \cdot 10^4$ cells/per well in Dulbecco's modified Eagle's medium supplemented with 10% FCS and allowed to adhere. The cells were subjected to 48 h of growth arrest in medium containing 0% FCS then treated with 1 mL of the various conditioned media collected from control PECs. PEC serum-free medium was obtained as follows: at the time of initiating PA-SMC growth arrest, PECs were seeded in 24-well plates at a density of $5 \cdot 10^4$ cells per well and were allowed to adhere and to grow in supplemented MCDB 131 as described above, for 24 h. The PECs were then subjected to 24 h of growth arrest in MCDB 131 medium with 0.2% FCS, with or without 5 ng/mL of TGF-β in the presence or absence of anti-ENG antibody. The medium was removed and used for PA-SMC incubation for 48 h, after which the PA-SMCs were counted.

Effect of TGF-β on cytokine induction in PECs. PECs were seeded and synchronized as previously described. The cells were either untreated or treated for 4 h with 5 ng/mL of TGF-β in the presence or absence of anti-ENG antibody. The PECs were then used for QRT-PCR.

Studies in mice

Chronic hypoxia model. ENG-deficient (*Eng*$^{+/-}$)[7] and wild-type (*Eng*$^{+/+}$) transgenic C57BL6 mice were exposed to chronic hypoxia (10% O_2) in a ventilated chamber (500-L volume, Flufrance) or to normoxia for 3 weeks. The hypoxic environment was established by flushing the chamber with a mixture of room air and nitrogen (10% oxygen, 90% diazote (N_2) and recirculating the gas. Carbon dioxide was removed using soda lime granules, and excess humidity was prevented by cooling the recirculation circuit. The chamber environment was monitored using an oxygen analyzer.

Assessment of pulmonary hypertension in mice. Mice were anesthetized with intraperitoneal sodium pentobarbital (4 mg/100 g). After incision of the abdomen, a pressure transducer was inserted into the RV and RV systolic pressure (RVSP) was recorded, as previously described [8]. To assess RV hypertrophy, the RV was dissected from the left ventricle and septum, and the ratio of RV weight over the weight of the left ventricle and septum (LV+S) was computed (Fulton's index).

The lungs were removed, fixed, and processed for paraffin embedding. The percentage of muscularized vessels was calculated as previously described [8]. Briefly, in each mouse, 60 intra-acinar arteries at a size lower than 80 μm were categorized as non-muscularized (NM), partially muscularized (PM) or fully muscularized (M) to assess the degree of muscularization. The lungs were also removed and stored at −80°C for QRT-PCR.

Immunohistochemistry. Paraffin sections (5 μm) of lung specimens were mounted on Superfrost Plus slides (Fisher Scientific, Illkirch, France). The slides were dewaxed in 100% toluene, and the sections were progressively rehydrated by immersion in decreasing ethanol concentrations (100%, 95%, and 70%) and, finally, in distilled water. Endogenous peroxidase activity was blocked with H_2O_2 in methanol (0.3% v/v) for 10 minutes. After three washes with phosphate buffer saline (PBS), the sections were preincubated in PBS supplemented with 3% (w/v) BSA for 30 min then incubated overnight at 4°C with antibodies. Mouse PECs were stained with goat polyclonal anti-PECAM-1 antibody (Santa Cruz) diluted 1:200 and macrophages were stained with rat anti-mouse F4/80 (AbD Serotec, Düsseldorf, Germany) diluted 1:400. The sections were then exposed for 30 min to biotin-labeled anti-goat secondary antibodies (Dako, Trappes, France) diluted 1:200 in the same buffer then to streptavidin-biotin horseradish peroxidase solution. For F4/80 staining, the sections were exposed to anti-rat HRP (Santa Cruz) diluted 1:200 in PBS. Peroxidase staining was carried out using 3,3′-diaminobenzidine tetrahydrochloride dihydrate (DAB, Sigma) and hydrogen peroxide. Finally, the sections were stained with hematoxylin and eosin. Vascular density and macrophage infiltration were assessed in 10 selected fields and stored as digital field images. The results were expressed as vessel number and macrophage number per 100 alveoli.

Statistical analysis

All data are reported as mean±SEM. Statistical significance was tested using ANOVA or the nonparametric Mann-Whitney test. *P* values <0.05 were considered statistically significant.

Results

Pulmonary and cell expression of TGF-β/TGF-β receptors in patients with iPAH and controls

TGF-β protein levels were increased in serum and lung tissue homogenates from patients with iPAH, compared to controls (Figure 1A and B). TGF-β mRNA levels were also higher in cultured PA-SMCs from iPAH patients compared to those from controls (Figure 1C).

Compared to controls, lung tissue and PECs from iPAH patients had higher levels of ENG and ALK1 mRNA and proteins

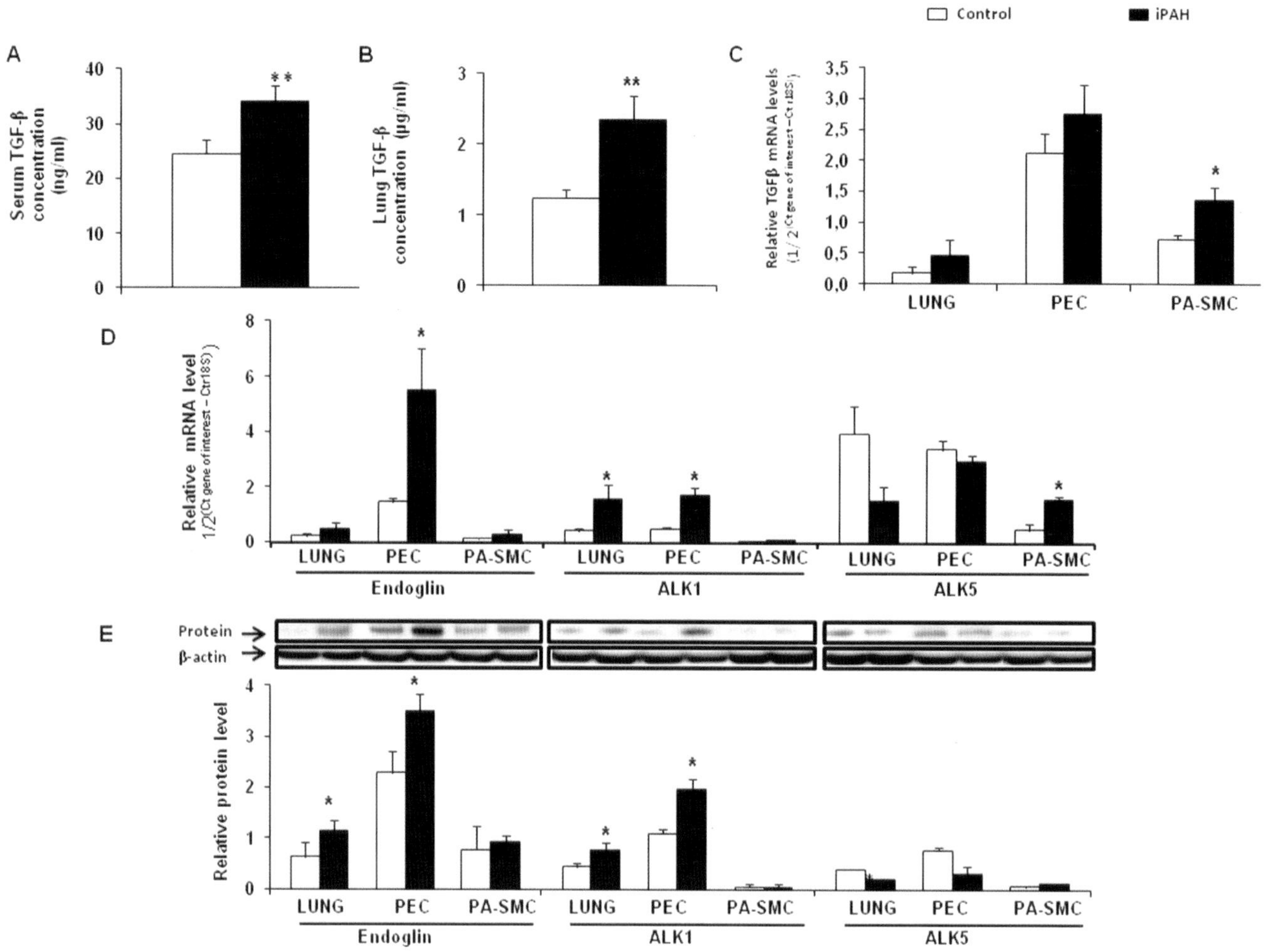

Figure 1. The open bars indicate the results in controls and the closed bars in patients with idiopathic pulmonary hypertension (iPAH). TGF-β was assayed using an ELISA in serum and lung homogenates (controls, n = 15; iPAH patients, n = 14) (**A** and **B**). (**C**) TGF-β mRNA measured in pulmonary endothelial cells (PECs) and pulmonary-artery smooth-muscle cells (PA-SMCs; controls, n = 7; iPAH patients, n = 7). (**D**) TGF-β receptor expression: *ALK1, ALK5*, and *ENG* mRNA measured in PECs and PA-SMCs (controls, n = 7; iPAH patients, n = 7). (**E**): ENG, ALK1, and ALK5 protein expression in LUNG, PECs and PA-SMCs. Protein levels were normalized for β-actin (controls, n = 7; iPAH patients, n = 7). Values are mean ± SEM. **P*<0.05 and ***P*<0.01 compared with controls.

(Figure 1D, E, F). ENG protein was also increased in serum and PEC supernatants from patients with iPAH (data not shown). In contrast, in PA-SMCs from both groups, ENG expression was very low and ALK1 was not detected (Figure 1D, and E). ALK5 MRNA levels were increased in iPAH PA-SMCs, but we did not detect any increase of ALK5 protein levels in the lungs, PEC and PA-SMC from patients with iPAH (Figure 1D, and E).

Differential effects of TGF-β on the Smad signaling pathway in human PECs

Because PECs have been shown to express highly ALK1 and ENG and moderatelyALK5, we evaluated the effects of TGF-β treatment on Smad1/5/8 and Smad2/3 phosphorylation in these cells. Increasing concentrations of TGF-β (0, 5, and 50 ng/mL) induced phosphorylation of Smad1/5/8 in PECs from patients with iPAH and, to a lesser extent, from controls. The maximal effect was observed at 5 ng/mL of TGF-β (Figure 2A). Phosphorylation of Smad2/3 was not detected at this concentration, but a weak signal was observed at 50 ng/mL of TGF-β and remained similar in the two groups (Figure 2B).

PA-SMC growth in response to medium from cultured PECs treated with TGF β

Serum-free medium from cultured PECs from controls was added to PA-SMCs from the same individuals cultured without serum. This produced a marked increase in PA-SMC proliferation compared to the basal condition. When the PECs were treated with 5 ng/mL of TGF-β, the conditioned medium had a stronger effect on PA-SMCs. This effect was completely inhibited when TGF-β was combined with anti-ENG antibody (Figure 2C). TGF-β 5 ng/mL added directly to PA-SMCs had no effect (data not shown).

Effect of TGF-β on PEC paracrine factors influencing PA-SMC growth

Compared to the basal condition, control PECs exposed to TGF-β 5 ng/mL induced a marked increase in the expression of *ET-1, PDGFb*, and *FGF2* mRNAs (Figure 3 A, C and D). These increases did not occur when PECs were exposed to TGF-β (5 ng/mL) combined with the anti-ENG antibody. TGF-β (5 ng/mL)

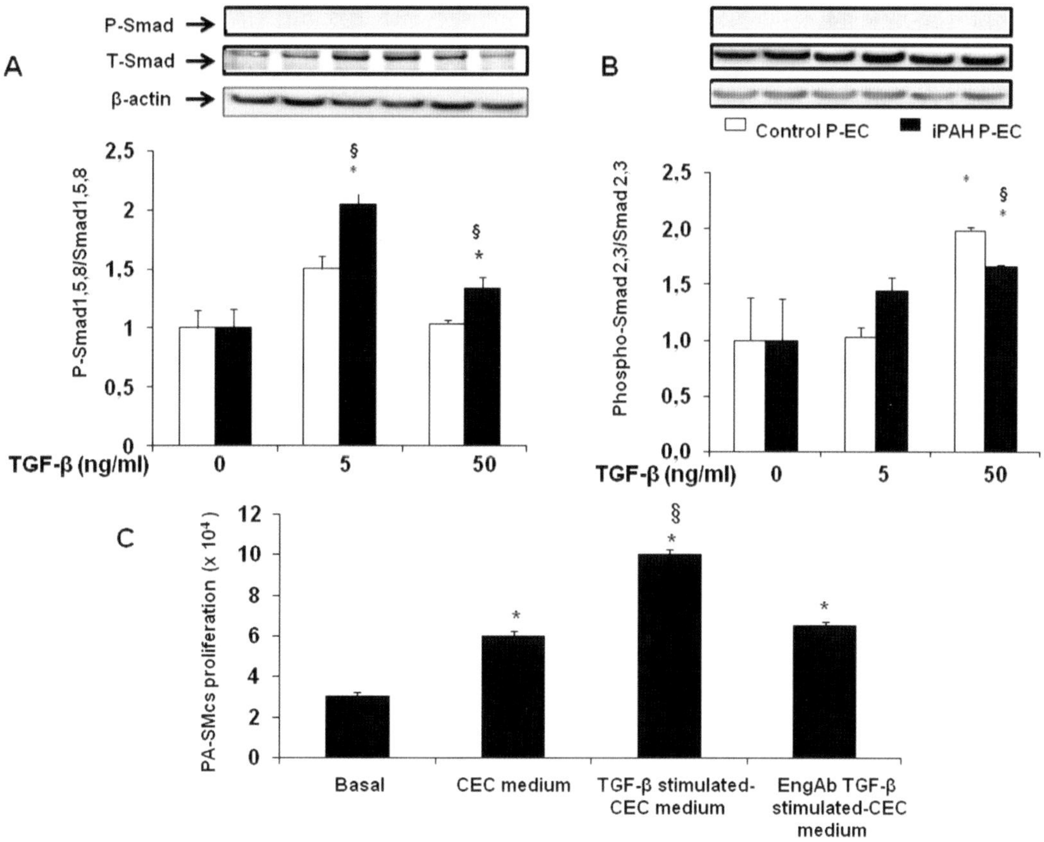

Figure 2. Effect of increasing TGF-β doses on Smad 1,5,8 and Smad 2,3 phosphorylation, respectively, in pulmonary endothelial cells (PECs) from controls and from patients with idiopathic pulmonary hypertension (iPAH) (**A** and **B**). Protein levels were normalized for β-actin. Values are means±SEM normalized for results without TGF-β. *$P<0.05$ compared to relevant controls without TGF-β, §$P<0.05$ compared to control PECs under the same conditions. (**C**) Growth of pulmonary-artery smooth-muscle cells (PA-SMCs) from controls in response to serum-free media derived from cultured PECs from controls and stimulated by TGF-β with or without anti-ENG antibody (ENG Ab).Values are mean±SEM. *$P<0.05$ compared to basal condition, §$P<0.05$ compared to PA-SMCs stimulated with PEC medium.

had no effect on mRNA levels of *PDGFa*, *EGF*, *MCP1*, or *IL-6* expressed by PECs (Figure 3 B, E, F and G).

Evaluation of chronic hypoxia-induced pulmonary hypertension in $Eng^{+/-}$ and wild-type mice

Four groups of 8-week-old mice (8 $Eng^{+/-}$ and 5 $Eng^{+/+}$ mice) were established, with balanced numbers of males and females in each genotype group. The mice were exposed to chronic hypoxia (10% O_2) or normoxia for 3 weeks. PAH was assessed based on RVSP, RV/(LV+S), and distal-artery muscularization after 3 weeks.

In normoxia, RVSP, RV/LV+S, and distal-artery muscularization were not significantly different between $Eng^{+/-}$ and wild-type mice (Figures 3A, B and C). After 3 weeks of chronic hypoxia, the increases in RVSP, RV/LV+S, and distal pulmonary artery muscularization were smaller in the $Eng^{+/-}$ mice than in the wild-type mice (Figure 4) ($P<0.05$).

Evaluation of vascularization and inflammation in $Eng^{+/-}$ and wild-type mice exposed to 3 weeks of chronic hypoxia

In normoxia, vessel density was significantly lower in the $Eng^{+/-}$ mice compared to the wild-type mice ($P<0.02$). Exposure to chronic hypoxia for 3 weeks did not affect the pulmonary vessel number in the $Eng^{+/-}$ or wild-type mice (Figure 5A and B). In normoxia, pulmonary macrophage infiltrates were more marked in the $Eng^{+/-}$ mice than in the wild-type mice. Chronic hypoxia induced pulmonary macrophage infiltration in the wild-type mice but not in the $Eng^{+/-}$ mice (Figure 5C and D).

Growth factors and Cytokine profile induced by chronic hypoxia in $Eng^{+/-}$ and wild-type mice

We evaluated the expression of genes coding for ET-1, growth factors, and inflammatory mediators previously shown to play a key role in PAH progression and pulmonary arteriole remodeling. Chronic hypoxia (10% O_2) induced an increase in mRNA levels of *preproET-1*, which remained lower in $Eng^{+/-}$ than in wild-type mice. Similarly, *PDGFb* and FGF2 induction in response to chronic hypoxia was less marked in lungs from $Eng^{+/-}$ mice than from wild-type animals. In contrast, the increase in MCP-1 and IL-6 mRNA levels under hypoxia was more marked in $Eng^{+/-}$ mice than in the wild-type mice, whereas no significant differences occurred for *PDGFa* (Figure 6B–G).

Discussion

The main findings from this study are as follows: (i) compared to control specimens, lung tissue and PECs from patients with iPAH expressed increased amounts of ALK1 and ENG located predominantly on endothelial cells; (ii) compared to controls,

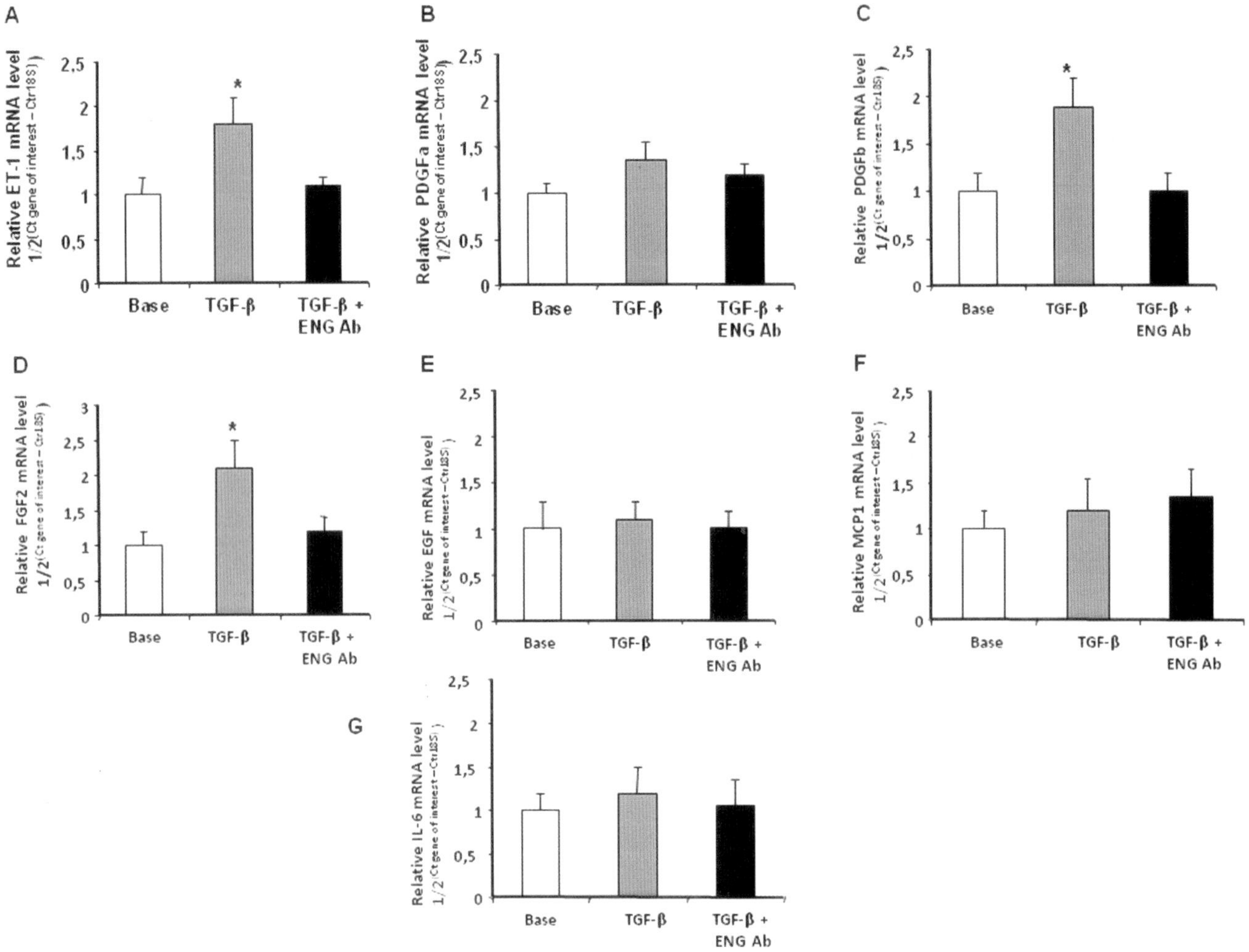

Figure 3. Effect of pulmonary endothelial cells (PECs) from controls incubated with TGF-β with or without anti-ENG antibody (ENG Ab) on mRNA expression of A) *preproET-1*, (B) *PDGFa*, (C) *PDGFb*, (D) *FGF2*, (E) *EGF*, (F) *MCP-1*, and (G) *IL-6*. Values are mean±SEM.*$P<0.05$ compared to PECs without TGF-β treatment.

patients with iPAH had higher serum and lung TGF-β levels; (iii) PECs from patients with iPAH exhibited Smad1/5/8 phosphorylation in response to increasing doses of TGF-β; (iv) medium from PECs treated with TGF-β markedly increased PA-SMC growth, and this effect seemed related to induction by TGF-β of *ET-1*, *PDGFb*, and *FGF2* expression in PECs and disappeared in the presence of anti-ENG antibody; and (v) ENG-deficient mice were partly protected against chronic hypoxia-induced PAH to wild-type mice, a finding that seemed related to decreased expression of PDGFa, PDGFb, and FGF2, three factors playing a key role in vascular remodeling and in the development of human and experimental PAH.

ALK1 and *ENG* mutations have been associated with HHT and, to a lesser extent, heritable PAH [2], two familial vascular dysplasias with apparently opposite phenotypes. Thus, HHT is characterized by dilated vessels, telangiectasia, and arteriovenous malformations in the lung, liver, and brain. In the lungs, the arteriovenous malformations can result in right-to-left shunts, leading to severe cyanosis and dyspnea, and potentially to the development of pulmonary vascular remodeling with PAH. Various physiological factors, such as blood flow (shear stress) or pressure (cyclic strain), have been shown to trigger the vessel remodeling process, which involves PA-SMC proliferation and extracellular matrix protein synthesis and accumulation. Taken in concert, these data highlight the importance of the TGF-β/ALK1/ENG signaling pathway in maintaining vascular integrity.

Increased expression of TGF-β and its receptors ALK1 and ENG led to an increase in TGF-β/ALK1/ENG signaling activity in lung tissue and PECs from iPAH patients. Several studies have assessed the contribution of TGF-β to PAH, which remains debated. A recent study found decreased pulmonary TGF-β mRNA expression in PAH patients [9], contrasting with increases in TGF-β1 [10] or TGF-β isoforms 2 and 3 in previous studies [11]. These discrepancies may be ascribable to differences in measurement techniques: the previous studies relied on mRNA analysis [9] or TGF-β protein measurement in pulmonary arteries [10,11], whereas we measured both lung and serum TGF-β protein contents. Upregulation of TGF-β has also been reported in several animal models of PAH [12,13], and decreased TGF-β signaling related to dominant negative TGF-β type II receptor (TGF-βRII) overexpression [12,14] or anti-TGF-β antibody [15] protects against PAH. Over the last 10 years, the importance of ALK1 and ENG in the pathogenesis of PAH has been established, notably by the identification of gene mutations [2,16]. More recently, a nonsense mutation of Smad8, a component of the TGF-β/ALK1/ENG signaling pathway, was described in a

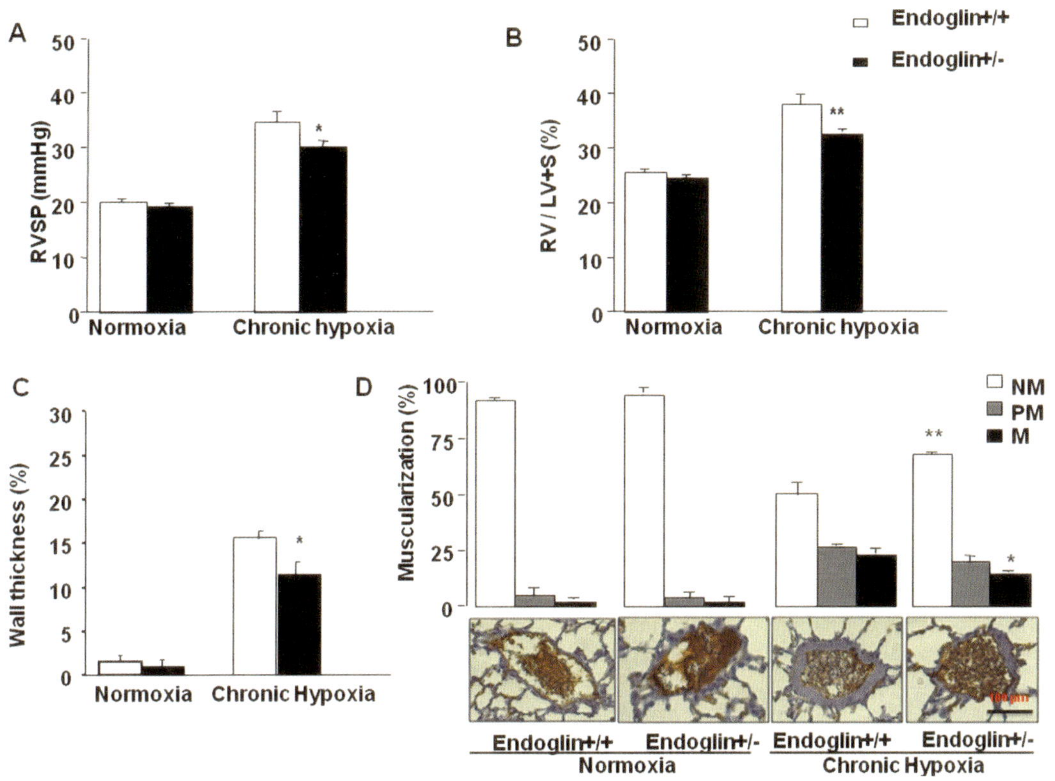

Figure 4. Mouse right ventricular (RV) systolic pressure (RVSP, mm Hg) (**A**). (**B**) RV hypertrophy reflected by the RV/(left ventricle+septum) weight ratio. (**C**) Percentage of lung vessel thickness. (**D**) Percentages of nonmuscularized (NM), partially muscularized (PM), and fully muscularized (M) lung vessels (top panel). Representative images for muscularization of distal pulmonary arteries (bottom panel). Values are mean±SEM. *$P<0.05$ and **$P<0.01$ compared with wild-type mice under the same conditions.

patient with iPAH [17]. Data on the role for the TGF/ALK1 pathway in experimental models are conflicting. Thus, ALK1 was upregulated in monocrotaline-induced PAH [18], TGF-β and ALK1 where increased in a lamb model of congenital heart disease [19], whereas ALK1 and ENG were downregulated in another study [20]. Although it has been shown that Eng+/− and Alk1+/− mice spontaneously develop pulmonary hypertension based on the age [9]. Here, we found ALK1 and ENG overexpression in lungs from iPAH patients. In keeping with an earlier study [9], we found no significant change in *ALK5* mRNA expression in lungs from iPAH patients. In pulmonary arteries, PECs seem to be the main target of TGF-β, notably in iPAH. Thus, PECs from iPAH patients exhibited ALK1 and ENG overexpression without changes in ALK5 expression.

ENG was previously shown to play a pivotal role not only in the balance between TGF-β/ALK1 and TGF-β/ALK5 signaling [21], but also in determining the endothelial-cell growth potential. Here, we showed that PEC medium stimulated PA-SMC growth and that this effect was more marked when the PECs were previously incubated with low-dose TGF-β. These results support our previous finding that cultured PECs constitutively produce and release growth-promoting factors that act on PA-SMCs [5]. We also showed that PEC treatment with TGF-β induced overexpression of *ET-1*, *PDGFb*, and *FGF2*, three factors that may play a key role in PA-SMC growth and PAH development [22–24]. There are several reports that ALK1 activation by TGF-β or by bone morphogenetic protein (BMP)-9 induces the production of the vasoconstricting and mitogenic compound endothelin (ET)-1 [25,26]. Recent studies also indicate that TGF-β induces endothelial IL-6 secretion [27], myofibroblast proliferation [28], and leukocyte migration [29], which are involved in the pathogenesis of PAH [23]. On the other hand, TGF-β-treated PECs from patients with iPAH showed a more sensitive activation of the Smad1/5/8 and, to a lesser degree, Smad2/3 signaling pathways, suggesting a predominance of the TGF-β/ALK1/Smad1/5/8 signaling pathways in these cells.

In the second part of our study, we investigated the consequences of ENG deficiency on PH development in mice. Because $Eng^{-/-}$ mice die during embryogenesis due to defects in vascular and cardiac maturation [7], we used engineered $Eng^{+/-}$ mice, previously described as an experimental model of HHT [7]. ENG deficiency in our $Eng^{+/-}$ mice partly prevented the development of chronic hypoxia-induced PH, as assessed based on RVSP, RV/(LV+S), and pulmonary arteriolar remodeling, compared with wild-type mice. Seeing that endoglin is determinant in the control of vascular density and that vessel numbers were inversely related to the severity of pulmonary hypertension, here we tried to establish a link between the degree of PH and vascular density in mice after exposure to chronic hypoxia. Our results show that, despite the reduction of the pulmonary vascular density, the $Eng^{+/-}$ mice were protected against the development of chronic hypoxic PH. Ardelean et al reported decrease of lung microvascular density and right ventricular hypertrophy in $Eng^{+/-}$ mice [30]. The discrepancy between the results could be due to background or age difference. In addition, $Eng^{+/-}$ mice exhibited increased pulmonary macrophage infiltration. This inflammation has been described as a potential precipitant of vascular bleeding in HHT [7] but may also be important in the pathogenesis of PAH

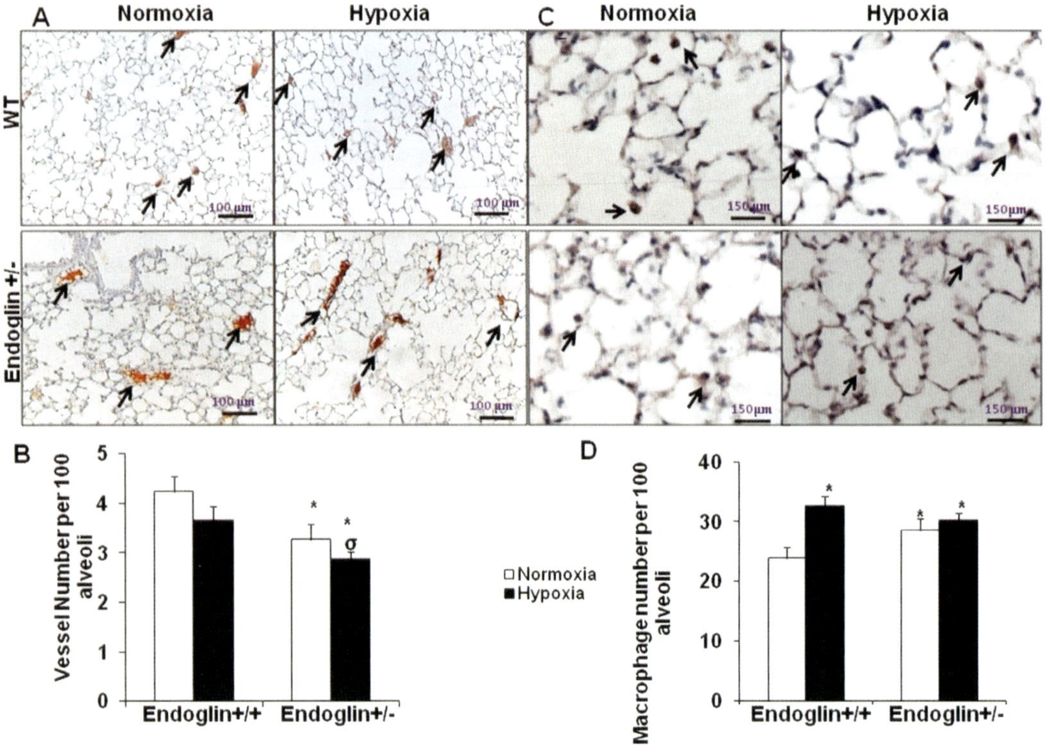

Figure 5. Mouse lung PECAM-1 immunostaining (**A**). (**B**) Number of vessels per 100 alveoli. (**C**) Mouse lung F4/80 immunostaining. (**D**) Number of macrophages per 100 alveoli. Values are mean±SEM. *$P<0.02$ compared with wild-type mice exposed to normoxia and $^{\sigma}P<0.02$ compared with wild-type mice exposed to hypoxia.

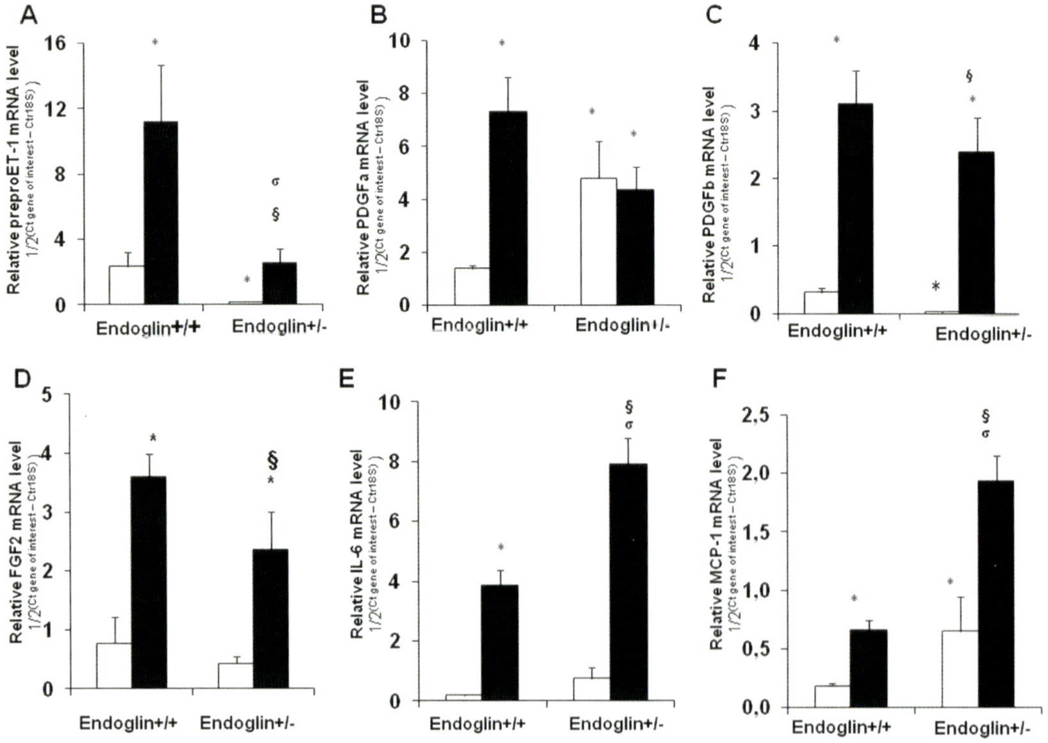

Figure 6. Mouse lung relative mRNA levels of (A) ***preproET-1*****, (B)** ***PDGFa*****, (C)** ***PDGFb*****, (D)** ***FGF2*****, (E)** ***IL-6*****, and (F)** ***MCP-1*** **in normoxia (open bars) versus hypoxia (closed bars).** Values are mean±SEM.*$P<0.05$ compared to wild-type mice exposed to normoxia, $^{\S}P<0.05$ compared to $Eng^{+/-}$ mice exposed to normoxia, and $^{\sigma}P<0.05$ compared to wild-type mice exposed to hypoxia.

[22]. However, $Eng^{+/-}$ mice were partly protected against hypoxia-induced PH compared to wild-type mice, suggesting that this underlying inflammatory phenotype did not exacerbate the effects of chronic hypoxia. Nevertheless, IL-6 and MCP-1, two cytokines previously implicated in PAH [22], were expressed at higher levels, both in normoxic and in hypoxic $Eng^{+/-}$ mice. The higher expression levels of these cytokines were in accordance with the degree of macrophage infiltration, which was more marked in lungs from $Eng^{+/-}$ mice.

We investigated the mechanism by which $Eng^{+/-}$ mice were partially protected against hypoxic PH and we measured growth factors involved in the development of human and experimental PAH. In keeping with previous data on PAH [23], chronic hypoxia was associated with increased *preproET-1* expression in both genotypes but the increase was significantly smaller in $Eng^{+/-}$ mice than in wild-type mice.

Because PA-SMC hyperplasia is among the main pathological changes in patients with PAH, we focused on the consequence of ENG deficiency in growth factor production in our experimental PAH model. Chronic hypoxia exposure was followed by increases in lung levels of PDGFb and FGF2 mRNA, but the levels of both growth factors remained significantly lower in $Eng^{+/-}$ mice than in wild-type mice. These *in vivo* results were consistent with the *in vitro* findings obtained using human PECs. These last data suggest that the protective effect against chronic hypoxic PH may be related to alterations in the PDGFb and FGF2 pathways. Indeed, previous studies showed that both growth factors played a key role in human and experimental PAH. The production of these growth factors or their receptors is increased in human PAH [22,24,31,32]. Furthermore, inhibiting PDGFb or FGF2 synthesis using SiRNA or receptor antagonists protects and/or reverses PAH in experimental models.

Our study establishes a key role for the TGF-β/ALK1/ENG signaling pathway in PAH and suggests that TGF-β may act upstream to pathways that are crucial in PAH in both humans and rodents, such as the Endothelin1, PDGFb, and FGF2 pathways.

Author Contributions

Conceived and designed the experiments: SE FL RN MH. Performed the experiments: BG SE OM MI FL LD. Analyzed the data: BG MI SE FL GS EF PD. Contributed reagents/materials/analysis tools: BG FL LD SE MI. Wrote the paper: SE BG MI.

References

1. Galie N, Hoeper MM, Humbert M, Torbicki A, Vachiery JL, et al. (2009) Guidelines for the diagnosis and treatment of pulmonary hypertension: the Task Force for the Diagnosis and Treatment of Pulmonary Hypertension of the European Society of Cardiology (ESC) and the European Respiratory Society (ERS), endorsed by the International Society of Heart and Lung Transplantation (ISHLT). Eur Heart J 30: 2493–2537.
2. Machado RD, Eickelberg O, Elliott CG, Geraci MW, Hanaoka M, et al. (2009) Genetics and genomics of pulmonary arterial hypertension. J Am Coll Cardiol 54: S32–42.
3. Massague J (1998) TGF-beta signal transduction. Annu Rev Biochem 67: 753–791.
4. Goumans MJ, Lebrin F, Valdimarsdottir G (2003) Controlling the angiogenic switch: a balance between two distinct TGF-b receptor signaling pathways. Trends Cardiovasc Med 13: 301–307.
5. Eddahibi S, Guignabert C, Barlier-Mur AM, Dewachter L, Fadel E, et al. (2006) Cross talk between endothelial and smooth muscle cells in pulmonary hypertension: critical role for serotonin-induced smooth muscle hyperplasia. Circulation 113: 1857–1864.
6. Eddahibi S, Humbert M, Fadel E, Raffestin B, Darmon M, et al. (2001) Serotonin transporter overexpression is responsible for pulmonary artery smooth muscle hyperplasia in primary pulmonary hypertension. J Clin Invest 108: 1141–1150.
7. Torsney E, Charlton R, Diamond AG, Burn J, Soames JV, et al. (2003) Mouse model for hereditary hemorrhagic telangiectasia has a generalized vascular abnormality. Circulation 107: 1653–1657.
8. Eddahibi S, Hanoun N, Lanfumey L, Lesch KP, Raffestin B, et al. (2000) Attenuated hypoxic pulmonary hypertension in mice lacking the 5-hydroxytryptamine transporter gene. J Clin Invest 105: 1555–1562.
9. Rajkumar R, Konishi K, Richards TJ, Ishizawar DC, Wiechert AC, et al. (2010) Genomewide RNA expression profiling in lung identifies distinct signatures in idiopathic pulmonary arterial hypertension and secondary pulmonary hypertension. Am J Physiol Heart Circ Physiol 298: H1235–1248.
10. Selimovic N, Bergh CH, Andersson B, Sakiniene E, Carlsten H, et al. (2009) Growth factors and interleukin-6 across the lung circulation in pulmonary hypertension. Eur Respir J 34: 662–668.
11. Botney MD, Bahadori L, Gold LI (1994) Vascular remodeling in primary pulmonary hypertension. Potential role for transforming growth factor-beta. Am J Pathol 144: 286–295.
12. Ambalavanan N, Nicola T, Hagood J, Bulger A, Serra R, et al. (2008) Transforming growth factor-beta signaling mediates hypoxia-induced pulmonary arterial remodeling and inhibition of alveolar development in newborn mouse lung. Am J Physiol Lung Cell Mol Physiol 295: L86–95.
13. Long L, Crosby A, Yang X, Southwood M, Upton PD, et al. (2009) Altered bone morphogenetic protein and transforming growth factor-beta signaling in rat models of pulmonary hypertension: potential for activin receptor-like kinase-5 inhibition in prevention and progression of disease. Circulation 119: 566–576.
14. Chen YF, Feng JA, Li P, Xing D, Zhang Y, et al. (2006) Dominant negative mutation of the TGF-beta receptor blocks hypoxia-induced pulmonary vascular remodeling. J Appl Physiol 100: 564–571.
15. Megalou AJ, Glava C, Oikonomidis DL, Vilaeti A, Agelaki MG, et al. (2010) Transforming growth factor-beta inhibition attenuates pulmonary arterial hypertension in rats. Int J Clin Exp Med 3: 332–340.
16. Girerd B, Montani D, Coulet F, Sztrymf B, Yaici A, et al. (2010) Clinical outcomes of pulmonary arterial hypertension in patients carrying an ACVRL1 (ALK1) mutation. Am J Respir Crit Care Med 181: 851–861.
17. Shintani M, Yagi H, Nakayama T, Saji T, Matsuoka R (2009) A new nonsense mutation of SMAD8 associated with pulmonary arterial hypertension. J Med Genet 46: 331–337.
18. Ramos MF, Lame MW, Segall HJ, Wilson DW (2008) Smad signaling in the rat model of monocrotaline pulmonary hypertension. Toxicol Pathol 36: 311–320.
19. Mata-Greenwood E, Meyrick B, Steinhorn RH, Fineman JR, Black SM (2003) Alterations in TGF-beta1 expression in lambs with increased pulmonary blood flow and pulmonary hypertension. Am J Physiol Lung Cell Mol Physiol 285: L209–221.
20. Zakrzewicz A, Kouri FM, Nejman B, Kwapiszewska G, Hecker M, et al. (2007) The transforming growth factor-beta/Smad2,3 signalling axis is impaired in experimental pulmonary hypertension. Eur Respir J 29: 1094–1104.
21. Lebrin F, Goumans MJ, Jonker L, Carvalho RL, Valdimarsdottir G, et al. (2004) Endoglin promotes endothelial cell proliferation and TGF-beta/ALK1 signal transduction. EMBO J 23: 4018–4028.
22. Hassoun PM, Mouthon L, Barbera JA, Eddahibi S, Flores SC, et al. (2009) Inflammation, growth factors, and pulmonary vascular remodeling. J Am Coll Cardiol 54: S10–19.
23. Humbert M, Morrell NW, Archer SL, Stenmark KR, MacLean MR, et al. (2004) Cellular and molecular pathobiology of pulmonary arterial hypertension. J Am Coll Cardiol 43: 13S–24S.
24. Izikki M, Guignabert C, Fadel E, Humbert M, Tu L, et al. (2009) Endothelial-derived FGF2 contributes to the progression of pulmonary hypertension in humans and rodents. J Clin Invest 119: 512–523.
25. Castanares C, Redondo-Horcajo M, Magan-Marchal N, ten Dijke P, Lamas S, et al. (2007) Signaling by ALK5 mediates TGF-beta-induced ET-1 expression in endothelial cells: a role for migration and proliferation. J Cell Sci 120: 1256–1266.
26. Star GP, Giovinazzo M, Langleben D (2010) Bone morphogenic protein-9 stimulates endothelin-1 release from human pulmonary microvascular endothelial cells: a potential mechanism for elevated ET-1 levels in pulmonary arterial hypertension. Microvasc Res 80: 349–354.
27. Chen Q, Chen L, Liu B, Vialli C, Stone P, et al. (2010) The role of autocrine TGFbeta1 in endothelial cell activation induced by phagocytosis of necrotic trophoblasts: a possible role in the pathogenesis of pre-eclampsia. J Pathol 221: 87–95.
28. Jiang BH, Tardif JC, Sauvageau S, Ducharme A, Shi Y, et al. (2010) Beneficial effects of atorvastatin on lung structural remodeling and function in ischemic heart failure. J Card Fail 16: 679–688.
29. Burton VJ, Ciuclan LI, Holmes AM, Rodman DM, Walker C, et al. (2011) Bone morphogenetic protein receptor II regulates pulmonary artery endothelial cell barrier function. Blood 117: 333–341.

30. Ardelean DS, Yin M, Jerkic M, Peter M, Ngan B, et al. (2014) Anti-VEGF therapy reduces intestinal inflammation in Endoglin heterozygous mice subjected to experimental colitis. Angiogenesis.
31. Perros F, Dorfmuller P, Montani D, Hammad H, Waelput W, et al. (2012) Pulmonary Lymphoid Neogenesis in Idiopathic Pulmonary Arterial Hypertension. Am J Respir Crit Care Med.
32. Tu L, Dewachter L, Gore B, Fadel E, Dartevelle P, et al. (2011) Autocrine fibroblast growth factor-2 signaling contributes to altered endothelial phenotype in pulmonary hypertension. Am J Respir Cell Mol Biol 45: 311–322.

12

Inhalation of the BK_{Ca}-Opener NS1619 Attenuates Right Ventricular Pressure and Improves Oxygenation in the Rat Monocrotaline Model of Pulmonary Hypertension

Marc Revermann[1,2]*, Skevi Neofitidou[1], Thomas Kirschning[1], Manuel Schloss[2], Ralf P. Brandes[2], Christian Hofstetter[1]

1 Department of Anesthesiology and Critical Care Medicine, University Hospital Mannheim, Faculty of Medicine, University of Heidelberg, Heidelberg, Germany, **2** Institute for Cardiovascular Physiology, Medical Faculty of the Goethe-University Frankfurt, Frankfurt, Germany

Abstract

Background: Right heart failure is a fatal consequence of chronic pulmonary hypertension (PH). The development of PH is characterized by increased proliferation of vascular cells, in particular pulmonary artery smooth muscle cells (PASMCs) and pulmonary artery endothelial cells. In the course of PH, an escalated right ventricular (RV) afterload occurs, which leads to increased perioperative morbidity and mortality. BK_{Ca} channels are ubiquitously expressed in vascular smooth muscle cells and their opening induces cell membrane hyperpolarization followed by vasodilation. Moreover, BK activation induces anti-proliferative effects in a multitude of cell types. On this basis, we hypothesized that treatment with the nebulized BK channel opener NS1619 might be a therapy option for pulmonary hypertension and tested this in rats.

Methods: (1) Rats received monocrotaline injection for PH induction. Twenty-four days later, rats were anesthetized and NS1619 or the solvent was administered by inhalation. Systemic hemodynamic parameters, RV hemodynamic parameters, and blood gas analyses were measured before as well as 30 and 120 minutes after inhalation. (2) Rat PASMCs were stimulated with PDGF-BB in the presence and absence of NS1619. AKT, ERK1 and ERK2 activation were investigated by western blot analyses, and relative cell number was determined 48 hours after stimulation.

Results: Inhalation of a 12 μM and 100 μM NS1619 solution significantly reduced RV pressure without affecting systemic arterial pressure. Blood gas analyses demonstrated significantly reduced carbon dioxide and improved oxygenation in NS1619-treated animals pointing towards a considerable pulmonary shunt-reducing effect. In PASMC's, NS1619 (100 μM) significantly attenuated PASMC proliferation by a pathway independent of AKT and ERK1/2 activation.

Conclusion: NS1619 inhalation reduces RV pressure and improves oxygen supply and its application inhibits PASMC proliferation *in vitro*. Hence, BK opening might be a novel option for the treatment of pulmonary hypertension.

Editor: Tohru Fukai, University of Illinois at Chicago, United States of America

Funding: The Medical Faculties of Mannheim and Frankfurt and the B. Braun foundation supported the work. The funders had no role in study design, data collection and analysis, decision to publish, or preparation of the manuscript.

Competing Interests: The authors have declared that no competing interest exist.

* E-mail: marc.revermann@umm.de

Introduction

Pulmonary hypertension (PH) is a serious disease with a fatal progressive course and a risk of perioperative morbidity and mortality. Although pharmacological treatment improved in recent years, the survival of patients suffering from PH is limited by right heart failure and arrhythmias [1]. Current PH treatment strategies rely on vasodilatory and anti-proliferative agents, e.g. prostaglandin-analogues, phosphodiesterase type 5 inhibitors and endothelin-receptor antagonists [2]. Since drugs which exclusively dilate the pulmonary vasculature are not available yet, inhalative application of vasoactive compounds is a promising approach to bring on selective pulmonary vasodilation with few systemic side effects. However, although some inhalatively applicable drugs have been developed, PH is still a therapeutic challenge with problematic prognosis. Thus, new therapeutic strategies to improve the survival of patients suffering from this disease are still required.

An ideal drug for PH therapy has to fulfil the following two requirements: 1. Improvement of right ventricular performance. 2. Checking the disease's long-term progression by limiting the uncontrolled pulmonary arterial vascular cell proliferation, particularly pulmonary artery smooth muscle cell (PASMC) proliferation.

Right ventricular dysfunction and failure are the limiting factors concerning the prognosis of pulmonary hypertension. Right ventricular (RV) afterload, contractility and relaxation are parameters, which characterize right ventricular function. Here, determination of appropriate parameters, such as RV pressure, dP/dt_{max}, and dP/dt_{min} help to assess RV function.

In this regard, the velocity of pressure rise (dP/dt_{max}) is a parameter which is dependent on right ventricular contractility and right ventricular afterload, whereas dP/dt_{min} is a parameter which is useful for determination of ventricular relaxation.

Moreover, right ventricular oxygen demand-supply-ratio is an objective of PH treatment. Concerning the latter, right ventricular myocardial oxygen demand depends on right ventricular work, which in turn mainly depends on the right ventricular afterload. Additionally, PH is usually characterized by an increased pulmonary shunt volume, which results in a reduced oxygenation state and general hypoxemia.

Potassium ion channels are involved in numerous cardiovascular functions. In vascular cells their opening leads to hyperpolarization of the cell membrane and induces a multitude of changes in the cellular activity. In endothelial cells hyperpolarization increases calcium influx and enhances endothelial NO synthase activation [3], and in smooth muscle cells hyperpolarization induces relaxation by reducing the open probability of L-type calcium channels [4]. This in turn provokes vasodilation and decreases the activity of – at least partly – pro-proliferative calcium dependent mitogen activated protein (MAP) kinases.

The BK channel is a calcium-sensitive potassium ion channel, which is ubiquitously expressed in blood vessels, especially in endothelial and vascular smooth muscle cells [3,5]. Among the family of calcium-dependent potassium channels, BK channels show the most substantial potassium efflux. Since potassium channels modulate the vascular tone [6] and the cellular proliferative state [7], we investigated the impact of the BK channel opener NS1619 on right ventricular and systemic hemodynamic performance and blood gases in the rat monocrotaline PH model as well as on PASMC proliferation in cell culture.

Materials and Methods

Animals and Study Protocol

Animal experiments were performed in accordance with the National Institutes of Health Guidelines on the Use of Laboratory Animals. Both the University Animal Care Committee and the Federal Authorities for Animal Research of the Regierungspräsidium Darmstadt (Hessen, Germany) approved the study protocol. Male Sprague-Dawley rats (300–350 g body weight) were obtained from Charles River Laboratories (Sulzfeld, Germany). Rats were exposed to Monocrotaline (Sigma, Deishofen, Germany), which was dissolved in HCl (0.1 mol/l), adjusted to pH 7.4 with NaOH solution (0.1 mol/l) and administered as a single subcutaneous injection (60 mg/kg body weight) as described previously [8]. After twenty-four days, rats (440,8±33,72 g body weight) were randomized to the different study groups. After anesthesia with pentobarbital (Narcoren, Merial, Halbergmoos, Germany; 50 mg/kg, i.p.) plus fentanyl (Janssen-Cilag, Neuss, Germany; 0.05 mg/kg, i.p.), rats were weighed and then placed supine on a heating pad. A tracheotomy was performed, and a 14-gauge cannula (inner diameter 2.0 mm, outer diameter 2.5 mm, Abbott, Wiesbaden, Germany) was inserted to ventilate the animals with an infant ventilator (Stephanie, Stephan, Gackenbach, Germany). The following parameters were used in a pressure-controlled ventilation protocol: initial maximum pressure 16 cm H2O; positive endexpiratory pressure 4 cm H2O; respiratory rate 30 breaths/min; time inspiratory/expiratory: 1/1; FiO2 0.21. Body temperature was monitored by a rectal probe and kept constant at 37.0–38.0°C throughout the experiment. Fluid-filled polyurethane catheters (inner diameter 0.58 mm, outer diameter 0.96 mm, SIMS Portex, Hythe, UK) were inserted in the right femoral vein for infusion of anesthetics and in the right femoral artery for invasive blood pressure measurement and withdrawal of blood samples, respectively. After anesthetic dosage titration, anesthesia was maintained by continuous intravenous infusion of pentobarbital (5–10 mg/kg/hr) and fentanyl (2.5–5 μg/kg/hr). With the help of a skin incision the right jugular vein was exposed and a catheter (Millar, 2F; ADInstruments, Spechbach, Germany) was inserted into the vessel and advanced to the right ventricle. Inspiratory pressure levels were adjusted to achieve standardized basal carbon dioxide values (34–46 mmHg). Afterwards, no further changes of the lung ventilator settings were performed. Systemic arterial and right ventricular pressure curves and their derivatives, and body temperature were recorded permanently using a data acquirement system (Powerlab; ADInstruments, Germany). Volume reagibility parameters were calculated as follows: Systolic blood pressure variation (SPV) = $bp_{sys}max - bp_{sys}min/bp_{sys}mean$, pulse pressure variation (PPV) = PPmax − PPmin/PPmean, relative stroke volume variation (SVV) = $RR_{integral}$ max – $RR_{integral}$ min/RR $_{integral}$ mean. Following the principles of pulse contour analysis we determined the changes of the integral below the arterial pressure curve and describe the changes of that area as "relative stroke volume" (rSV) or as "relative stroke volume variation" (rSVV).

Thirty-one rats were randomized. Four animals were excluded because of technical, respectively experimental problems (e.g. catheter dislocation). Only rats with overt pulmonary hypertension (RVSP values 35–75 mmHg) were included in the study. Three of the remaining twenty-seven animals were excluded because their RVSP was not within the target range. The RVSP of healthy male Sprague Dawley rats is approximately 25 mmHg [9]. Data were continuously recorded and statistical analysis was performed for data average of a 60 seconds period once hemodynamic steady state was reached for 3 minutes. Blood gas analyses of animals with initial normocapnia ($PaCO_2$ 34–46 mmHg) were recorded (Radiometer ABL 80 flex, Radiometer GmbH, Willich, Deutschland) before, 30 and 120 minutes after compound nebulization and statistical analysed.

Nebulization

For the nebulization, NS1619 (Sigma, Deishofen, Germany) was dissolved in Dimethyl Sulfoxide (DMSO; Sigma, Deishofen, Germany) and expanded with sodium chloride solution, resulting in 3 ml of 100 μM (100 μM group) and 12.5 μM (12 μM group) NS1619 solutions. These solutions were applied by an integrated nebulizer (multisonic infracontrol, Schill, Probstzella, Germany) which produced particles with a median size of 2.0 μm and an intrapulmonary deposition fraction of 3.8% (manufacturer information) for a three-minute period.

3-(4,5-Dimethylthiazol-2-yl)-2,5-diphenyltetrazolium Bromide Pulmonary Arterial Smooth Muscle Cells Proliferation Assay

Rat pulmonary artery smooth muscle cells (PASMCs) were seeded in multiwell plates in cell culture medium (8%FCS) after isolating them from rat pulmonary arteries as described previously [8]. When a subconfluent growth state was reached, culture medium was replaced by a 8% FCS containing medium, and NS1619 (100 μmol/l final concentration; Sigma-Aldrich, Germany) or the solvent (DMSO) were added to subgroups. Their proliferation was subsequently stimulated by platelet-derived growth factor-BB (PDGF-BB; 20–30 ng/ml). After two days, the cell number was determined by the MTT test. In brief, the plates were washed and (3-(4,5-dimethylthiazol-2-yl)-2,5-diphenyltetrazolium bromide (MTT, Sigma) was added. After an incubation period of two hours (37°C, 5% CO_2), acidified isopropanol was added to dissolve the precipitated formazan. Absorbance was determined by a spectrophotometer (550 nm wavelength; Wallac Victor; EG&G Wallac, Freiburg, Germany).

Immunoblotting

For the western blot analysis rat PASMCs were isolated from rat pulmonary arteries and seeded in 3.5 cm dishes until they reached a nearly confluent growth state. PASMCs were starved for 24 hours (0.1% BSA) and afterwards stimulated with PDGF-BB (10 ng/ml) in the absence or presence of NS1619 (100 µmol/l; 120 minutes preincubation, Sigma-Aldrich, Germany). After four and eight minutes, respectively, the cells were frozen in liquid nitrogen and subsequently scraped in triton-X-100 lysis buffer. Protein concentration was determined by Bradford assay. Extracted protein samples were boiled in a Laemmli buffer and 50 µg of each sample was separated by sodium dodecyl sulfate–polyacrylamide gel electrophoresis (SDS–PAGE; 10%) and transferred onto nitrocellulose membrane as described previously [8]. Proteins were detected using primary antibodies against p-ERK1, p-ERK2, ERK1, ERK2 and p-AKT (Cell Signaling, Danvers, USA;1:1.000 each antibody) and appropriate secondary antibodies labeled with infrared dyes and visualized using the Odyssey infrared imaging system (Li-COR Biosciences, Bad Homburg, Germany). Densitometry was carried out using the integrated Odyssey software.

Data and Statistical Analysis

Statistical analyses were performed by using Kolmogorov-Smirnov normality test and analysis of variance (ANOVA), followed by Tukey-corrected Fisher's LSD test and the unpaired t-test for normal distributed data and Kruskal-Wallis test with Dunn's post test or, where appropriate, the Mann-Whitney test, for nonparametric distributed data. A P value of less than 0.05 was considered statistically significant.

Results

Inhalation of NS1619

In this study, we explored whether the BK channel opener NS1619 could affect hemodynamics with focussing on the right ventricle as its failure is the life-threatening consequence of PH. To minimize systemic side effects and optimize the drug's concentration in the target organ, NS1619 or the solvent were applied by inhalation. As the current study investigates both, a possible biologic effect of inhaled NS1619 on cardiopulmonary function in principle, and a possible dose dependency, we performed two separate statistical analyses: 1. Dose-dependent effects were examined by comparing all three study groups. 2. General NS1619-dependent effects were examined by comparing all NS1619-treated animals ($\sum$NS1619 = $\sum$) with the control group.

The basic values for each of the parameter recorded did not differ significantly between the three groups (Solvent, 12 µM NS1619, 100 µM NS1619) (**Table 1**).

Inhalation of NS1619 Reduces Right Ventricular Afterload

Twenty-four days after the monocrotaline challenge, PH was established. This was shown by an elevated average right ventricular systolic pressure (RVSP) of 50,8 mmHg and an average right ventricular mean pressure (RVMP) of 23 mmHg (**Table 1**). 120 minutes after inhalation, the NS1619 treatment reduced right ventricular pressure significantly (**Figure 1**). Accordingly, right ventricular myocardial work, defined by the product of heart rate and right ventricular afterload (RVSP), decreased in animals treated with 100 µM NS1619 and in the $\sum$NS1619 group. Right ventricular maximum velocity of the pressure slope (dP/dt_{max}) were significantly attenuated in the 12 µM group 120 minutes after inhalation. The maximum velocity of the pressure drop (dP/dt_{min}), on the other hand, increased after inhalation of NS1619 and reached statistical significance in the 12 µM group as well as in the pooled NS1619 group compared to control animals (**Figure 1**).

Inhalation of NS1619 does not Affect Systemic Hemodynamic Parameters

30 and 120 minutes after inhalation, the results for heart rate, arterial systolic, mean and diastolic blood pressure did not differ between subjects receiving NS1619 or subjects receiving the solvent (**Table 2**).

Inhalation of NS1619 does not Affect Predictors of Fluid Responsiveness

To explore possible alterations of fluid responsiveness predictors, which are more difficult to determine than systemic arterial blood pressure, we determined the changes of relative stroke volume (rSV), relative stroke volume variation (rSVV), systolic pressure variation (SPV) and pulse pressure variation (PPV). Concerning these parameters, there was no significant difference between NS1619 treated and control animals (**Table 3**).

Inhalation of NS1619 does not Affect Left Ventricular Hemodynamic Parameters

For estimating left ventricular work, the product of heart rate and systolic arterial blood pressure was calculated. Here, no significant difference between the three groups was found. Furthermore, the analysis of the blood pressure curve's dP/dt_{max}, which depends on left ventricular contractility and vascular compliance, did not show significant variation after NS1619 inhalation. To assess the cardiac output the product of heart rate and the integral below the arterial blood pressure curve was calculated. No compound-dependent alteration was found (**Table 4**).

NS1619 Inhalation Reduces Dissolved Carbon Dioxide and Increases Dissolved Oxygen in the Blood

For evaluating the impact of BK channel opener on gas exchange and oxygen supply, blood gas analyses were performed before as well as 30 and 120 minutes after inhalation. Initial values of blood gas analyses did not differ between the three groups investigated. 120 minutes after inhalation of NS1619, carbon dioxide levels were significantly reduced in animals which were treated with NS1619 (**Figure 2**). On the other hand, the oxygen level was considerably increased 30 and 120 minutes after NS1619 inhalation. This effect reached high significance level after 120 minutes (**Figure 2;** $p<0.05$). Also, 120 minutes after inhalation, pH was significantly increased in the pooled NS1619 group, indicating the development of a respiratory alkalosis. Base excess and bicarbonate values did not differ significantly between the three groups.

The BK_{Ca} Channel Opener NS1619 Reduces Pulmonary Artery Smooth Muscle Cell (PASMC) Proliferation

To test the hypothesis that BK channel opening affects PASMC proliferation, we investigated the effect of NS1619 on PDGF-induced PASMC proliferation *in vitro* (**Figure 3**). The platelet-derived growth factor (PDGF-BB) was applied as stimulus as it is a well-known contributor to formation of some PH subspecies, in

Table 1. Basic values.

Parameter	Solvent	12 μM NS1619	100 μM NS1619
RVSP (mmHg)	51,59±3,868	48,54±2,388	51,78±2,958
RVMP (mmHg)	22,65±1,697	23,06±1,088	23,66±2,148
RVDP (mmHg)	2,466±1,200	4,143±1,322	2,629±1,504
Heart rate * RVSP	19863±1439	18514±1621	17875±1109
dP/dt $_{max}$ (mmHg * s^{-1})	1913±122,7	2043±251,6	1619±162,8
dP/dt $_{min}$ (mmHg * s^{-1})	−1824±115,8	−1723±162,2	−1523±139,1
heart rate (bpm)	387,3±14,73	378,7±22,35	345,8±9,934
bp sys (mmHg)	149,4±5,292	148,7±5,031	163,3±10,76
bp mean (mmHg)	111,9±4,868	108,6±5,447	131,0±9,340
bp dia (mmHg)	98,78±4,670	85,66±5,017	110,8±7,863
rSVV	0,1712±0,01687	0,2048±0,04766	0,1667±0,02251
SPV	0,1594±0,01857	0,1602±0,03862	0,09328±0,01192
rSV (mmHg* s)	16,88±1,051	17,28±1,902	19,86±3,363
PPV	0,2026±0,02420	0,1761±0,04488	0,1622±0,02647
Heart rate * rSV (min^{-1} *mmHg*s)	6446±289,1	6313±328,0	6757±1039
Heart rate * RR sys (min^{-1} * mmHg)	57947±3102	55948±2694	56143±3292
dP/dt $_{max}$ (mmHg xs^{-1})	3367±286,4	3430±353,9	3312±346,2
PaO_2 (mmHg)	80,73±3,136	69,27±2,089	72,83±4,362
$PaCO_2$ (mmHg)	40,39±1,481	41,17±1,486	40,67±1,430
HCO_3^- (mmol/l)	24,84±0,5464	24,48±0,8220	25,63±1,119
Base excess (mmol/l)	0,6000±0,6541	0,06667±0,6839	1,117±1,364
pH	7,408±0,01601	7,392±0,00654	7,412±0,02535

The basic values for each of the parameter recorded did not differ significantly between the three groups (Solvent, 12 μM NS1619, 100 μM NS1619).

particular development of pulmonary arterial hypertension (PAH). In fact, 100 μM NS1619 attenuated PDGF-dependent PASMC proliferation significantly (**Figure 3A**).

The Antiproliferative Effect of NS1619 is Independent of MAP Kinases

Since mitogen-activated protein kinases ERK1, ERK2 and AKT are important elements of PDGF's intracellular signaling pathway, we performed western blot analyses to find out whether those kinases mediate the anti-proliferative effect of NS1619. Accordingly, in cultured PASMC's, activation of ERK1, ERK2 and AKT was investigated by measuring the phosphorylation state four and eight minutes after the PDGF-BB challenge (**Figure 3B**). Phosphorylation of ERK1, ERK2 and AKT significantly increased four minutes after PDGF stimulation (**Figure 3C;** *: $p<0.05$). In the period between four and eight minutes after stimulation, ERK1 and ERK2 phosphorylation increased time-dependently (*:$p<0.05$) whereas AKT phosphorylation increased by trend within this period. NS1619 (100 μmol/l) did not affect ERK1, ERK2 and AKT activation state after PDGF-BB challenge (**Figure 3B,C**).

Discussion

The present study focused on the acute effect of nebulized BK channel opening agent NS1619 on the cardiopulmonary system, i.e. pharmacologically induced changes of right ventricular performance, systemic hemodynamic parameters, and blood gas exchange of rats with experimentally induced pulmonary hypertension. Additionally, we investigated the impact of the BK channel opening compound on pulmonary arterial smooth muscle cell proliferation *in vitro*.

NS1619 reduced right ventricular afterload without affecting systemic hemodynamic parameters. Blood gas analyses revealed an increase of dissolved oxygen and a decrease of dissolved carbon dioxide and development of a respiratory alkalosis after pharmacological BK opening.

Potassium channel generate the basis of the cellular resting membrane potential in numerous cell types and are involved in organization of the contractile tone of vascular smooth muscle cells [10–13]. Calcium-dependent BK_{Ca} channels occur ubiquitously in the vascular system and conduct ionic currents that mediate membrane hyperpolarization causing vasodilation [6]. They are regulated by calcium, but also by a number of other factors, such as cellular membrane potential and channel phosphorylation [6], and have recently been detected in pulmonary artery smooth muscle cells [14,] [15].

Since NS1619 is described as a vasodilating and anti-proliferative compound, we investigated its impact in the rat monocrotaline model of pulmonary hypertension. To do so, NS1619 was administered by inhalation as this application modality is preferable to systemic application concerning reduced systemic side effects and high local concentrations at the target site [16]. Accordingly, the failing right ventricle is very sensitive to low systemic arterial blood pressure.

In this context, systemic BK ion channel opening may attenuates the protective Euler-Liljestrand mechanism by causing an increased pulmonary shunt volume followed by impaired oxygenation.

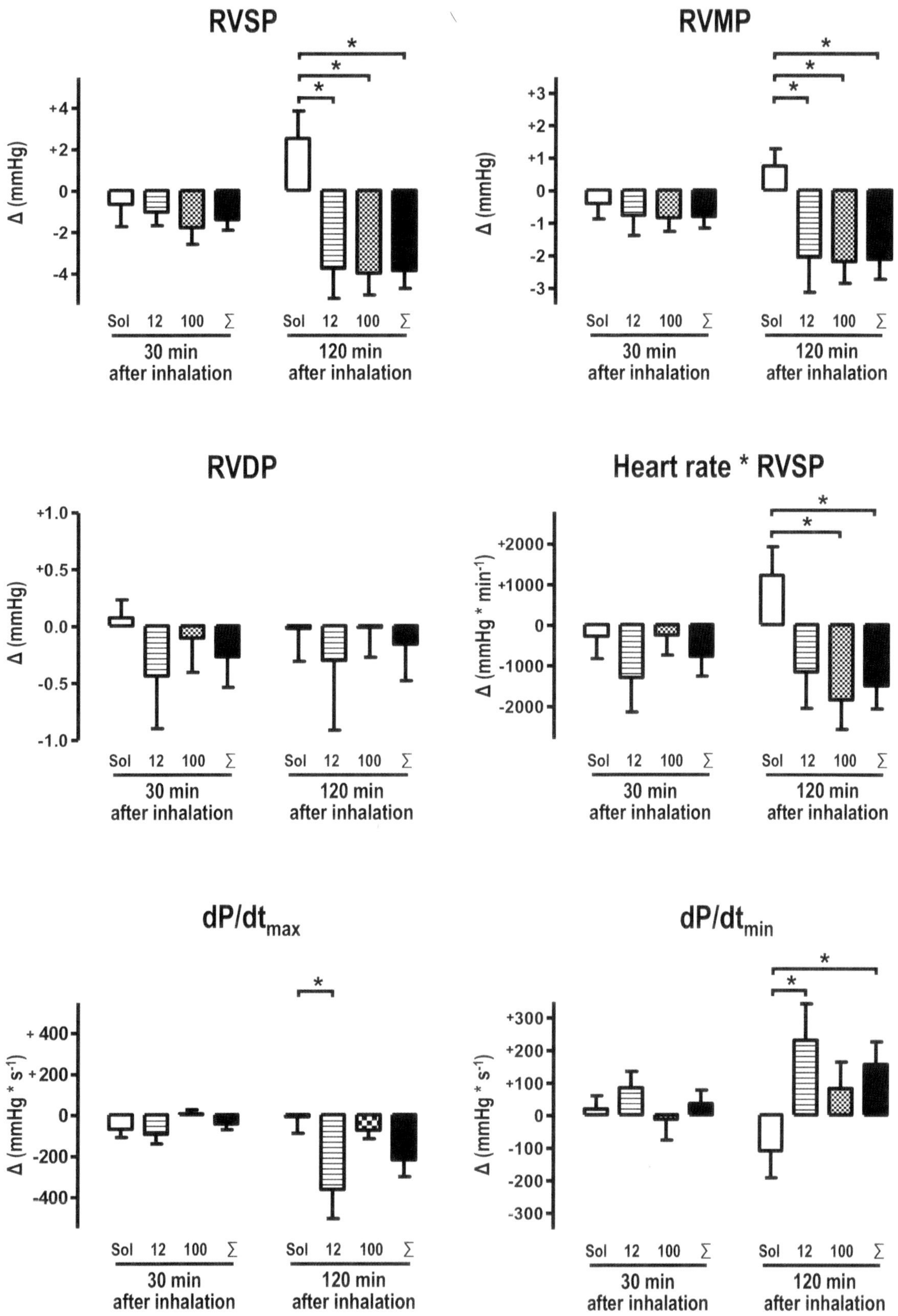

Figure 1. NS1619 reduces right ventricular pressure. Inhalation of 12 μM and 100 μM NS1619 significantly attenuates monocrotaline-induced right ventricular hypertension in comparison to solvent-treated animals 120 minutes after inhalation. In detail, right ventricular systolic pressure (RVSP) and right ventricular mean pressure (RVMP) were reduced in both NS1619 groups and consecutively in the cumulative ∑NS1619 versus solvent calculation. As a result of the reduced RVSP, the approximated right ventricular work, which is characterized by the product of heart rate and RVSP is attenuated in the 100 μM and the ∑NS1619 group, too. Right ventricular maximum velocity of the pressure slope (dP/dt_{max}) were

significantly attenuated in the 12 μM group 120 minutes after inhalation. Moreover, 12 μM NS1619 as well as the ∑NS1619 group exhibit a significant diminishment of the right ventricular relaxation velocity by an increase of the dP/dt_{min}-slope. Data obtained after inhalation were subtracted from individual basis values and individual value differences (Δ) were calculated for each animal and time point. RVDP: right ventricular diastolic pressure, dP/dt_{max}: maximum contraction velocity (Solvent: n = 10; 12 μM: n = 7, 100 μM: n = 7; ∑NS1619: n = 14;*: $p<0.05$).

In the present study inhalative application of NS1619 did not affect heart rate, systemic arterial pressure and volume state indicating parameters, like pulse pressure variation and systolic pressure variation.

Two hours after solvent inhalation, compared to the baseline measurements, right ventricular systolic pressure (RVSP) and right ventricular mean pressure (RVMP) were increased in control animals indicating a successive mismatch of ventilation-perfusion ratio in artificially ventilated animals.

The latter effect seemed to be compensated by NS1619 inhalation, which is characterized by a significant RVSP and RVMP reduction in NS1619-treated animals. The delayed achievement of a significance level could be explained by the long diffusion distance and the diminished relaxation potential of the multilayered vascular medial layer. Interestingly, right ventricular rate-pressure product is attenuated in NS1619-treated animals, presumably resulting in a reduced right ventricular oxygen demand.

Some well known pulmonary vascular dilators, like NO and prostaglandins, could activate BK channel activity via cGMP and cAMP dependent protein kinase phosphorylation [17]'[18–20]. Accordingly, the established PH therapy strategies are at least partially dependent on BK activation.

For this reason, direct activation of a primary pharmacological target in PH therapy was a goal of this study. Neither of the NS1619 concentrations chosen for the *in vivo* study part, produced significantly different results. This may be accounted for by a pharmacological ceiling effect, which apparently already occurred at 12 μM. Thus, an increase from 12 to 100 μM did not improve either hemodynamic performance or ventilation-perfusion-ratio.

Two hours after inhalation we observed a decrease of the right ventricular maximum velocity of the pressure slope (dP/dt_{max}) in the 12 μM group. This effect could be caused by a decreased afterload, which has been reported previously and indicate a reduced right ventricular work in consequence of PH treatment [21–23]. Accordingly, we observed an increase of the relaxation velocity (dP/dt_{min}), which frequently accompanies a treatment-induced dP/dt_{max} reduction [21–23]. The reduced right ventricular lusitropy, characterized by dP/dt_{min} increase, was found in the 12 μM group and in the pooled NS1619 group. To our knowledge, there is no immediate connection of BK channels and the three main lusitropy mediating cardiomyocytical enzyme systems (Calcium ATPase, Na-Ca exchanger and the sarcoplasmic reticulum calcium ATPase, SERCA) observed so far and, additionally, BK channels are supposed to be absent from the cardiac myocyte sarcolemmal membrane [24]. This indicates that afterload reduction influences right ventricular lusitropy, perhaps mediated by a diminished sympathoadrenergic drive following RV pressure relief. Furthermore, the demonstrated acute attenuation of right ventricular rate-pressure-product could be caused by a reduced adrenergic stimulation of SERCA leading to an increase of dP/dt_{min}.

Two hours after inhalation, carbon dioxide plasma level was significantly reduced and corresponding oxygen plasma level was significantly increased in NS1619-treated animals. Besides a putative bronchodilatory effect of NS1619 [25]' [26], this phenomenon is possibly due to reduction of pulmonary arterio-venous shunt volume. Here, a disproportional oxygen increase over carbon dioxide decrease could be either caused by carbon dioxide replenishment from bicarbonate and/or a consequence of the reduced pulmonary shunt volume. Since we were not able to take mixed-venous blood samples, shunt calculation with the help of the Berggren formula could not be applied. However, we assume that the net oxygenation rise is due to pulmonary shunt reduction which may underlines the beneficial impact of NS1619 on PH disease.

Intracellular calcium augments smooth muscle cell contraction and stimulates cell proliferation [27] which could be mediated by calcium-dependent ras-activation resulting in phosphorylation and activation of mitogen activated protein kinases, such as ERK1 (p44), ERK2 (p42) and AKT [28,29]. BK channel activation reduces intracellular calcium concentration via smooth muscle cell membrane hyperpolarization and consecutive inhibition of l-type calcium channels [30]. Pulmonary vascular remodeling is – at least partially - initiated or mediated by the platelet derived growth factor (PDGF) [31–34]. In this regard, PDGF antagonism is possibly a promising treatment strategy, especially for humans suffering from pulmonary arterial hypertension (PAH/group I, WHO PH classification) [34]. This in mind, we used PDGF as stimulus for pulmonary artery smooth muscle cell (PASMC)

Table 2. Systemic hemodynamic parameters.

	Solv.	12 μM	100 μM	∑ NS1619	Solv. vs. ∑ NS1619	Solvent	12 μM	100 μM	∑ NS1619	Solv. vs. ∑ NS1619
heart rate (bpm)	−0,9±8,6	−19,2±17,3	+6,9±6,7	−6,2±9,6	P = 0,70	+4,2±6,7	+5,6±11,1	−9,5±13,7	−1,9±8,7	P = 0,61
bp sys (mmHg)	−2,2±5,1	−4,7±5,9	+0,9±5,6	−1,9±4,0	P = 0,96	−0,0±10,0	−5,1±7,1	−1,7±9,1	−3,4±5,6	P = 0,75
bp mean (mmHg)	+0,6±2,7	+0,0±4,0	+3,2±4,1	+1,6±2,8	P = 0,79	+2,3±8,8	−0,4±6,6	+1,0±9,2	+0,3±5,5	P = 0,84
bp dia (mmHg)	+0,7±2,7	+0,7±3,6	+3,7±3,2	+2,2±2,4	P = 0,68	+2,0±8,9	+2,0±6,3	+2,2±7,9	+2,1±4,8	P = 0,99
	(Δ) 30 min after inhalation					**(Δ) 120 min after inhalation**				

Heart rate, systolic (bp sys), mean (bp mean), diastolic (bp dia) arterial blood pressure were determined before (basis) as well as 30 and 120 minutes after inhalation of two different NS1619 concentrations, respectively solvent. Data obtained after inhalation were subtracted from individual basis values and individual value differences (Δ) were calculated for each animal and time point. None of the parameters investigated were affected by NS1619 inhalation in a significant manner. According to the character of the study as "a proof of principle", pooled NS1619 (∑NS1619) data was compared with the control group (Solvent = Solv.). No NS1619-dependent effect on systemic hemodynamic parameters was discovered.

Table 3. Intravascular volume parameters.

	Solvent	12 μM	100 μM	∑ NS1619	Solv. vs. ∑ NS1619	Solvent	12 μM	100 μM	∑ NS1619	Solv. vs. ∑ NS1619
rSVV	+0,00±0,01	−0,03±0,04	−0,01±0,02	−0,02±0,02	P = 0,44	+0,02±0,02	+0,01±0,03	−0,04±0,02	+0,02±0,02	P = 0,18
SPV	−0,01±0,02	+0,03±0,04	+0,01±0,01	+0,02±0,02	P = 0,31	+0,02±0,02	+0,05±0,03	+0,01±0,01	+0,03±0,02	P = 0,76
rSV (mmHg* s)	+0,04±0,52	+2,93±3,02	−0,22±0,74	+1,35±1,56	P = 0,50	+0,49±1,20	−0,58±0,97	+0,28±1,42	−0,15±0,84	P = 0,66
PPV	+0,01±0,01	+0,08±0,08	−0,01±0,01	+0,04±0,04	P = 0,38	+0,03±0,03	+0,09±0,04	−0,00±0,02	+0,05±0,03	P = 0,72
	(Δ) 30 min after inhalation					**(Δ) 120 min after inhalation**				

For the investigation of fluid responsive parameters were calculated: relative stroke volume (rSV) characterized by the area under the arterial blood pressure curve, systolic pressure variation (SPV), relative stroke volume variation (rSVV), and pulse pressure variation (PPV). No NS1619-dependent effect on these parameters was discovered. Data obtained after inhalation were subtracted from individual basis values and individual value differences (Δ) were calculated for each animal and time point.

proliferation *in vitro*, which represents a cellular model for PAH initiation *in vivo* [35]. However, recently published data indicates that PDGF inhibition ameliorates exercise capacity and hemodynamics in PAH patients but without affecting mortality and functional class affiliation [36].

In the present study, 100 μmol/l NS1619 reduced PDGF-induced PASMC proliferation reliably and significantly. According to other studies, 30 to 100 μmol/l NS1619 generates a general anti-proliferative effect, which has been shown in diverse cellular types [37–39]. Also, recently published data concerning the effect of NS1619 on vascular smooth muscle cell proliferation underlines the impact of BK channel activation on vascular remodeling [39]. Since intracellular calcium content is reduced after BK channel-mediated hyperpolarization, our hypothesis was that the calcium dependent ras/ERK/AKT pathways perhaps convey the anti-proliferative effect and performed cell culture experiments without detecting an alteration of ERK1, ERK2 and AKT phosphorylation depending on NS1619 exposure. Concerning this matter, we can only speculate whether anti-proliferative properties of NS1619 are due to mitochondrial membrane effects. Here, it has been reported that the opening of mitochondrial potassium channels has a benefit in the context of ischemic and anesthetic cardiac preconditioning [40–42]. Moreover, potassium channel opening has been proposed for mediating smooth muscle cell proliferation reduction and apoptosis induction, which, in turn, could be an essential mechanism for reducing pulmonary vascular wall remodeling in PAH [43,44].

Limitations

- Initially we wanted to investigate the effect of NS1619 in two PH models, namely in the MCT model and in the thromboxane-analogue U46619-induced PH model. But although we applied U46619 doses up to 6000 ng/100 g/min, which was sixfold higher than described previously [45], we were not able to induce a robust right ventricular hypertension. Instead of that, we observed a massive bronchial obstruction and so we stopped this study section.
- Although the monocrotaline model of PH is well established, the results obtained in this animal model have to be considered carefully because of the different features of vascular remodeling in rats and humans. In humans, endothelium-derived vascular alterations, like plexiform lesions, are pathognomonic for pulmonary arterial hypertension whereas MCT-treated animals show mainly medial layer alterations [46]. Because of the problematic expression of BK channels in cultured endothelial cells [47], we focused on the effect of NS1619 on PASMCs.

Table 4. Left ventricular work.

	Solvent	12 μM	100 μM	∑ NS1619	Solv. vs. ∑ NS1619	Solvent	12 μM	100 μM	∑ NS1619	Solv. vs. ∑ NS1619
Heart rate *		+643±	+140±						+8±	
rSV	+29±154	668	231	+392±345	P = 0,41	+276±481	−8±386	+25±532	316	P = 0,63
(min^{-1} *mmHg*s)										
Heart rate *							–	–		
RR sys	−966±2433	−4232±	+1719±	−1257±2395	P = 0,93	+452±406	1100±3788	1299±4684	−1199±	P = 0,74
(min^{-1} * mmHg)		3948	2513						2894	
dP/dt $_{max}$	−201±377	−570±	−157±	−364±235	P = 0,70	−633±457	−454±451	−548±444	−501±	P = 0,80
(mmHg xs^{-1})		341	329						304	
	(Δ) 30 min after inhalation					**(Δ) 120 min after inhalation**				

Left ventricular work was estimated as the product of heart rate (HR) and systolic arterial pressure (bp sys). Relative cardiac output was estimated as the product of heart rate and relative stroke volume (integral of the arterial curve). dP/dt $_{max}$ of the arterial pressure curve did not show a NS1619-dependent variation. Data obtained after inhalation were subtracted from individual basis values and individual value differences (Δ) were calculated for each animal and time point. (Solvent: n = 10; 12 μM: n = 7, 100 μM: n = 7; ∑NS1619: n = 14;*: $p < 0.05$).

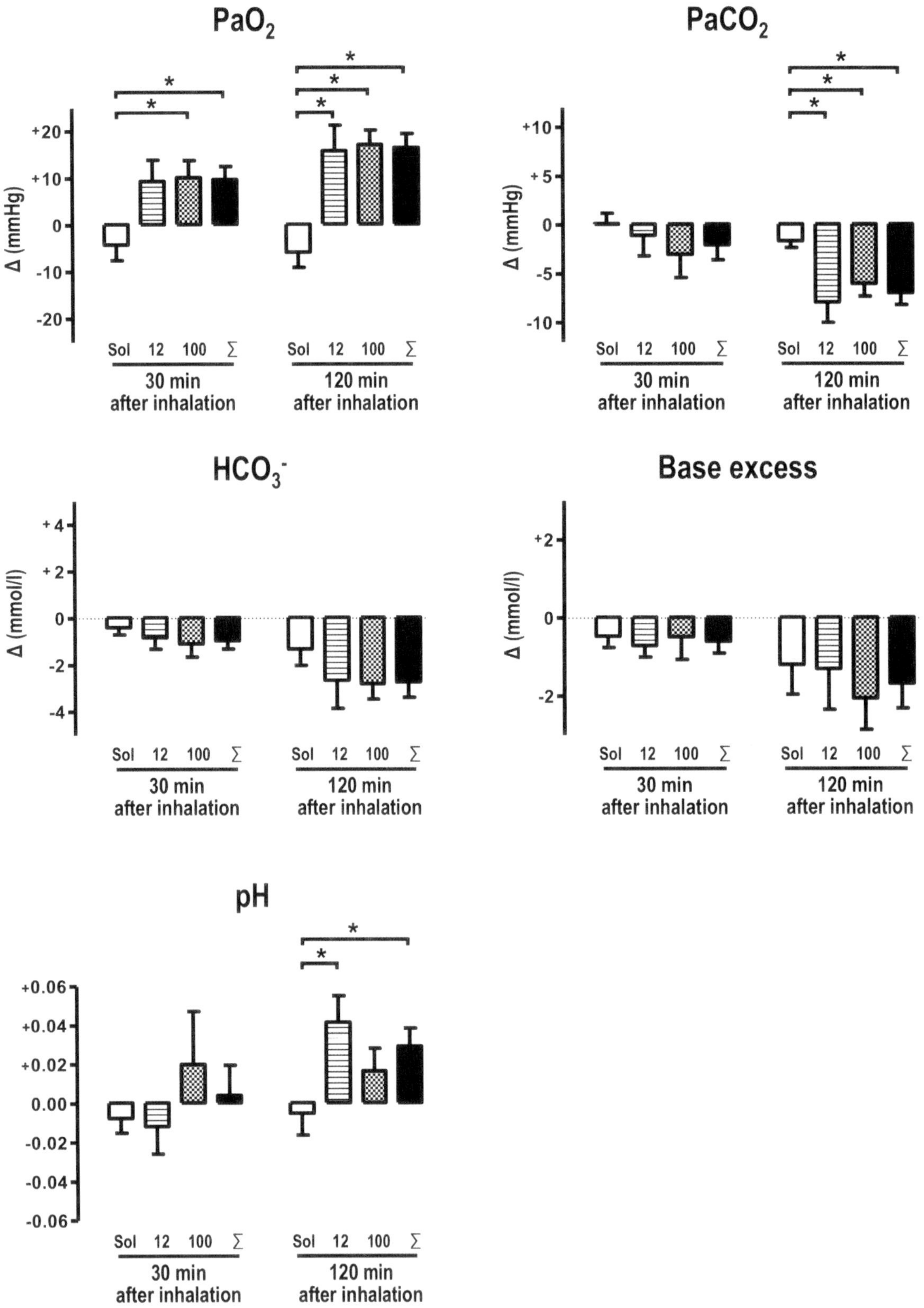

Figure 2. Blood gas analyses. 12 μM and 100 μM NS1619 improved oxygenation (PaO_2) considerably 120 minutes after inhalation and 100 μM and ∑NS1619 data exhibits a significant increase already 30 minutes after NS1619 inhalation. Carbon dioxide levels ($PaCO_2$) were attenuated 120 minutes after NS1619 inhalation. 12 μM and ∑NS1619 data demonstrate an elevated pH 120 minutes after inhalation. Base excess (BE) and bicarbonate concentration were not altered significantly by NS1619 although HCO_3^- was attenuated in NS1619 treated animals at least by trend. Data obtained after inhalation were subtracted from individual basis values and individual value differences (Δ) were calculated for each animal and time point. (Solvent: n = 8; 12 μM: n = 6, 100 μM: n = 6, ∑NS1619: n = 12; *: $p < 0.05$).

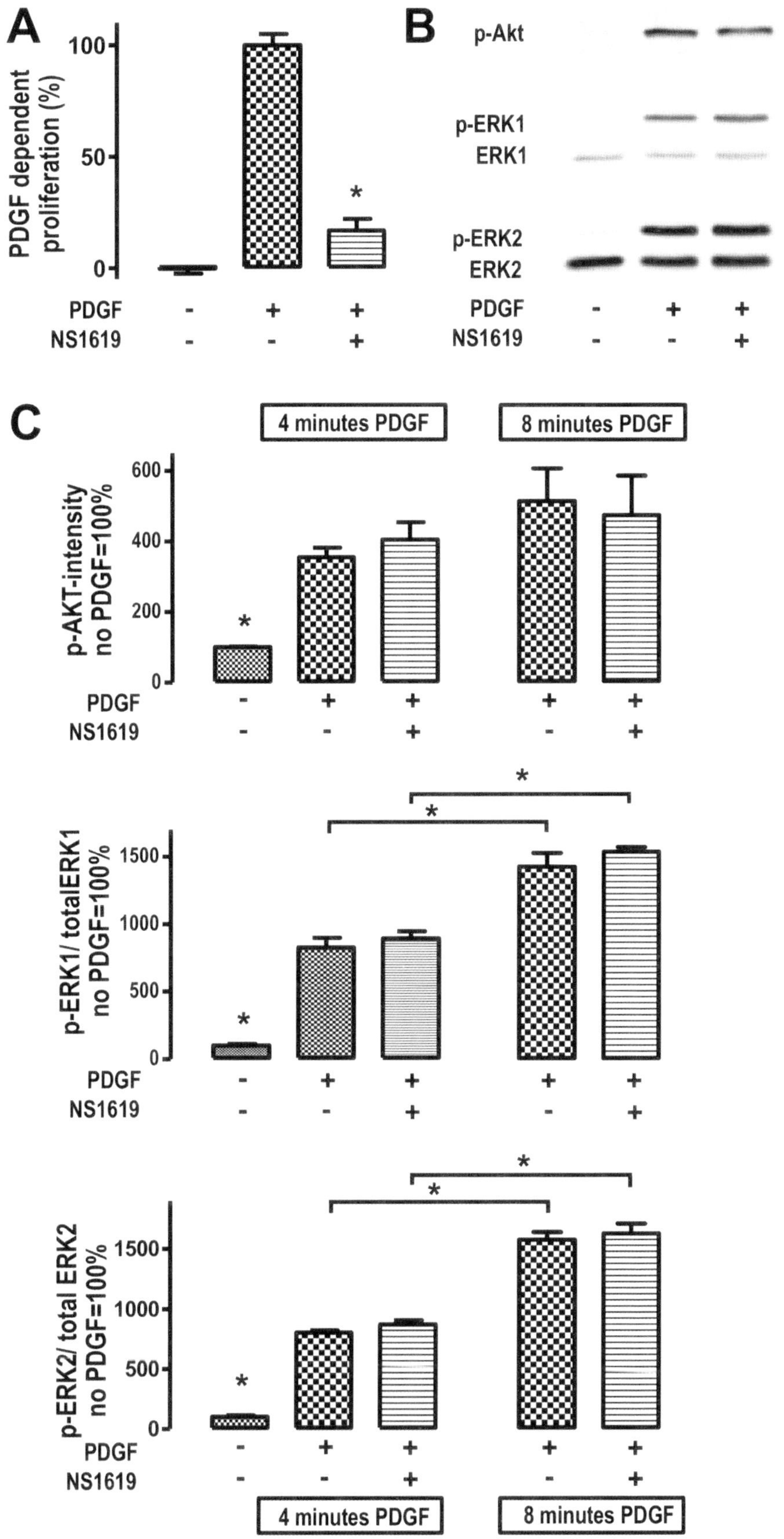

Figure 3. NS1619 attenuates PDGF-induced PASMC proliferation. (A) BK channel opening agent NS1619 (100 μmol/l) reduces PDGF-induced PASMC proliferation (n = 21 each column; * $p < 0.05$). (B,C) In cultured PASMCs, phosphorylation state of protein kinases ERK1, ERK2 and AKT increased

significantly 4 minutes after PDGF-BB stimulation (n = 3–6, *:p<0.05). Afterwards, phosphorylation states of ERK1 and ERK2 significantly increased within the period between 4 and 8 minutes after PDGF stimulation (n = 3–6; *:p<0.05) whereas AKT phosphorylation state rose by trend. BK channel opening by NS1619 (100 µmol/l) treatment does not affect phosphorylation of any kinase analysed.

Conclusion

Our study demonstrates that BK channel opening by NS1619 might be an option for treating pulmonary hypertension. Its inhalation reduces right ventricular work and improves myocardial oxygenation. The topical application of NS1619 attenuates PASMC proliferation in cell culture. As a next step, further research work needs to be conducted for investigating the effect of repetitive NS1619 inhalations on the course of PH disease.

Author Contributions

Conceived and designed the experiments: MR CH. Performed the experiments: MR SN TK MS. Analyzed the data: MR SN RPB CH. Contributed reagents/materials/analysis tools: RPB CH. Wrote the paper: MR RPB CH.

References

1. Badesch DB, Champion HC, Sanchez MA, Hoeper MM, Loyd JE, et al. (2009) Diagnosis and assessment of pulmonary arterial hypertension. J Am Coll Cardiol 54: S55–S66. S0735-1097(09)01214-5 [pii];10.1016/j.jacc.2009.04.011 [doi].
2. Barst RJ, Gibbs JS, Ghofrani HA, Hoeper MM, McLaughlin VV, et al. (2009) Updated evidence-based treatment algorithm in pulmonary arterial hypertension. J Am Coll Cardiol 54: S78–S84. S0735-1097(09)01223-6 [pii];10.1016/j.jacc.2009.04.017 [doi].
3. Vang A, Mazer J, Casserly B, Choudhary G (2010) Activation of endothelial BKCa channels causes pulmonary vasodilation. Vascul Pharmacol 53: 122–129. S1537-1891(10)00088-1 [pii];10.1016/j.vph.2010.05.001 [doi].
4. Edwards G, Niederste-Hollenberg A, Schneider J, Noack T, Weston AH (1994) Ion channel modulation by NS 1619, the putative BKCa channel opener, in vascular smooth muscle. Br J Pharmacol 113: 1538–1547.
5. Bonnet S, Archer SL (2007) Potassium channel diversity in the pulmonary arteries and pulmonary veins: implications for regulation of the pulmonary vasculature in health and during pulmonary hypertension. Pharmacol Ther 115: 56-69. S0163-7258(07)00076-9 [pii];10.1016/j.pharmthera.2007.03.014 [doi].
6. Brayden JE, Nelson MT (1992) Regulation of arterial tone by activation of calcium-dependent potassium channels. Science 256: 532–535.
7. Blackiston DJ, McLaughlin KA, Levin M (2009) Bioelectric controls of cell proliferation: ion channels, membrane voltage and the cell cycle. Cell Cycle 8: 3519–3528. 9888 [pii].
8. Revermann M, Barbosa-Sicard E, Dony E, Schermuly RT, Morisseau C, et al. (2009) Inhibition of the soluble epoxide hydrolase attenuates monocrotaline-induced pulmonary hypertension in rats. J Hypertens 27: 322–331.
9. Dahal BK, Cornitescu T, Tretyn A, Pullamsetti SS, Kosanovic D, et al. (2010) Role of epidermal growth factor inhibition in experimental pulmonary hypertension. Am J Respir Crit Care Med 181: 158–167. 200811-1682OC [pii];10.1164/rccm.200811-1682OC [doi].
10. Archer SL, Souil E, Dinh-Xuan AT, Schremmer B, Mercier JC, et al. (1998) Molecular identification of the role of voltage-gated K+ channels, Kv1.5 and Kv2.1, in hypoxic pulmonary vasoconstriction and control of resting membrane potential in rat pulmonary artery myocytes. J Clin Invest 101: 2319–2330. 10.1172/JCI333 [doi].
11. Zhao YJ, Wang J, Rubin LJ, Yuan XJ (1998) Roles of K+ and Cl- channels in cAMP-induced pulmonary vasodilation. Exp Lung Res 24: 71–83.
12. Barnes PJ, Liu SF (1995) Regulation of pulmonary vascular tone. Pharmacol Rev 47: 87–131.
13. Nelson MT, Quayle JM (1995) Physiological roles and properties of potassium channels in arterial smooth muscle. Am J Physiol 268: C799–C822.
14. Bonnet S, Savineau JP, Barillot W, Dubuis E, Vandier C, et al. (2003) Role of Ca(2+)-sensitive K(+) channels in the remission phase of pulmonary hypertension in chronic obstructive pulmonary diseases. Cardiovasc Res 60: 326–336. S0008636303005273 [pii].
15. Bae YM, Park MK, Lee SH, Ho WK, Earm YE (1999) Contribution of Ca2+-activated K+ channels and non-selective cation channels to membrane potential of pulmonary arterial smooth muscle cells of the rabbit. J Physiol 514 (Pt 3): 747–758.
16. Nagaoka T, Fagan KA, Gebb SA, Morris KG, Suzuki T, et al. (2005) Inhaled Rho kinase inhibitors are potent and selective vasodilators in rat pulmonary hypertension. Am J Respir Crit Care Med 171: 494–499. 200405-637OC [pii];10.1164/rccm.200405-637OC [doi].
17. White RE, Kryman JP, El-Mowafy AM, Han G, Carrier GO (2000) cAMP-dependent vasodilators cross-activate the cGMP-dependent protein kinase to stimulate BK(Ca) channel activity in coronary artery smooth muscle cells. Circ Res 86: 897–905.
18. Bolotina VM, Najibi S, Palacino JJ, Pagano PJ, Cohen RA (1994) Nitric oxide directly activates calcium-dependent potassium channels in vascular smooth muscle. Nature 368: 850–853. 10.1038/368850a0 [doi].
19. Barman SA, Zhu S, Han G, White RE (2003) cAMP activates BKCa channels in pulmonary arterial smooth muscle via cGMP-dependent protein kinase. Am J Physiol Lung Cell Mol Physiol 284: L1004–L1011. 10.1152/ajplung.00295.2002 [doi];00295.2002 [pii].
20. Montani D, Chaumais MC, Guignabert C, Gunther S, Girerd B, et al. (2013) Targeted therapies in pulmonary arterial hypertension. Pharmacol Ther. S0163-7258(13)00207-6 [pii];10.1016/j.pharmthera.2013.10.002 [doi].
21. Carlino C, Tobias JD, Schneider RI, Heller RL, Alpert MA, et al. (2010) Pulmonary hemodynamic response to acute combination and monotherapy with sildenafil and brain natriuretic peptide in rats with monocrotaline-induced pulmonary hypertension. Am J Med Sci 339: 55–59. 10.1097/MAJ.0b013e3181c078d7 [doi].
22. Falcao-Pires I, Goncalves N, Henriques-Coelho T, Moreira-Goncalves D, Roncon-Albuquerque R, et al. (2009) Apelin decreases myocardial injury and improves right ventricular function in monocrotaline-induced pulmonary hypertension. Am J Physiol Heart Circ Physiol 296: H2007–H2014. 00089.2009 [pii];10.1152/ajpheart.00089.2009 [doi].
23. Cui B, Cheng YS, Dai DZ, Li N, Zhang TT, et al. (2009) CPU0213, a non-selective ETA/ETB receptor antagonist, improves pulmonary arteriolar remodeling of monocrotaline-induced pulmonary hypertension in rats. Clin Exp Pharmacol Physiol 36: 169–175. CEP5044 [pii];10.1111/j.1440-1681.2008.05044.x [doi].
24. Xu W, Liu Y, Wang S, McDonald T, Van Eyk JE, et al. (2002) Cytoprotective role of Ca2+- activated K+ channels in the cardiac inner mitochondrial membrane. Science 298: 1029–1033. 10.1126/science.1074360 [doi];298/5595/1029 [pii].
25. Dimitropoulou C, White RE, Ownby DR, Catravas JD (2005) Estrogen reduces carbachol-induced constriction of asthmatic airways by stimulating large-conductance voltage and calcium-dependent potassium channels. Am J Respir Cell Mol Biol 32: 239–247. 2004-0331OC [pii];10.1165/rcmb.2004-0331OC [doi].
26. Bowring NE, Arch JR, Buckle DR, Taylor JF (1993) Comparison of the airways relaxant and hypotensive potencies of the potassium channel activators BRL 55834 and levcromakalim (BRL 38227) in vivo in guinea-pigs and rats. Br J Pharmacol 109: 1133–1139.
27. Short AD, Bian J, Ghosh TK, Waldron RT, Rybak SL, et al. (1993) Intracellular Ca2+ pool content is linked to control of cell growth. Proc Natl Acad Sci U S A 90: 4986–4990.
28. Lang F, Foller M, Lang KS, Lang PA, Ritter M, et al. (2005) Ion channels in cell proliferation and apoptotic cell death. J Membr Biol 205: 147–157. 10.1007/s00232-005-0780-5 [doi].
29. Cook SJ, Lockyer PJ (2006) Recent advances in Ca(2+)-dependent Ras regulation and cell proliferation. Cell Calcium 39: 101–112. S0143-4160(05)00206-X [pii];10.1016/j.ceca.2005.10.014 [doi].
30. Dick GM, Tune JD (2010) Role of potassium channels in coronary vasodilation. Exp Biol Med (Maywood) 235: 10–22. 235/1/10 [pii];10.1258/ebm.2009.009201 [doi].
31. Perros F, Montani D, Dorfmuller P, Durand-Gasselin I, Tcherakian C, et al. (2008) Platelet-derived growth factor expression and function in idiopathic pulmonary arterial hypertension. Am J Respir Crit Care Med 178: 81–88. 200707-1037OC [pii];10.1164/rccm.200707-1037OC [doi].
32. Humbert M, Monti G, Fartoukh M, Magnan A, Brenot F, et al. (1998) Platelet-derived growth factor expression in primary pulmonary hypertension: comparison of HIV seropositive and HIV seronegative patients. Eur Respir J 11: 554–559.
33. Schermuly RT, Dony E, Ghofrani HA, Pullamsetti S, Savai R, et al. (2005) Reversal of experimental pulmonary hypertension by PDGF inhibition. J Clin Invest 115: 2811–2821. 10.1172/JCI24838 [doi].
34. Ghofrani HA, Seeger W, Grimminger F (2005) Imatinib for the treatment of pulmonary arterial hypertension. N Engl J Med 353: 1412–1413. 353/13/1412 [pii];10.1056/NEJMc051946 [doi].
35. Pullamsetti S, Krick S, Yilmaz H, Ghofrani HA, Schudt C, et al. (2005) Inhaled tolafentrine reverses pulmonary vascular remodeling via inhibition of smooth muscle cell migration. Respir Res 6: 128. 1465-9921-6-128 [pii];10.1186/1465-9921-6-128 [doi].
36. Hoeper MM, Barst RJ, Bourge RC, Feldman J, Frost AE, et al. (2013) Imatinib mesylate as add-on therapy for pulmonary arterial hypertension: results of the

randomized IMPRES study. Circulation 127: 1128–1138. CIRCULATIONAHA.112.000765 pii];10.1161/CIRCULATIONAHA.112.000765 [doi].

37. Chang H, Ma YG, Wang YY, Song Z, Li Q, et al. (2011) High glucose alters apoptosis and proliferation in HEK293 cells by inhibition of cloned BK Ca channel. J Cell Physiol 226: 1660–1675. 10.1002/jcp.22497 [doi].
38. Han X, Xi L, Wang H, Huang X, Ma X, et al. (2008) The potassium ion channel opener NS1619 inhibits proliferation and induces apoptosis in A2780 ovarian cancer cells. Biochem Biophys Res Commun 375: 205–209. S0006-291X(08)01494-0 [pii];10.1016/j.bbrc.2008.07.161 [doi].
39. Costa RS, Assreuy J (2005) Multiple potassium channels mediate nitric oxide-induced inhibition of rat vascular smooth muscle cell proliferation. Nitric Oxide 13: 145–151. S1089-8603(05)00076-5 [pii];10.1016/j.niox.2005.05.010 [doi].
40. Xu W, Liu Y, Wang S, McDonald T, Van Eyk JE, et al. (2002) Cytoprotective role of Ca2+- activated K+ channels in the cardiac inner mitochondrial membrane. Science 298: 1029–1033. 10.1126/science.1074360 [doi];298/5595/1029 [pii].
41. Bentzen BH, Osadchii O, Jespersen T, Hansen RS, Olesen SP, et al. (2009) Activation of big conductance Ca(2+)-activated K (+) channels (BK) protects the heart against ischemia-reperfusion injury. Pflugers Arch 457: 979–988. 10.1007/s00424-008-0583-5 [doi].
42. Redel A, Lange M, Jazbutyte V, Lotz C, Smul TM, et al. (2008) Activation of mitochondrial large-conductance calcium-activated K+ channels via protein kinase A mediates desflurane-induced preconditioning. Anesth Analg 106: 384–91, table. 106/2/384 [pii];10.1213/ane.0b013e318160650f [doi].
43. Yun J, Park H, Ko JH, Lee W, Kim K, et al. (2010) Expression of Ca2+ -activated K+ channels in human dermal fibroblasts and their roles in apoptosis. Skin Pharmacol Physiol 23: 91–104. 000265680 [pii];10.1159/000265680 [doi].
44. Krick S, Platoshyn O, McDaniel SS, Rubin LJ, Yuan JX (2001) Augmented K(+) currents and mitochondrial membrane depolarization in pulmonary artery myocyte apoptosis. Am J Physiol Lung Cell Mol Physiol 281: L887–L894.
45. Aranda M, Bradford KK, Pearl RG (1999) Combined therapy with inhaled nitric oxide and intravenous vasodilators during acute and chronic experimental pulmonary hypertension. Anesth Analg 89: 152–158.
46. Tuder RM, Abman SH, Braun T, Capron F, Stevens T, et al. (2009) Development and pathology of pulmonary hypertension. J Am Coll Cardiol 54: S3–S9. S0735-1097(09)01212-1 [pii];10.1016/j.jacc.2009.04.009 [doi].
47. Sandow SL, Grayson TH (2009) Limits of isolation and culture: intact vascular endothelium and BKCa. Am J Physiol Heart Circ Physiol 297: H1–H7. 00042.2009 [pii];10.1152/ajpheart.00042.2009 [doi].

13

Early Treatment with Fumagillin, an Inhibitor of Methionine Aminopeptidase-2, Prevents Pulmonary Hypertension in Monocrotaline-Injured Rats

Daniel J. Kass[1] *, Eileen Rattigan[2], Rehan Kahloon[1], Katrina Loh[3], Liyang Yu[1], Asaf Savir[3], Mark Markowski[3], Anjali Saqi[4], Revathi Rajkumar[5], Ferhaan Ahmad[5,6], Hunter C. Champion[1,5,6]

1 Division of Pulmonary, Allergy, and Critical Care Medicine, Department of Medicine, University of Pittsburgh School of Medicine and the Dorothy P. and Richard P. Simmons Center for Interstitial Lung Disease, Pittsburgh, Pennsylvania, United States of America, **2** Department of Cardiology, Geisinger Health System, Wilkes-Barre, Pennsylvania, United States of America, **3** Division of Pulmonary, Allergy, and Critical Care Medicine, Department of Medicine, Columbia University College of Physicians and Surgeons, New York, New York, United States of America, **4** Department of Pathology, Columbia University College of Physicians and Surgeons, New York, New York, United States of America, **5** Department of Medicine, Cardiovascular Institute, University of Pittsburgh School of Medicine, Pittsburgh, Pennsylvania, United States of America, **6** Vascular Medicine Institute, University of Pittsburgh School of Medicine, Pittsburgh, Pennsylvania, United States of America

Abstract

Pulmonary Hypertension (PH) is a pathophysiologic condition characterized by hypoxemia and right ventricular strain. Proliferation of fibroblasts, smooth muscle cells, and endothelial cells is central to the pathology of PH in animal models and in humans. Methionine aminopeptidase-2 (MetAP2) regulates proliferation in a variety of cell types including endothelial cells, smooth muscle cells, and fibroblasts. MetAP2 is inhibited irreversibly by the angiogenesis inhibitor fumagillin. We have previously found that inhibition of MetAP2 with fumagillin in bleomycin-injured mice decreased pulmonary fibrosis by selectively decreasing the proliferation of lung myofibroblasts. In this study, we investigated the role of fumagillin as a potential therapy in experimental PH. *In vivo*, treatment of rats with fumagillin early after monocrotaline injury prevented PH and right ventricular remodeling by decreasing the thickness of the medial layer of the pulmonary arteries. Treatment with fumagillin beginning two weeks after monocrotaline injury did not prevent PH but was associated with decreased right ventricular mass and decreased cardiomyocyte hypertrophy, suggesting a direct effect of fumagillin on right ventricular remodeling. Incubation of rat pulmonary artery smooth muscle cells (RPASMC) with fumagillin and MetAP2-targeting siRNA inhibited proliferation of RPASMC *in vitro*. Platelet-derived growth factor, a growth factor that is important in the pathogenesis of PH and stimulates proliferation of fibroblasts and smooth muscle cells, strongly increased expression of MetP2. By immunohistochemistry, we found that MetAP2 was expressed in the lesions of human pulmonary arterial hypertension. We propose that fumagillin may be an effective adjunctive therapy for treating PH in patients.

Editor: Martin R J. Kolb, McMaster University, Canada

Funding: This work was funded in part by a peer-reviewed grant administered by the Entelligence Scholars in Pulmonary Hypertension and funded by Actelion Pharmaceuticals. This work was also funded by National Institutes of Health (NIH) grants UL1 RR024156 and 5P30 ES009089-11. The funders had no role in study design, data collection and analysis, decision to publish, or preparation of the manuscript.

Competing Interests: This work was funded in part by a peer-reviewed grant administered by the Entelligence Scholars in Pulmonary Hypertension and funded by Actelion Pharmaceuticals. This work was also funded by NIH grants UL1 RR024156 and 5P30 ES009089-11.

* E-mail: kassd2@upmc.edu

Introduction

Pulmonary Hypertension (PH) is a pathophysiologic condition defined by a mean pulmonary arterial pressure >25 mmHg at rest [1] and is characterized by hypoxemia, exercise limitation, and in many cases, death [2]. PH occurs in a variety of clinical situations and is associated with a broad spectrum of histological patterns and abnormalities [3]. While idiopathic pulmonary arterial hypertension (IPAH) is rare (15 per one million [4]), PH complicates and worsens the prognosis of many systemic diseases including chronic obstructive pulmonary disease, idiopathic pulmonary fibrosis (IPF), human immunodeficiency virus infection, systemic sclerosis (SSc), and liver cirrhosis (reviewed in [5]). A shared pathologic feature of PH and diseases such as IPF or SSc is the expansion of the mesenchymal cell compartment in the lung. The lesions of PH are characterized to various degrees, depending on the particular etiology, by the accumulation of endothelial cells, smooth muscle cells, and fibroblasts in the pulmonary vasculature (reviewed in [6]). Altered rates of proliferation and apoptosis in mesenchymal cells lead to thickened and narrowed vessels resulting ultimately, in increased pulmonary arterial pressures and right ventricular strain [6]. In human PH (reviewed in [7]) and in experimental models of PH [3,8,9], smooth muscle and endothelial cells actively proliferate, leading to occlusion of the pulmonary arteries and the stigmata of PH. Therapies that prevent the accumulation of these cells in the pulmonary arterial bed would be predicted to impact positively both quality-of-life and survival in PH. The currently available vasodilatory therapies for IPAH do enhance survival [10,11] but do not significantly address the root pathological lesions of PH: the accumulation of fibroblasts, smooth muscle and endothelial cells.

Methionine aminopeptidase-2 (MetAP2) is a metalloprotease that functions in the regulation of fibroblast [12], smooth muscle [13], and endothelial cell [14] proliferation. The enzymatic function of MetAP2 is to cleave the N-terminal methionine off polypeptides, a process that is necessary for many downstream, post-translational modifications of certain proteins [15,16]. Fumagillin is a fungal metabolite [17] that irreversibly inactivates the enzymatic activity of MetAP2 [18,19]. Fumagillin and its analogues are potent inhibitors of proliferation and have advanced into clinical trials as angiogenesis inhibitors in multiple cancers. There is accumulating evidence that fumagillin may be an effective therapy in animal models of fibrosis. We have previously found that fumagillin decreased bleomycin-induced pulmonary fibrosis in mice by selective inhibition of myofibroblast replication [12]. In addition, the fumagillin analogue TNP-470 has been found to inhibit both liver fibrosis [20] and peritoneal fibrosis [21] in animal models. The role of fumagillin in PH has not previously been explored. We hypothesized that inhibition of MetAP2 with fumagillin would prevent the accumulation of smooth muscle cells in the pulmonary vasculature that leads to PH.

Materials and Methods

This protocol was approved by the Institutional Animal Care and Use Committees and the Institutional Review Boards of both Columbia University and the University of Pittsburgh. At Columbia University the relevant protocols are: IRB-AAAE4847, Expression of MetAP2 in Pulmonary Hypertension and IACUC-AAAB0235, Modification of Smooth Muscle Cell Proliferation with Fumagillin. At the University of Pittsburgh, the relevant protocols are: IRB-08020021, Genetics, Transcriptional Genomics, and Pharmacogenomics of Pulmonary Hypertension and IACUC-1009954, Modification of Smooth Muscle Cell Proliferation with Fumagillin.

Reagents

Monocrotaline, fumagillin, bromodeoxyuridine (BrdU), and monoclonal antibodies against α-smooth muscle actin (clone 1A4) were obtained from Sigma (St Louis, MO). SYBR Green dye and Rabbit IgG against MetAP2, and Alexa Fluor 488–conjugated goat anti-mouse IgG were from Invitrogen (Carlsbad, CA). Monoclonal antibody (mAb) against bromodeoxyuridine (BrdU) (clone BMC 9318) was from Roche (Indianapolis, IN). Platelet-Derived Growth Factor (PDGF) was purchased from R&D Systems (Minneapolis, MN). Rabbit polyclonal antibodies against Ki67 and von Willebrand Factor were obtained from Neomarkers (Fremont, CA). A mouse monoclonal antibody directed against rat CD45 (clone OX-1) was obtained from AbdSerotec (Raleigh, NC). A goat antibody directed against CD31 (PECAM-1, cat# M-20) was from Santa Cruz Biotechnology (Santa Cruz, CA). MetAP2- and non-targeting siRNA oligonucleotides were purchased from Dharmacon (Lafayette, CO). Hiperfect and primers specific for human MetAP2 and PPIA were from Qiagen (Valencia, CA).

Monocrotaline-Induced Pulmonary Hypertension

Male Sprague-Dawley Rats (Harlan, Indianapolis, IA) were purchased at 250 grams of mass. Monocrotaline was dissolved in 0.5N hydrochloric acid, and the pH was slowly adjusted to 7.4 with 0.2N sodium hydroxide. A single subcutaneous injection of monocrotaline (60 mg/kg) or vehicle control was administered on day 0. Fumagillin was dissolved in dimethyl sulfoxide (DMSO) at 10 mg/ml, and then further diluted in RPMI 1640 pH 8.0 to a final concentration of 10% DMSO. Beginning three days (early) or two weeks (late) after monocrotaline injury, fumagillin (0.5 mg/kg) was administered by inhalation. Under isoflurane anesthesia, a gel-loading pipet tip was gently inserted into the nares of the rat, a volume of 125 microliters was slowly introduced, and the volume was inhaled. This dosage of fumagillin and route of administration was chosen, rather than the more commonly used higher doses in rodents (20–100 mg/kg [22,23,24,25]), because intranasal delivery afforded localized pulmonary, rather than systemic delivery. Drug or vehicle control was administered every other day for the duration of the experiment. Animals were weighed weekly. Animals were sacrificed at four or five weeks after monocrotaline injury.

Measurement of Right Ventricular Systolic Blood Pressure

At four weeks after monocrotaline injury, animals were anesthetized with a combination of ketamine and xylazine. The right internal jugular vein was exposed and a 2-French catheter (Millar Instruments, Houston, TX) was introduced and advanced to the right ventricle. Pressure measurements were transduced using PowerLab 4/30 from ADI Instruments (Colorado Springs, CO).

Measurement of Hemodynamics and Echocardiography

At five weeks after MCT injury, animals were brought to the phenotyping core of the Vascular Medicine Institute of the University of Pittsburgh. Central venous access was obtained via internal jugular venous cannulation using sterile PE-50 tubing. To obtain *in vivo* hemodynamic measurements, rats were anesthetized with a mixture of ketamine (100 mg/kg) and acepromazine (5 mg/kg). The rats were then ventilated by the insertion of a tracheal cannula attached to a rodent ventilator (Harvard Apparatus, South Natick, MA) set to 90 breaths/min with a tidal volume of 8 ml/kg body weight. The chest was opened with a midline incision and then a four-electrode pressure-volume catheter (Scisence Inc., London, Ontario, Canada) was placed through the right ventricular apex to record chamber volume by admittance and pressure micromanometry as described previously analyzed using customized acquisition software (IOX2; Emka, Falls Church, VA) [26,27]. Direct Doppler velocities of the pulmonary arterial flow were obtained using a 20 MHz ultrasound probe and analyzed using customized software (Doppler signal processing workstation; DSPW; Indus Instruments, Houston, TX). A silk tie was loosely placed around the inferior vena cava (IVC), and a transient decrease in preload was achieved by a gentle constriction of the tie to obtain ESPVR. A family of pressure-volume loops was generated to allow for the evaluation of the right ventricular end-systolic pressure volume relationship (Ees) and ventricular-arterial coupling (Ees/Ea).

Measurement of Cardiomyocyte Cross-Sectional Area and Vessel Thickness

Sections of the free wall of the right ventricle were fixed in 10% neutral buffered formalin. Five μm sections of paraffin-embedded tissue were cut and routine hematoxylin and eosin staining was performed. The section was scanned by a blinded reviewer for cells cut in cross section. Cross-sectional area was measured using an Olympus CH2 microscope with a DP25 camera and DP2-BSW software (Tokyo, Japan). Modified Movat's pentachrome staining was performed on paraffin-embedded samples of rat lung sections using a kit from Electron Microscopy Services (Hatfield, PA). The pulmonary vessels <250 μm were identified by morphological features and their proximity to airways. Twenty-five vessels in cross-sectional diameter were assessed for each rat sample by a blinded reader. Medial diameter of the vessel wall was measured by determining the distance between the internal and external elastic laminae, stained black by the Movat stain. The widest diameter of the vessel was used. The percent medial thickness is reported as percentage of the medial diameter to the diameter of the entire vessel. Measurements were made at 400× magnification using an Olympus DP25 microscope camera.

Rat Pulmonary Artery Smooth Muscle Cell Culture and Immunoblotting

Rat pulmonary artery smooth muscle cells (RPASMC) were provided generously by Dr. Brian Zuckerbraun, University of Pittsburgh. The isolation of RPASMC has been described elsewhere [28]. Cells were cultured in low-glucose DMEM:F-12 (1:1) supplemented with 4 mM glutamine (Glutamax, from Invitrogen). Cells were used between the fourth and eighth passages. For immunoblotting, cells were plated in 24-well plates. On the next day, cells were cultured in serum-free DMEM:F12 overnight. On the next day, cells were stimulated with PDGF at 10 ng/mL. 24 h after the addition of PDGF, cells were lysed in RIPA buffer (150 mM NaCl, 1% NP-40, 0.25% sodium deoxycholate, 0.1% sodium dodecyl sulfate (SDS), 1 mM EDTA, 5 mM PMSF, 50 μg/ml leupeptin, 50 μg/ml aprotinin, 50 mM Tris-HCl, pH 7.4), and subjected to SDS-polyacrylamide gel electrophoresis and immunoblotting with a rabbit polyclonal antibody against MetAP2 and a goat polyclonal against β-actin as previously described [12]. Quantification of band intensity was performed with ImageJ software (http://rsb.info.nih.gov/ij/).

Cell Proliferation Assays

RPASMC were washed and incubated in DMEM:F12 without FBS for 24 h to synchronize the cells in G0 [29]. To release RPASMC from G0 arrest, the media were then replaced with DMEM:F12 + 10% FBS supplemented with fumagillin 20 nM dissolved in DMSO or vehicle control. RPASMC were also grown with or without PDGF at 10 ng/mL and incubated for 24, 48, and 72 h. To facilitate counting cells, RPASMC were fixed in 3.7% formaldehyde, permeabilized in 0.2% Triton X-100, and stained with the DNA-sensitive dye SYBR green (Invitrogen). SYBR green fluorescence was quantitated with a plate-reading spectrofluorimeter. We have found and published previously that SYBR green fluorescence intensity correlated with cell counts in a hemacytometer. All data represent fold changes in cell number following background subtraction [29].

For quantification of BrdU incorporation, RPASMC were plated in 24-well plates on glass coverslips. Cells were washed and incubated in DMEM:F12 without FBS for 24 h to synchronize the cells in G0 [29]. The media were then replaced with DMEM:F12+10% FBS supplemented with fumagillin dissolved in DMSO or vehicle control, with or without PDGF at 10 ng/mL and incubated for an additional 48 h. Cells were pulsed with BrdU 10 μM for the final 30 minutes. Cells were fixed in 3.7% formaldehyde and permeabilized in 0.2% Triton X-100. To expose the incorporated BrdU, we incubated the fixed cells with 100 U/ml DNase for 60 min at 37°C. Cells were processed for immunofluorescence using a monoclonal antibody against BrdU followed by Alexa Fluor 488–conjugated goat anti-mouse IgG and counterstaining with DAPI. Cells were visualized with a Nikon Eclipse TE200 microscope (Nikon, Tokyo, Japan) equipped with epifluorescence. At least 15 fields were selected at random, and BrdU+ cells were enumerated and scored as a percentage of all cells present/high-power field (hpf). About 1500 cells were counted per experiment.

Transfection of siRNA

RPASMC were plated in DMEM/F12 and 10% fetal bovine serum on day 0, and were transfected with 37.5 ng of siRNA oligonucleotides specific for rat MetAP2 or non-targeting controls using Hiperfect (Qiagen) on days 0 and 1. Cells were then incubated in the presence of fumagillin 20 nM or vehicle control for 36 hours. Cells were processed for immunoblotting or determination of BrdU incorporation as noted above.

Immunostaining of Rat and Human Lung

Human lung tissues from patients with Idiopathic Pulmonary Arterial Hypertension (IPAH, World Health Organization, class I) or normal controls were obtained from the Columbia University Tissue Bank. Normal lung was obtained from histologically normal appearing lung distant from resected lung cancers [29]. All diagnoses were rendered by a dedicated lung pathologist according to standard American Thoracic Society criteria. For immunohistochemistry, sections were deparaffinized with xylene followed by rehydration through graded ethanol series. Antigen retrieval with 10 mM sodium citrate was performed for Ki67, MetAP2, and von Willebrand Factor. For brightfield microscopy, antigens were developed with the Vectastain ABC Universal kit (Vector Labs, Burlingame, CA). Diaminobenzidine (brown) and Vector SG (gray) were used for double-labelling experiments. Sections were counterstained with Harris' hematoxylin, dehydrated through graded alcohol series, and mounted with Permount (Fisher, Fairlawn, NJ). Sections were visualized using an Olympus CHS microscope and images were photographed with an Olympus DP25 camera (Olympus, Tokyo, Japan). Ki67+ cells were counted as the number of positively-staining nuclei per vessel per high power field (hpf). Immunostaining for CD45 was performed on cryosections of lungs from rats. CD45+ cells were quantified as the number of positively-staining cells per hpf. Immunofluorescent staining on human lung was performed on paraffin-embedded tissue with rhodamine- and Cy5-conjugated secondary antibodies (Jackson Immunoresearch, West Grove, PA). Nuclei were counterstained with DAPI. Black and white images were photographed on the TE200 Nikon Eclipse, processed, and pseudocolored using Adobe Photoshop.

Terminal Deoxynucleotidyl Transferase dUTP Nick End Labeling (TUNEL)

Five μm sections of formalin-fixed, paraffin-embedded lung and heart tissues were cut, deparaffinized, and rehydrated through graded ethanol series. Sections were then prepared with proteinase K pre-treatment. TUNEL staining was then performed employing the ApopTag Peroxidase kit (Millipore, Billerica, MA). TUNEL+ cells were counted as the number of positively-staining nuclei per high power field.

Quantitative RT-PCR

The preparation of samples of cDNA from lungs of patients with pulmonary arterial hypertension (PAH) or normal controls has been described elsewhere [30]. Quantitative RT-PCR was performed, and data were analyzed on the Applied Biosystems 7500 (Carlsbad, CA). Primers specific for human MetAP2 and the endogenous control PPIA were obtained from Qiagen and used according to the manufacturer's recommendations.

Statistics

Data were analyzed by one-way ANOVA followed by Bonferroni's *post-hoc* test (unless otherwise stated) using GraphPad Prism 5 (GraphPad Software, La Jolla, CA).

Results

Inhibition of MetAP2 by Fumagillin Prevents PH in MCT-Injured Rats

We have previously found that delivery of fumagillin to bleomycin-injured mice decreased pulmonary fibrosis by a selective reduction in the number of accumulated fibroblasts in the lung parenchyma. In this study, we sought to expand on our previous findings and determine if treatment of rats with fumagillin would attenuate PH in an animal model where smooth muscle and fibroblast accumulation was a prominent feature. We chose to test the efficacy of fumagillin in the monocrotaline (MCT) model of PH. MCT was injected subcutaneously on day 0, followed by treatment with fumagillin or vehicle control beginning either on day 3 (early treatment), or day 14 (late treatment), after MCT injury. Treatment continued every other day for the duration of the experiment. Animals were weighed weekly as a measure of overall health. All animals gained weight every week for the first four weeks of the experiment (Figure 1A). Between the fourth and fifth weeks, MCT-injured animals, treated with the vehicle all lost nearly 20 grams (Figure 1B). In contrast, MCT-injured rats, treated with fumagillin beginning on day 3 continued to gain weight at a rate similar to uninjured animals. Animals treated with fumagillin beginning 14 days after MCT lost significantly less weight at week 5 than MCT-injured animals treated with the vehicle. These data suggest that treatment with fumagillin initiated at 3 d protected animals from weight loss induced by MCT injury. When fumagillin treatment was initiated at 14 d, we observed attenuated weight loss in response to MCT injury suggesting at least partial protection.

Next, we assessed the effects of fumagillin treatment on MCT-injured animals using physiologic and histopathologic measures of PH. On day 28 after injury, right ventricular systolic blood pressure (RVSP) was determined (Figure 2A). RVSP was determined by catheterization of the right internal jugular vein. Average RVSP was less than 25 mmHg in uninjured animals treated with fumagillin or the vehicle control. In MCT-injured, vehicle-treated animals, the average RVSP was 66 mmHg. However, in the MCT-injured animals treated with fumagillin early after injury, the average RVSP was significantly reduced at 28 mmHg. In contrast, animals treated with the vehicle or fumagillin beginning at 14 d after MCT exhibited similarly elevated RVSPs (63 vs. 69 mmHg, respectively). Thus, only early treatment with fumagillin prevented MCT-induced pulmonary hypertension. Treatment of animals with fumagillin beginning at 14 d after MCT injury did not prevent PH.

We next determined the effect of fumagillin on heart size in MCT-injured rats. At five weeks after MCT injury, the hearts and lungs were excised and prepared for gross and histopathologic analysis. We measured the mass of the right ventricle normalized to the mass of the left ventricle and the interventricular septum (Figure 2B). Compared to uninjured controls, the ratio of RV mass to LV mass increased 2.5-fold with MCT injury and treatment with the vehicle. Early treatment with fumagillin attenuated the increase in right ventricular mass induced by MCT injury. Surprisingly, late treatment with fumagillin, beginning 14 d after MCT injury, also attenuated right ventricular remodeling induced by MCT despite RVSPs as high as the vehicle-treated and MCT-injured rats. These data suggest that fumagillin treatment as early as three days and as late as 14 days after MCT injury prevents RV remodeling due to PH.

Fumagillin Treatment Preserves Right Ventricular Function in MCT-Injured Rats

The decreased weight loss exhibited by MCT-injured animals treated with fumagillin late and the decrease in the RV size in these animals in the presence of elevated RVSP suggested to us that fumagillin may offer a direct protective effect on the hearts of animals injured with MCT. We next measured hemodynamics in animals both injured with MCT and treated with fumagillin (Figure 3). Measures of systolic function, including cardiac output and ejection fraction, between uninjured animals treated with the vehicle or fumagillin were identical (data not shown). We found that early treatment with fumagillin significantly increased RV ejection fraction (RVEF) 2.4-fold compared to vehicle-treated, MCT-injured controls (Figure 3A). The mean RVEF was lower in the late fumagillin-treated animals compared to the early treatment, but

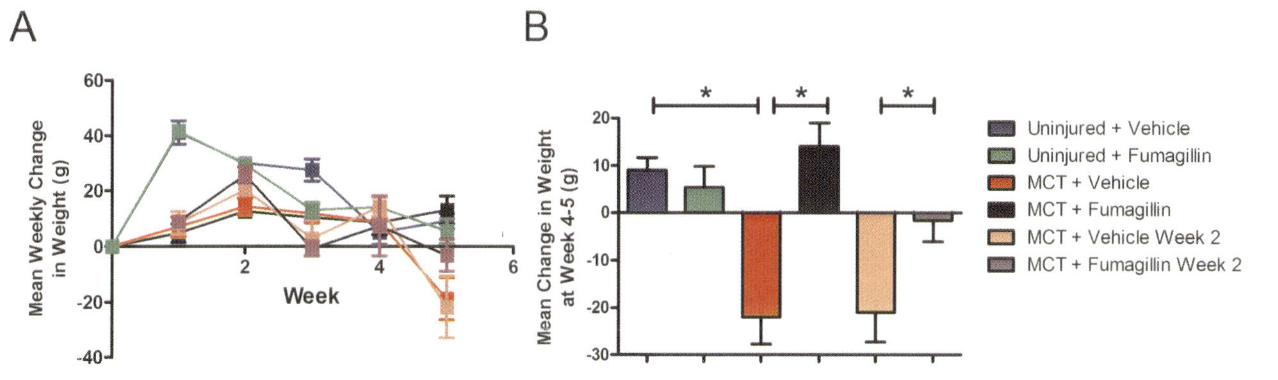

Figure 1. Early Fumagillin Treatment is Associated with Growth in Monocrotaline-Injured Rats. Rats were injected with monocrotaline (MCT) as described in Materials and Methods. Treatment with fumagillin or vehicle controls was initiated on the third day or 14th day after injury and continued every other day for the duration of the experiment. Animals were weighed weekly. At weeks 1–4, all MCT-injured animals gained weight at a similar rate (A). Panel (B) represents the data shown in panel (A) at week 5. MCT-injured rats treated with the vehicle lost nearly 20 g compared with the early fumagillin-treated animals that continued to gain weight at a rate similar to uninjured animals (*$P<0.05$, MCT+fumagillin v MCT+vehicle, n = 6 per group). In the MCT-injured animals treated with fumagillin starting at week 2, animals exhibited decreased weight loss compared with the MCT-injured animals treated with the vehicle (*$P<0.05$ MCT+fumagillin week 2 v. MCT + Vehicle, week 2). Data were analyzed by one-way ANOVA followed by the Bonferroni post-hoc test.

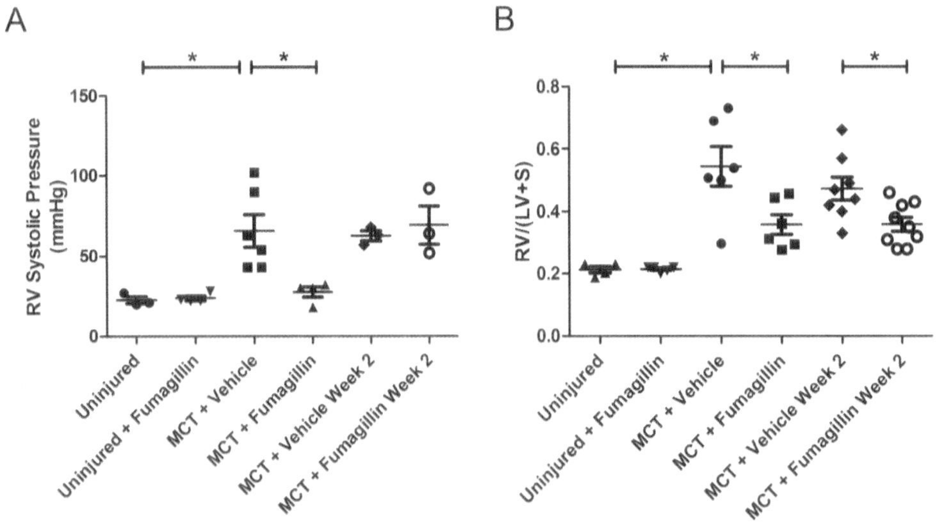

Figure 2. Fumagillin Prevents Pulmonary Hypertension and Right Ventricular Hypertrophy in MCT-Injured Rats. Rats were injected with MCT and treated with fumagillin or vehicle control as described in Materials and Methods. After four weeks, animals were killed, and direct right ventricular pressure was measured (A). MCT injury significantly increased RV systolic BP, which is prevented by early, but not late, treatment with fumagillin (*$P<0.05$, one-way ANOVA followed by Bonferroni's post hoc test). (B) Measurement of right ventricular mass normalized to left ventricular mass (RV/LV+S). Five weeks after MCT injury, hearts were excised, fixed in formalin, and the masses of the RV and the LV+septum were determined. MCT-injured animals treated with the vehicle exhibited a significant increase in RV mass, which was prevented in both early and late fumagillin-treated animals (*$P<0.05$, ANOVA followed by Bonferroni's post-hoc test).

this difference was not statistically significant. We next measured minimum dP/dt as a measurement of diastolic function in the RV (Figure 3B). We observed a similar trend: early treatment with fumagillin in MCT-injured animals was associated with a statistically significant 1.7-fold improvement in minimum dP/dt as compared to vehicle-treated, MCT-injured controls. Similar to RVEF, min dP/dt was lower in the late fumagillin-treated animals compared to the early treatment, but this difference too was not statistically significant. Early treatment with fumagillin was also associated with a significant reduction in RV end-diastolic pressure (RVEDP) (Figure 3C), a measure of RV failure, in comparison to MCT-injured and vehicle-treated controls. Early treatment with fumagillin also led to a significant increase in the ratio of RV end-systolic volume to stroke volume (Ees/Ea) (Figure 3D), a measure of right ventricular and pulmonary artery coupling [31]. Again, late treatment was associated with measurements that were intermediate between vehicle treatment and early fumagillin treatment. Thus, treatment with fumagillin is associated with improved hemodynamics in MCT-injured animals. The most significant improvements in hemodynamics were observed in animals treated early with fumagillin after MCT injury.

Fumagillin Inhibits Cardiac Myocyte Hypertrophy in MCT-Induced PH

Because we found that late treatment with fumagillin decreased RV mass in the presence of high pulmonary arterial pressures, we next measured the cross-sectional diameter of cardiac myocytes in animals injured with MCT and treated with the vehicle or with late fumagillin (14 d after MCT) (Figure 4). No significant difference in cardiac myocyte diameter was found between uninjured animals treated with the vehicle or with fumagillin. After MCT injury, myocyte diameter in vehicle-treated animals significantly increased 2.3-fold compared to the uninjured control. Late treatment with fumagillin significantly attenuated the increase in myocyte diameter induced by MCT by 76%. Thus fumagillin has a direct effect on the cardiomyocyte hypertrophy in MCT-injured animals.

Late Fumagillin Does Not Affect Capillary Number in the Right Ventricles of MCT-Injured Rats

To investigate further the effect of fumagillin on the hearts of MCT-injured animals, we performed immunohistochemistry for CD31 (PECAM) to quantify the number of capillaries in the hearts of these animals (Figure 5). We found that vehicle treatment in MCT-injured animals was associated with an increase in the number of capillaries compared to vehicle-treated uninjured controls. Early treatment with fumagillin resulted in a borderline reduction in capillary number, but late treatment with fumagillin did not affect capillary number in the heart in comparison to the MCT-injured, vehicle-treated controls. These data suggest that late treatment of MCT-injured animals with fumagillin does not impair right ventricular neoangiogenesis in response to pulmonary hypertension.

Fumagillin Decreases Apoptosis in the Right Ventricles of MCT-Injured Rats

We next examined histologic sections of the right ventricles of MCT-injured animals to determine if fumagillin affected the rate of apoptosis in injured hearts. We performed terminal deoxynucleotidyl transferase dUTP nick end labeling (TUNEL) on rat hearts following MCT injury and treatment at different time points with fumagillin (Figure 6). Following MCT injury, there was a significant increase in the number of apoptotic cells in the vehicle-treated animals that was blocked by either early or late treatment with fumagillin.

Early Treatment with Fumagillin Decreases Medial Thickness of the Pulmonary Arteries

Next, we examined histologic sections of the lung from MCT-injured animals to determine the effects of fumagillin treatment on the pulmonary vasculature. We hypothesized that fumagillin would directly block accumulation of smooth muscle cells in MCT-injured rats. Routine hematoxylin and eosin staining was performed on lung sections from uninjured and MCT-injured animals (Figure 7A–D).

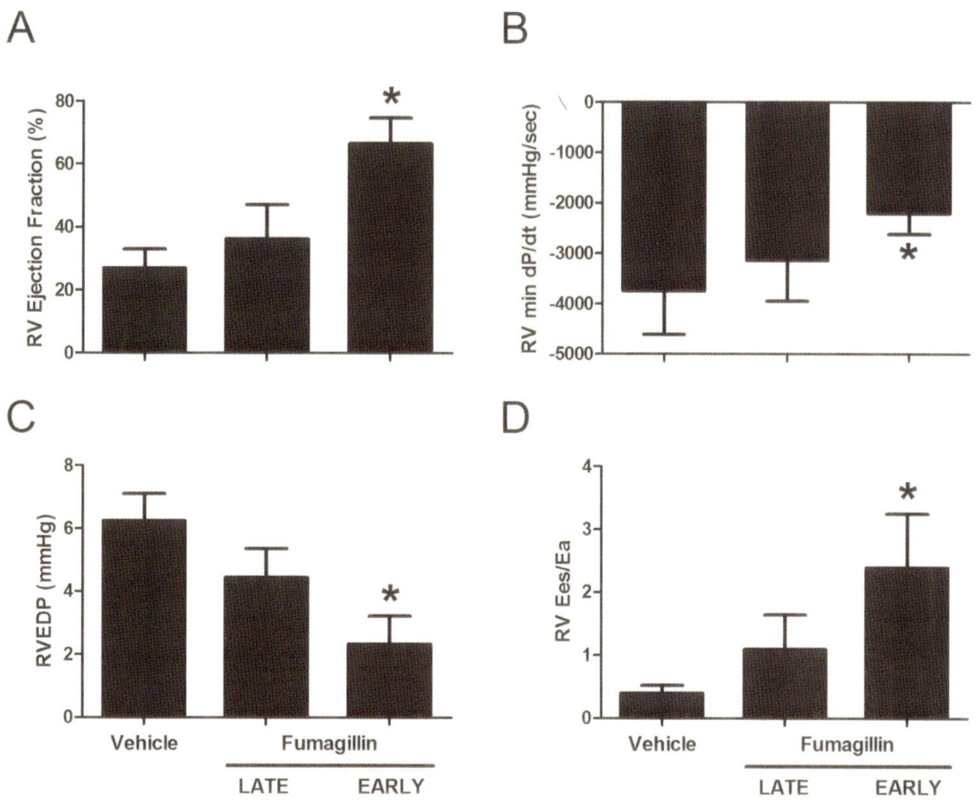

Figure 3. Treatment of monocrotaline-injured rats with fumagillin leads to improved right ventricular function. Rats were injected with MCT and treated with fumagillin or vehicle control beginning at 3 d or 14 d after MCT injury as described in Materials and Methods. At five weeks after MCT injury, animals were prepared for echocardiography and measurement of invasive hemodynamics as described in Materials and Methods: (A) right ventricular ejection fraction, (B) right ventricular minimum dP/dt, (C) right ventricular end-diastolic pressure, and (D) the ratio of right ventricular to pulmonary artery elastance, Ees/Ea. Note stepwise improvement in these hemodynamic parameters as fumagillin treatment is delivered late vs. early (**P*<0.05, MCT+early fumagillin v. MCT+vehicle, by t-test n = 4−7 animals per group).

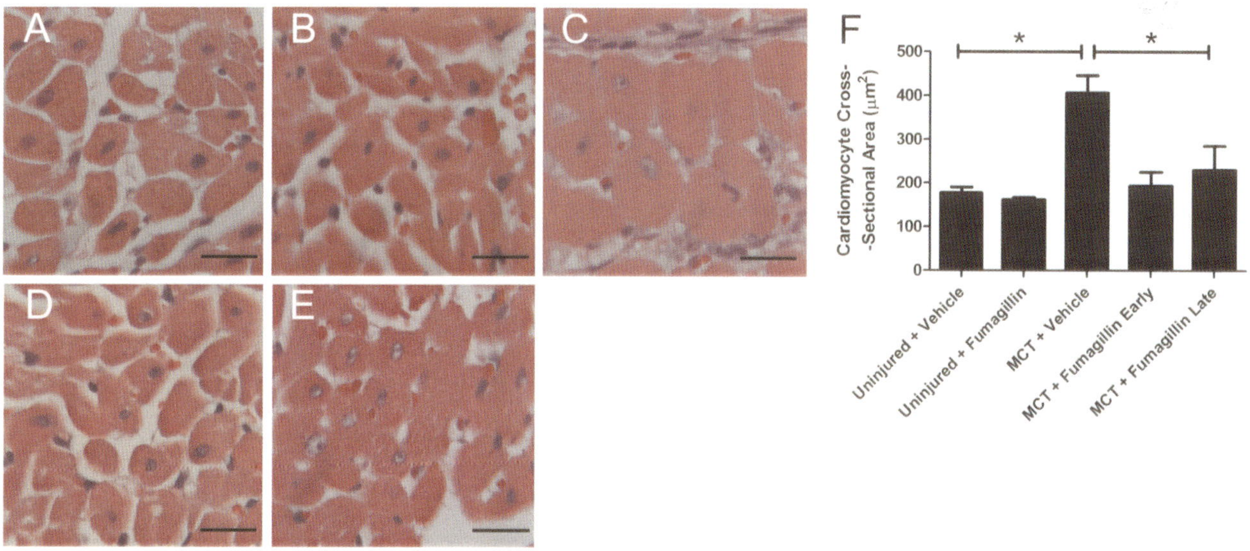

Figure 4. Late treatment with fumagillin inhibits RV cardiomyocyte hypertrophy. Rats were injected with MCT and treated with fumagillin or vehicle control beginning at 14 d after MCT injury as described in Materials and Methods. At five weeks after MCT injury, animals were killed and the free wall of the right ventricles were prepared for histology: (A) Uninjured + vehicle, (B) uninjured + fumagillin, (C) MCT + vehicle, week 2, (D) MCT + fumagillin early, and (E) MCT + fumagillin late (magnification ×400, bar = 20 μm). The area of cardiomyocytes cut in cross section was measured as described in Materials and Methods (F). MCT injury led to a significant increase in cardiomyocyte cross-sectional area, which was attenuated by treatment with fumagillin (**P*<0.05, one-way ANOVA, followed by Bonferroni's post-hoc test).

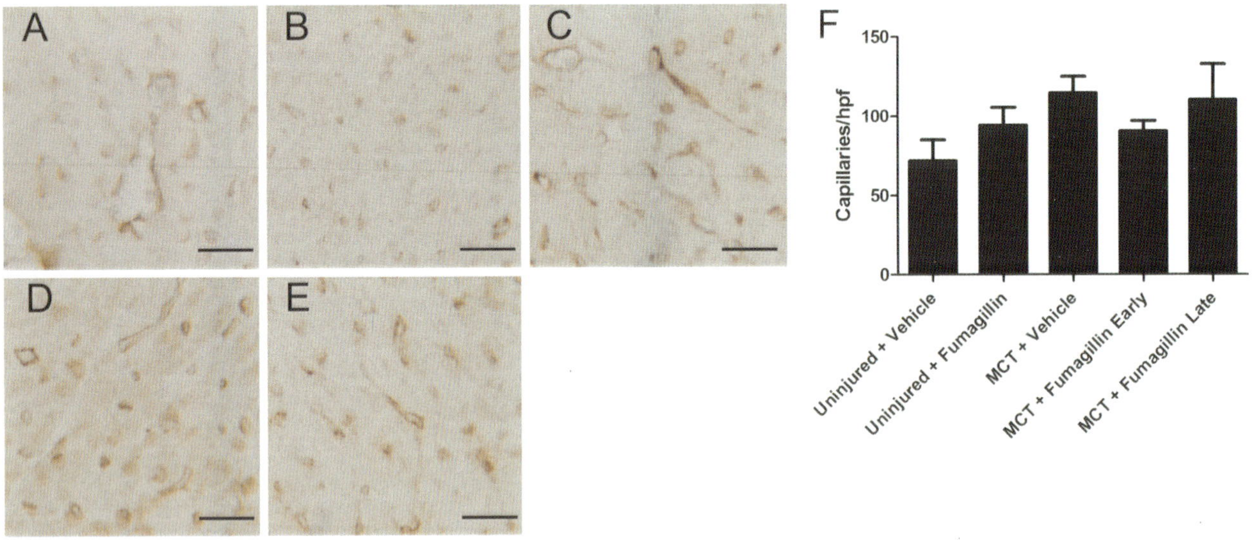

Figure 5. Treatment with fumagillin is not associated with differences in capillary density in MCT-injured animals. Rats were injected with MCT and treated with fumagillin or vehicle control beginning at 14 d after MCT injury as described in Materials and Methods. At five weeks after MCT injury, animals were killed and the free wall of the right ventricles were prepared for immunostaining for PECAM: (A) Uninjured + vehicle, (B) uninjured + fumagillin, (C) MCT + vehicle, week 2, and (D) MCT + fumagillin early, and (E) MCT + fumagillin late (magnification ×400, bar = 20 μm). The number of microvessels was counted per hpf as described in Materials and Methods (F). No significant differences in the number of microvessels were detected in fumagillin-treated animals compared to vehicle controls (data analyzed by one-way ANOVA, followed by Bonferroni's post-hoc test, n = 3–5 animals per group).

MCT injury was associated with severe lung injury including architectural distortion and the prominent accumulation of foamy macrophages. In MCT-injured, vehicle-treated animals, significant thickening of the medial layer was observed in all vessels. Some vessels in the vehicle-treated MCT-injured animals were also occluded. In the MCT-injured, early fumagillin-treated animals, the medial layers were thickened, but all vessels observed remained patent. We also performed double-label immunohistochemistry for α-smooth muscle actin (α-SMA) to mark smooth muscle cells and myofibroblasts, and von Willebrand Factor (vWF) to mark endothelial cells (*inset*, Figure 7C, D). In MCT-injured, vehicle-treated animals, there was significant thickening of the medial layer with endothelial cells appearing bunched, and some vessels exhibited extensive muscularization. In contrast, in early fumagillin-treated animals, vessels again were mildly thickened but widely patent. We measured vessel thickness employing Movat staining in the pulmonary vasculature as described in Materials and Methods (Figure 7E–G). Representative Movat images are shown in Figure S1. In all vessels measuring less than 250 μm and in the vessels measuring less than 50 and 30 μm in cross-sectional diameter, MCT injury and vehicle treatment was associated with significant vessel thickening, which was attenuated by early

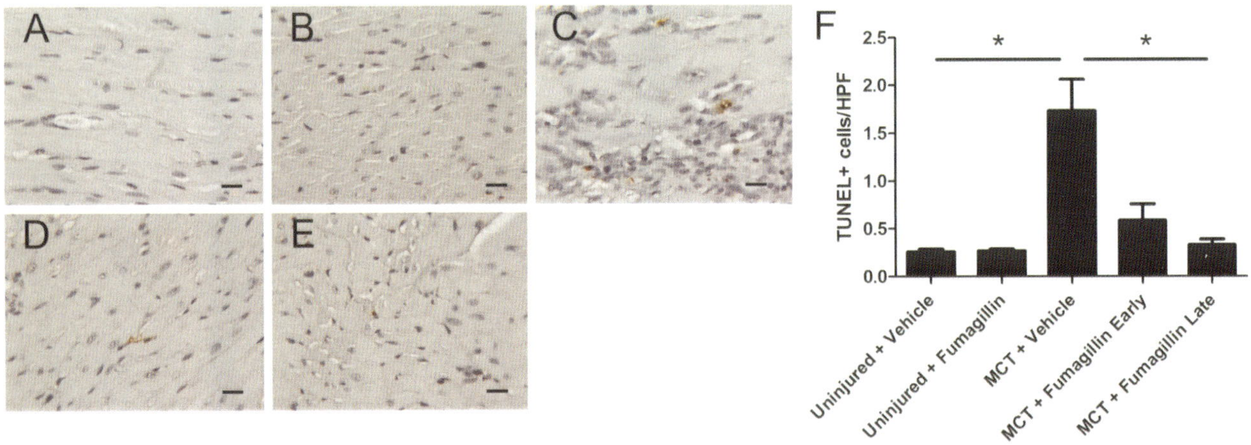

Figure 6. Treatment with fumagillin decreases the number of apoptotic cells in rat hearts. Rats were injected with MCT and treated with fumagillin or vehicle control beginning at 14 d after MCT injury as described in Materials and Methods. At five weeks after MCT injury, animals were killed and the free wall of the right ventricles were prepared for TUNEL staining: (A) Uninjured + vehicle, (B) uninjured + fumagillin, (C) MCT + vehicle, week 2, (D) MCT + fumagillin early, and (E) MCT + fumagillin late (magnification ×400, bar = 20 μm). The number of TUNEL+ cells in the right ventricles were increased by MCT injury but attenuated by fumagillin treatment (F) (*$P<0.05$, one-way ANOVA, followed by Bonferroni's post-hoc test, n = 3–5 animals per group).

treatment with fumagillin. In the animals receiving late fumagillin therapy, there was no significant difference in vessel thickness between fumagillin- and vehicle-treated animals. These data show that early fumagillin treatment is associated with decreased thickening of the medial layer of the pulmonary arteries in MCT-injured animals. Because late fumagillin treatment did not decrease thickening of the medial layers of the pulmonary vasculature, these data also suggest that the accumulation of cells in the medial layer in MCT-injured animals is an event that occurs within the first 14 days after MCT injury [32].

Fumagillin Treatment Decreases the Accumulation of CD45+ Cells after Monocrotaline Injury

To understand the effect of fumagillin on inflammation in MCT-injured lungs, we quantified the number of CD45+ cells in the lungs (Figure 8). No significant differences were detected between uninjured animals treated either with the vehicle or fumagillin. After MCT injury, we observed a large reduction in the number of CD45+ cells. Many of the CD45+ cells in the MCT-injured animals appeared to be foamy macrophages. In MCT-injured animals, fumagillin decreased the accumulation of CD45+ cells by 34% compared to vehicle treatment. Thus, fumagillin was associated with reduced inflammation following MCT injury.

MetAP2 Inhibition by Fumagillin Suppresses Proliferation in Rat PA Smooth Muscle Cells

Because we found decreased thickening of the pulmonary arteries in MCT-injured rats with fumagillin, we reasoned that fumagillin may inhibit the proliferation of smooth muscle cells directly. We have previously found that inhibition of MetAP2 by fumagillin, or that silenced expression of MetAP2 by short interfering RNA (siRNA), decreased proliferation of rat lung fibroblasts *in vitro* [12]. In this section, we tested the hypothesis that fumagillin, via MetAP2, would inhibit the proliferation of RPASMC *in vitro*. The effect of fumagillin on rat PASMC, a cell type that is actively proliferating in experimental PH [9], is unknown. We incubated primary RPASMC in serum-free medium, as described in Materials and Methods, to synchronize cells in G0. The cells were then released from growth arrest by addition of serum, and were incubated with or without PDGF, a pro-proliferative growth factor in smooth muscle cells [9], in the presence of fumagillin or vehicle control (Figure 9A). Cells were grown for one, two, and three days after the addition of serum. Cell number was determined by total SYBR Green intensity as measured by a fluorimetric plate reader. After the addition of serum, cell number increased in all conditions by day 1. By days 2 and 3, the increases in RPASMC number in the vehicle conditions were suppressed by fumagillin. Compared to RPASMC grown with the vehicle control, there were nearly 25% fewer cells

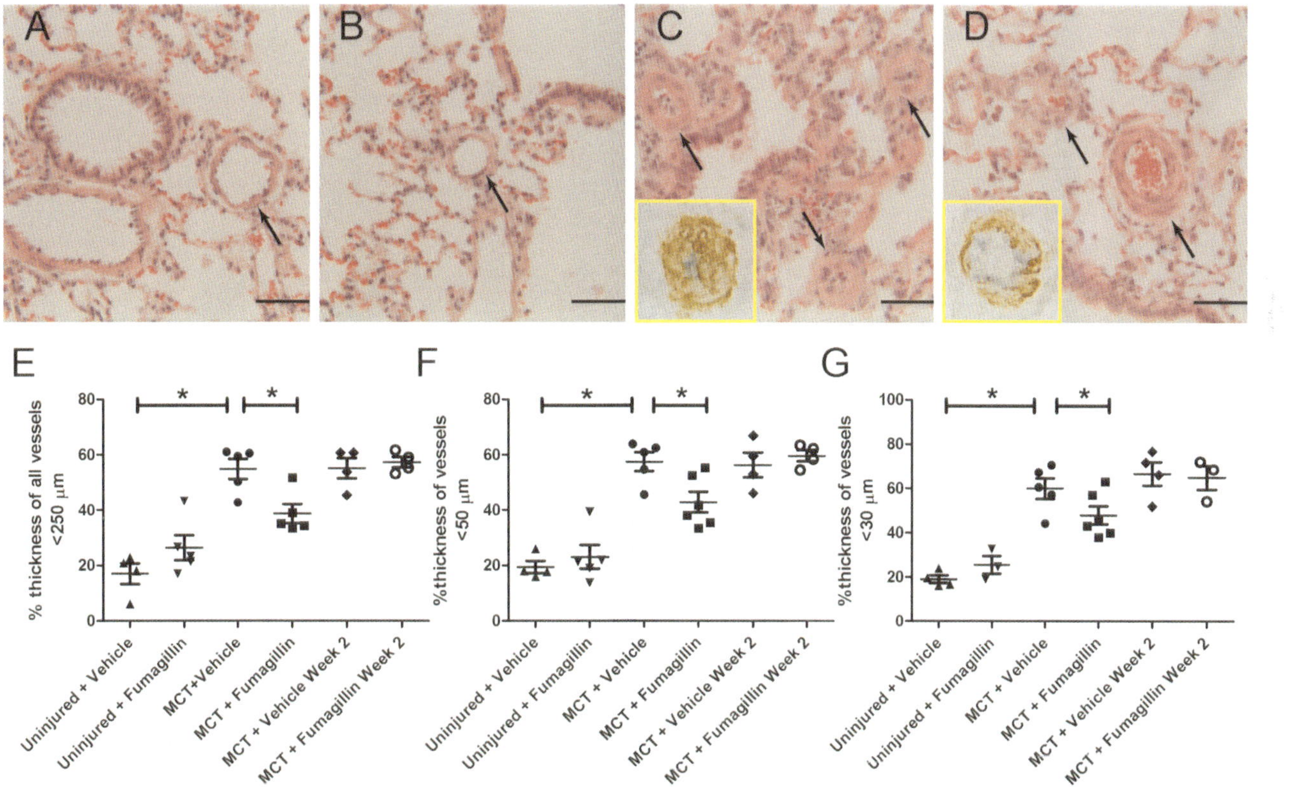

Figure 7. Fumagillin Protects Rats from PA thickening in MCT-injured Rats. Rats were injected with MCT and underwent treatment with fumagillin or vehicle control as described in Materials and Methods. Animals were killed on day 35 after injury, and the lungs were processed for histology. Hematoxylin and eosin staining of lungs from (A) uninjured, vehicle-treated (B) uninjured, fumagillin-treated, (C) MCT-injured, vehicle treated, or (D) MCT-injured, early fumagillin treated. Arrows point to thickened pulmonary arteries (×100 magnification, scale bar = 50 μm). Inset images are 400× magnification and show immunohistochemistry for α-SMA (brown) and vWF (gray) as described in Materials and Methods. Pulmonary artery thickness was measured by Movat staining as described in Materials and Methods (Representative images are shown in Figure S1) (E) All vessels <250 μm, (H) vessels <50 μm, (I) vessels <30 μm. *$P<0.05$, n = 4–6 animals). Data were analyzed by one-way ANOVA followed by the Bonferroni post-hoc test.

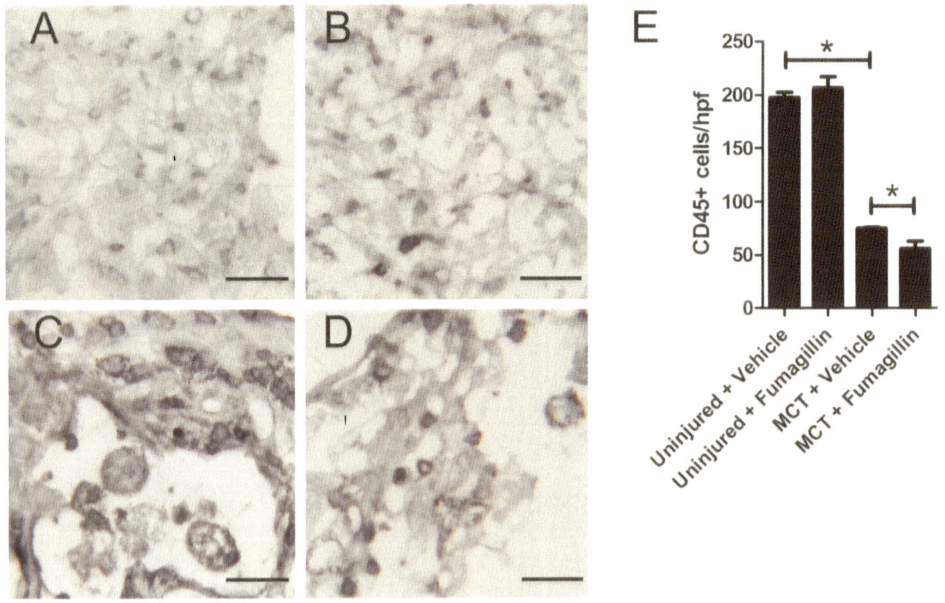

Figure 8. Fumagillin treatment decreases the number of inflammatory cells following monocrotaline injury. Immunohistochemistry was performed for common leukocyte antigen (CD45). CD45+ cells were quantified per high power field (hpf) as described in Materials and Methods. MCT injury was associated with a significant decrease in the number of CD45+ cells in the lung. Early treatment with fumagillin decreased CD45+ cells in the lung by 25% (*$P<0.05$ by ANOVA, n = 3–4 animals per group).

incubated with fumagillin at days 2 and 3 after the addition of serum. Compared to RPASMC grown with the vehicle and PDGF, the addition of fumagillin decreased RPASMC number by nearly 33% at days 2 and 3 after the addition of serum. We also determined the rate of BrdU incorporation of RPASMC grown in the presence of fumagillin or vehicle control (Figure 9B–C). Cells grown in the presence of serum and fumagillin exhibited less BrdU incorporation than cells grown in the presence of serum and the vehicle. The apparent IC50 for the growth inhibition of fumagillin of RPASMC grown in the presence of serum is in the range of 2 nM, which is similar to published data in different cell types [12,33]. Cells grown in the presence of serum, PDGF, and fumagillin also exhibited decreased BrdU incorporation compared to the vehicle control. Thus, fumagillin directly inhibits proliferation of RPASMC *in vitro*.

To determine if MetAP2 expression is necessary for proliferation, we incubated RPASMC in the presence of MetAP2-targeting short-interfering RNA (siRNA). Immunoblotting revealed suppression of MetAP2 expression in the absence of fumagillin (Figure 9D). In the presence of non-targeting RNA oligonucleotides and the vehicle, there was no inhibition of proliferation as measured by BrdU incorporation (Figure 9E). When incubated with MetAP2-targeting siRNA, RPASMC proliferation was inhibited. Incubation of fumagillin-treated cells where MetAP2 expression was suppressed by siRNA did not lead to any additional growth inhibition. These data support the hypothesis that MetAP2 expression is necessary for proliferation in RPASMC, and that the anti-proliferative effect of fumagillin is specific for MetAP2.

PDGF Increases MetAP2 in Rat PA Smooth Muscle Cells

Several growth factors that induce proliferation of smooth muscle cells and fibroblasts have been implicated in the pathogenesis of PH. One such growth factor is platelet-derived growth factor (PDGF) [9,34]. We previously found that PDGF induced expression of MetAP2 in primary rat lung fibroblasts *in vitro* [12]. The effect of PDGF on MetAP2 expression in RPASMC is unknown. We hypothesized that MetAP2 expression would be increased downstream of PDGF. To test this, we used cultured RPASMC as a model system for thickening of vascular media in PH. RPASMC were cultured in the absence of serum with or without PDGF (Figure 10). Immunoblotting for MetAP2 revealed a nearly six-fold increase in MetAP2 protein expression in response to PDGF. Thus, PDGF, a pro-proliferative growth factor that is critical for the development of PH in animals [9,35] and possibly in humans [9,36] increased MetAP2 protein expression in RPASMC.

The Effect of Fumagillin on the Proliferation and Death of Cells in the Pulmonary Arteries in MCT-Injured Rats

Because we observed that fumagillin decreased proliferation of RPASMC *in vitro*, we hypothesized that fumagillin treatment might specifically decrease proliferation of cells in the medial layer of pulmonary arteries in MCT-injured rats directly. And because fumagillin has well-known effects on endothelial cell proliferation [14], we also quantified the number of Ki67+ endothelial cells in the pulmonary arteries. We stained for the proliferation marker Ki67 [37] in lung sections from MCT-injured animals treated with fumagillin or vehicle at 28 days after MCT injury (Figure 11). Double staining for the smooth muscle marker, α-SMA, the endothelial cell marker, vWF, and Ki67 are shown in Figure S2. By visual inspection, abundant staining for Ki67 was present in the pulmonary arteries from MCT-injured, vehicle-treated animals compared to the pulmonary arteries of MCT-injured, early fumagillin-treated rats. Fewer Ki67+ cells were quantified in the animals treated with fumagillin three days after MCT injury compared to the vehicle controls, but this difference did not reach statistical significance. We also quantified Ki67+ cells in the medial layer of the pulmonary arteries in injured animals at two weeks following injury and found a similar trend to decreased Ki67

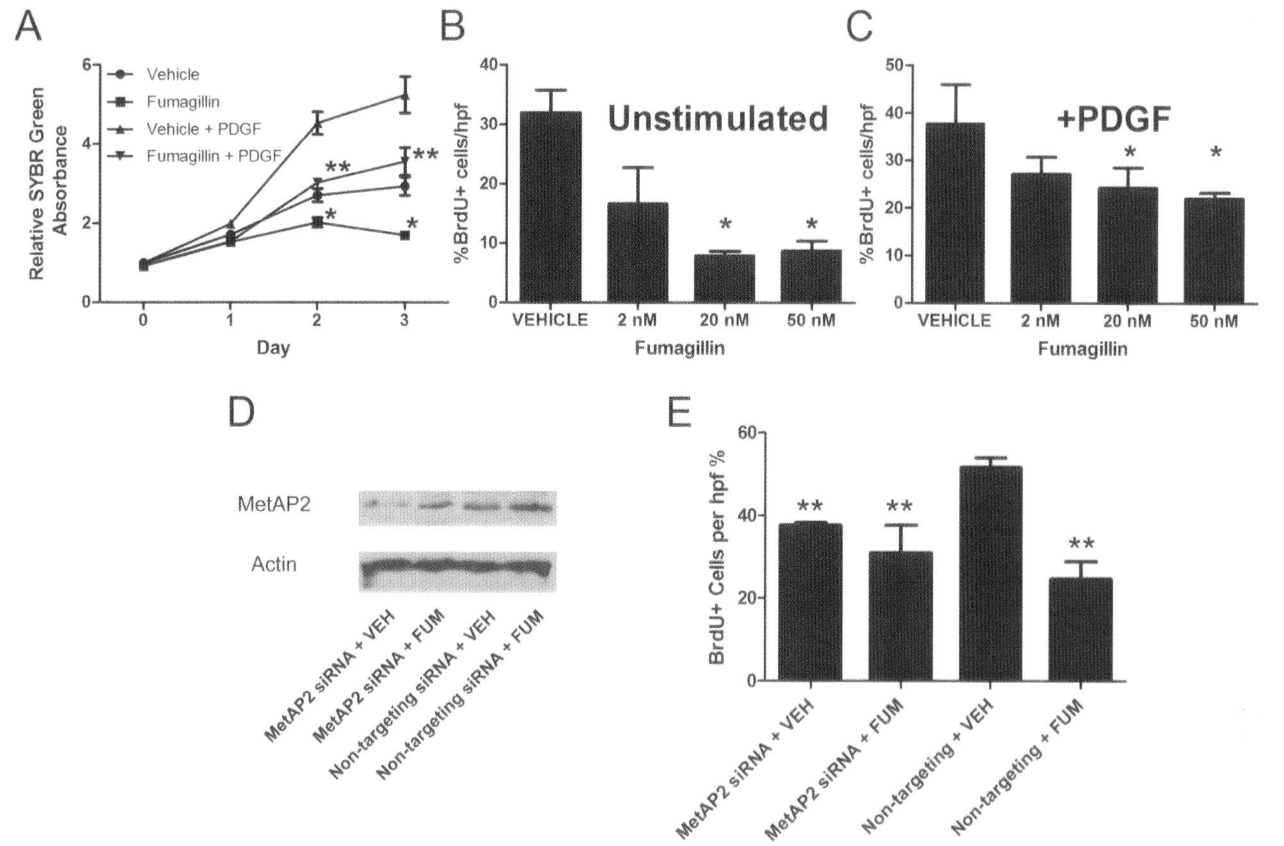

Figure 9. Fumagillin and Silencing of MetAP2 Expression Inhibit Proliferation of RPASMC *in vitro*. (A) Primary RPASMC were serum-starved in basal medium for 24 h to synchronize all cells in G0. Cells were then released from G0 by addition of 10% FBS supplemented with or without PDGF (10 ng/mL) or fumagillin (20 nM). Cells were fixed after 0, 1, 2, and 3 days of culture and then stained with SYBR Green as described in Materials and Methods. Fluorescent intensity, which correlates with relative cell number, was measured by a fluorimetric plate reader. Data represent mean + SEM, n = 4. At days 2 and 3, fumagillin significantly reduced cell number in cells incubated in the absence of PDGF (*$P<0.01$) or in the presence of PDGF (**$P<0.001$). (B–C) RPASMC were incubated in the absence of serum followed by addition of serum (B) or serum with PDGF (10 ng/mL) (C) with or without fumagillin at the indicated concentrations. Cells were incubated for an additional 48 h and pulsed with BrdU for the final 30 minutes then fixed. BrdU+ cells were quantified as described in Materials and Methods. Data represent mean + SEM. Data analyzed by ANOVA followed by Tukey's multiple comparison test (*$P<0.05$, fumagillin v vehicle AND fumagillin + PDGF v. vehicle + PDGF). (D) Immunoblotting for MetAP2 of RPASMC cultured in the presence of 10% serum and exposed to MetAP2-targeting siRNA (lanes 1 and 2) or non-targeting RNA oligonucleotides (lanes 3 and 4). Cells in lanes 1 and 3 were incubated with the vehicle control, and cells in lanes 2 and 4 were incubated with fumagillin 20 nM. Note the increased band intensity of MetAP2 in the fumagillin conditions. (E) Incorporation of BrdU in RPASMC during silencing of MetAP2 gene expression by siRNA. During suppression of MetAP2 gene expression, BrdU incorporation was decreased 27% compared to the non-targeting control (**$P<0.05$, ANOVA followed by Neuman-Keuls post-hoc test compared to Non-targeting + VEH). In the presence of fumagillin, silencing of MetAP2 did not lead to additional inhibition of proliferation.

positivity in fumagillin-treated animals (*data not shown*). Furthermore, we found no significant differences in the number of Ki67+ endothelial cells in MCT-injured animals treated either with fumagillin or the vehicle. Thus, at four weeks after injury, there is no significant difference in the number of Ki67+ proliferating cells in the medial layer of the pulmonary arteries from MCT-injured rats treated with fumagillin compared to the vehicle control. We also performed terminal deoxynucleotidyl transferase dUTP nick end labeling (TUNEL) in parallel and found no significant differences in the number of TUNEL+ cells in animals that were treated with fumagillin or the vehicle (*data not shown*).

MetAP2 Expression in Human and Rat PH

Having shown efficacy of fumagillin, a MetAP2 inhibitor, in a rat model of PH, we sought to determine if MetAP2, the target of fumagillin, is expressed in human disease. We performed immunohistochemistry for MetAP2 on multiple samples of lungs from patients with IPAH and from MCT-injured rats (Figure 12). MetAP2 staining was present in multiple cell types including endothelial cells and cells in the medial layer of the pulmonary vasculature. Very mild staining was present in the non-immune control. Double staining for the smooth muscle marker, α-SMA, the endothelial cell marker, vWF, and MetAP2 are shown in Figure S3. These results support the hypothesis that the cells in the pathologic lesions of human pulmonary arterial hypertension express MetAP2.

To determine if MetAP2 gene expression is increased in the lungs of patients with pulmonary arterial hypertension, we performed quantitative RT-PCR on lung samples from patients with IPAH (n = 6) compared to normal controls (n = 6). No significant difference in MetAP2 gene expression was detected between IPAH and normal controls (*data not shown*).

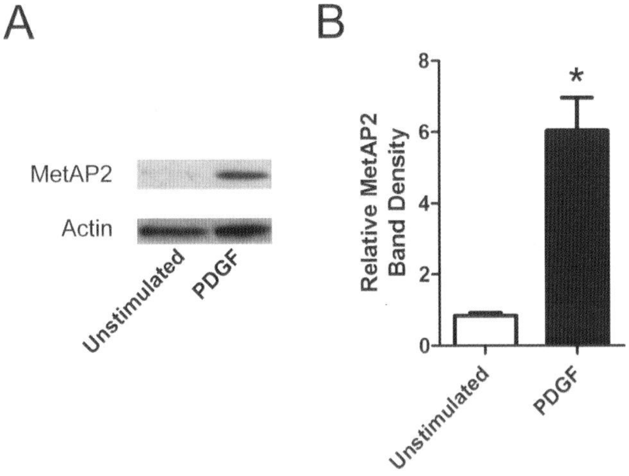

Figure 10. PDGF Increases MetAP2 in Rat Pulmonary Artery Smooth Muscle Cells. RPASMC were incubated in basal medium with 0.5% FBS. Cells were then stimulated with PDGF (10 ng/mL) for 18 hours. Cells were lysed in detergent and subjected to SDS-PAGE and immunoblotting for MetAP2 and Actin. (A) A representative immunoblot showing an increase in MetAP2 expression by PDGF. (B) Quantitative densitometry was performed as described in Materials and Methods and expressed as fold-increase compared to cells incubated in the absence of PDGF (mean + SEM, n = 3,*$P<0.03$). Data were analyzed by paired t-test.

Discussion

In this study, we tested the hypothesis was that fumagillin would prevent MCT-induced pulmonary hypertension by a direct anti-proliferative effect on rat pulmonary artery smooth muscle cells. We did indeed find that early treatment with fumagillin did prevent MCT-induced PH, but we discovered that the protective mechanism of fumagillin in MCT injury is far more complex than a simple effect on smooth muscle cell proliferation. We found that animals treated early with fumagillin did exhibit decreased vessel thickness. While fumagillin, and knockdown of its pharmacologic target MetAP2, did inhibit proliferation *in vitro*, we did not observe significant differences in the number of Ki67+ smooth muscle cells *in vivo*. We did uncover an anti-inflammatory effect of fumagillin following MCT injury, as we found fewer CD45+ leukocytes in the lungs of MCT-injured, fumagillin-treated animals compared to controls. But perhaps our most surprising observation was that late treatment of MCT-injured animals with fumagillin disconnected RV remodeling from PH.

The MCT-injured, late fumagillin-treated animals exhibited both decreased RV mass and decreased right ventricular cardiac myocyte cross-sectional area compared to the MCT-injured vehicle controls. We did not detect any clear differences between the number of capillaries in MCT-injured animals treated with fumagillin late or the vehicle suggesting that the effect of fumagillin in the heart was not a result of altered neoangiogenesis. We did find significantly reduced apoptosis in the heart of MCT-injured animals treated with fumagillin compared with the vehicle controls. We suggest that the effect of fumagillin on the myocardium is at least partially protective. MCT-injured rats treated with fumagillin beginning 14 d after injury exhibited decreased weight loss compared to the vehicle controls. While we found that MCT-injured animals treated late with fumagillin exhibited decreased cardiomyocyte hypertrophy compared to the MCT-injured, vehicle-treated controls, we did not detect significant differences in RV ejection fraction, RV end-diastolic pressure, RV minimum dP/dt, and Ees/Ea between these groups. We suggest that the risk of type II error in these observations is high. The measurement of these hemodynamic parameters in mechanically-ventilated animals following thoracotomy proved to be challenging. Because the intra-operative mortality of this procedure was high, the number of MCT-injured and vehicle-treated animals with adequate hemodynamic data was low. Little is known about the effects of fumagillin on the myocardium. Previous data support the efficacy of the fumagillin analogue TNP-470 in combination with cyclosporine in preventing myocardial arteriosclerosis after heart transplant in rats [38]. Our data lend further support to a growing body of literature that suggests that RV failure in PH is not solely explained by RV pressure afterload [39,40]. Pulmonary artery banding studies have shown that there is RV hypertrophy with sustained PH but is associated with preserved RV function [41,42]. In this model, the effects of MetAP2 inhibition, or off-target effects, by fumagillin on neurohormonal or growth factor signaling known to be important in right ventricular remodeling in MCT injury remain unknown. Further study of fumagillin will be necessary to elucidate the molecular mechanisms that govern right ventricular hypertrophy in animal models of PH.

What about the effect of fumagillin on endothelial cell proliferation? We found no effect of fumagillin on the number of microvessels in the heart following MCT injury or on proliferation of large vessel endothelial cells. It should be noted that a recent study found that the fumagillin analogue, TNP-470, when delivered subcutaneously at 30 mg/kg in MCT-injured animals, beginning at 21 d after injury, prevented the protective effects of estrogen by inhibition of pulmonary neoangiogenesis [43]. In addition, TNP-470 suppressed the "protective" cardiomyocyte hypertrophy in aorta-constricted mice expressing active heat shock transcription factor 1 (HSF1), an effect that the authors attribute to decreased angiogenesis [44]. The discrepancies between the effects of fumagillin and TNP-470 in MCT injury may be an effect of the dose of fumagillin that we employed, the route of administration, or the timing of fumagillin treatment. Our data suggest that the protective effects of fumagillin in MCT injury are certainly complex and involve effects of fumagillin on other cell types including inflammatory cells, smooth muscle cells, and cardiomyocytes.

The finding that fumagillin decreased both MCT-induced PH (this study) and bleomycin-induced pulmonary fibrosis [12]

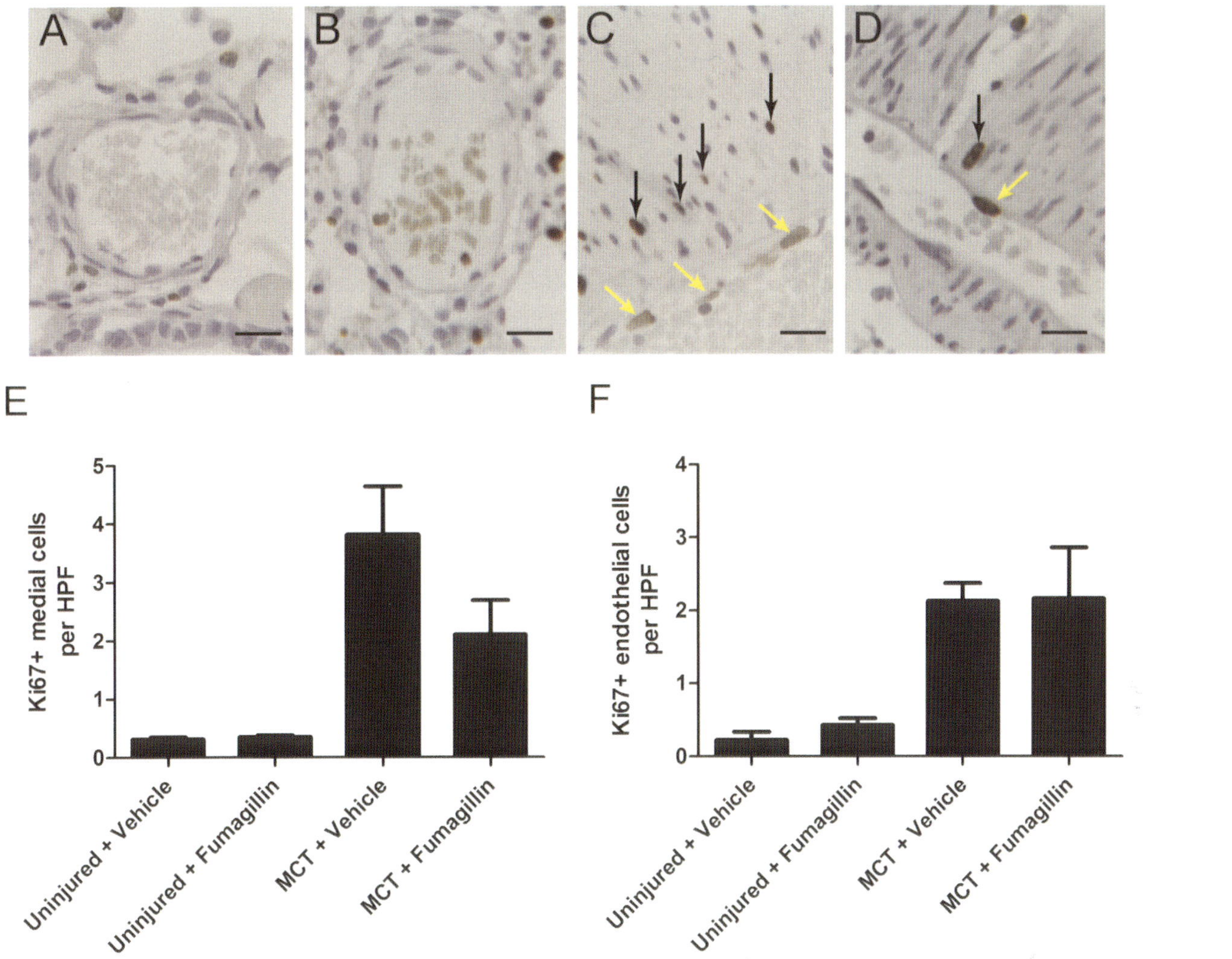

Figure 11. Quantification of Ki67 Staining in Rat Pulmonary Arteries. Immunohistochemistry for Ki67 was performed on rat lung sections from animals injured with MCT treated with or without fumagillin. Images of pulmonary arteries are shown (A) uninjured + vehicle (B) uninjured + fumagillin (C) MCT + vehicle and (D) MCT + fumagillin (Magnification ×400, bar = 20 µm). Black arrows point to Ki67+ nuclei in the medial layer of pulmonary arteries and yellow arrows point to Ki67+ nuclei in endothelial cells. Magnification ×400, inset line 20 mm. (E) Ki67+ nuclei in the medial layer (n = 4–6 per group) and (F) Ki67+ nuclei in endothelial cells of the pulmonary arteries (n = 4 per group) were quantified per hpf as described in Materials and Methods. MCT injury resulted in a nearly 15-fold increase in the number of Ki67+ nuclei in medial cells per vessel per hpf in the MCT-injured vehicle-treated lung. The increase in the number of Ki67+ nuclei was decreased nearly 30% with fumagillin treatment, but this difference did not reach statistical significance. Similarly, MCT significantly increased the number of endothelial cells staining positively for Ki67 nearly tenfold. However, no differences in the number of Ki67+ nuclei were detected after fumagillin treatment.

suggests that fumagillin may be effective in treating so-called "secondary" PH, that is World Health Organization Class III, PH, which is associated with hypoxemic diseases such as IPF. Further studies will be necessary to determine if fumagillin is efficacious in attenuating both pulmonary fibrosis and PH in animal models of secondary PH.

Why use MCT injury as a model for PH? Many correctly note that MCT injury is not associated with the plexiform lesion, the histopathologic hallmark of idiopathic pulmonary arterial hypertension in humans [3]. Moreover multiple agents have been shown to prevent MCT-induced PH, including agents that are associated with PH in humans [3]. Many cases of human PH are advanced at the time of diagnosis. Anti-proliferative approaches, such as fumagillin, for example, may have clinical utility, perhaps in conjunction with currently available therapies, in preventing disease progression. Perhaps most critical to developing any therapy for pulmonary hypertension is to determine the effect of the compound on the right ventricle. Death in PH is due to failure of the right ventricle. MCT injury, as opposed to chronic hypobaric hypoxia, is associated with significant PH, RV strain, and failure [3]. Further studies will be necessary to determine if fumagillin is effective in preventing cardiac remodeling in other animals of PH.

Our data show that MetAP2 expression is increased by PDGF in RPASMC *in vitro*. We suggest that MetAP2 exerts a permissive effect on RPASMC proliferation. But how does fumagillin inhibit proliferation of RPASMC? The enzymatic function of MetAP2 is to cleave the N-terminal methionine from nascent polypeptides during protein synthesis [15]. The removal of methionine is essential for further N-terminal modifications, for example acetylation by N-α-acetyltransferase and myristoylation of glycine by N-myristoyltransferase [16]. Growth inhibition induced by TNP-470 is dependent on p21 and p53 [33]. How the inhibition of the enzymatic function of MetAP2 leads to p21 induction is not

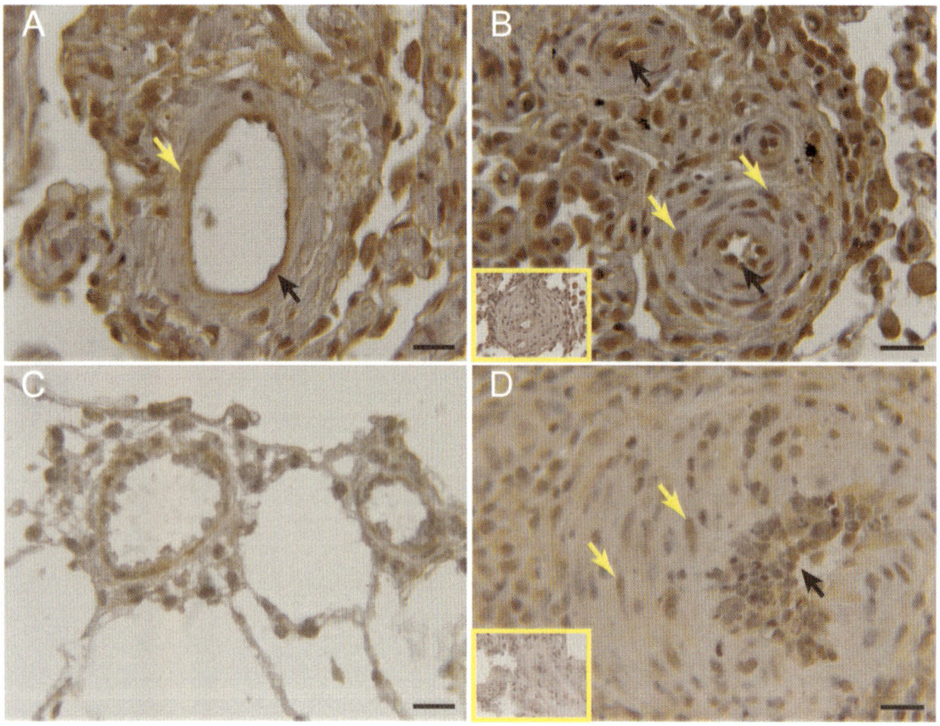

Figure 12. Detection of MetAP2 in human and rat lungs. Immunohistochemistry for MetAP2 was performed on formalin-fixed paraffin-embedded samples. Sections were counterstained with hematoxylin. Representative sections are shown, n = 3: (A) normal human lung (B) Pulmonary arterial hypertension (*inset* non-immune rabbit IgG) (C) normal rat lung (D) MCT-injured rat lung (*inset* non-immune rabbit IgG). Magnification ×400, bar = 20 μm. Note staining for MetAP2 in endothelial cells (black arrows) and cells in the medial layer (yellow arrows).

clear [33]. Incorrect processing of a protein's N-terminus can theoretically result in aberrant biological functions and lead to a cell stress response [45]. Although the current study has implicated the enzymatic activity of MetAP2 in promoting proliferation, MetAP2 has other recognized non-enzymatic functions. It was first characterized in 1988 as a 67 kDa protein that binds to eukaryotic initiation factor-2α (eIF2-α), protecting it from phosphorylation and thus maintaining active protein synthesis [15]. Pharmacologic inhibition of MetAP2 by fumagillin-type compounds does not affect the ability of MetAP2 to protect eIF2-α from phosphorylation [46]. While our *in vitro* data support a specific effect of fumagillin for MetAP2, we also cannot exclude MetAP2-independent effects of fumagillin *in vivo* [47].

Fumagillin, and its analogues, have advanced into clinical trials in different malignancies [48,49,50]. Dose-limiting neurotoxicity has limited the application of fumagillin-like treatments in clinical practice. Typically these fumagillin doses reach ranges of 20–100 mg/kg. We chose intranasal delivery, at a significantly lower dosage (0.5 mg/kg). We found no efficacy of fumagillin delivered by intraperitoneal injection at 0.5 mg/kg (*data not shown*). Although use of the intranasal route for the delivery of fumagillin or its analogues has not been described in human clinical trials, the potential for delivery of high local concentrations of MetAP2 inhibitors might be expected to minimize neurotoxicity. Further studies will be required to determine the safety, effectiveness, and pharmacokinetics of inhaled fumagillin in human lung diseases.

Supporting Information

Figure S1 Movat staining of the pulmonary vasculature in MCT-injured rats. Rats were injected with MCT and underwent treatment with fumagillin or vehicle control as described in Materials and Methods. Pulmonary artery thickness was measured by Movat staining as described in Materials and Methods. Representative images of vessels with similar luminal diameters are shown: (A) Uninjured + vehicle, (B) uninjured + fumagillin, (C) MCT + vehicle early, (D) MCT + fumagillin early, (E) MCT + vehicle late, and (F) MCT + fumagillin late (magnification ×400, bar = 20 μm).

Figure S2 Double-label immunohistochemistry for Ki67, vWF, and α-SMA. Double staining for Ki67 (brown) and the endothelial cell marker, von Willebrand Factor (gray). Yellow arrows point to a vWF+/Ki67+ cell. (B) Double staining for Ki67 (gray) and the smooth muscle cell marker, αSMA (brown). Yellow arrows point to an α-SMA+/Ki67+ cell. Inset image is the non-immune control for α-SMA (magnification ×400, bar = 20 μm).

Figure S3 Immunofluorescent detection of MetAP2 and smooth muscle and endothelial cell markers. Immunofluorescence for MetAP2 and α-smooth muscle actin (αSMA) and von Willebrand Factor (vWF) was performed on formalin-fixed paraffin-embedded samples. (A) MetAP2, (B) αSMA, (C) DAPI, and (D) merged image showing MetAP2 positivity in αSMA+ cells. (E) MetAP2, (F) vWF, (G) DAPI, and (H) merged image. White arrows point out MetAP2+ and vWF+ cells. Images A′–H′ show the corresponding non-immune controls (magnification ×400, bar = 50 μm).

Author Contributions

Conceived and designed the experiments: DJK EMR HCC. Performed the experiments: DJK EMR RK KL LY MCM A. Saqi A. Savir RR FA. Analyzed the data: DJK HCC. Contributed reagents/materials/analysis tools: DJK EMR RK KL YL A. Savir MCM A. Saqi RR FA HCC. Wrote the paper: DJK.

References

1. Badesch DB, Champion HC, Sanchez MA, Hoeper MM, Loyd JE, et al. (2009) Diagnosis and assessment of pulmonary arterial hypertension. J Am Coll Cardiol 54: S55–66.
2. Halpern SD, Doyle R, Kawut SM (2008) The ethics of randomized clinical trials in pulmonary arterial hypertension. Proc Am Thorac Soc 5: 631–635.
3. Stenmark KR, Meyrick B, Galie N, Mooi WJ, McMurtry IF (2009) Animal models of pulmonary arterial hypertension: the hope for etiological discovery and pharmacological cure. Am J Physiol Lung Cell Mol Physiol 297: L1013–1032.
4. Humbert M, Sitbon O, Chaouat A, Bertocchi M, Habib G, et al. (2006) Pulmonary arterial hypertension in France: results from a national registry. Am J Respir Crit Care Med 173: 1023–1030.
5. Rubin LJ (2006) Pulmonary arterial hypertension. Proc Am Thorac Soc 3: 111–115.
6. Humbert M, Morrell NW, Archer SL, Stenmark KR, MacLean MR, et al. (2004) Cellular and molecular pathobiology of pulmonary arterial hypertension. J Am Coll Cardiol 43: 13S–24S.
7. Budhiraja R, Tuder RM, Hassoun PM (2004) Endothelial dysfunction in pulmonary hypertension. Circulation 109: 159–165.
8. Daley E, Emson C, Guignabert C, de Waal Malefyt R, Louten J, et al. (2008) Pulmonary arterial remodeling induced by a Th2 immune response. J Exp Med 205: 361–372.
9. Schermuly RT, Dony E, Ghofrani HA, Pullamsetti S, Savai R, et al. (2005) Reversal of experimental pulmonary hypertension by PDGF inhibition. J Clin Invest 115: 2811–2821.
10. Barst RJ, Galie N, Naeije R, Simonneau G, Jeffs R, et al. (2006) Long-term outcome in pulmonary arterial hypertension patients treated with subcutaneous treprostinil. Eur Respir J 28: 1195–1203.
11. McLaughlin VV, Sitbon O, Badesch DB, Barst RJ, Black C, et al. (2005) Survival with first-line bosentan in patients with primary pulmonary hypertension. Eur Respir J 25: 244–249.
12. Kass D, Bridges RS, Borczuk A, Greenberg S (2007) Methionine aminopeptidase-2 as a selective target of myofibroblasts in pulmonary fibrosis. Am J Respir Cell Mol Biol 37: 193–201.
13. Koyama H, Nishizawa Y, Hosoi M, Fukumoto S, Kogawa K, et al. (1996) The fumagillin analogue TNP-470 inhibits DNA synthesis of vascular smooth muscle cells stimulated by platelet-derived growth factor and insulin-like growth factor-I. Possible involvement of cyclin-dependent kinase 2. Circ Res 79: 757–764.
14. Yeh JR, Mohan R, Crews CM (2000) The antiangiogenic agent TNP-470 requires p53 and p21CIP/WAF for endothelial cell growth arrest. Proc Natl Acad Sci U S A 97: 12782–12787.
15. Datta B (2000) MAPs and POEP of the roads from prokaryotic to eukaryotic kingdoms. Biochimie 82: 95–107.
16. Turk BE, Griffith EC, Wolf S, Biemann K, Chang YH, et al. (1999) Selective inhibition of amino-terminal methionine processing by TNP-470 and ovalicin in endothelial cells. Chem Biol 6: 823–833.
17. Ingber D, Fujita T, Kishimoto S, Sudo K, Kanamaru T, et al. (1990) Synthetic analogues of fumagillin that inhibit angiogenesis and suppress tumour growth. Nature 348: 555–557.
18. Liu S, Widom J, Kemp CW, Crews CM, Clardy J (1998) Structure of human methionine aminopeptidase-2 complexed with fumagillin. Science 282: 1324–1327.
19. Sin N, Meng L, Wang MQ, Wen JJ, Bornmann WG, et al. (1997) The anti-angiogenic agent fumagillin covalently binds and inhibits the methionine aminopeptidase, MetAP-2. Proc Natl Acad Sci U S A 94: 6099–6103.
20. Wang YQ, Ikeda K, Ikebe T, Hirakawa K, Sowa M, et al. (2000) Inhibition of hepatic stellate cell proliferation and activation by the semisynthetic analogue of fumagillin TNP-470 in rats. Hepatology 32: 980–989.
21. Yoshio Y, Miyazaki M, Abe K, Nishino T, Furusu A, et al. (2004) TNP-470, an angiogenesis inhibitor, suppresses the progression of peritoneal fibrosis in mouse experimental model. Kidney Int 66: 1677–1685.
22. Katzenstein HM, Rademaker AW, Senger C, Salwen HR, Nguyen NN, et al. (1999) Effectiveness of the angiogenesis inhibitor TNP-470 in reducing the growth of human neuroblastoma in nude mice inversely correlates with tumor burden. Clin Cancer Res 5: 4273–4278.
23. Ohta Y, Watanabe Y, Tabata T, Oda M, Hayashi Y, et al. (1997) Inhibition of lymph node metastasis by an anti-angiogenic agent, TNP-470. Br J Cancer 75: 512–515.
24. Huang ZH, Fan YF, Xia H, Feng HM, Tang FX (2003) Effects of TNP-470 on proliferation and apoptosis in human colon cancer xenografts in nude mice. World J Gastroenterol 9: 281–283.
25. Brakenhielm E, Cao R, Gao B, Angelin B, Cannon B, et al. (2004) Angiogenesis inhibitor, TNP-470, prevents diet-induced and genetic obesity in mice. Circ Res 94: 1579–1588.
26. Burkhoff D, Mirsky I, Suga H (2005) Assessment of systolic and diastolic ventricular properties via pressure-volume analysis: a guide for clinical, translational, and basic researchers. Am J Physiol Heart Circ Physiol 289: H501–512.
27. Pacher P, Nagayama T, Mukhopadhyay P, Batkai S, Kass DA (2008) Measurement of cardiac function using pressure-volume conductance catheter technique in mice and rats. Nat Protoc 3: 1422–1434.
28. Zuckerbraun BS, Shiva S, Ifedigbo E, Mathier MA, Mollen KP, et al. (2009) Nitrite potently inhibits hypoxic and inflammatory pulmonary arterial hypertension and smooth muscle proliferation via xanthine oxidoreductase-dependent nitric oxide generation. Circulation 121: 98–109.
29. Bridges RS, Kass D, Loh K, Glackin C, Borczuk AC, et al. (2009) Gene expression profiling of pulmonary fibrosis identifies Twist1 as an antiapoptotic molecular "rectifier" of growth factor signaling. Am J Pathol 175: 2351–2361.
30. Rajkumar R, Konishi K, Richards TJ, Ishizawar DC, Wiechert AC, et al. (2010) Genomewide RNA expression profiling in lung identifies distinct signatures in idiopathic pulmonary arterial hypertension and secondary pulmonary hypertension. Am J Physiol Heart Circ Physiol 298: H1235–1248.
31. Champion HC, Michelakis ED, Hassoun PM (2009) Comprehensive invasive and noninvasive approach to the right ventricle-pulmonary circulation unit: state of the art and clinical and research implications. Circulation 120: 992–1007.
32. Lappin PB, Roth RA (1997) Hypertrophy and prolonged DNA synthesis in smooth muscle cells characterize pulmonary arterial wall thickening after monocrotaline pyrrole administration to rats. Toxicol Pathol 25: 372–380.
33. Zhang Y, Griffith EC, Sage J, Jacks T, Liu JO (2000) Cell cycle inhibition by the anti-angiogenic agent TNP-470 is mediated by p53 and p21WAF1/CIP1. Proc Natl Acad Sci U S A 97: 6427–6432.
34. Perros F, Montani D, Dorfmuller P, Durand-Gasselin I, Tcherakian C, et al. (2008) Platelet-derived growth factor expression and function in idiopathic pulmonary arterial hypertension. Am J Respir Crit Care Med 178: 81–88.
35. Balasubramaniam V, Le Cras TD, Ivy DD, Grover TR, Kinsella JP, et al. (2003) Role of platelet-derived growth factor in vascular remodeling during pulmonary hypertension in the ovine fetus. Am J Physiol Lung Cell Mol Physiol 284: L826–833.
36. Humbert M, Monti G, Fartoukh M, Magnan A, Brenot F, et al. (1998) Platelet-derived growth factor expression in primary pulmonary hypertension: comparison of HIV seropositive and HIV seronegative patients. Eur Respir J 11: 554–559.
37. Baisch H, Gerdes J (1990) Identification of proliferating cells by Ki-67 antibody. Methods Cell Biol 33: 217–226.
38. Denton MD, Magee C, Melter M, Dharnidharka VR, Sayegh MH, et al. (2004) TNP-470, an angiogenesis inhibitor, attenuates the development of allograft vasculopathy. Transplantation 78: 1218–1221.
39. Bogaard HJ, Natarajan R, Mizuno S, Abbate A, Chang PJ, et al. (2010) Adrenergic receptor blockade reverses right heart remodeling and dysfunction in pulmonary hypertensive rats. Am J Respir Crit Care Med 182: 652–660.
40. Bogaard HJ, Natarajan R, Henderson SC, Long CS, Kraskauskas D, et al. (2009) Chronic pulmonary artery pressure elevation is insufficient to explain right heart failure. Circulation 120: 1951–1960.
41. Faber MJ, Dalinghaus M, Lankhuizen IM, Bezstarosti K, Verhoeven AJ, et al. (2007) Time dependent changes in cytoplasmic proteins of the right ventricle during prolonged pressure overload. J Mol Cell Cardiol 43: 197–209.
42. Faber MJ, Dalinghaus M, Lankhuizen IM, Steendijk P, Hop WC, et al. (2006) Right and left ventricular function after chronic pulmonary artery banding in rats assessed with biventricular pressure-volume loops. Am J Physiol Heart Circ Physiol 291: H1580–1586.
43. Umar S, Iorga A, Matori H, Nadadur RD, Li J, et al. (2011) Estrogen Rescues Pre-existing Severe Pulmonary Hypertension in Rats. Am J Respir Crit Care Med.
44. Zou Y, Li J, Ma H, Jiang H, Yuan J, et al. (2011) Heat shock transcription factor 1 protects heart after pressure overload through promoting myocardial angiogenesis in male mice. J Mol Cell Cardiol 51: 821–829.
45. Warder SE, Tucker LA, McLoughlin SM, Strelitzer TJ, Meuth JL, et al. (2008) Discovery, identification, and characterization of candidate pharmacodynamic markers of methionine aminopeptidase-2 inhibition. J Proteome Res 7: 4807–4820.
46. Griffith EC, Su Z, Turk BE, Chen S, Chang YH, et al. (1997) Methionine aminopeptidase (type 2) is the common target for angiogenesis inhibitors AGM-1470 and ovalicin. Chem Biol 4: 461–471.
47. Kim S, LaMontagne K, Sabio M, Sharma S, Versace RW, et al. (2004) Depletion of methionine aminopeptidase 2 does not alter cell response to fumagillin or bengamides. Cancer Res 64: 2984–2987.
48. Herbst RS, Madden TL, Tran HT, Blumenschein GR Jr., Meyers CA, et al. (2002) Safety and pharmacokinetic effects of TNP-470, an angiogenesis inhibitor, combined with paclitaxel in patients with solid tumors: evidence for activity in non-small-cell lung cancer. J Clin Oncol 20: 4440–4447.

49. Kudelka AP, Levy T, Verschraegen CF, Edwards CL, Piamsomboon S, et al. (1997) A phase I study of TNP-470 administered to patients with advanced squamous cell cancer of the cervix. Clin Cancer Res 3: 1501–1505.

50. Tran HT, Blumenschein GR Jr., Lu C, Meyers CA, Papadimitrakopoulou V, et al. (2004) Clinical and pharmacokinetic study of TNP-470, an angiogenesis inhibitor, in combination with paclitaxel and carboplatin in patients with solid tumors. Cancer Chemother Pharmacol 54: 308–314.

Glycogen Synthase Kinase 3beta Contributes to Proliferation of Arterial Smooth Muscle Cells in Pulmonary Hypertension

Piotr Sklepkiewicz[1]†, Ralph Theo Schermuly[1,2]†, Xia Tian[1], Hossein Ardeschir Ghofrani[1], Norbert Weissmann[1], Daniel Sedding[3], Tarek Kashour[4], Werner Seeger[1,2], Friedrich Grimminger[1], Soni Savai Pullamsetti[1,2]*

1 Medical Clinic II/V, University Hospital, Giessen, Germany, **2** Max-Planck-Institute for Heart and Lung Research, Bad Nauheim, Germany, **3** Medical Clinic I, University Hospital, Giessen, Germany, **4** King Fahad Medical City, Riyadh, Saudi Arabia

Abstract

Rationale: Pulmonary arterial hypertension (PAH) is a rare progressive pulmonary vascular disorder associated with vascular remodeling and right heart failure. Vascular remodeling involves numerous signaling cascades governing pulmonary arterial smooth muscle cell (PASMC) proliferation, migration and differentiation. Glycogen synthase kinase 3beta (GSK3ß) is a serine/threonine kinase and can act as a downstream regulatory switch for numerous signaling pathways. Hence, we hypothesized that GSK3ß plays a crucial role in pulmonary vascular remodeling.

Methods: All experiments were done with lung tissue or isolated PASMCs in a well-established monocrotaline (MCT)-induced PAH rat model. The mRNA expression of Wnt ligands (Wnt1, Wnt3a, Wnt5a), upstream Wnt signaling regulator genes (Frizzled Receptors 1, 2 and secreted Frizzled related protein sFRP-1) and canonical Wnt intracellular effectors (GSK3ß, Axin1) were assessed by real-time polymerase chain reaction and protein levels of GSK3ß, phospho-GSK3ß (ser 9) by western blotting and localization by immunohistochemistry. The role of GSK3ß in PASMCs proliferation was assessed by overexpression of wild-type GSK3ß (WT) and constitutively active GSK3ß S9A by [^{3}H]-thymidine incorporation assay.

Results: Increased levels of total and phosphorylated GSK3ß (inhibitory phosphorylation) were observed in lungs and PASMCs isolated from MCT-induced PAH rats compared to controls. Further, stimulation of MCT-PASMCs with growth factors induced GSK3ß inactivation. Most importantly, treatment with the PDGFR inhibitor, Imatinib, attenuated PDGF-BB and FCS induced GSK3ß phosphorylation. Increased expression of GSK3ß observed in lungs and PASMC isolated from MCT-induced PAH rats was confirmed to be clinically relevant as the same observation was identified in human iPAH lung explants. Overexpression of GSK3ß significantly increased MCT-PASMCs proliferation by regulating ERK phosphorylation. Constitutive activation of GSK3ß (GSK3ß S9A, 9th serine replaced to alanine) inhibited MCT-PASMCs proliferation by decreasing ERK phosphorylation.

Conclusion: This study supports a central role for GSK3ß in vascular remodeling processes and suggests a novel therapeutic opportunity for the treatment of PAH.

Editor: Aernout Luttun, Katholieke Universiteit Leuven, Belgium

Funding: This work was supported by the Deutsche Forschungsgemeinschaft, Sonderforschungsbereich 547 "Kardiopulmonales Gefäßsystem", Projekt B11 and C6 (http://www.dfg.de/index.jsp). The funders had no role in study design, data collection and analysis, decision to publish, or preparation of the manuscript.

Competing Interests: The authors have declared that no competing interests exist.

* E-mail: soni.pullamsetti@mpi-bn.mpg.de

† These authors contributed equally to this work.

Introduction

Pulmonary arterial hypertension (PAH) is a progressive pulmonary vascular disorder with high morbidity and mortality [1,2]. The pulmonary vascular remodeling may typically involve numerous molecular signaling cascades governing endothelial dysfunction, neovascularization of small pulmonary arteries, pulmonary arterial smooth muscle cell (PASMC) and adventitial fibroblast (PAAF) migration and proliferation [3,4]. However, 3 of the currently approved therapies targeting vasoconstrictive/vasodilatory abnormalities in PAH, like endothelin, nitric oxide or prostacyclin, show beneficial effects and improved quality of life [5,6,7], but do not appear to reverse or modify disease progression.

To this end, in the last 5 years, enormous progress has been made by our group and authors in developing new anti-proliferative and pro-apoptotic therapeutic strategies to reverse the disease progression. The role of growth factors, tyrosine/serine-threonine kinase receptors in PAH has been extensively studied at the cellular, preclinical and clinical levels. Accumulation of growth factors such as platelet derived growth factor (PDGF), epidermal growth factor (EGF), fibroblast growth factor (FGF) and vascular endothelial growth factor (VEGF) and pro-survival factors like survivin in the pulmonary vasculature suggest categorizing this disease as a pseudo-malignant proliferative disorder [8,9,10,11,12]. In accordance, inhibition of anti-cancer compounds, Imatinib/STI571 (PDGFRß, C-kit, SDF-1), PKI166 (EGFR) and Sorafenib (multikinase inhibitor), prove effective in reversing vascular remodeling and improved survival in various experimental models of PAH [8,10,13]. These studies not only highlighted the importance of anti-cancer therapeutics in PAH but also open avenues to explore new intracellular signaling pathways in the PAH disease pathogenesis.

GSK3ß (Glycogen Synthase Kinase-3 beta) is a ubiquitously expressed, highly conserved serine/threonine protein kinase found in all eukaryotes. Although initially identified as a regulator of glycogen metabolism, GSK3ß can act as a downstream regulatory switch for numerous signaling pathways [14,15]. GSK3ß is constitutively active in unstimulated, resting cells, and is inactivated during cellular responses. Treatment of cells with a growth factors such as insulin, is shown to cause GSK3ß inactivation through a PI 3-kinase (PI3K)-dependent mechanism. PI3K-induced activation of PKB/Akt results in phosphorylation of ser 9 on GSK3ß, that inhibits GSK3ß activity [16,17]. Similarly, GSK3ß was shown to play a key inhibitory role in the Wnt signaling pathway [18]. This inactivation causes reduced phosphorylation of its substrates, such as ß-Catenin, c-Myc, endothelin, VEGF, survivin etc [19,20,21]. Thus, GSK3 by regulating several of its substrates participates in a wide spectrum of cellular processes, including glycogen metabolism, transcription, translation, cytoskeleton regulation, intracellular vesicular transport, cell cycle progression and apoptosis.

Recent evidences suggest that inactivation of GSK3ß can positively regulate proliferation and cell survival in many types of cancer and in vascular remodeling [22,23]. Hence we hypothesized that GSK3ß plays a crucial role in remodeling of vascular components during PAH. Our aims were at first to determinate expression profile of GSK3ß and its regulatory genes (Wnt ligands 1, 3a, 5a, Frizzled Receptor 1 and 2, sFRP-1 and Axin1) and quantify protein level changes and phosphorylation status in MCT-induced PAH rat lungs and in isolated PASMCs. Further, to assess the functional role of GSK3ß in PASMCs proliferation and down stream molecular mechanisms by overexpression of wild type and constitutively active mutant of GSK3ß.

Materials and Methods

Ethics Statement

The study protocol for human tissue donation was approved by the ethics committee (Ethik Kommission am Fachbereich Humanmedizin der Justus Liebig Universität Giessen) of the University Hospital Giessen (Giessen, Germany) in accordance with national law and with "Good Clinical Practice/International Conference on Harmonisation" guidelines (AZ 31/93). A written informed consent was obtained from each individual patient or the patient's next to kin.

The University Animal Care Committee and the Federal Authorities approved all animal studies for Animal Research of the Regierungspräsidium Giessen (Hessen, Germany) (Az. GI 20/10 Nr. 09/2010).

Materials

GSK3ß total, phospho-GSK3ß (ser 9), AKT, phospho-AKT antibodies were purchased from Cell Signaling (Denver, USA). Axin1, phospho-ERK1/2, ERK total and H1 histone antibodies were obtained from Santa Cruz (Heidelberg, Germany). GAPDH antibody was obtained from Novus (Littleton, USA). Dulbecco's Modified Eagle's medium, nutrient mixture F-12 (DMEM-F12), fetal calf serum (FCS), Streptomycin/Penicillin, Vitamins and non-essentials amino acids were obtained from Gibco (Karlsruhe, Germany). Platelet derived growth factor BB (PDGF-BB) was purchased from PeproTech (Hamburg, Germany). Wnt3A ligand was purchased from R&D Systems (Minneapolis, USA). PDGFRß inhibitor Imatinib (Gleevec) was obtained from Novartis (Switzerland). Im Prom reverse transcriptase and Taq polymerase PCR Kit were obtained from Promega (Mannheim, Germany). RIPA buffer was obtained from Santa Cruz (Heidelberg, Germany). ECL detection kit was obtained from Amersham Biosciences (Piscataway, USA). Histostain SP Rabbit Primary (AEC) was purchased from ZYMED Laboratories (Carlsbad, USA). MiniPrep Plasmid Isolation Kit was obtained from PeqLab (Erlangen, Germany) and MaxiPrep Plasmid Isolation Kit, PCR purification Kit was purchased from QIAGEN (Hilden, Germany), pGEMT-Easy vector Kit was obtained from Promega, (Mannheim, Germany), pcDNA3.1 Directional TOPO Expression Kit, Lipofectamine 2000, T4 Ligase, Platinum Taq DNA Polymerase High Fidelity, Platinum SYBR Green qPCR SuperMix-UDG was purchased from Invitrogen (Karlsruhe, Germany), restriction enzymes (BamHI, BsmI, EcoRV) was purchased from New England BioLabs (Frankfurt, Germany). Gel Extraction Kit was obtained from QIAGEN (Hilden, Germany), Opti-DMEM medium was purchased from Gibco (Karlsruhe, Germany).

Animal experiments

Experiments were performed on male CD rats of 300–350 g body weight (Charles River, Sulzfeld, Germany). Pulmonary arterial hypertension was induced by a single subcutaneous injection of monocrotaline (MCT, 60 mg/kg, Sigma, Deishofen, Germany), dissolved in 0.1 M NaOH, adjusted to pH 7.4 with 0.1 M HCl, as described previously [24]. In these experiments 3 study groups were used: healthy rats, MCT-injected rats sacrificed either 3 weeks or 5 weeks after injection.

Pulmonary arterial smooth muscle cells isolation

Rat PASMCs were isolated from pulmonary arteries using the explant method as described previously [8] and the characterization and purity was assessed as described [25]. Briefly, characterization of PASMCs was done using immunocytochemical staining for a-smooth muscle actin and desmin. The presence of endothelial cells and fibroblasts were excluded by staining for CD31 and FSP1. Further in order to determine the purity of PASMCs, flow cytometric analysis was performed with anti-desmin and anti-α-smooth muscle actin antibodies. Usually, the purity of isolated PASMCs is 91–94%. Cultures were maintained at 37°C in a humidified 5% CO_2/95% O_2 atmosphere. All experiments using PASMCs were performed between 2–4 passages. Expression analysis studies were done at early passages to minimize the influence of phenotypic alterations.

Cell culture

Primary rat PASMC's were maintained at 37°C in a humidified 5%CO_2/95%O_2 atmosphere. Cells were grown on 10 cm^2 dishes, 6 and 48-well plates in DMEM-F12 supplemented with 10% FCS, 5% streptomycin/penicillin, 5% glutamate. Cells were cultured from the time of isolation in 10% FCS medium and subsequently in experiments with 0.1% FCS medium supplemented with PDGF-BB (60 ng/ml) or Wnt3a (100 ng/ml) for 6 and 24 hrs. Additionally, PASMC's were stimulated with PDGF-BB (60 ng/

ml) for 6 hrs and 24 hrs and were also pretreated with 1 and 5 μM of the PDGFRβ inhibitor Imatinib (Gleevec) in the presence of 10% FCS.

Reverse transcriptase PCR and Real-Time PCR

Total RNA was isolated from tissue rat's lung homogenates and primary rat pulmonary arterial smooth muscle cells (PASMC) with Trizol® Reagent. The quantity and quality of RNA was determined by NanoDrop (PeqLab, Erlangen, Germany). Equal amounts of RNA from each sample were used as templates for reverse transcription reaction for generation of cDNA using Im Prom Reverse Transcriptase and Taq polymerase PCR Kit with oligo(dT)$_{18}$ primers according to the supplier's instructions. Later, quantitative Real-Time PCR analysis was performed as described previously [26]. Briefly, 1 μl cDNA was placed into 25 μl reaction volume containing Platinum SYBR Green qPCR SuperMix-UDG and sequence-specific oligonucleotide primers. The thermal cycle conditions used for all reactions were as follows: activation, 50°C for 2 min; denaturation, 95°C for 10 min; and cycle, 95°C for 10 s and 59°C for 30 s (40 times). Specific primers used for sequence detection both in tissue homogenates as well as in the cells were: Wnt1 (Forward 5′CTA CGT TGC TAC TGG CAC TGA C3′, Reverse 5′AGA CTC TTG GAA TCT GTC AGC AG3′), Wnt3a (Forward 5′ATT TGG AGG AAT GGT CTC TCG3′, Reverse 5′GCA GGT CTT CAC TTC GCA AC3′), Wnt5a (Forward 5′GCC ACT TGT ATC AGG ACC ACA3′, Reverse 5′GGC ATT TAC CAC TCC AGC AG3′), sFRP-1 (Forward 5′GCT AGA GAG GAG CCC TGA AAA T3′, Reverse 5′TGC ACT GTA TCC CTC TAT CTT GC3′), Frizzled 1 receptor (Forward 5′CGT ACT GAG TGG AGT GTG TTT TG3′, Reverse 5′TGA GCT TTT CCA GTT TCT CTG TC3′), Frizzled 2 receptor (Forward 5′GTG TAG AGC ACG GAG AAG ACG3′, Reverse 5′TAC CTG TTC ATC GGC ACA TC3′), Axin1 (Forward 5′CCA CAG AAA TAG TAG GCC ACA3′, Reverse 5′GGA GGA AGA AGA AAA GAG AGC3′), GSK3β (Forward 5′TCG CCA CTC GAG TAG AAG AAA3′, Reverse 5′ACT TTG TGA CTC AGG AGA ACT3′), PBGD (Forward 5′CAA GGT TTT CAG CAT CGC TAC3′, Reverse 5′ATG TCC GGT AAC GGC GGC3′).

Protein isolation and Western blotting

Lung tissue and PASMC's samples were homogenized using tissue homogenizer (for tissues only) or lysed in RIPA buffer (Santa Cruz) with addition of a protease inhibitor cocktail and PMSF. Tissue and cells lysates were equalized with SDS 5× sample buffer and electrophoretically separated on 10% polyacrylamide gels and transferred for 1 h on to nitrocellulose membranes. Subsequently membranes were blocked 1 h with 5% non-fat dry milk in Tris-buffered saline/0.1% Tween 20. After blocking, membranes were probed with primary antibodies diluted as follows: GSK3β total (1:1000), phospho-GSK3β (ser 9) (1:1000), AKT (1:1000), phospho-AKT (1:1000), Axin1 (1:500), phospho-ERK1/2 (1:1000), ERK total (1:1000), GAPDH (1:5000). Samples were normalized to GAPDH housekeeping gene and total protein of interest (when examining protein phosphorylation) and further quantification was performed. After primary antibody incubation, membranes were incubated with secondary goat anti-rabbit (1:30000) or rat anti-mouse (1:50000) HRP-conjugated antibodies (Sigma). Signals were then detected by ECL detection system and further quantified using specific software as described [27].

Immunohistochemistry

Paraffin-embedded lung sections were cut to 3 μm thickness by microtome and incubated 45 minutes at 65°C and subsequently deparaffinized in xylene three times, each 3 minutes. Samples were hydrated with 100% to 80% ethanol concentration washed with water and the antigen was unmasked by microwaving 20 minutes in the retrieval buffer. Sections were incubated in 3% hydrogen peroxide in methanol for 20 minutes at room temperature to block endogenous peroxidase activity, washed and blocked for 30 minutes in 2% bovine serum albumin. Then sections were probed overnight at 4°C with primary anti-rabbit antibody (GSK3β Cell Signaling, 1:50 dilution). After overnight incubation sections was washed with PBS and incubated with secondary biotinylated horse anti-rabbit IgG Antibody (Vector Laboratories) for 30 min, followed by incubation with the ABC reagent kit (avidin and biotinylated peroxidase, Vector Laboratories) for 30 min. Development of the target-bound peroxidase for detection of GSK3β was carried out with Vector NovaRed

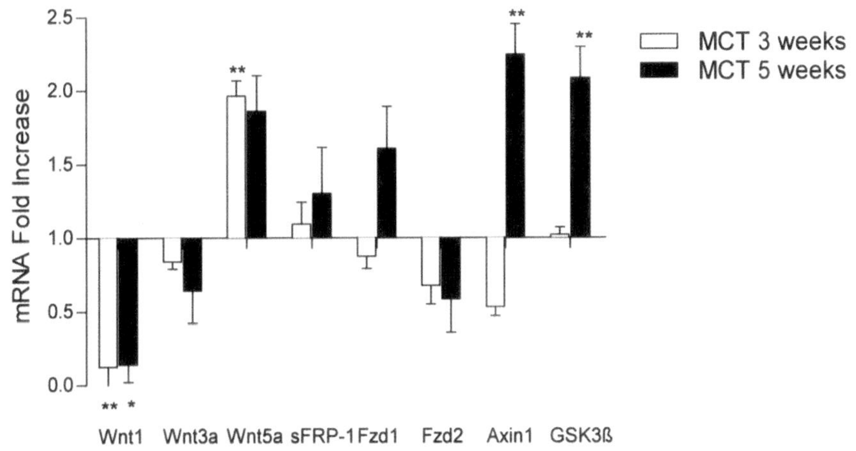

Figure 1. Expression of Wnt signaling upstream regulators of GSK3β in lung tissues of control and MCT-induced PAH rats. mRNA expression of Wnt1, Wnt3a, Wnt5a, Frizzled 1, Frizzled 2, sFRP-1, Axin 1 and GSK3β in lung homogenates from control and after 3 weeks (white bar) and 5 weeks (black bar) of MCT-induced PAH rats, as analyzed by quantitative real-time PCR. All values were given as the mean ± SEM (n = 3) and were normalized to Porphobilinogen deaminase (PBGD). Values were presented significant as *P<0.05, **P<0.01 *vs* control lungs. Healthy controls were set as 1 on X axis and expression profile from 3 and 5 weeks MCT were presented as fold of gene regulation.

substrate kit for peroxidase according to manufacturer's instruction (Vector Laboratories). Finally, sections were counterstained with haematoxylin (Zymed Laboratory, Cambridge, UK), mounted with VectaMount (Vector Laboratories) and visualized by light microscopy (bright-field microscopy).

Cloning

Human GSK3ß wild type full length insert was obtained on the human PASMCs cDNA template by PCR reaction using Platinum Taq DNA Polymerase High Fidelity with the following primers: Forward 5′CCT AAC ACC CCA ACA TAA AGA CA3′, Reverse 5′GTA ACT GGT GGT TTT TCC TGT GC3′. Human GSK3ß WT insert was subsequently ligated into the pGEMT-Easy Vector and then electroporated to the DH5α competent strain of *E.Coli*, becoming the template for following active GSK3ß mutant construction. Later GSK3ß full length and mutant constructs was transferred to mammalian pcDNA3.1 expression vector TOPO cloning system and transformed to JM-109 compentent *E.Coli* strain following heat shock procedure. After transformation constructs were digested with *Bam*HI and verified on a 0.7% agarose gel. Pure plasmid GSK3ß constructs were obtained using MaxiPrep Plasmid Isolation Kit in extensive amounts for subsequent transient transfection and further sent for sequencing to AGOWA GmbH sequencing service (Berlin, Germany).

Mutagenesis and Sequencing

Wild type pGEMT- GSK3ß was used as a template for creating mutants of GSK3ß which are S9A- constitutively active mutant of GSK3ß where serine 9 residue was substituted with alanine. To prepare constitutively active constructs of GSK3ß, point mutations were done with long template PCR technique with use of following mutagenesis primers: GSK3ß S9A (Sense 5′GGC CCA GAA CCA CCG CAT TCG CGG AGA GCT GCA A3′; Antisense 5′TTG CAG CTC TCC GCG AAT GCG GTG GTT CTG GGC C3′) in the following set up (95°C-90 s; 95°C-30 s; 62°C-30 s; 68°C-900 s; 68°C-1200 s; 4°C). Digestion of methylated template was done by 3 h incubation in 37°C with use of *Dpn*I

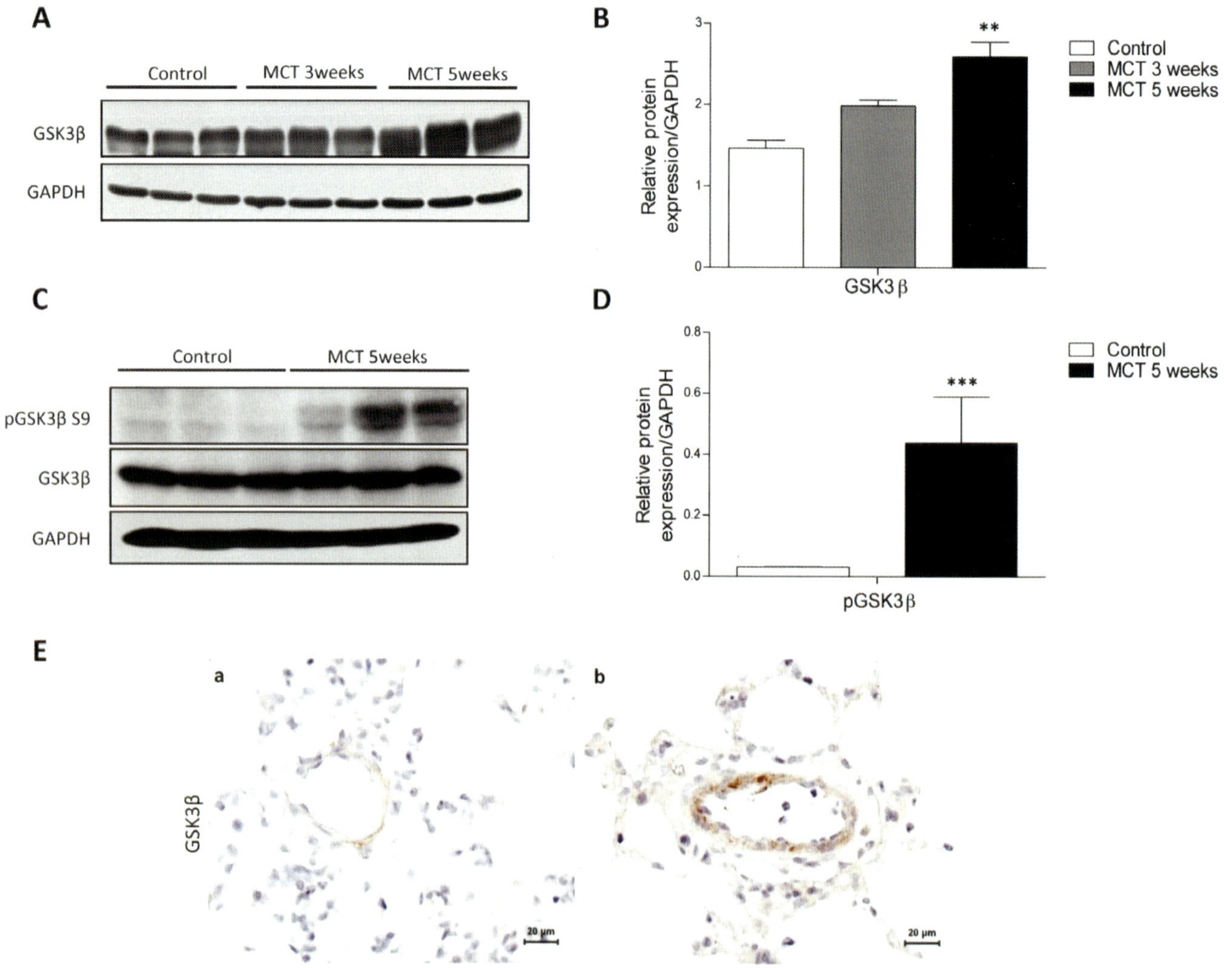

Figure 2. Increased GSK3ß and its phosphorylated form in MCT-induced PAH rat lungs. Protein expression as analyzed by (**A**) western blotting and subsequent (**B**) densitometric quantification of GSK3ß in control (white bar) and after 3 weeks (grey bar) and 5 weeks (black bar) of MCT-induced PAH in rats. Phosphorylation analysis by (**C**) western blotting and subsequent (**D**) densitometric quantification of pGSK3ß (serine 9) in control (white bar) and 5 weeks (black bar) lungs of MCT-induced PAH in rats. GAPDH was used as a loading control. Values were presented significant as $^{**}P<0.01$, $^{***}P<0.001$ *vs* control lungs. All values were expressed as mean ± SEM (n = 3). (**E**) Immunohistochemical localization of GSK3β in the healthy lungs (a) and lungs 5 weeks after MCT injury (b). Magnification 40×.

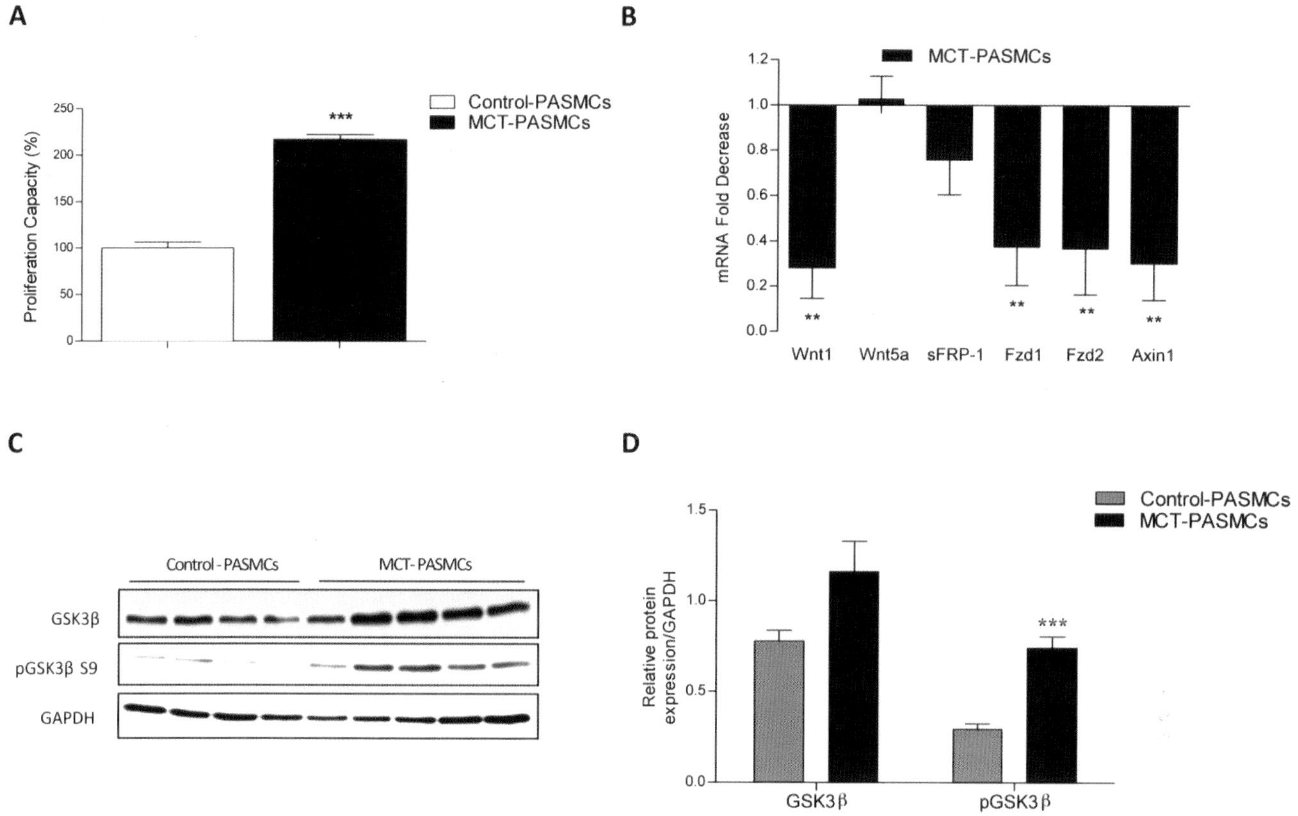

Figure 3. Increased GSK3ß and its phosphorylated form in primary PASMCs isolated from lungs of control and MCT-induced PAH rats. (**A**) Proliferation capacity of primary rat MCT-PASMCs compared to healthy control-PASMCs isolated from rat lungs 5 weeks post MCT injury in 10% FCS conditioned media was assessed by [3H]-thymidine incorporation (n = 5). Data were obtained as counts per minute (cpm) and normalized to the amount of cells per well. All values were expressed as the percentage of proliferation capacity (mean ± SEM). Values were presented significant as *** P<0.001 *vs* control. (**B**) mRNA expression of Wnt1, Wnt3a (not expressed), Wnt5a, Frizzled 1, Frizzled 2, sFRP-1, Axin 1 and GSK3ß in primary control PASMCs and PASMCs from MCT-induced PAH rats isolated from the lungs 5 weeks after MCT injection, as analyzed by quantitative real-time PCR. Rat PASMC were maintained in culture media supplemented with 10% FCS. All values were normalized to Porphobilinogen deaminase (PBGD) and were presented as fold of gene regulation with a control set as 1. Values were presented significant as **P<0.01 *vs* control PASMCs. All values were expressed as mean ± SEM (n = 4). Protein expression as analyzed by (**C**) western blotting and subsequent (**D**) densitometric quantification of total GSK3ß/GAPDH, phosphorylation of GSK3ß at serine 9 residue (pGSK3ß S9/total GSK3ß) in primary PASMCs isolated from control (grey bar) and MCT-induced PAH rats (black bar). GAPDH was used as a loading control. All values were expressed as mean ± SEM (Control PASMCs, n = 4; MCT-PASMCs n = 5). Values were presented significant as ***P<0.001 *vs* control PASMCs. Both mRNA and protein were isolated from healthy control- and MCT-PASMCs at passage 3 in 10% FCS conditioned media.

enzyme. Subsequently precipitated plasmid was transformed to JM-109 strain of *E.Coli* and produced in extensive amounts for subsequent transfections.

Transient transfection of PASMCs with pcDNA3.1 TOPO-GSK3β construct

PASMCs were plated in 6 or 48-well plates until they reach 60 to 80% confluence at the time of transfection. Empty pcDNA3.1 vector and pcDNA3.1-GSK3ß construct (GSK3ß WT, S9A) were mixed with Opti-DMEM F12 medium and combined with Lipofectamine 2000 transfection reagent and added to cultured MCT PASMCs for 6 hrs as described [28]. After this time cells were washed with PBS and stimulated with 10% FCS to allow cell recovery for next 18 hrs and later depending on further assays adequately stimulated with 0.1 or 10% FCS supplied DMEM F12 medium.

Proliferation Assay

For assessment of proliferation, rat PASMCs from passage 2 were seeded in 48-well plates. Primary cells were starved by incubation for 24 hrs in DMEM containing 0.1% FCS. Subsequently, they were stimulated with 10% FCS/DMEM or PDGF-BB (60 ng/ml) to induce cell cycle reentry. During the last 4 hrs of the stimulation period, cells were pulsed with 1.5 µCi per well [^{3}H] thymidine (Amersham Pharmacia Biotech Ltd). The [^{3}H] thymidine content of cell lysates was determined by scintillation counting as described previously [8]. Data were expressed as counts per minute (cpm) and normalized to the amount of cells per well. In our study all of [3H] thymidine uptake experiments were carried out on 48-well plates and the amount of PASMCs seeded on one well was around 30,000.

Patient characteristics

Human lung tissue was obtained from donors and iPAH patients undergoing lung transplantation. Donor lung tissue was from non-transplanted lung tissue of transplant donors. Donor lungs were explanted according to a standard European explant protocol (Eurotransplant), using cold perfused with preservation buffer and stored inflated on ice until use. Non-transplanted donor lung was not transplanted because i) the complete lung would not

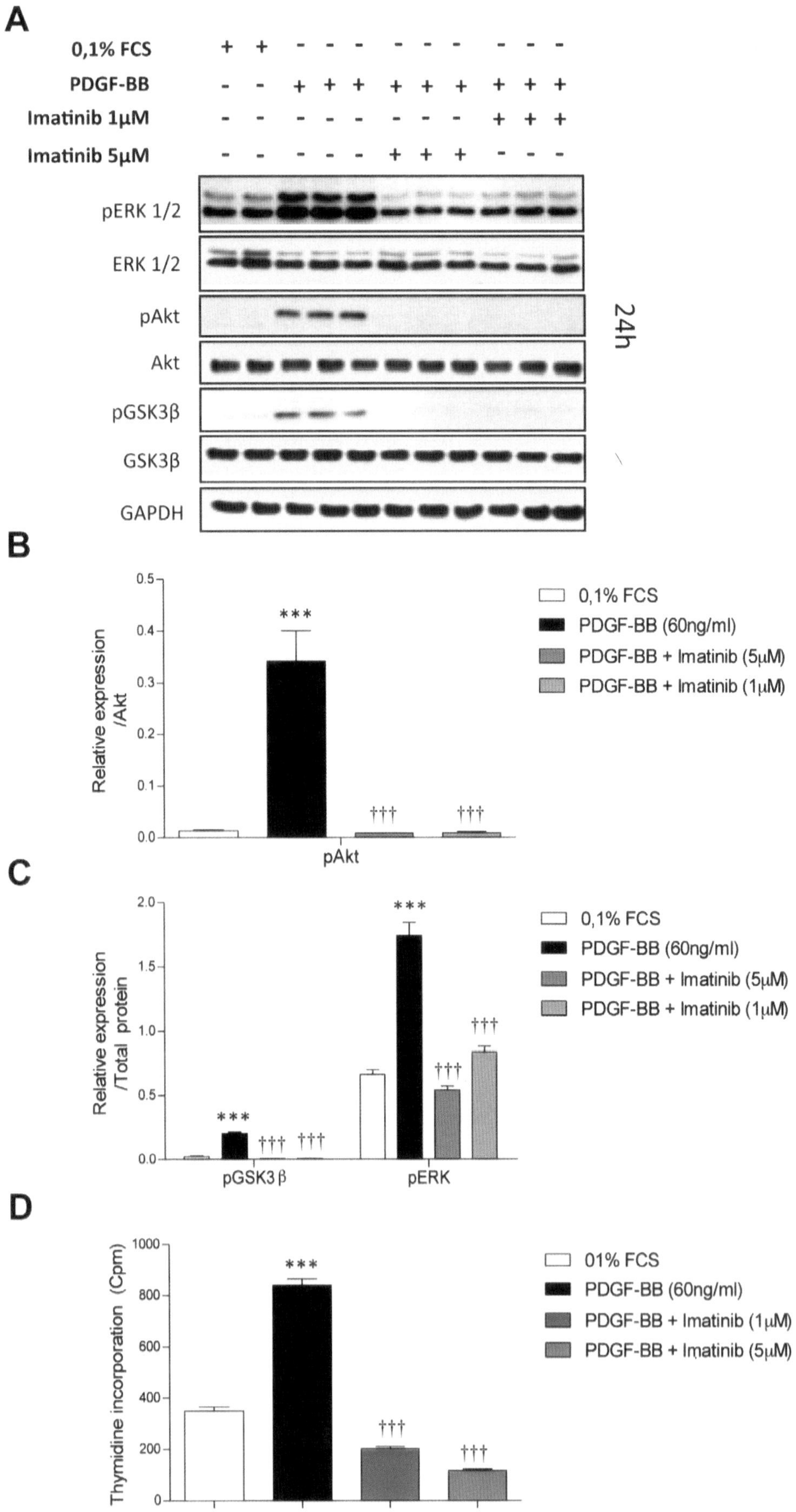
A
0,1% FCS
PDGF-BB
Imatinib 1μM
Imatinib 5μM
pERK 1/2
ERK 1/2
pAkt
Akt
pGSK3β
GSK3β
GAPDH
24h
B
Relative expression /Akt
pAkt
0,1% FCS
PDGF-BB (60ng/ml)
PDGF-BB + Imatinib (5μM)
PDGF-BB + Imatinib (1μM)
C
Relative expression /Total protein
pGSK3 β
pERK
0,1% FCS
PDGF-BB (60ng/ml)
PDGF-BB + Imatinib (5μM)
PDGF-BB + Imatinib (1μM)
D
Thymidine incorporation (Cpm)
01% FCS
PDGF-BB (60ng/ml)
PDGF-BB + Imatinib (1μM)
PDGF-BB + Imatinib (5μM)

Figure 4. PDGF regulates GSK3β, Akt, ERK phosphorylation and proliferation in primary rat MCT-PASMCs. (**A**) Western blot analysis and subsequent (**B, C**) quantification of Akt, GSK3ß, ERK and phosphorylation status in primary rat MCT-PASMCs stimulated with PDGF-BB (60 ng/ml) alone or in combination with two doses of Imatinib (1 and 5 μM) for 24 hrs. GAPDH was used as reference loading control. (**D**) Proliferation of primary rat MCT-PASMCs was assessed by [3H]-thymidine incorporation (n = 6). Data were expressed as counts per minute (cpm) and normalized to the amount of cells per well. All values were expressed as mean ± SEM. Values were presented significant as *** P<0.001 *vs* control, ††† P<0.001 *vs* PDGF-BB.

fit into the recipient thorax and a part was resected or ii) due to on site decision of the transplant surgeon not to use the lung, based on edema, pulmonary thrombi or obvious pneumonia. In either case, lung tissue was snap-frozen directly after transplantation.

Results

GSK3β is dysregulated in total lung homogenates of monocrotaline-induced pulmonary arterial hypertension in rats

Expression of Wnt ligands (Wnt1, Wnt3a, and Wnt5a) and Wnt signaling upstream regulator genes (Frizzled1 and 2 receptors and sFRP-1) and intracellular effectors (Axin1 and GSK3β) were investigated in pulmonary hypertensive rat lungs, 3 and 5 weeks after MCT injury. Real-time RT-PCR demonstrated a decrease in Wnt canonical ligands (Wnt1 and Wnt3a) with no significant changes in Frizzled receptors expression in 5 weeks of MCT-PAH rat lungs (Figure 1). Parallel increase in mRNA expression of GSK3ß and Axin1 was observed (Figure 1). Western blotting demonstrated a significant increase in total GSK3ß expression in MCT lungs 3 and 5 weeks post MCT injury (Figure 2A, B) as well as significant increase in its phosphorylation in 5 weeks MCT-PAH rat lungs (Figure 2C, D). However, phosphorylation of GSK3ß was not altered 3 weeks after MCT treatment (data not shown). Immunohistochemical analysis suggested an immunoreactivity of GSK3ß was observed in the medial layer of pulmonary arteries of both 5 weeks MCT-PAH rat lungs and control PAH rat lungs (Figure 2E).

Increased GSK3ß and it's phosphorylated form in pulmonary arterial smooth muscle cells isolated from MCT-PAH rats

Interestingly PASMCs isolated from the rat lungs 5 weeks after MCT injury displays much stronger proliferative phenotype as compared to healthy control-PASMCs in 10% FCS condition (Figure 3A) and PDGF-BB (60 ng/ml) supplemented media (Figure S1). Therefore, we tested the expression profile of GSK3ß-related genes (Figure 3B) in these hyper-proliferative PASMCs. Similarly to the mRNA level in the lungs after MCT injury we found a decrease in canonical Wnt1 (Figure 3B). On the other hand, reduction in Frizzled receptor 2 is significant in isolated MCT-PASMCs, but not in MCT injured lungs as compared to healthy controls (Figure 3B). Additionally, we observed discrepancies in Axin 1 mRNA expression level which was significantly upregulated in lungs 5 weeks after MCT injury, but its mRNA level was significantly reduced in MCT-PASMCs. Downregulation of upstream regulators of GSK3ß and GSK3ß itself (Figure S2), on mRNA level, in MCT-PASMCs as compared to healthy controls (Figure 3B) suggests dysregulation of canonical Wnt signaling pathway. Interestingly, further analysis of GSK3ß and its phosphorylated form at serine 9 residue in primary isolated pulmonary arterial smooth muscle cells (PASMCs) revealed an increase in total protein expression of GSK3ß and significant increase in its phosphorylated (inactivated) form in PASMCs isolated from MCT-PAH rats compared to control rats (Figure 3C, D).

Growth factors signaling regulates GSK3ß phosphorylation in primary rat PASMCs

To investigate upstream regulators of GSK3ß, quiescent PASMCs were stimulated with PDGF-BB (60 ng/ml) for 6 (Figure S3) and 24 hrs (Figure 4) or 10% FCS (Figure 5) for 24 hrs. In addition, to verify the specificity of PDGF-BB mediated signaling, primary rat PASMCs were also simultaneously treated with Imatinib (1 and 5 μM). Proteins from untreated and stimulated cells were isolated and western blotting for AKT, GSK3ß, phospho-AKT and phospho-GSK3ß ser 9 and ERK and phospho-ERK were performed.

Interestingly, in all cases PDGF-BB and 10% FCS stimulation caused a significant increase in phospho-AKT and phospho-GSK3ß (Ser 9) in combination with significant activation of ERK (Figure 4A–C, 5A–C, Figure S3). The increased phosphorylation of AKT, GSK3ß at ser 9 site and ERK observed after stimulation with growth factors were significantly abrogated by Imatinib treatment (Figure 4A–C, 5A–C, Figure S3). Decreased phosphorylation status of AKT, GSK3β and ERK after Imatinib treatment were accompanied with significant decrease in proliferation capacity of these cells after 24 hrs stimulation with PDGF-BB as well as 10% FCS (Figure 4D, 5D). This suggest that GSK3β is a possible crucial player in growth factors signaling and abnormal proliferation of PASMCs in experimental PAH.

Overexpression of GSK3β and phosphorylation deficiency of GSK3β influences PASMCs proliferation

To further evaluate the contribution of GSK3ß to vascular remodeling processes, we generated pcDNA 3.1 TOPO-cloning constructs carrying GSK3ß wild type (WT) cDNA and GSK3ß S9A (where serine at residue 9 is replaced to alanine) mutant. Sequence analysis performed on each construct confirmed the intended point mutations at specific sites in GSK3ß S9A (data not shown).

Transient overexpression of GSK3ß WT and GSK3ß S9A mutant in PASMCs resulted in a significantly enhancement of GSK3ß expression 24 hrs post transfection. Empty vector (EV) transfection caused no change in GSK3ß protein expression (Figure 6A). Importantly, serum stimulation did not cause GSK3ß phosphorylation in GSK3ß S9A mutant overexpressing cells while another tyrosine 216 residue was phosphorylated (Figure 6A). The gain of GSK3ß WT expression was coupled to a significantly increase of [^{3}H]-thymidine uptake as compared to cells transfected with either empty pcDNA3.1 vector or Lipofectamine 2000 reagent (LF2000) only, 24 hrs post serum stimulation (Figure 6B). On the other hand, GSK3ß S9A mutant expression decreased [^{3}H]-thymidine uptake, suggested that GSK3ß inactivation is involved in PASMCs proliferation (Figure 6B).

Overexpression of GSK3β and phosphorylation deficiency of GSK3β influences proliferation via ERK phosphorylation

Transient overexpression of GSK3ß WT significantly increased ERK phosphorylation compared to empty pcDNA3.1 vector transfection (Figure 7A, B). In contrary, GSK3ß S9A mutant

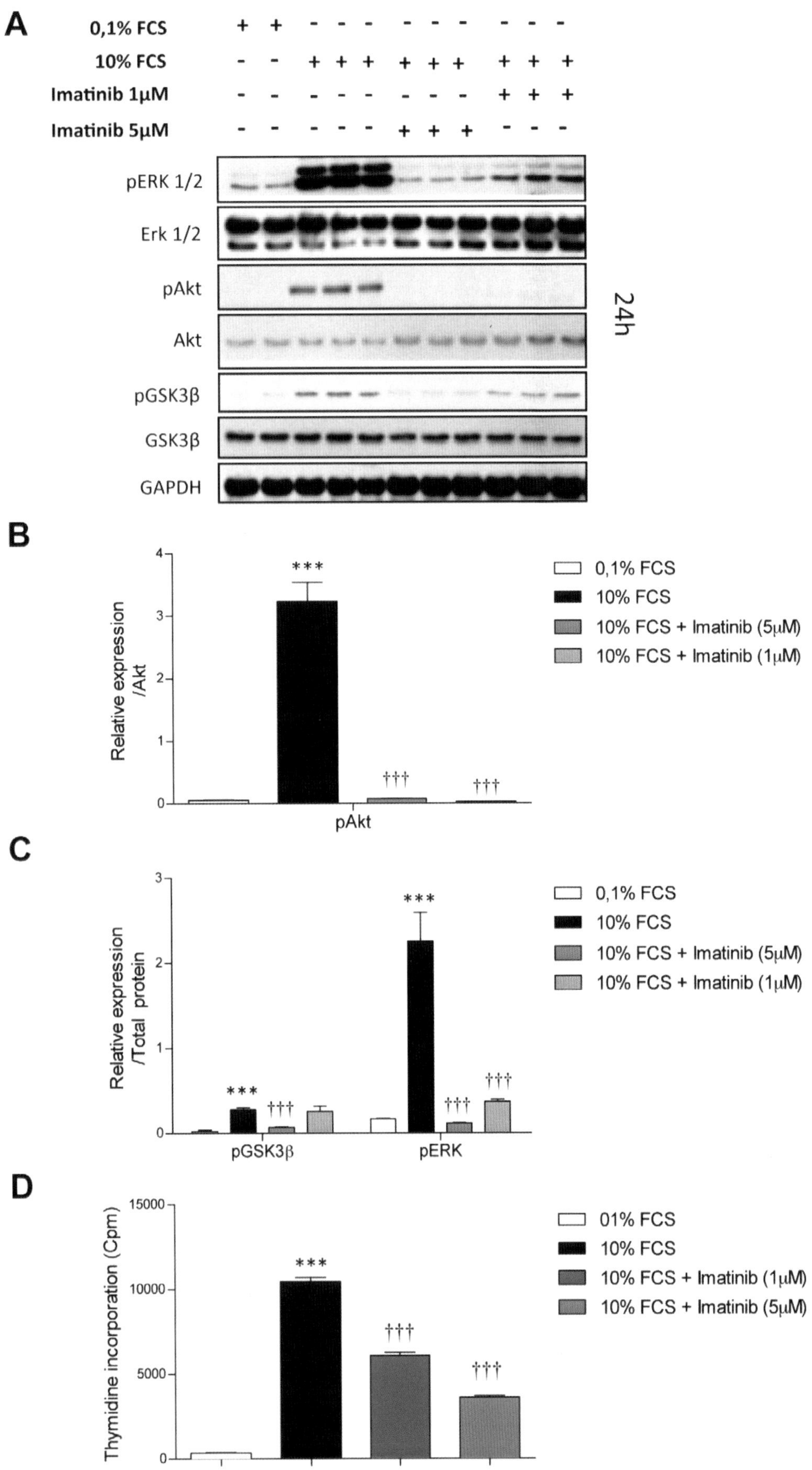
A
0,1% FCS
10% FCS
Imatinib 1µM
Imatinib 5µM
pERK 1/2
Erk 1/2
pAkt
Akt
pGSK3β
GSK3β
GAPDH
24h
B
Relative expression /Akt
pAkt
0,1% FCS
10% FCS
10% FCS + Imatinib (5µM)
10% FCS + Imatinib (1µM)
C
Relative expression /Total protein
pGSK3β
pERK
0,1% FCS
10% FCS
10% FCS + Imatinib (5µM)
10% FCS + Imatinib (1µM)
D
Thymidine incorporation (Cpm)
01% FCS
10% FCS
10% FCS + Imatinib (1µM)
10% FCS + Imatinib (5µM)

Figure 5. Serum regulates GSK3β, Akt, ERK phosphorylation and proliferation in primary rat MCT-PASMCs. (**A**) Western blot analysis and subsequent (**B, C**) quantification of Akt, GSK3ß, ERK and phosphorylation status in primary rat MCT-PASMCs stimulated with 10% FCS in combination with two doses of Imatinib (1 and 5 μM) for 24 hrs. GAPDH was used as reference loading control. (**D**) Proliferation of primary rat MCT-PASMCs was assessed by [^{3}H]-thymidine incorporation (n = 6). Data were expressed as counts per minute (cpm) and normalized to the amount of cells per well. All values were expressed as mean ± SEM. Values were presented significant as *** P<0.001 *vs* control, ††† P<0.001 *vs* 10% FCS.

decreased ERK1/2 phosphorylation, in serum induced proliferation of PASMCs (Figure 7A, B).

Increase in GSK3β protein levels in human PAH lung explants

Expression of GSK3ß was investigated also in iPAH patients lung explants. While mRNA levels of GSK3ß was not regulated in iPAH patient lungs (Figure S4), western blotting analysis showed significant upregulation of total GSK3ß protein in iPAH lung homogenates compared to healthy donor lung homogenates (Figure 8A, B).

Discussion

This study has 4 salient features. First, GSK3ß and the phosphorylated form of GSK3ß (inactivation) are increased in

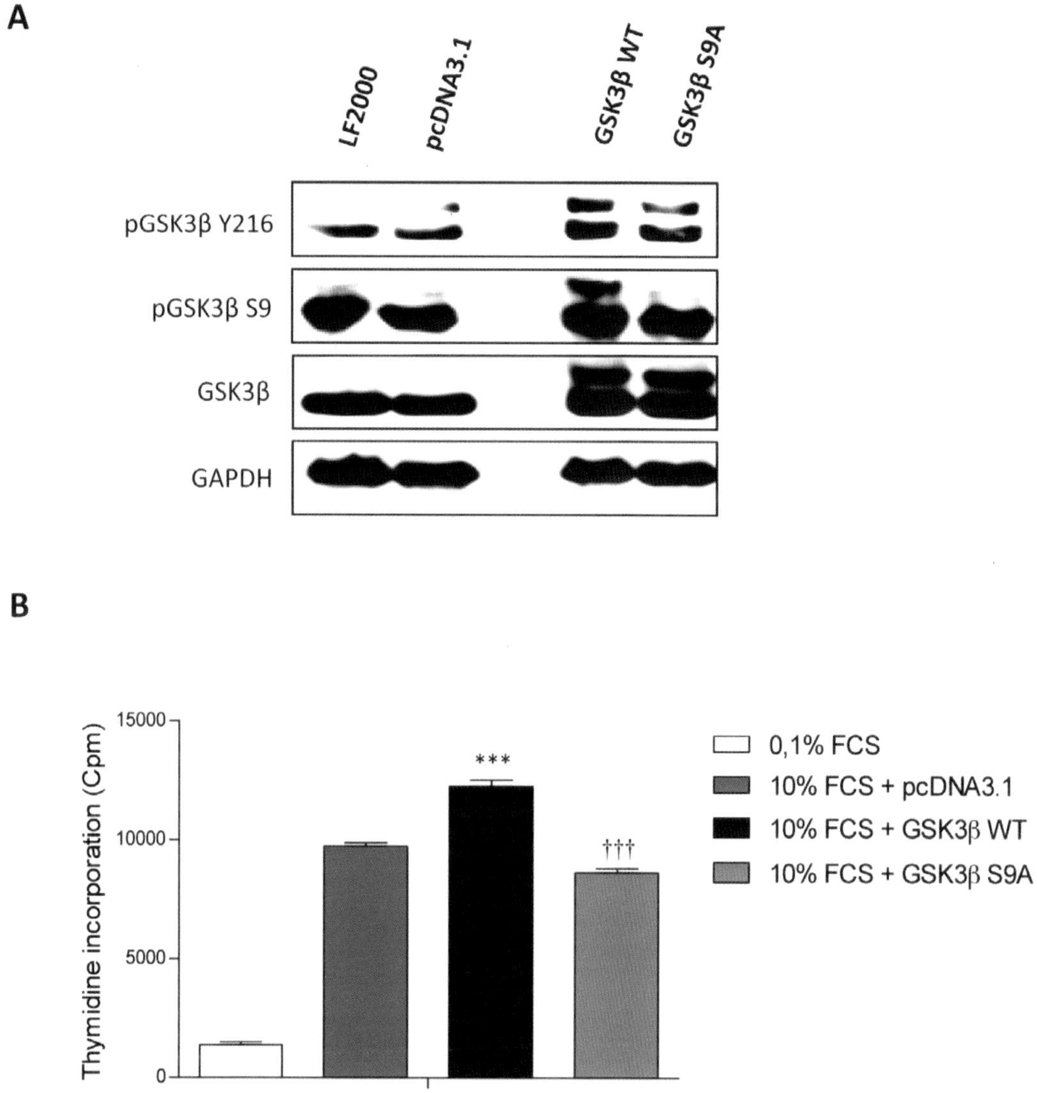

Figure 6. GSK3ß overexpression and S9A modification influences proliferation of primary rat PASMCs. (**A**) Primary rat PASMCs were transiently transfected with GSK3ß wild type (GSK3ß WT), constitutively active GSK3ß (GSK3ß S9A), empty vector (pcDNA3.1 TOPO). 24 hrs post transfection, expression and phosphorylation of GSK3ß were analyzed by western blotting. (**B**) Primary rat PASMCs transiently transfected with GSK3ß wild type (GSK3ß WT), constitutively active GSK3ß (GSK3ß S9A), empty vector (pcDNA3.1 TOPO) and proliferation was assessed after stimulation with 10% FCS for 24 hrs by [^{3}H]-thymidine incorporation. All values are expressed as mean ± SEM (n = 6, WT or S9A n = 12). Data were expressed as counts per minute (cpm) and normalized to the amount of cells per well. Values were presented significant as ***P<0.001 *vs* 0.1% Empty Vector pcDNA3.1 and ††† p<0.001 *vs* GSK3ß WT transfected cells.

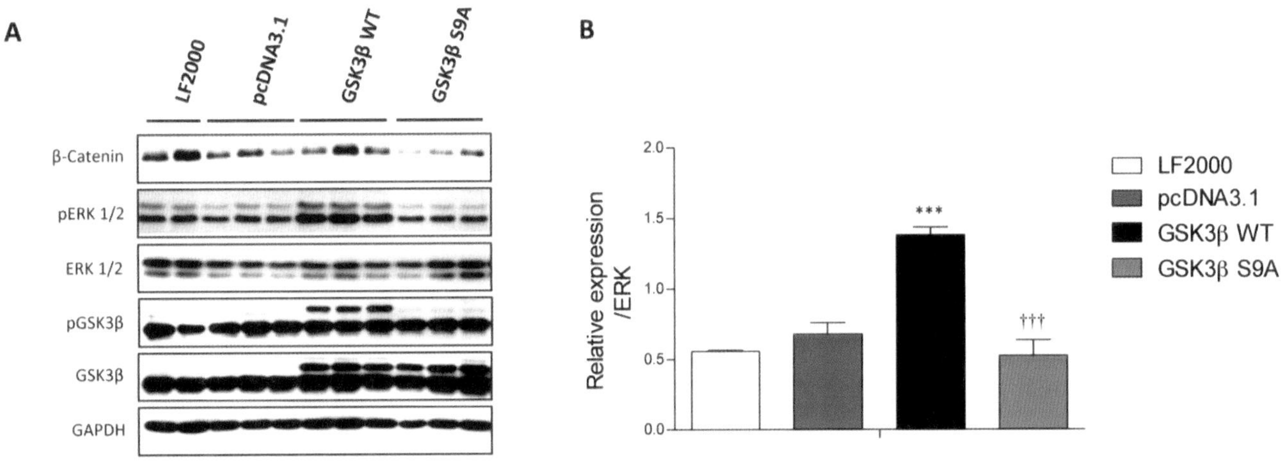

Figure 7. GSK3ß overexpression and S9A modification regulates ERK phosphorylation in primary rat PASMCs. (**A**) Primary rat PASMCs were transiently transfected with GSK3ß wild type (GSK3ß WT), constitutively active GSK3ß (GSK3ß S9A), empty vector (pcDNA3.1 TOPO). 24 hrs post transfection, expression and phosphorylation of GSK3ß and ERK were analyzed by western blotting followed by (**B**) densitometric quantification. All values are expressed as mean ± SEM (n = 4). Values were presented significant as ***P<0.001 *vs* 0.1% Empty Vector pcDNA3.1 and ††† p<0.001 *vs* GSK3ß WT transfected cells.

MCT lungs and PASMCs isolated from monocrotaline induced pulmonary arterial hypertensive rats compared to control rats. Second, both PDGF and FCS stimulation induced GSK3ß phosphorylation (inactivation) in PASMCs. Third, treatment with the PDGFR inhibitor, Imatinib, attenuated growth factors-induced GSK3ß and ERK phosphorylation. Fourth, overexpression of wild type and constitutively activate form of GSK3ß (GSK3ß S9A; 9th serine replaced to alanine) influenced serum induced MCT-PASMCs proliferation by regulating ERK phosphorylation. This study supports a central role for GSK3ß in vascular remodeling processes and suggests a novel therapeutic opportunity for the treatment of pulmonary hypertension.

The dynamic process of pulmonary vascular remodeling involves numerous molecular signaling cascades governing PASMCs proliferation, differentiation and migration [4,29]. We hypothesized that GSK3ß signaling plays a critical regulatory role in pulmonary vascular remodeling. In accord with our hypothesis, we demonstrated significant increase in total GSK3ß expression levels as well as its phosphorylation status in lungs and PASMCs in response to MCT injury and total GSK3ß in human iPAH lung explants. Interestingly, the increase in GSK3ß and its phosphorylated form, observed in primary PASMCs isolated from MCT-PAH rats as well as in rat and human lungs, suggest that aberrant GSK3ß signaling may trigger the proliferative phenotype of PASMCs. In line with this notion, aberrant GSK3ß signaling was recently implicated in various vascular- and fibro-proliferative diseases [23,30,31].

GSK3ß remains increased and inactivated 5 weeks after MCT injury, which is accompanied by decreases in mRNA expression of canonical Wnt ligands (Wnt1 and Wnt3a) and an increase in non-canonical Wnt5a ligand, 3 and 5 weeks after MCT injury. However, GSK3ß was downregulated at the mRNA level in MCT-PASMCs compared to control-PASMCs. We assume that downregulation of GSK3ß mRNA levels concurrent with upregulation of protein expression may occur when a protein's half-life is increased due to stabilization-components involved with the protein's normal turnover may be disrupted. It is also possible that the protein may become stabilized through protein-protein interactions. Additionally, this can be explained by transcriptional repression when high levels of proteins accumulate. Furthermore as delineated in our study, GSK3ß phosphorylation is regulated by growth factors, i.e. PDGF-BB that were highly upregulated in PAH. Hence we believe that GSK3ß is clearly dependent on multiple lines of regulation in addition to the phosphorylation state of GSK3ß [32,33,34].

In our study, upregulation of non-canonical [35,36] Wnt5a mRNA in MCT-lungs is in line with previously published data, showing involvement of non-canonical Wnt signaling in human IPAH [37]. Moreover, downstream targets of the non-canonical Wnt pathway, like Rho-kinases or calcium signaling, were shown to significantly contribute to PASMCs proliferation and vasoconstriction and demonstrated therapeutic potential in pulmonary hypertension [38,39,40].

Our data indicate that MCT-PASMCs are hyper-proliferative in the presence of FCS and PDGF compared to control-PASMCs. Interestingly, our results showed that PDGF and FCS stimulation on MCT-PASMCs, acting via PI3-kinase-dependent activation of AKT, causes GSK3ß (Ser 9) phosphorylation and GSK3ß inactivation followed by ERK activation, which is potentially suppressed by Imatinib. A similar role of growth factors, such as PDGF, IGF and EGF, mediated GSK3ß inactivation was described previously [41,42]. Furthermore, several kinases were also shown to be capable of mediating ser 9 phosphorylation, including AKT, PKA, PKC and Wnts [16,32,43]. Considering the crucial role of PDGF signaling in pulmonary vascular remodeling [8,9], the increased presence of growth factors signaling in human and experimental PAH [8,10,13] and PDGF and FCS mediated alteration of GSK3ß activity, collectively suggests GSK3ß plays an important role in the pathogenesis of PAH.

The effects of GSK3ß are also regulated by Wnt signaling pathway protein complex formation, a process involved in modulating ß-Catenin levels [18,44]. Future studies are needed to study the regulation of canonical Wnt signaling and the multitude of factors regulating ß-Catenin expression in the pathogenesis of pulmonary hypertension. Albeit recent studies suggest that recruitment of both canonical and non-canonical Wnt pathways promote pulmonary arterial endothelial cell proliferation, survival, and migration. In addition, it was demonstrated that both canonical and non-canonical Wnt pathways are required for BMP-2-mediated angiogenesis in

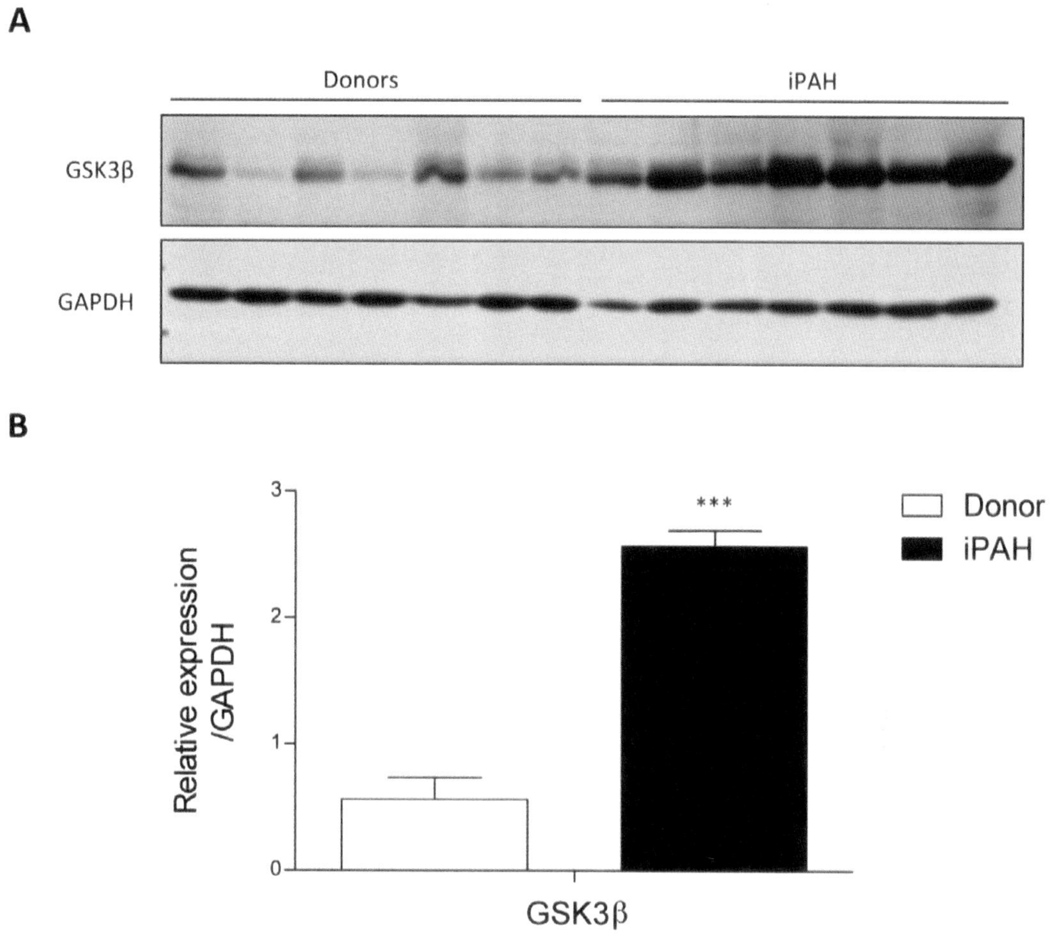

Figure 8. Increased GSK3ß and its phosphorylated form in human lungs of healthy donor and iPAH patients. (**A**) Protein expression as analyzed by western blotting and subsequent (**B**) densitometric quantification of GSK3ß and in human lungs of healthy donor and iPAH patients. GAPDH was used as a loading control. Values were presented significant as ***P<0.001 *vs* control lungs. All values were expressed as mean ± SEM (n = 7).

severe combined immunodeficient (SCID) mice [45]. These findings may help better understand the pathogenesis of pulmonary hypertension, a disease that featured with the loss of small precapillary arteries.

In the present study, overexpression of GSK3ß significantly increased expression of GSK3ß that was accompanied by increased proliferation capacity of MCT-PASMCs proliferation after FCS stimulation. Constitutive activation of GSK3ß significantly reduced expression of phospho-GSK3ß and PASMCs proliferation. This effect can be due to GSK3ß phosphorylation of a diverse group of substrates or by inhibition of transcription factor activation such as p53, CREB and ß-Catenin [17,18,19]. In addition, GSK3ß constitutively activation (S9A) has also been shown to directly effects cyclin D1 expression, independent of ß-Catenin [46]. Here, we show that overexpression of wild-type GSK3ß significantly influenced the proliferation capacity of MCT-PASMCs via regulating phosphorylation of ERK. In a recent study by Wang *et al.*, it was shown that GSK3ß acts as a negative regulator of ERK in human colon cancer cells [47]. Our study shows that constitutive activation of GSK3ß significantly reduced phospho-GSK3ß levels and PASMCs proliferation that was accompanied by a significant decrease in ERK phosphorylation. These results collectively suggest that modification of GSK3ß can significantly influence highly dysregulated growth factors signaling associated with abnormal proliferation of PASMCs in PAH.

Although mRNA levels of GSK3ß is downregulated in MCT-PASMCs and in human iPAH patient lungs, along with other canonical Wnt signaling dependent genes we found that protein levels of GSK3ß increased in a time dependent fashion with disease progression in the MCT-induced PAH model (lungs and MCT-PASMCs) and also in explanted iPAH patient lungs, suggesting a role for GSK3ß in disease progression, potentially independent of canonical Wnt signaling. Recently a crucial role for GSK3ß in systemic vascular remodeling was reported [48,49]. Authors demonstrated for the first time *in vivo* that active GSK3ß gene transfer results in a significant reduction in neointima formation in the restenosis model of balloon injury in rat carotid arteries. These effects were attributable, at least in part to the ability of GSK3ß to inhibit smooth muscle proliferation and to promote sustained apoptosis. This concept was extended to demonstrate that GSK3ß plays a significant role in VSMCs proliferation and apoptosis in vascular remodeling after balloon injury [49]. Similarly, in our study the inactivation of GSK3β by serine 9 phosphorylation was observed 5 weeks after MCT injury in rats, both in PASMCs and lung homogenates. This suggest that the introduction of active GSK3β (S9A) may also prove beneficial for regression of vascular remodeling in experimental PAH.

To our knowledge this is the first study to demonstrate that GSK3ß is significantly altered in the pathogenesis of experimental as well as human PAH and the regulatory role for GSK3ß in pulmonary arterial smooth muscle cell proliferation. This study supports a central role for GSK3ß in vascular remodeling processes and suggests a novel therapeutic opportunity for the treatment of pulmonary arterial hypertension.

Supporting Information

Figure S1 MCT-PASMCs display significant increase of PDGF-BB-induced proliferation capacity as compared to healthy control-PASMCs. Proliferation capacity of primary rat MCT-PASMCs compared to healthy control PASMCs isolated from rat lungs 5 weeks post MCT injury in 10% FCS conditioned media was assessed by [3H]-thymidine incorporation (n = 5). Data were obtained as counts per minute (cpm) and normalized to the amount of cells per well. All values were expressed as percentage of proliferation capacity (mean ± SEM). Values were presented significant as *** P<0.001 *vs* control.

Figure S2 Expression of GSK3β in rat MCT-PASMCs. mRNA expression of GSK3β in MCT-PASMCs after 5 weeks of MCT-induced PAH rats, as analyzed by quantitative real-time PCR. All values were given as the mean ± SEM (n = 3) and were normalized to Porphobilinogen deaminase (PBGD). Values were presented significant as *P<0.05, *vs* PASMCs isolated from healthy rat lungs. Healthy controls were set as 1 on X axis and expression profile from 5 weeks MCT-PASMCs were presented as fold of gene regulation.

Figure S3 PDGF regulates GSK3β, Akt and ERK phosphorylation in primary rat MCT-PASMCs. (**A**) Western blot analysis and subsequent (**B, C**) quantification of Akt, GSK3ß and ERK phosphorylation status in primary rat MCT-PASMCs stimulated with PDGF-BB (60 ng/ml) alone or in combination with two doses of Imatinib (1 and 5 μM) for 6 hrs. All values were expressed as mean ± SEM (n = 4). Values were presented significant as *** P<0.001 *vs* control, ††† P<0.001 *vs* PDGF-BB. GAPDH was used as reference loading control.

Figure S4 GSK3β is not significantly regulated in iPAH patient lungs on mRNA level. mRNA expression of GSK3ß in donor lungs and iPAH patient lungs as analyzed by quantitative real-time PCR. All values were normalized to Porphobilinogen deaminase (PBGD) and determined as fold of gene regulation. All values were expressed as mean ± SEM (n = 8).

Author Contributions

Conceived and designed the experiments: PS RTS FG WS SSP. Performed the experiments: PS XT. Analyzed the data: PS SSP. Contributed reagents/materials/analysis tools: DS NW HAG TK. Wrote the paper: PS RTS SSP.

References

1. Rubin LJ (2006) Pulmonary arterial hypertension. Proc Am Thorac Soc 3: 111–115.
2. D'Alonzo GE, Barst RJ, Ayres SM, Bergofsky EH, Brundage BH, et al. (1991) Survival in patients with primary pulmonary hypertension. Results from a national prospective registry. Ann Intern Med 115: 343–349.
3. Humbert M, Morrell NW, Archer SL, Stenmark KR, MacLean MR, et al. (2004) Cellular and molecular pathobiology of pulmonary arterial hypertension. J Am Coll Cardiol 43: 13S–24S.
4. Rabinovitch M (2008) Molecular pathogenesis of pulmonary arterial hypertension. J Clin Invest 118: 2372–2379.
5. Rubin LJ, Badesch DB, Barst RJ, Galie N, Black CM, et al. (2002) Bosentan therapy for pulmonary arterial hypertension. N Engl J Med 346: 896–903.
6. Barst RJ, Rubin LJ, Long WA, McGoon MD, Rich S, et al. (1996) A comparison of continuous intravenous epoprostenol (prostacyclin) with conventional therapy for primary pulmonary hypertension. The Primary Pulmonary Hypertension Study Group. N Engl J Med 334: 296–302.
7. Galie N, Ghofrani HA, Torbicki A, Barst RJ, Rubin LJ, et al. (2005) Sildenafil citrate therapy for pulmonary arterial hypertension. N Engl J Med 353: 2148–2157.
8. Schermuly RT, Dony E, Ghofrani HA, Pullamsetti S, Savai R, et al. (2005) Reversal of experimental pulmonary hypertension by PDGF inhibition. J Clin Invest 115: 2811–2821.
9. Perros F, Montani D, Dorfmuller P, Durand-Gasselin I, Tcherakian C, et al. (2008) Platelet-derived growth factor expression and function in idiopathic pulmonary arterial hypertension. Am J Respir Crit Care Med 178: 81–88.
10. Merklinger SL, Jones PL, Martinez EC, Rabinovitch M (2005) Epidermal growth factor receptor blockade mediates smooth muscle cell apoptosis and improves survival in rats with pulmonary hypertension. Circulation 112: 423–431.
11. Wedgwood S, Devol JM, Grobe A, Benavidez E, Azakie A, et al. (2007) Fibroblast growth factor-2 expression is altered in lambs with increased pulmonary blood flow and pulmonary hypertension. Pediatr Res 61: 32–36.
12. McMurtry MS, Archer SL, Altieri DC, Bonnet S, Haromy A, et al. (2005) Gene therapy targeting survivin selectively induces pulmonary vascular apoptosis and reverses pulmonary arterial hypertension. J Clin Invest 115: 1479–1491.
13. Klein M, Schermuly RT, Ellinghaus P, Milting H, Riedl B, et al. (2008) Combined tyrosine and serine/threonine kinase inhibition by sorafenib prevents progression of experimental pulmonary hypertension and myocardial remodeling. Circulation 118: 2081–2090.
14. Grimes CA, Jope RS (2001) The multifaceted roles of glycogen synthase kinase 3beta in cellular signaling. Prog Neurobiol 65: 391–426.
15. Doble BW, Woodgett JR (2003) GSK-3: tricks of the trade for a multi-tasking kinase. J Cell Sci 116: 1175–1186.
16. van Weeren PC, de Bruyn KM, de Vries-Smits AM, van Lint J, Burgering BM (1998) Essential role for protein kinase B (PKB) in insulin-induced glycogen synthase kinase 3 inactivation. Characterization of dominant-negative mutant of PKB. J Biol Chem 273: 13150–13156.
17. Pap M, Cooper GM (1998) Role of glycogen synthase kinase-3 in the phosphatidylinositol 3-Kinase/Akt cell survival pathway. J Biol Chem 273: 19929–19932.
18. Sakanaka C, Weiss JB, Williams LT (1998) Bridging of beta-catenin and glycogen synthase kinase-3beta by axin and inhibition of beta-catenin-mediated transcription. Proc Natl Acad Sci U S A 95: 3020–3023.
19. Fiol CJ, Williams JS, Chou CH, Wang QM, Roach PJ, et al. (1994) A secondary phosphorylation of CREB341 at Ser129 is required for the cAMP-mediated control of gene expression. A role for glycogen synthase kinase-3 in the control of gene expression. J Biol Chem 269: 32187–32193.
20. Welsh GI, Miller CM, Loughlin AJ, Price NT, Proud CG (1998) Regulation of eukaryotic initiation factor eIF2B: glycogen synthase kinase-3 phosphorylates a conserved serine which undergoes dephosphorylation in response to insulin. FEBS Lett 421: 125–130.
21. Morisco C, Seta K, Hardt SE, Lee Y, Vatner SF, et al. (2001) Glycogen synthase kinase 3beta regulates GATA4 in cardiac myocytes. J Biol Chem 276: 28586–28597.
22. Shakoori A, Ougolkov A, Yu ZW, Zhang B, Modarressi MH, et al. (2005) Deregulated GSK3beta activity in colorectal cancer: its association with tumor cell survival and proliferation. Biochem Biophys Res Commun 334: 1365–1373.
23. Wang X, Xiao Y, Mou Y, Zhao Y, Blankesteijn WM, et al. (2002) A role for the beta-catenin/T-cell factor signaling cascade in vascular remodeling. Circ Res 90: 340–347.
24. Schermuly RT, Pullamsetti SS, Kwapiszewska G, Dumitrascu R, Tian X, et al. (2007) Phosphodiesterase 1 upregulation in pulmonary arterial hypertension: target for reverse-remodeling therapy. Circulation 115: 2331–2339.
25. Lai YJ, Pullamsetti SS, Dony E, Weissmann N, Butrous G, et al. (2008) Role of the prostanoid EP4 receptor in iloprost-mediated vasodilatation in pulmonary hypertension. Am J Respir Crit Care Med 178: 188–196.
26. Pullamsetti S, Krick S, Yilmaz H, Ghofrani HA, Schudt C, et al. (2005) Inhaled tolafentrine reverses pulmonary vascular remodeling via inhibition of smooth muscle cell migration. Respir Res 6: 128.
27. Pullamsetti S, Kiss L, Ghofrani HA, Voswinckel R, Haredza P, et al. (2005) Increased levels and reduced catabolism of asymmetric and symmetric dimethylarginines in pulmonary hypertension. FASEB J 19: 1175–1177.
28. Savai R, Schermuly RT, Voswinckel R, Renigunta A, Reichmann B, et al. (2005) HIF-1alpha attenuates tumor growth in spite of augmented vascularization in an A549 adenocarcinoma mouse model. Int J Oncol 27: 393–400.
29. Arciniegas E, Frid MG, Douglas IS, Stenmark KR (2007) Perspectives on endothelial-to-mesenchymal transition: potential contribution to vascular

remodeling in chronic pulmonary hypertension. Am J Physiol Lung Cell Mol Physiol 293: L1–8.

30. Bentley JK, Deng H, Linn MJ, Lei J, Dokshin GA, et al. (2009) Airway smooth muscle hyperplasia and hypertrophy correlate with glycogen synthase kinase-3(beta) phosphorylation in a mouse model of asthma. Am J Physiol Lung Cell Mol Physiol 296: L176–184.
31. Chilosi M, Poletti V, Zamo A, Lestani M, Montagna L, et al. (2003) Aberrant Wnt/beta-catenin pathway activation in idiopathic pulmonary fibrosis. Am J Pathol 162: 1495–1502.
32. Goode N, Hughes K, Woodgett JR, Parker PJ (1992) Differential regulation of glycogen synthase kinase-3 beta by protein kinase C isotypes. J Biol Chem 267: 16878–16882.
33. Ali A, Hoeflich KP, Woodgett JR (2001) Glycogen synthase kinase-3: properties, functions, and regulation. Chem Rev 101: 2527–2540.
34. George SJ, Beeching CA (2006) Cadherin:catenin complex: a novel regulator of vascular smooth muscle cell behaviour. Atherosclerosis 188: 1–11.
35. Mikels AJ, Nusse R (2006) Purified Wnt5a protein activates or inhibits beta-catenin-TCF signaling depending on receptor context. PLoS Biol 4: e115.
36. Miller JR, Hocking AM, Brown JD, Moon RT (1999) Mechanism and function of signal transduction by the Wnt/beta-catenin and Wnt/Ca2+ pathways. Oncogene 18: 7860–7872.
37. Laumanns IP, Fink L, Wilhelm J, Wolff JC, Mitnacht-Kraus R, et al. (2009) The noncanonical WNT pathway is operative in idiopathic pulmonary arterial hypertension. Am J Respir Cell Mol Biol 40: 683–691.
38. Chen XY, Dun JN, Miao QF, Zhang YJ (2009) Fasudil hydrochloride hydrate, a Rho-kinase inhibitor, suppresses 5-hydroxytryptamine-induced pulmonary artery smooth muscle cell proliferation via JNK and ERK1/2 pathway. Pharmacology 83: 67–79.
39. Li F, Xia W, Yuan S, Sun R (2009) Acute inhibition of Rho-kinase attenuates pulmonary hypertension in patients with congenital heart disease. Pediatr Cardiol 30: 363–366.
40. Zhang S, Dong H, Rubin LJ, Yuan JX (2007) Upregulation of Na+/Ca2+ exchanger contributes to the enhanced Ca2+ entry in pulmonary artery smooth muscle cells from patients with idiopathic pulmonary arterial hypertension. Am J Physiol Cell Physiol 292: C2297–2305.
41. Tsakiridis T, Tsiani E, Lekas P, Bergman A, Cherepanov V, et al. (2001) Insulin, insulin-like growth factor-I, and platelet-derived growth factor activate extracellular signal-regulated kinase by distinct pathways in muscle cells. Biochem Biophys Res Commun 288: 205–211.
42. Shin HS, Lee HJ, Nishida M, Lee MS, Tamura R, et al. (2003) Betacellulin and amphiregulin induce upregulation of cyclin D1 and DNA synthesis activity through differential signaling pathways in vascular smooth muscle cells. Circ Res 93: 302–310.
43. Fang X, Yu SX, Lu Y, Bast RC, Jr., Woodgett JR, et al. (2000) Phosphorylation and inactivation of glycogen synthase kinase 3 by protein kinase A. Proc Natl Acad Sci U S A 97: 11960–11965.
44. Rubinfeld B, Albert I, Porfiri E, Fiol C, Munemitsu S, et al. (1996) Binding of GSK3beta to the APC-beta-catenin complex and regulation of complex assembly. Science 272: 1023–1026.
45. de Jesus Perez VA, Alastalo TP, Wu JC, Axelrod JD, Cooke JP, et al. (2009) Bone morphogenetic protein 2 induces pulmonary angiogenesis via Wnt-beta-catenin and Wnt-RhoA-Rac1 pathways. J Cell Biol 184: 83–99.
46. Diehl JA, Cheng M, Roussel MF, Sherr CJ (1998) Glycogen synthase kinase-3beta regulates cyclin D1 proteolysis and subcellular localization. Genes Dev 12: 3499–3511.
47. Wang Q, Zhou Y, Wang X, Evers BM (2006) Glycogen synthase kinase-3 is a negative regulator of extracellular signal-regulated kinase. Oncogene 25: 43–50.
48. Bonnet S, Paulin R, Sutendra G, Dromparis P, Roy M, et al. (2009) Dehydroepiandrosterone reverses systemic vascular remodeling through the inhibition of the Akt/GSK3-{beta}/NFAT axis. Circulation 120: 1231–1240.
49. Park KW, Yang HM, Youn SW, Yang HJ, Chae IH, et al. (2003) Constitutively active glycogen synthase kinase-3beta gene transfer sustains apoptosis, inhibits proliferation of vascular smooth muscle cells, and reduces neointima formation after balloon injury in rats. Arterioscler Thromb Vasc Biol 23: 1364–1369.

Endothelin-1 Augments Na^+/H^+ Exchange Activity in Murine Pulmonary Arterial Smooth Muscle Cells via Rho Kinase

Clark Undem, Eon J. Rios, Julie Maylor, Larissa A. Shimoda*

Division of Pulmonary and Critical Care Medicine, Department of Medicine, Johns Hopkins School of Medicine, Baltimore, Maryland, United States of America

Abstract

Excessive production of endothelin-1 (ET-1), a potent vasoconstrictor, occurs with several forms of pulmonary hypertension. In addition to modulating vasomotor tone, ET-1 can potentiate pulmonary arterial smooth muscle cell (PASMC) growth and migration, both of which contribute to the vascular remodeling that occurs during the development of pulmonary hypertension. It is well established that changes in cell proliferation and migration in PASMCs are associated with alkalinization of intracellular pH (pH_i), typically due to activation of Na^+/H^+ exchange (NHE). In the systemic vasculature, ET-1 increases pH_i, Na^+/H^+ exchange activity and stimulates cell growth via a mechanism dependent on protein kinase C (PKC). These results, coupled with data describing elevated levels of ET-1 in hypertensive animals/humans, suggest that ET-1 may play an important role in modulating pH_i and smooth muscle growth in the lung; however, the effect of ET-1 on basal pH_i and NHE activity has yet to be examined in PASMCs. Thus, we used fluorescent microscopy in transiently (3–5 days) cultured rat PASMCs and the pH-sensitive dye, BCECF-AM, to measure changes in basal pH_i and NHE activity induced by increasing concentrations of ET-1 (10^{-10} to 10^{-8} M). We found that application of exogenous ET-1 increased pH_i and NHE activity in PASMCs and that the ET-1-induced augmentation of NHE was prevented in PASMCs pretreated with an inhibitor of Rho kinase, but not inhibitors of PKC. Moreover, direct activation of PKC had no effect on pH_i or NHE activity in PASMCs. Our results indicate that ET-1 can modulate pH homeostasis in PASMCs via a signaling pathway that includes Rho kinase and that, in contrast to systemic vascular smooth muscle, activation of PKC does not appear to be an important regulator of PASMC pH_i.

Editor: Rory Edward Morty, University of Giessen Lung Center, Germany

Funding: This work was supported by grants from the National Institutes of Health (HL-67919, HL-73859 and HL-07963) and by a Scientist Development Grant from the American Heart Association (AHA9930255N). The funders had no role in study design, data collection and analysis, decision to publish, or preparation of the manuscript.

Competing Interests: The authors have declared that no competing interests exist.

* E-mail: shimodal@welch.jhu.edu

Introduction

Pulmonary hypertension can result from a variety of etiologies, including genetic mutations, environmental factors (i.e, anorexigens), and hypoxia due to chronic lung diseases [1–3]. In all cases, increased muscularization of the vasculature and enhanced vasomotor tone contribute to the elevation in pulmonary arterial pressure. The exact mechanisms underlying the pathogenesis of PASMC growth are not known, but studies have shown that increased intracellular pH (pH_i) accompanies cell proliferation in systemic [4–6] and pulmonary [7] vascular smooth muscle cells.

In mammalian cells, pH_i homeostasis is maintained in large part by several membrane bound transporters, including the Na^+-HCO_3^- co-transporter, Na^+-dependent Cl^-/HCO_3^- exchange, Na^+-independent Cl^-/HCO_3^- exchange and Na^+/H^+ exchange, all of which have been shown to be functionally present and contribute to control of pH_i in vascular smooth muscle [8–12]. In PASMCs, the use of Na^+/H^+ exchanger (NHE) antagonists revealed that this transporter plays a significant role in regulating resting pH_i [11], [13]. Na^+/H^+ exchangers are plasma membrane spanning proteins that use the transmembrane Na^+ gradient to extrude protons. Many stimuli, including acute [10] and chronic hypoxia [13] and growth factors [7] induce PASMC alkalinization. The increase in pH_i observed in response to chronic hypoxia or platelet-derived and epidermal growth factor was demonstrated to require activation of NHE activity [7], [13]. Moreover, inhibition of Na^+/H^+ exchange with amiloride analogs or selective knockdown of NHE isoform 1 (NHE1) prevents PASMC proliferation in response to growth factors and attenuated vascular remodeling and pulmonary hypertension in rodents exposed to chronic hypoxia, respectively [7], [14], [15]. The results from these studies indicate that enhanced NHE activity in response to growth factors is an important component in modulating pH_i and PASMC growth.

Since its discovery in 1988 [16], ET-1 has emerged as a strong candidate in mediating the development and progression of pulmonary hypertension. ET-1 is one of the most potent and abundant endothelial-derived constricting factors identified to date, and has mitogenic and anti-apoptotic properties [17–21]. Three isoforms of endothelin (ET-1, ET-2, ET-3) have been identified, of which ET-1 is the most widely distributed, and thus, the most widely studied. ET-1 was initially identified as a secretory product from aortic endothelial cells [16] and is primarily produced in, and secreted from, vascular endothelium. ET-1 levels are markedly increased in almost all forms of pulmonary hypertension, and ET-1 receptor antagonists prevent and partially reverse the development of hypoxic pulmonary hypertension in animal models [22–30] and are now used clinically in the management of many forms of pulmonary hypertension [31]. While ET-1 was shown to increase pH_i, NHE activity and cell growth in systemic vascular smooth muscle [32], the effects of ET-1 on PASMC pH homeostasis are unknown.

Two endothelin receptor subtypes have been identified and characterized: ET_A and ET_B, both of which mediate proliferation in PASMCs [33]. Once ET-1 binds to its surface receptor, a complex signaling process is set in motion. In general, endothelin receptors are G-protein coupled to the phospholipase C cascade, leading to increased $[Ca^{2+}]_i$ and activation of protein kinase C (PKC) and Rho kinase (ROCK) [34–37]. That PKC activation leads to increased NHE activity has been well documented in systemic vascular smooth muscle [38–41], and in several cell types the action of ET-1 on Na^+/H^+ exchange was confirmed to require PKC [42–44].

Despite the fact that overwhelming evidence suggests that alterations in pH_i and Na^+/H^+ exchange are necessary for vascular smooth muscle cell growth, and that ET-1 levels are elevated pulmonary hypertension patients and animal models of pulmonary hypertension, the effect of ET-1 on basal pH_i and NHE activity has yet to be examined in PASMCs. Thus, in this study, we used fluorescent microscopy to measure basal pH_i and NHE activity to test the hypothesis that challenge with ET-1 would lead to PKC-dependent activation of NHE activity and a consequent alkaline shift in pH_i in PASMCs.

Methods

Ethics Statement

All procedures were performed in strict accordance with the recommendations in the Guide for the Care and Use of Laboratory Animals of the National Institutes of Health and were approved by the Animal Care and Use Committee of The Johns Hopkins University School of Medicine (Protocol number MO06M161).

Cell Isolation and Culture

The method for obtaining single PASMCs has been described previously [13]. Briefly, adult, male C57/B6 mice were anesthetized with sodium pentobarbital (65 mg/kg i.p.), and under deep anesthesia the heart and lungs removed and transferred to a petri dish containing HEPES-buffered salt solution (HBSS) containing (in mmol/L): 130 NaCl, 5 KCl, 1.2 $MgCl_2$, 1.5 $CaCl_2$, 10 N-[2-hydroxyethyl]piperazine-N'-[2-ethanesulfonic acid] (HEPES) and 10 glucose, with pH adjusted to 7.2 with 5 mol/L NaOH. Intrapulmonary arteries (100–400 µm outer diameter) were isolated and cleaned of connective tissue. After disrupting the endothelium by gently rubbing the luminal surface with a cotton swab, the arteries were allowed to recover for 30 min in cold (4°C) HBSS, followed by 20 min in reduced-Ca^{2+} (20 µmol/L $CaCl_2$) HBSS at room temperature. The tissue was digested in reduced-Ca^{2+} HBSS containing collagenase (type I; 1750 U/ml), papain (9.5 U/ml), bovine serum albumin (2 mg/ml) and dithiothreitol (1 mmol/L) at 37°C for 10 minutes. Following digestion, single smooth muscle cells were dispersed by gentle trituration with a wide-bore transfer pipette in Ca^{2+}-free HBSS and the cell suspension was placed on 25 mm glass cover slips. PASMCs were cultured under normoxic conditions in SmBm complete media (Lonza) supplemented with 10% fetal calf serum for 2–4 days and placed in serum-free media 24 hr before experiments. The identity of the cells under study was confirmed as smooth muscle by elongated, spindle morphology (Fig 1A), and positive staining for both smooth muscle specific α-actin (SMA) and heavy chain myosin (HCM) (Fig 1B). For immunofluorescence, cells were grown on glass coverslips, fixed with 10% formalin, washed with PBS, permeabilized with 0.5% Triton-X and blocked with 20% goat serum. Cells were then incubated with monoclonal antibodies against SMA (Sigma-Aldrich) or HCM (Abcam), followed by fluorescent secondary antibody (CY3; Molecular Probes) and the nuclear dye, YO-PRO. Random fields were examined to achieve a minimum total cell count of 100 per animal, and the number of cells exhibiting SMA/HCM positivity calculated as a percent of total cell number.

Intracellular pH Measurements

PASMCs were placed in a laminar flow cell chamber perfused with HBSS with pH adjusted to 7.4. pH_i was measured in cells incubated with the membrane permeant (acetoxymethyl ester) form of the pH-sensitive fluorescent dye 2′,7′-bis(carboxyethyl)-5(6)-carboxyfluorescein (BCECF-AM) for 60 min at 37°C under an atmosphere of 20% O_2-5% CO_2. Cells were then washed with HBSS for 15 min at 37°C to remove extracellular dye and allow complete de-esterification of cytosolic dye. Ratiometric measurement of BCECF fluorescence was performed on a workstation

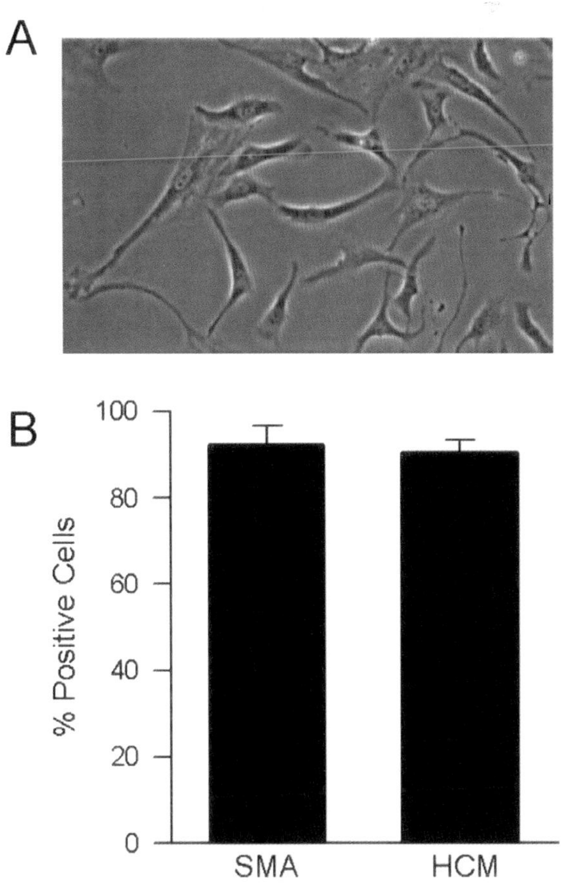

Figure 1. Characterization of murine pulmonary arterial smooth muscle cells (PASMCs). A) Representative phase contrast image showing morphology of murine PASMCs. **B)** Bar graph showing mean±SEM values (n = 3-4 isolations) for the percent of cells staining positive for the smooth muscle cell markers smooth muscle specific α-actin (SMA) and heavy chain myosin (HCM).

(Intracellular Imaging Inc, Cincinnati, OH) consisting of a Nikon TSE 100 Ellipse inverted microscope with epi-fluorescence attachments. The light beam from a xenon arc lamp was filtered by interference filters at 490 and 440 nm, and focused onto the PASMCS under examination via a 20× fluorescence objective (Super Fluor 20, Nikon). Light emitted from the cell at 530 nm was returned through the objective and detected by an imaging camera. An electronic shutter (Sutter Instruments) was used to minimize photobleaching of dye. Protocols were executed and data collected on-line with InCyte software (Intracellular Imaging Inc). pH_i was estimated from *in situ* calibration after each experiment. Cells were perfused with a solution containing (in mmol/L): 105 KCl, 1 $MgCl_2$, 1.5 $CaCl_2$, 10 glucose, 20 HEPES-Tris and 0.01 nigericin to allow pH_i to equilibrate to external pH. A two point calibration was created from fluorescence measured as pH_i was adjusted with KOH from 6.5 to 7.5. Intracellular H^+ ion concentration ($[H^+]_i$) was determined from pH_i using the formula: $pH_i = -\log([H^+]_i)$.

Experimental Protocols

Effect of ET-1and PMA on basal pH_i. Baseline pH_i was measured for five minutes in PASMCs under control conditions. Values were averaged to obtain a mean value for each cell. The effect of agonists on baseline pH_i was then determined by monitoring pH_i for an additional 10 min in the same cells during exposure to ET-1 (10^{-10} to 10^{-8} M) or phorbol 12-myristate 13-acetate (PMA; 1 μmol/L). Each concentration was tested on a separate coverslip of cells.

Effect of antagonists on basal pH_i. The effect of antagonists on basal pH_i was determined in HBSS-perfused cells. After obtaining a stable baseline for 5 min, cells were then perfused with antagonists for 10 min. For Y-27632, cells were pretreated for 30 min to allow complete cell penetration and ROCK inhibition. Thus, the effect of Y-27632 on basal pH_i was determined by comparing baseline in paired coverslips (control and Y-27632-treated). To determine the effect of antagonists on the ET-1-induced increase in pH_i, cells were then challenged for 10 min with 10^{-8} mol/L ET-1 in the presence of antagonist.

Effect of ET-1on Na^+/H^+ exchange. A standard ammonia pulse technique was used to measure NHE activity (Figure 2A). PASMCs loaded with BCECF were perfused at a rate of 1 mL/min with Solution 1 containing (in mmol/L): 130 NaCl, 5 KCl, 1$MgCl_2$, 1.5 $CaCl_2$, 10 glucose and 20 HEPES with pH adjusted to 7.4 with NaOH at 37°C. Baseline pH_i was measured for 2 min before cells were briefly exposed to NH_4Cl (ammonium pulse) by perfusing with Solution 2 containing (in mmol/L): 110 NaCl, 20 NH_4Cl, 5 KCl, 1$MgCl_2$, 1.5 $CaCl_2$, 10 glucose, 20 HEPES at a pH of 7.4 using NaOH for 3 min. The ammonium pulse caused alkalinization due to influx of NH_3 and buffering of intracellular H^+ (Fig 2A). Washout of NH_4Cl in the absence of extracellular Na^+ using a Na^+- and NH_4^+- free solution containing (in mmol/L): 130 choline chloride, 5 KCl, 1$MgCl_2$, 1.5 $CaCl_2$, 10 glucose and 20 HEPES at a pH of 7.4 using KOH for 10 min results in acidification due to rapid diffusion and washout of NH_3. The external solution was then switched back to Na^+-containing Solution 1 for 10 min. Re-addition of extracellular Na^+ allows activation of Na^+/H^+ exchange and recovery from acidification to basal levels. The rate of Na^+-dependent recovery from intracellular acidification (change in pH over 2 min) corresponds to NHE activity.

Drugs and Solutions

ET-1 was obtained from American Peptides (Sunnyvale, CA). Y-27632 and GF 102903X were obtained from Calbiochem (La

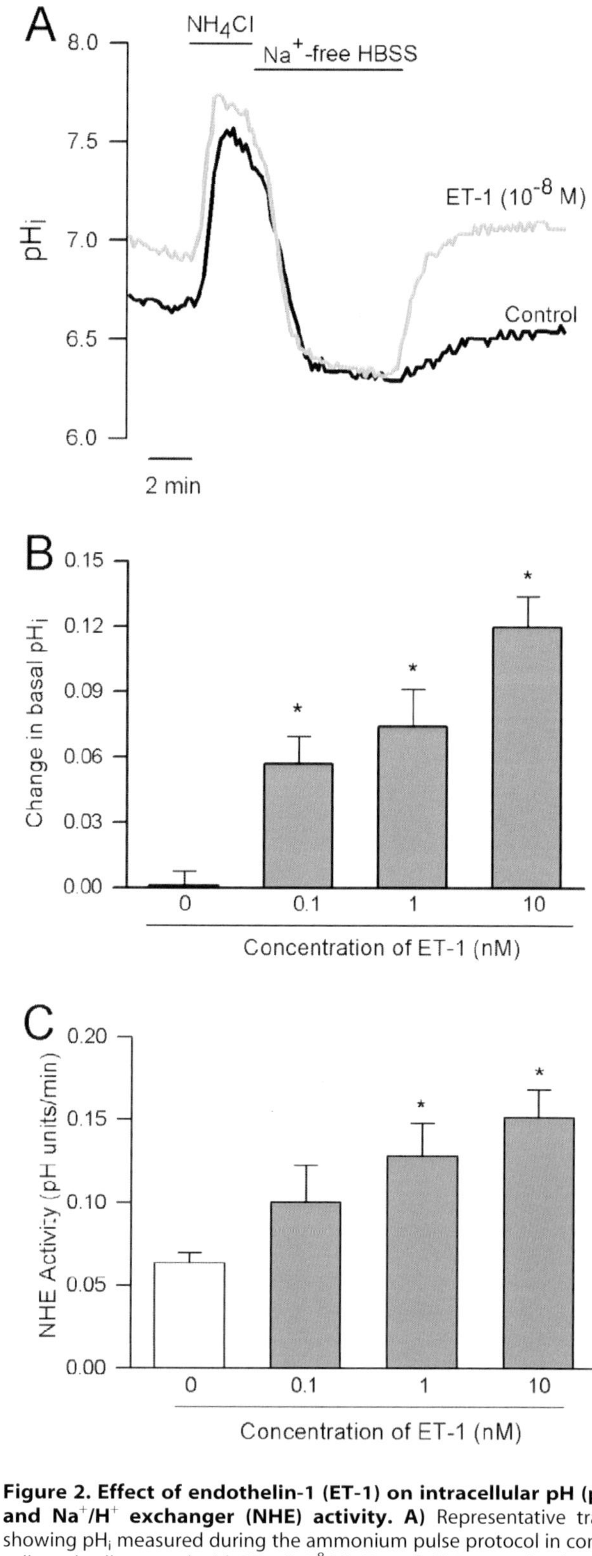

Figure 2. Effect of endothelin-1 (ET-1) on intracellular pH (pH_i) and Na^+/H^+ exchanger (NHE) activity. A) Representative traces showing pH_i measured during the ammonium pulse protocol in control cells and cells treated with ET-1 (10^{-8} M). **B and C)** Bar graphs showing mean±SEM values for **B)** the change (Δ) in baseline pH_i (n = 3-6) and **C)** NHE activity (n = 5-15) induced by different concentrations of ET-1. * indicates significant difference from control (0 nmol/L ET-1)

Jolla, CA). All other reagents were obtained from Sigma Aldrich (St. Louis, MO). ET-1 (10^{-5} mol/L in deionized H_2O) was made up in a stock solution, divided into aliquots, and stored at −20°C until used. Stock solutions of Y-27632 (10 mmol/L in deionized H_2O) and PMA (0.1 mmol/L in deionized H_2O) were made, aliquotted, and stored at 0°C until used. GF 109203X (GFX; 10 mmol/L in DMSO), and staurosporine (Stauro; 10 mmol/L in DMSO) were made up in a stock solution and stored at 4°C. A stock solution of 5-(N,N-Dimethyl)amiloride hydrochloride (DMA; 10 mmol/L in deionized H_2O) was made and used on the day of the experiment. All stock solutions were diluted to working concentrations in perfusate on the day of experiment.

Data Analysis

All values are expressed as mean ± SEM. In each experiment, data was collected from up to 30 cells, and the values averaged to obtain a single value for each experiment. Cells isolated from different animals were used in each experiment, thus, "n" refers to both the number of experiments as well as number of animals from which cells were derived. Although presented as pH_i values in the text and figures, pH values were converted to $[H^+]_i$ prior to running statistics. Change in pH_i (ΔpH_i) was computed by subtracting the average basal pH_i, determined from 1 min of data collected immediately prior to beginning challenge, from the average of five data points at the peak of the response. For each agonist (ET-1 and PMA), all data were compared against a single control group as a single analysis using a one-way ANOVA with a Holm-Sidak *post hoc* test to determine differences between groups. In some cases, a one-sample t-test was used to determine whether the change in pH_i observed after treatment was statistically different from zero (i.e., value for the ΔpH_i is significantly different from the test value of 0). A P value <0.05 was accepted as statistically significant.

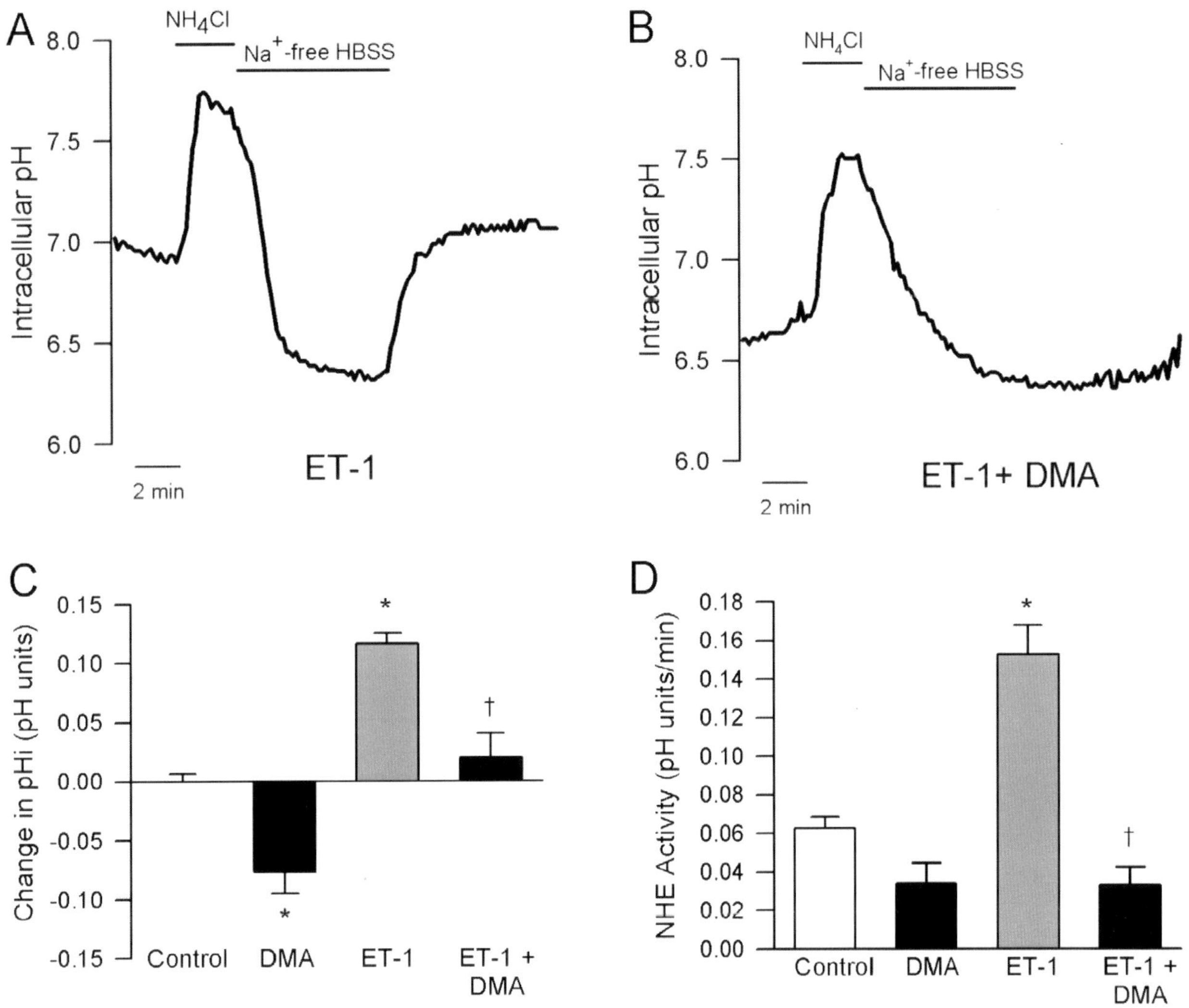

Figure 3. Effect of dimethyl amiloride (DMA; 1 μmol/L) on intracellular pH (pH_i) and Na^+/H^+ exchanger (NHE) activity. A and B) Representative traces showing pH_i measured during the ammonium pulse protocol in cells treated with ET-1 (10^{-8} M) in the **A)** absence and **B)** presence of DMA. **C and D)** Bar graphs showing mean±SEM values for **C)** the change (Δ) in baseline pH_i (n = 3-6) and **D)** NHE activity (n = 5-15) in control (Con) cells or in cells treated with DMA alone (n = 4 for pH_i and n = 6 for NHE activity), ET-1 (10^{-8} M; n = 5 for pH_i and n = 11 for NHE activity) and ET-1 + DMA (n = 6 for pH_i and n = 5 for NHE activity). * indicates significant difference from control; †indicates significant difference from ET-1 alone.

Results

Effect of ET-1 on pH_i and NHE Activity

When monitored over 10 min, basal pH_i was stable and no significant change in pH_i was observed. However, application of ET-1 caused concentration-dependent increases in pH_i (Fig 2B), with an average change of greater than 0.1 pH units at 10^{-8} mol/L ET-1, a concentration that we previously found caused maximal contraction in pulmonary arteries [45], [46]. The ammonium pulse technique was used to measure the effect of ET-1 on NHE activity (Fig 2A). PASMCs were exposed to different concentrations of ET-1 for 15 min before beginning the ammonium pulse. Consistent with the effects of ET-1 on baseline pH_i, the rate of Na^+-dependent recovery from acid-loading (NHE activity), measured during the first 2 min after re-addition of Na^+, was greater in the presence of ET-1 (Fig 2C). Although increases in NHE activity were observed at all concentrations of ET-1 tested, with a greater than 2-fold increase in NHE activity at 10 nmol/L, the difference with 0.1 nmol/L ET-1 did not quite reach statistical significance.

Although perfusion of cells with bicarbonate-free extracellular solution should eliminate contributions of the Cl^-/HCO_3^- exchangers to regulation of pH_i, we verified that the increase in basal pH_i was due to increased NHE activity by repeating experiments in the presence of DMA (1 μmol/L), a NHE inhibitor (Fig 3A and B). Consistent with the known role of NHE in regulating pH_i in PASMCs, DMA caused a significant reduction in basal pH_i (Fig 3C). When applied in the presence of DMA, the ET-1-induced increase in basal pH_i was greatly reduced, with only a small, statistically insignificant increase in pH_i observed (Fig 3C). DMA also reduced NHE activity under control conditions (Fig 3D), although the reduction did not quite reach statistical significance ($P = 0.06$), and completely prevented the ET-1-induced increase in NHE activity.

Role of PKC in Mediating the ET-1-induced Increase in NHE Activity

PKC activation has been shown to enhance NHE activity in a variety of cell types, including vascular smooth muscle [38–41]. To determine whether the increase in PASMC pH_i and NHE activity in response to ET-1 was due to activation of PKC, cells were pretreated with two different PKC inhibitors: Stauro (50 nmol/L), a relatively nonselective PKC inhibitor, and GFX (30 nmol/L), a selective PKC inhibitor with greater affinity for Ca^{2+}-dependent isoforms [47]. Neither inhibitor had a significant effect on basal

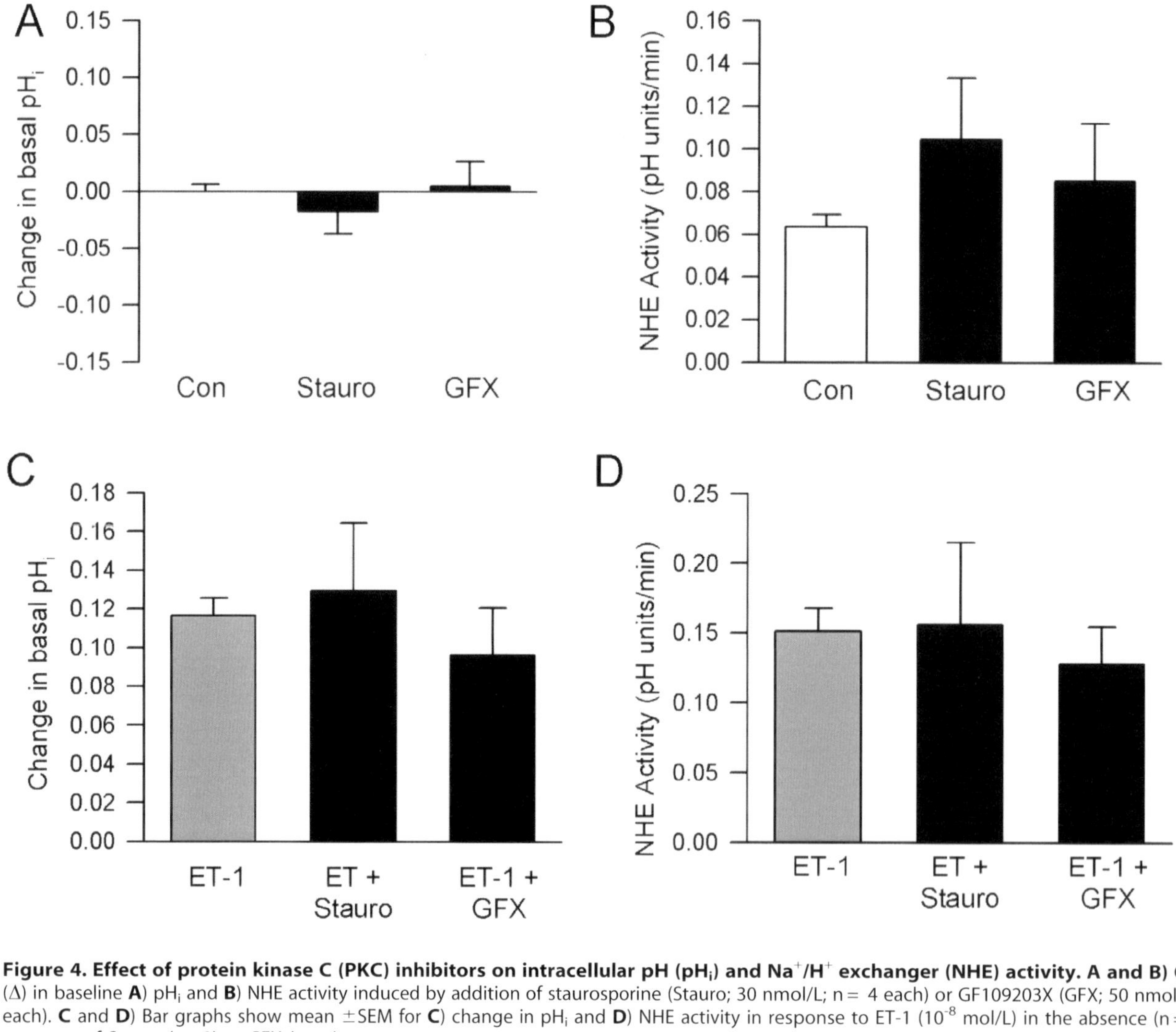

Figure 4. Effect of protein kinase C (PKC) inhibitors on intracellular pH (pH_i) and Na^+/H^+ exchanger (NHE) activity. A and B) Change (Δ) in baseline **A)** pH_i and **B)** NHE activity induced by addition of staurosporine (Stauro; 30 nmol/L; n = 4 each) or GF109203X (GFX; 50 nmol/l; n = 4 each). **C** and **D)** Bar graphs show mean ±SEM for **C)** change in pH_i and **D)** NHE activity in response to ET-1 (10^{-8} mol/L) in the absence (n = 11) or presence of Stauro (n = 3) or GFX (n = 4).

pH_i (Fig 4A) or NHE activity (Fig 4B). Surprisingly, inhibiting PKC with either Stauro or GFX could not prevent the ET-1-induced increase in pH_i (Fig 4C) or NHE activity (Fig 4D).

Effect of PMA on pH_i and NHE Activity

Since PKC inhibition failed to block ET-1-induced changes in pH_i and NHE activity, we tested whether PKC activation could stimulate NHE activity in PASMCs by challenging cells with PMA (500 nmol/L) (Fig 5A and B). Although we previously showed this concentration of PMA to be sufficient to induce Ca^{2+} influx and reduce K_V currents in PASMCs [37], [48], since this concentration of PMA appeared to have no observable effect on either baseline pH_i or NHE activity, we increased the concentration of PMA to 1 µmol/L. Perfusion with 1 µmol/L PMA for 15 min had no effect on basal pH_i (Fig 5C). Moreover, NHE activity was similar in control and PMA-treated cells (Fig 5D).

Role of ROCK in Mediating ET-1-induced PKC Activation

Since our results appeared to rule out a role for PKC in mediating the ET-1-induced activation of NHE activity, we next tested whether ROCK was involved using the ROCK inhibitor, Y-27632 (10 µmol/L). In order to allow sufficient time for Y-273632 to enter the cells, cells were pretreated with Y-27632 for 30 min prior to beginning experiments. Incubation with Y-27632 had no effect on basal pH_i (Fig 6A). When cells were challenged with ET-1 (10^{-8} mol/L) in the presence of Y-27632, no significant increase in pH_i was observed (Fig 6B). Consistent with the lack of effect of Y-27632 on basal pH_i, ROCK inhibition did not alter NHE activity (Fig 6C); however, pretreatment with Y-27632 completely prevented the ET-1-induced increase in NHE activity.

Discussion

In this study, we demonstrated that acute exposure to ET-1 increased NHE activity in PASMCs, leading to a rapid alkaline

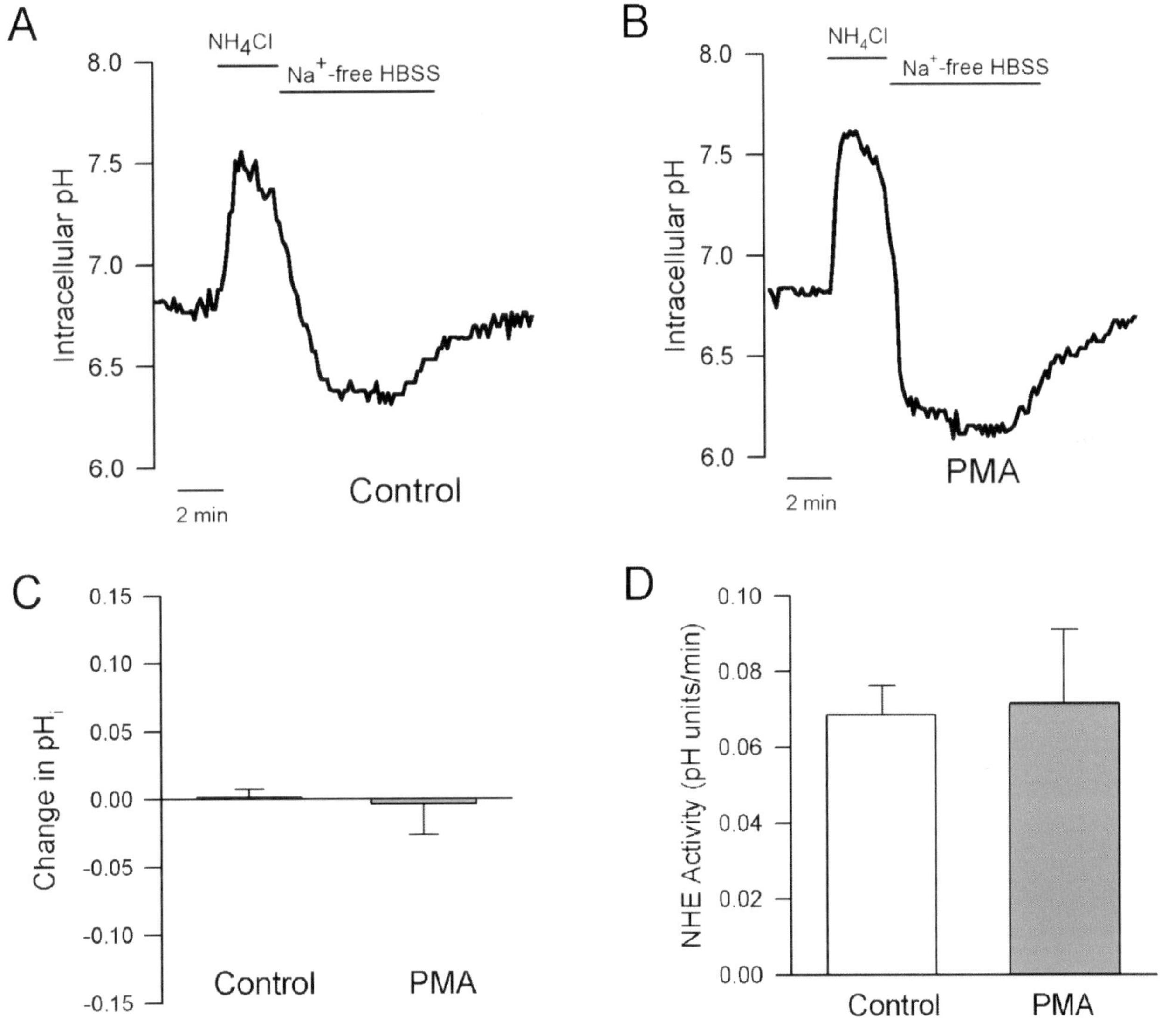

Figure 5. Effect of PKC activation on intracellular pH (pH_i) and Na^+/H^+ exchanger (NHE) activity. Representative traces show pH_i measured during ammonium pulse in the **A)** absence and **B)** presence of PMA (1 µmol/L). **C and D)** Bar graphs show mean±SEM for **C)** the change (Δ) in baseline pH_i (n = 7) and **D)** NHE activity (n = 8) in response to PMA.

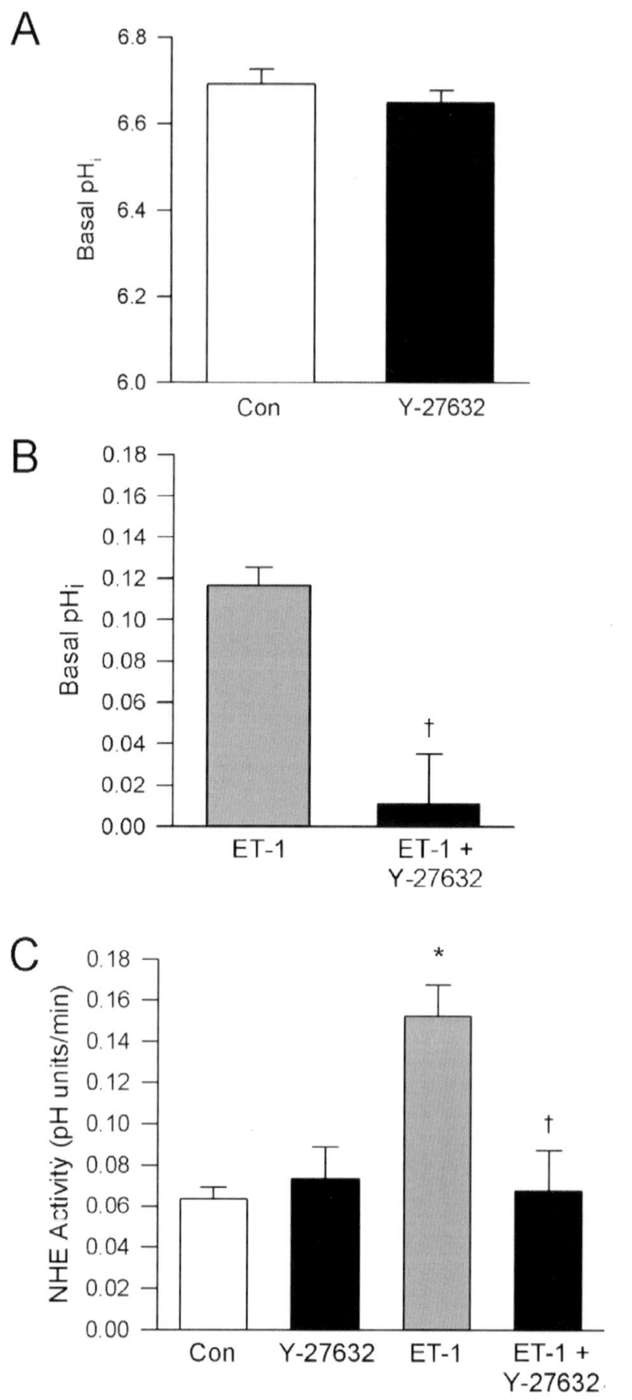

Figure 6. Effect of ROCK inhibition on intracellular pH (pH_i) and Na^+/H^+ exchanger (NHE) activity. A) Bar graph showing mean±''' SEM values for basal pH_i measured in cells in the absence (n=4) or presence (n=4) of Y-27632 (10 μmol/L; 30 min). **B)** Bar graph shows mean±SEM values for the change (Δ) in baseline pH_i in response to ET-1 (10^{-8} mol/L) in the absence (n=5) and presence (n=3) of Y-27632. **C)** Bar graph showing mean±SEM for NHE activity in cells challenged with ET-1 in the absence (n=11) and presence (n=5) of Y-27632. * indicates significant difference from control; †indicates significant difference from ET-1 alone.

shift in pH_i. The enhancement of NHE activity in response to ET-1 was dependent on ROCK activation, but did not appear to involve activation of PKC (Fig 7). In contrast to previous results reported in systemic vascular smooth muscle [39–41], [49], [50], activation of PKC did not stimulate NHE activity or increase pH_i in PASMCs.

Our results confirm previous observations [10], [11], [13] that NHE contributes to the regulation of resting pH_i in PASMCs, although our data suggest that NHE activity is low under basal conditions, since DMA caused only a small reduction (<0.1 unit) in resting pH_i levels. DMA reduced, but did not completely eliminate, basal NHE activity, perhaps due to incomplete inhibition; it is possible that higher concentrations of DMA could have resulted in complete inhibition of NHE activity and a greater reduction in basal pH_i. Nonetheless, our data is consistent with previously reported results demonstrating a reduction in pH_i with DMA or EIPA [11], [13]. Moreover, we found that neither PKC nor ROCK inhibition altered resting pH_i or NHE activity, indicating a lack of phosphorylation-dependent activation of NHE in PASMCs under control conditions.

Application of ET-1 increased both pH_i and NHE activity in a concentration-dependent manner. The ET-1-induced increase in pH_i that we observed in PASMCs is in line with the alkalinizing effect of ET-1 on basal pH_i reported in cultured systemic vascular smooth muscle cells [32], [51], [52]. Since the current study was focused on delineating the effects of ET-1 on NHE activity, experiments were performed in CO_2- and bicarbonate-free solutions, eliminating the effects of the Cl^-/HCO_3^- exchangers. Determining whether the activity of these exchangers is also altered in the presence of ET-1 or contributes to either enhanced or diminished alkalinization in response to ET-1 will require further investigation.

In previous studies, the modulation of pH_i by ET-1 was inhibited by EIPA and Stauro [32], [51], indicating that ET-1 increased the activity of the Na^+/H^+ exchanger through a PKC-dependent mechanism. Since PKC activation is a well-recognized consequence of ET receptor activation [53–56], and given previous reports supporting PKC-dependent enhancement of NHE activity [38–41], we hypothesized that the effects of ET-1 in PASMCs would also be prevented or reduced with PKC inhibition. However, somewhat surprisingly, two structurally unrelated PKC inhibitors failed to block the effects of ET-1 on pH_i and NHE activity in PASMCs. Although it might be argued that the lack of effect of GFX could be attributed to a role for non-

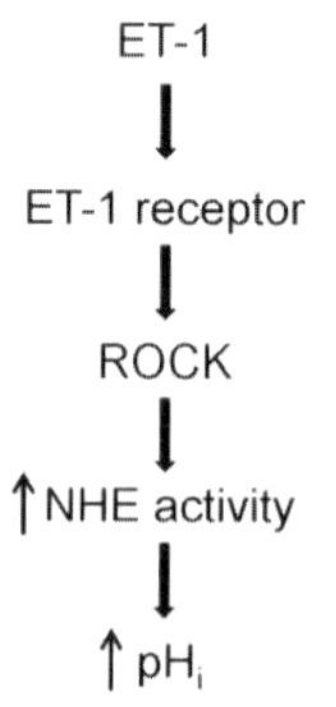

Figure 7. Schematic illustrating the effect of endothelin-1 (ET-1) on intracellular pH (pH_i) in pulmonary arterial smooth muscle cells. ET-1 binds to surface receptors, leading to activation of Rho kinase (ROCK). ROCK activation in turn results in enhanced Na^+/H^+ exchanger (NHE) activity, increased H^+ efflux and an alkaline shift in pH_i.

Ca^{2+}-dependent isoforms of PKC [47], Stauro is not selective for specific isoforms of PKC and was also unable to prevent or reduce the effects of ET-1, further confirming that PKC activation is not required for stimulation of NHE activity by ET-1. It is unlikely that the lack of effect of these inhibitors was due to insufficient inhibition of PKC activity, as we have previously shown that these concentrations applied for the same duration of time attenuated the effect of ET-1 on K_V currents [48], intracellular Ca^{2+} mobilization [37] and contraction [45], [46] in pulmonary vascular smooth muscle. Experiments in which PKC was directly activated in PASMCs further ruled out a role for PKC, as PMA altered neither pH_i nor Na^+-dependent recovery from acid-loading. These results clearly demonstrate that unlike vascular smooth muscle from systemic sources, PKC activation does not lead to enhanced NHE activity in PASMCs. The reason why is unclear, but it is unlikely that PMA did not activate PKC since the concentrations of PMA used in this study were 2-fold greater than those we previously found activated PKC-dependent Ca^{2+} influx and reduced K_V currents in PASMCs within a similar time-frame [37], [48].

Since PKC activation did not appear to mediate the effects of ET-1 on NHE activity in PASMCs, we next focused on the role of ROCK. Binding of ET-1 to either ET_A or ET_B receptors leads to activation of ROCK in a variety of cell types [55], [57], including PASMCs [58], and ROCK has been implicated as a possible regulator of NHE activity [59–61]. We found that inhibiting ROCK prevented both the ET-1-induced increase in NHE activity and the associated alkaline shift in pH_i, indicating that ROCK activation by ET-1 acutely enhanced NHE activity in PASMCs, most likely due to phosphorylation of one or more known phosphorylation-sensitive sites in the cytoplasmic C-terminal tail region.

It should be noted that the current experiments were performed in PASMCs isolated from normoxic animals and studied under normoxic conditions. In PASMCs isolated from chronically hypoxic rats, we have shown that ET-1-induced activation of ROCK was downstream of PKC activation [37]. However, this does not appear to be the case in PASMCs from normoxic animals since inhibiting PKC and ROCK differentially blocked the effects of ET-1 on pH_i and NHE activity. While these results suggest that there may be alterations in ET-1 signaling pathways during chronic hypoxia, whether this is due to activation of different receptors (i.e., ET_A versus ET_B), or indicates that the receptors are coupled to different downstream signaling mechanisms, remains to be determined. Future experiments are also needed to establish whether ET-1 still exerts an acute stimulatory effect on NHE activity in cells from chronically hypoxic animals and, if so, delineate the signaling pathways involved.

It is well-recognized that ET-1 can play a role in the pathogenesis of pulmonary hypertension. In addition to its vasoconstrictive properties, ET-1 also stimulates DNA synthesis and proliferation in PASMCs [33], [62], [63]. Investigation in mice [64] and rats [65] showed that hypoxia induces elevated levels of preproendothelin mRNA as well as ET-1 mRNA in pulmonary tissue. In addition, mRNA levels of ET receptors are elevated in pulmonary tissue after 48 h at 10% O_2 [66], [67]. The active role of ET-1 in the development of pulmonary hypertension is further supported by studies that have shown inhibition and even reversal of pulmonary hypertension in chronically hypoxic animals treated with ET_A-receptor antagonists [23], [25], [27], [28], [68], [69]. Clinical studies of pulmonary hypertensive patients also describe elevated plasma levels of ET-1 when compared to normotensive individuals and show higher ET-1 levels in the arterial circuit when compared to the venous circuit pointing to the possibility of a pulmonary origin of ET-1 [70]. Our current data further confirms a role for ET-1 in modulating NHE activity in PASMCs and provides an additional link between ET-1 and the development of pulmonary hypertension.

In summary, we demonstrated that acute challenge with exogenous ET-1 enhances NHE activity in PASMCs via a mechanism involving ROCK activation. Unlike other cell types, PKC activation does not appear to be involved in the regulation of NHE activity and pH_i in PASMCs. Since ET-1 can induce PASMC proliferation and enhanced NHE activity has been shown to play a central role in cell growth responses, our results may provide additional insight into the mechanism by which ET-1 modulates PASMCs growth under both physiological and pathologic conditions.

Author Contributions

Conceived and designed the experiments: LAS EJR CU. Performed the experiments: LAS EJR CU JM. Analyzed the data: LAS EJR CU JM. Wrote the paper: LAS CU JM.

References

1. Machado RD, Eickelberg O, Elliott CG, Geraci MW, Hanaoka M, et al. (2009) Genetics and genomics of pulmonary arterial hypertension. J Am Coll Cardiol. 54:S32–42.
2. Davies RJ, Morrell NW (2008) Molecular mechanisms of pulmonary arterial hypertension: role of mutations in the bone morphogenetic protein type II receptor. Chest. 134: 1271–7.
3. Abenhaim L, Moride Y, Brenot F, Rich S, Benichou J, et al. (1996) Appetite-suppressant drugs and the risk of primary pulmonary hypertension. International Primary Pulmonary Hypertension Study Group. N Engl J Med. 335: 609–16.
4. Bobik A, Grooms A, Little PJ, Cragoe EJ Jr, Grinpukel S (1991) Ethylisopropylamiloride-sensitive pH control mechanisms modulate vascular smooth muscle cell growth. Am J Physiol. 260:C581–8.
5. LaPointe MS, Batlle DC (1994) Na^+/H^+ exchange and vascular smooth muscle proliferation. Am J Med Sci. 307 Suppl 1:S9–16.
6. Mitsuka M, Nagae M, Berk BC (1993) Na^+-H^+ exchange inhibitors decrease neointimal formation after rat carotid injury. Effects on smooth muscle cell migration and proliferation. Circ Res. 73: 269–75.
7. Quinn DA, Dahlberg CG, Bonventre JP, Scheid CR, Honeyman T, et al. (1996) The role of Na^+/H^+ exchange and growth factors in pulmonary artery smooth muscle cell proliferation. Am J Respir Cell Mol Biol. 14: 139–45.
8. Aalkjaer C, Cragoe EJ Jr (1988) Intracellular pH regulation in resting and contracting segments of rat mesenteric resistance vessels. J Physiol. 402: 391–410.
9. Aalkjaer C, Peng HL (1997) pH and smooth muscle. Acta Physiol Scand. 161: 557–66.
10. Madden JA, Ray DE, Keller PA, Kleinman JG (2001) Ion exchange activity in pulmonary artery smooth muscle cells: the response to hypoxia. Am J Physiol Lung Cell Mol Physiol. 280:L264–71.
11. Quinn DA, Honeyman TW, Joseph PM, Thompson BT, Hales CA, et al. (1991) Contribution of Na^+/H^+ exchange to pH regulation in pulmonary artery smooth muscle cells. Am J Respir Cell Mol Biol. 5: 586–91.
12. Neylon CB, Little PJ, Cragoe EJ Jr, Bobik A (1990) Intracellular pH in human arterial smooth muscle. Regulation by Na^+/H^+ exchange and a novel 5-(N-ethyl-N-isopropyl)amiloride-sensitive Na^+- and HCO_3 dependent mechanism. Circ Res. 67: 814–25.
13. Rios EJ, Fallon M, Wang J, Shimoda LA (2005) Chronic hypoxia elevates intracellular pH and activates Na^+/H^+ exchange in pulmonary arterial smooth muscle cells. Am J Physiol Lung Cell Mol Physiol. 289(5):L867–74.
14. Quinn DA, Du HK, Thompson BT, Hales CA (1998) Amiloride analogs inhibit chronic hypoxic pulmonary hypertension. Am J Respir Crit Care Med. 157: 1263–8.
15. Yu L, Quinn DA, Garg HG, Hales CA (2008) Deficiency of the NHE1 gene prevents hypoxia-induced pulmonary hypertension and vascular remodeling. Am J Respir Crit Care Med. 177: 1276–84.
16. Yanagisawa M, Kurihara H, Kimura S, Goto K, Masaki T (1988) A novel peptide vasoconstrictor, endothelin, is produced by vascular endothelium and modulates smooth muscle Ca^{2+} channels. J Hypertens Suppl. 6:S188–91.
17. Biswas P, Roy A, Gong R, Yango A, Tolbert E, et al. (2005) Hepatocyte growth factor induces an endothelin-mediated decline in glomerular filtration rate. Am J Physiol Renal Physiol. 288:F8–15.

18. Raymond MN, Bole-Feysot C, Banno Y, Tanfin Z, Robin P (2006) Endothelin-1 inhibits apoptosis through a sphingosine kinase 1-dependent mechanism in uterine leiomyoma ELT3 cells. Endocrinology. 147: 5873–82.
19. Kawanabe Y, Hashimoto N, Masaki T (2002) Extracellular Ca^{2+} influx and endothelin-1-induced intracellular mitogenic cascades in rabbit internal carotid artery vascular smooth muscle cells. J Cardiovasc Pharmacol. 40: 307–14.
20. Mukherjee R, Apple KA, Squires CE, Kaplan BS, McLean JE, et al. (2006) Protein kinase C isoform activation and endothelin-1 mediated defects in myocyte contractility after cardioplegic arrest and reperfusion. Circulation. 114:I308–13.
21. Gallelli L, Pelaia G, D'Agostino B, Cuda G, Vatrella A, et al. (2005) Endothelin-1 induces proliferation of human lung fibroblasts and IL-11 secretion through an ET_A receptor-dependent activation of MAP kinases. J Cell Biochem. 96: 858–68.
22. Frasch HF, Marshall C, Marshall BE (1999) Endothelin-1 is elevated in monocrotaline pulmonary hypertension. Am J Physiol. 1999;276:L304–10.
23. Galie N, Manes A, Branzi A (2004) The endothelin system in pulmonary arterial hypertension. Cardiovasc Res. 61: 227–37.
24. Rubens C, Ewert R, Halank M, Wensel R, Orzechowski HD, et al. (2001) Big endothelin-1 and endothelin-1 plasma levels are correlated with the severity of primary pulmonary hypertension. Chest. 120: 1562–9.
25. DiCarlo VS, Chen SJ, Meng QC, Durand J, Yano M, et al. (1995) ET_A-receptor antagonist prevents and reverses chronic hypoxia-induced pulmonary hypertension in rat. Am J Physiol. 269:L690–7.
26. Nakanishi K, Tajima F, Nakata Y, Osada H, Tachibana S, et al. (1999) Expression of endothelin-1 in rats developing hypobaric hypoxia-induced pulmonary hypertension. Lab Invest. 79: 1347–57.
27. Bialecki RA, Fisher CS, Abbott BM, Barthlow HG, Caccese RG, et al. (1999) ZD1611, an orally active endothelin-A receptor antagonist, prevents chronic hypoxia-induced pulmonary hypertension in the rat. Pulm Pharmacol Ther. 12: 303–12.
28. Bonvallet ST, Zamora MR, Hasunuma K, Sato K, Hanasato N, et al. (1994) BQ123, an ET_A-receptor antagonist, attenuates hypoxic pulmonary hypertension in rats. Am J Physiol. 266:H1327–31.
29. Cody RJ, Haas GJ, Binkley PF, Capers Q, Kelley R (1992) Plasma endothelin correlates with the extent of pulmonary hypertension in patients with chronic congestive heart failure. Circulation. 85: 504–9.
30. Stelzner TJ, O'Brien RF, Yanagisawa M, Sakurai T, Sato K, et al. (1992) Increased lung endothelin-1 production in rats with idiopathic pulmonary hypertension. Am J Physiol. 262:L614–20.
31. Stenmark KR, Rabinovitch M (2010) Emerging therapies for the treatment of pulmonary hypertension. Pediatr Crit Care Med. 11:S85–90.
32. Lonchampt MO, Pinelis S, Goulin J, Chabrier PE, Braquet P (1991) Proliferation and Na^+/H^+ exchange activation by endothelin in vascular smooth muscle cells. Am J Hypertens. 4: 776–9.
33. Davie N, Haleen SJ, Upton PD, Polak JM, Yacoub MH, et al. (2002) ET_A and ET_B receptors modulate the proliferation of human pulmonary artery smooth muscle cells. Am J Respir Crit Care Med. 165: 398–405.
34. Rodriguez-Vita J, Ruiz-Ortega M, Ruperez M, Esteban V, Sanchez-Lopez E, et al. (2005) Endothelin-1, via ET_A receptor and independently of transforming growth factor-beta, increases the connective tissue growth factor in vascular smooth muscle cells. Circ Res. 97: 125–34.
35. Hersch E, Huang J, Grider JR, Murthy KS (2004) Gq/G13 signaling by ET-1 in smooth muscle: MYPT1 phosphorylation via ET_A and CPI-17 dephosphorylation via ET_B. Am J Physiol Cell Physiol. 287:C1209–18.
36. Luscher TF (1992) Endothelin: systemic arterial and pulmonary effects of a new peptide with potent biologic properties. Am Rev Respir Dis. 146:S56–60.
37. Luke T, Maylor J, Undem C, Sylvester JT, Shimoda LA (2012) Kinase dependent activation of voltage-gated Ca^{2+} channels by ET-1 in pulmonary arterial myocytes during chronic hypoxia. Am J Physiol Lung Cell Mol Physiol. 302(10):L1128–39.
38. Lucchesi PA, Berk BC (1995) Regulation of sodium-hydrogen exchange in vascular smooth muscle. Cardiovasc Res. 29: 172–7.
39. Berk BC, Taubman MB, Cragoe EJ Jr, Fenton JW 2nd, Griendling KK. (1990) Thrombin signal transduction mechanisms in rat vascular smooth muscle cells. Calcium and protein kinase C-dependent and -independent pathways. J Biol Chem. 265: 17334–40.
40. Touyz RM, Schiffrin EL (1997) Growth factors mediate intracellular signaling in vascular smooth muscle cells through protein kinase C-linked pathways. Hypertension. 30: 1440–7.
41. Ebata S, Muto S, Okada K, Nemoto J, Amemiya M, et al. (1999) Aldosterone activates Na^+/H^+ exchange in vascular smooth muscle cells by nongenomic and genomic mechanisms. Kidney Int. 56: 1400–12.
42. Koliakos G, Befani C, Paletas K, Kaloyianni M (2007) Effect of endothelin on sodium/hydrogen exchanger activity of human monocytes and atherosclerosis-related functions. Ann N Y Acad Sci. 1095: 274–91.
43. Walter R, Helmle-Kolb C, Forgo J, Binswanger U, Murer H (1995) Stimulation of Na^+/H^+ exchange activity by endothelin in opossum kidney cells. Pflugers Arch. 430: 137–44.
44. Guntupalli J, DuBose TD Jr (1994) Effects of endothelin on rat renal proximal tubule Na^+-Pi cotransport and Na^+/H^+ exchange. Am J Physiol. 266:F658–66.
45. Weigand LA, Sylvester JT, Shimoda LA (2006) Mechanisms of Endothelin-1-Induced Contraction in Pulmonary Arteries from Chronically Hypoxic Rats. Am J Physiol Lung Cell Mol Physiol. 290:L284-L290.
46. Shimoda LA, Sylvester JT, Booth GM, Shimoda TH, Meeker S, et al. (2001) Inhibition of voltage-gated K^+ currents by endothelin-1 in human pulmonary arterial myocytes. Am J Physiol Lung Cell Mol Physiol. 281:L1115–22.
47. Martiny-Baron G, Kazanietz MG, Mischak H, Blumberg PM, Kochs G, et al. (1993) Selective inhibition of protein kinase C isozymes by the indolocarbazole Go 6976. J Biol Chem. 268: 9194–7.
48. Shimoda LA, Sylvester JT, Sham JS (1998) Inhibition of voltage-gated K^+ current in rat intrapulmonary arterial myocytes by endothelin-1. Am J Physiol. 274:L842–53.
49. Muto S, Ebata S, Okada K, Saito T, Asano Y (2000) Glucocorticoid modulates Na^+/H^+ exchange activity in vascular smooth muscle cells by nongenomic and genomic mechanisms. Kidney Int. 57: 2319–33.
50. Mitsuka M, Berk BC (1991) Long-term regulation of Na^+-H^+ exchange in vascular smooth muscle cells: role of protein kinase C. Am J Physiol. 260:C562–9.
51. Danthuluri NR, Brock TA (1990) Endothelin receptor-coupling mechanisms in vascular smooth muscle: a role for protein kinase C. J Pharmacol Exp Ther. 254: 393–9.
52. Hubel CA, Highsmith RF (1995) Endothelin-induced changes in intracellular pH and Ca^{2+} in coronary smooth muscle: role of Na^+-H^+ exchange. Biochem J. 310 (Pt 3): 1013–20.
53. He JQ, Pi Y, Walker JW, Kamp TJ (2000) Endothelin-1 and photoreleased diacylglycerol increase L-type Ca^{2+} current by activation of protein kinase C in rat ventricular myocytes. J Physiol. 524 Pt 3: 807–20.
54. Bouallegue A, Daou GB, Srivastava AK (2007) Endothelin-1-induced signaling pathways in vascular smooth muscle cells. Curr Vasc Pharmacol. 5: 45–52.
55. Ivey ME, Osman N, Little PJ (2008) Endothelin-1 signalling in vascular smooth muscle: pathways controlling cellular functions associated with atherosclerosis. Atherosclerosis. 199: 237–47.
56. Griendling KK, Tsuda T, Alexander RW (1989) Endothelin stimulates diacylglycerol accumulation and activates protein kinase C in cultured vascular smooth muscle cells. J Biol Chem. 264: 8237–40.
57. Woodsome TP, Polzin A, Kitazawa K, Eto M, Kitazawa T (2006) Agonist- and depolarization-induced signals for myosin light chain phosphorylation and force generation of cultured vascular smooth muscle cells. J Cell Sci. 119: 1769–80.
58. Homma N, Nagaoka T, Morio Y, Ota H, Gebb SA, et al. (2007) Endothelin-1 and serotonin are involved in activation of RhoA/Rho kinase signaling in the chronically hypoxic hypertensive rat pulmonary circulation. J Cardiovasc Pharmacol. 50: 697–702.
59. Yang X, Huang HC, Yin H, Alpern RJ, Preisig PA (2007) RhoA required for acid-induced stress fiber formation and trafficking and activation of NHE3. Am J Physiol Renal Physiol. 293:F1054–64.
60. Tominaga T, Ishizaki T, Narumiya S, Barber DL (1998) p160ROCK mediates RhoA activation of Na-H exchange. Embo J. 17: 4712–22.
61. Tominaga T, Barber DL (1998) Na-H exchange acts downstream of RhoA to regulate integrin-induced cell adhesion and spreading. Mol Biol Cell. 9: 2287–303.
62. Janakidevi K, Fisher MA, Del Vecchio PJ, Tiruppathi C, Figge J, et al. (1992) Endothelin-1 stimulates DNA synthesis and proliferation of pulmonary artery smooth muscle cells. Am J Physiol. 263:C1295–301.
63. Wedgwood S, Dettman RW, Black SM (2001) ET-1 stimulates pulmonary arterial smooth muscle cell proliferation via induction of reactive oxygen species. Am J Physiol Lung Cell Mol Physiol. 281:L1058–67.
64. Aversa CR, Oparil S, Caro J, Li H, Sun SD, et al. (1997) Hypoxia stimulates human preproendothelin-1 promoter activity in transgenic mice. Am J Physiol. 273:L848–55.
65. Elton TS, Oparil S, Taylor GR, Hicks PH, Yang RH, et al. (1992) Normobaric hypoxia stimulates endothelin-1 gene expression in the rat. Am J Physiol. 263:R1260–4.
66. Li H, Chen SJ, Chen YF, Meng QC, Durand J, et al. (1994) Enhanced endothelin-1 and endothelin receptor gene expression in chronic hypoxia. J Appl Physiol. 77: 1451–9.
67. Li H, Elton TS, Chen YF, Oparil S (1994) Increased endothelin receptor gene expression in hypoxic rat lung. Am J Physiol. 266:L553–60.
68. Chen SJ, Chen YF, Opgenorth TJ, Wessale JL, Meng QC, et al. (1997) The orally active nonpeptide endothelin A-receptor antagonist A-127722 prevents and reverses hypoxia-induced pulmonary hypertension and pulmonary vascular remodeling in Sprague-Dawley rats. J Cardiovasc Pharmacol. 29: 713–25.
69. Eddahibi S, Raffestin B, Clozel M, Levame M, Adnot S (1995) Protection from pulmonary hypertension with an orally active endothelin receptor antagonist in hypoxic rats. Am J Physiol. 268: H828–35.
70. Stewart DJ, Levy RD, Cernacek P, Langleben D (1991) Increased plasma endothelin-1 in pulmonary hypertension: marker or mediator of disease? Ann Intern Med. 114: 464–9.

Complement C3 Deficiency Attenuates Chronic Hypoxia-Induced Pulmonary Hypertension in Mice

Eileen M. Bauer[1], Han Zheng[1], Suzy Comhair[4,5], Serpil Erzurum[4,5], Timothy R. Billiar[1], Philip M. Bauer[1,2,3]*

1 Department of Surgery, University of Pittsburgh School of Medicine, Pittsburgh, Pennsylvania, United States of America, 2 Department of Pharmacology and Chemical Biology, University of Pittsburgh School of Medicine, Pittsburgh, Pennsylvania, United States of America, 3 Vascular Medicine Institute, University of Pittsburgh School of Medicine, Pittsburgh, Pennsylvania, United States of America, 4 Department of Pathobiology, Lerner Research Institute, Cleveland Clinic, Cleveland, Ohio, United States of America, 5 Respiratory Institute, Cleveland Clinic, Cleveland, Ohio, United States of America

Abstract

Background: Evidence suggests a role of both innate and adaptive immunity in the development of pulmonary arterial hypertension. The complement system is a key sentry of the innate immune system and bridges innate and adaptive immunity. To date there are no studies addressing a role for the complement system in pulmonary arterial hypertension.

Methodology/Principal Findings: Immunofluorescent staining revealed significant C3d deposition in lung sections from IPAH patients and C57Bl6/J wild-type mice exposed to three weeks of chronic hypoxia to induce pulmonary hypertension. Right ventricular systolic pressure and right ventricular hypertrophy were increased in hypoxic vs. normoxic wild-type mice, which were attenuated in C3−/− hypoxic mice. Likewise, pulmonary vascular remodeling was attenuated in the C3−/− mice compared to wild-type mice as determined by the number of muscularized peripheral arterioles and morphometric analysis of vessel wall thickness. The loss of C3 attenuated the increase in interleukin-6 and intracellular adhesion molecule-1 expression in response to chronic hypoxia, but not endothelin-1 levels. In wild-type mice, but not C3−/− mice, chronic hypoxia led to platelet activation as assessed by bleeding time, and flow cytometry of platelets to determine cell surface P-selectin expression. In addition, tissue factor expression and fibrin deposition were increased in the lungs of WT mice in response to chronic hypoxia. These pro-thrombotic effects of hypoxia were abrogated in C3−/− mice.

Conclusions: Herein, we provide compelling genetic evidence that the complement system plays a pathophysiologic role in the development of PAH in mice, promoting pulmonary vascular remodeling and a pro-thrombotic phenotype. In addition we demonstrate C3d deposition in IPAH patients suggesting that complement activation plays a role in the development of PAH in humans.

Editor: Masuko Ushio-Fukai, University of Illinois at Chicago, United States of America

Funding: This work was supported by National Institutes of Health grants HL085134 (PMB), HL081064 (SE), HL60917 (SE) and by a Pilot Project Program in Hemostasis and Vascular Biology grant from the University of Pittsburgh Vascular Medicine Institute (PMB). The funders had no role in study design, data collection and analysis, decision to publish, or preparation of the manuscript.

Competing Interests: The authors have declared that no competing interests exist.

* E-mail: bauerpm@upmc.edu

Introduction

Pulmonary arterial hypertension (PAH) is a progressive disease characterized by increased pulmonary vascular resistance and pulmonary arterial pressure leading to right heart failure [1]. The pathogenesis of PAH is complex involving pulmonary vasoconstriction, remodeling of the pulmonary vascular wall, and *in situ* thrombosis [2]. It is becoming increasingly recognized that immune system activation and inflammation play important roles in the pathogenesis of PAH [3].

The complement system is a key sentry of innate immunity acting as a first line of defense against injurious stimuli and invading pathogens [4]. It may be activated by the classical, alternative or lectin pathways. All three pathways converge at the level of C3 cleavage and activation leading to the production of opsonins (C3b), the membrane attack complex (C5b-9) [5], and anaphylatoxins (C3a and C5a). The anaphylatoxins are particularly interesting as potential effectors in PAH because they recruit inflammatory cells, cause degranulation of mast cells, increase vascular permeability and stimulate pulmonary vascular smooth muscle contraction [6,7,8]. In addition, complement components C3 and C4a have been implicated as biomarkers of idiopathic pulmonary hypertension [9,10]. To date, however, there are no studies exploring a role for complement activation in PAH. In this study we utilized C3−/− mice to explore the role of complement in chronic hypoxia (CH)-induced PAH in mice.

Methods

Ethics Statement

Human tissue and cell samples were obtained in compliance with Cleveland Clinic and University of Pittsburgh institutional review board guidelines as previously described [11,12,13,14]. Animal studies were approved by the University of Pittsburgh

Institutional Animal Care and Use Committee (University of Pittsburgh Animal Assurance # A3187-01).

Mice

C57Bl/6J (stock #000664) and C3 −/− mice (stock #003641) were purchased from Jackson Laboratories. C3 −/− mice are reported by the Jackson Laboratories to be backcrossed to the C57BL/6J background for 7 generations. All experiments were performed on age-matched male mice between 8–10 weeks old.

Materials

Complement component C3d antibody (AF2655), complement component C5a antibody (AF2150) and recombinant mouse complement component C5a (2150-C5) were from R&D Systems. Recombinant human complement C3a (204881) and recombinant human complement C5a (234397) were from Calbiochem. Tissue factor antibody (SATF-IG) was from Affinity Biologicals.

Chronic hypoxia-induced pulmonary hypertension

Pulmonary hypertension was induced by housing mice under chronic hypoxic conditions ($FiO_2 = 0.10$, normobaric) for three weeks with age matched mice in normoxia serving as control.

Measurement of right ventricular systolic pressure (RVSP)

Mice were anesthetized with sodium pentobarbital (50 mg/kg i.p.) and ventilated via tracheotomy with room air (175 breaths/min, 175 µl tidal volume). Body temperature was monitored and regulated with a rectal probe and heating pad. Right ventricular systolic pressure (RVSP) was determined by placing a 1F solid state pressure transducing catheter (Millar Instruments Inc., Houston, TX) directly into the RV. Data were acquired using a PowerLab data acquisition system and LabChart Pro software (AD Instruments).

RV hypertrophy (RVH)

RVH was determined by the ratio of the weight of the RV to the left ventricle plus septum (Fulton index) as previously described [15].

Pulmonary vascular remodeling

Lung sections were stained against smooth muscle alpha actin antibody (1:100, DAKO) after deparaffinization and antigen retrieval. Pulmonary vascular remodeling was assessed by counting the number of partially and fully muscularized peripheral arterioles (35–100 mm) per high power field (200× total magnification). For each mouse, more than 20 high power fields were analyzed in multiple lung sections. Wall thickness of muscularized vessels was determined by measuring the thickness at 4 points on pulmonary arterioles using the Java-based image processing program: Image J (NIH).

Cultured Cells

Human pulmonary artery smooth muscle cells (hPASMC) [16] and human aortic smooth muscle cells (hASMC) [17] were isolated as previously described. hPASMC were grown in DMEM/F12 media supplemented with 10% FBS and penicillin/streptomycin and were maintained at 37°C and 5% CO_2. hASMC were maintained in SMC growth medium (Cell Applications, San Diego, CA). Cells were used between passage 4–9.

Cell Proliferation

Proliferation of hASMC and hPASMC was determined by measuring [^{3}H]-incorporation as previously described [18]. Briefly, cells were serum starved for 24 h in 12-well plates and treated with either 10 or 100 nM Human C3a or C5a with or without PDGF (10 ng/ml,Sigma P4056) for 24 h. During the last 16 hrs 0.2 µCi [^{3}H]thymidine was added. After the incubation period cells were washed twice with ice-cold PBS, and 1 ml of ice-cold 10% trichloroacetic acid (Sigma T0699) was added to each well for a 30-min incubation at 4°C, after which each well was washed with 1 ml of ice-cold 10% trichloroacetic acid. To each well 0.5 ml of 0.4 N NaOH, 0.1% (wt/vol) SDS was added, and the plates were incubated for 1 h at room temperature. The contents of each well were then transferred to 7 ml scintillation vials containing 4.5 ml of Pico-Fluor-15 scintillation mixture (ICN) and counted in a liquid scintillation spectrometer.

Bleeding Time

Mice were anesthetized with isoflurane and a cut was made 3 mm from the tip of the tail. After transection, the tail was placed in a beaker filled with 37°C phosphate buffered saline, and bleeding time was recorded. After bleeding succession another 30 sec was waited for possible rebleeding. Bleeding was stopped at 10 min and all tails were cauterized.

Immunohistochemistry

After sacrifice, mice were perfused intracardially with phosphate buffered saline to clear the vasculature of blood. After perfusing

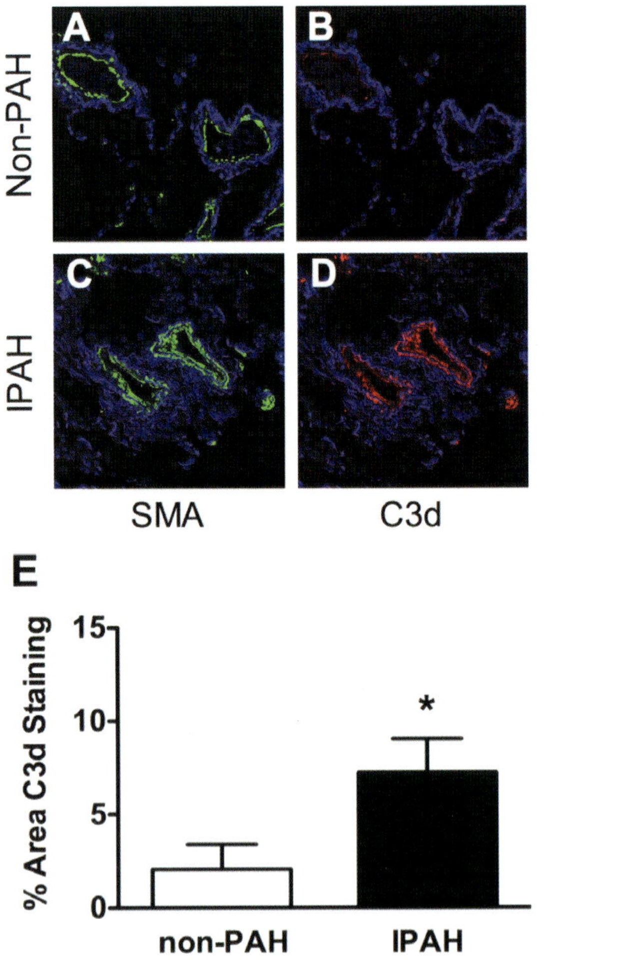

Figure 1. C3d deposition in human PAH. (A–D) Lung sections from non-PAH or IPAH patients (n = 3) were stained with α-C3d and α-SMA antibody and counterstained with DAPI to detect nuclei. Images shown are representative (E) Quantification of C3d staining in non-PAH and IPAH patients. Bars represent the mean ± SD (n = 4). *$P<0.05$.

the lungs via the trachea with 4% paraformaldehyde the trachea was tied off, the lungs excised, and kept for an additional 24 hrs in paraformaldehyde at 4°C. The tissue was paraffin embedded and sectioned (5 μm) by the University of Pittsburgh Research Histology Laboratory. Sections were warmed for 60 min at 56°C followed by deparaffinization in Xylene (3 times 3 min) and rehydrated to PBS (100% Ethanol 2×3 min, 90% Ethanol 1×3 min, 70% Ethanol 1×3 min and PBS 1×3 min). All slides were treated for antigen retrieval in citrate buffer followed by blocking and staining for either smooth muscle-α-actin (1:100 DAKO), fibrin (Nordic Immunology, polyclonal goat), Von Willebrand Factor (Santa Cruz, polyclonal rabbit), C3d (R&D Systems, goat) following manufacturer's recommendations and appropriate HRP- or fluorescently-labeled secondary antibodies. For morphometric analysis, the Vectastin Elite ABC DAB kit was used to visualize smooth muscle actin staining and images captured by light microspcopy. Fluorescently-labeled antibodies were detected by confocal microscopy using an Olympus Fluoview 1000. For all immunohistochemical staining a no primary control was used to confirm the specificity of the staining.

Quantification of C3d and Fibrin Deposition

Percent area of C3d and fibrin deposition was quantified using computer-assisted image analysis (Adobe Photoshop 5.0, NIH Image J) with the observer blinded as to tissue source.

ELISA

ELISA for endothelin-1 and intracellular adhesion molecule-1 were performed as per the manufacturer's instructions (R&D Systems).

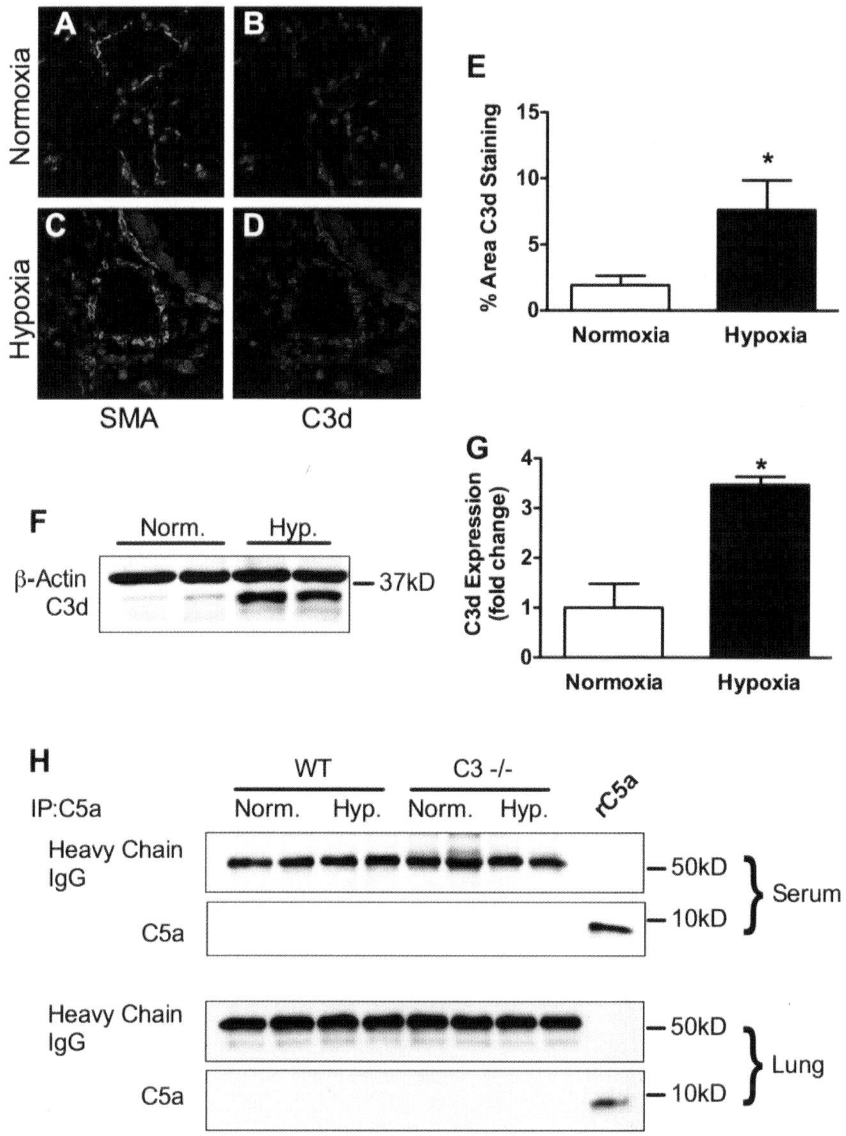

Figure 2. C3d deposition in chronic hypoxia-induced PH in mice. (A–D) Lungs from normoxic and hypoxic C57Bl/6J mice were stained with α-C3d and α-SMA antibody and counterstained with DAPI to detect nuclei(n = 4). (E) Quantification of C3d staining in WT vs. C3−/− mice in normoxia and hypoxia. Bars represent the mean ± SD (n = 4). **P*<0.05. (F) Representative Western blot for C3d in normoxic vs. hypoxic C57Bl/6J mice. (G) Quantification of Western blots for C3d in normoxic vs. hypoxic mice. Bars represent the mean ± SD (n = 4). **P*<0.05. (H) C5a was immunoprecipitated from lung or plasma of normoxic and hypoxic C57Bl/6J mice and analyzed by Western blot (rC5a = recombinant mouse C5a).

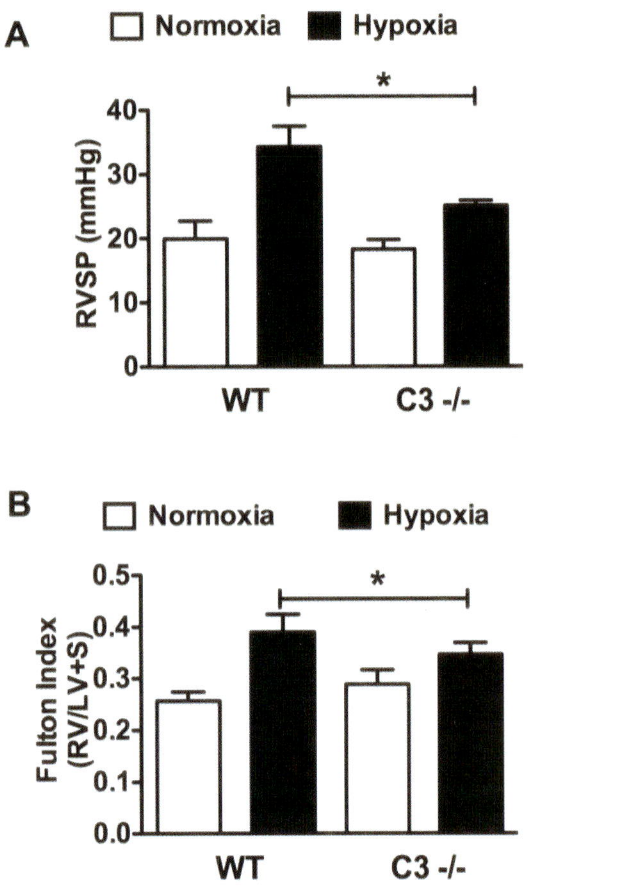

Figure 3. Genetic deletion of C3 attenuates CH-induced PAH in mice. WT or C3−/− mice were exposed to CH to induce PAH. After 3 weeks (A) RVSP and (B) RVH (Fulton index), were determined. Bars represent the mean ± SD (n = 8–12). *$P<0.05$.

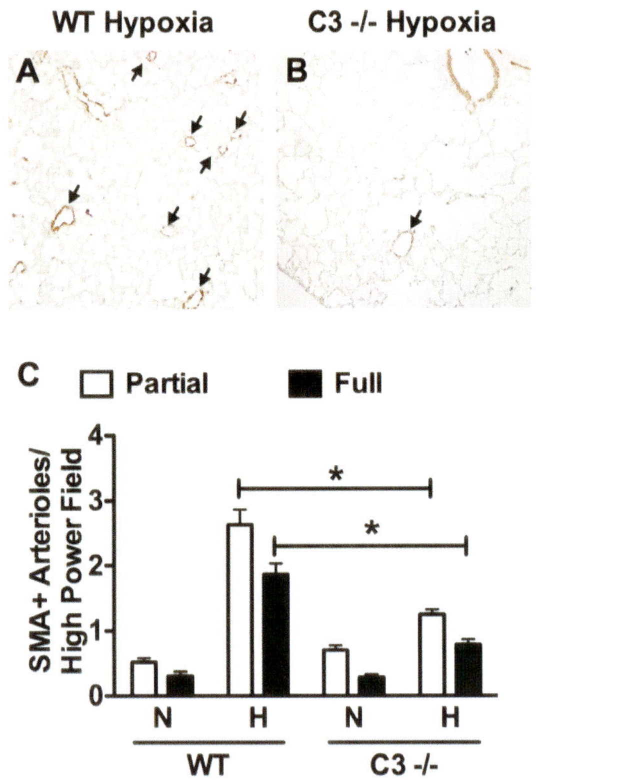

Figure 4. Loss of C3 attenuates muscularization of pulmonary arterioles in response to CH. (A–B) Representative photomicrographs of lungs stained against SMA from (A) hypoxic WT and (B) C3−/− mice. Arrows indicate muscularized arterioles. (C) Quantification of the number of partially and fully muscularized arterioles (<100 μm) per high power field (200× total magnification). Bars represent the mean ± SD (n = 4). *$P<0.05$.

Flow Cytometry

Mouse blood was obtained via cardiac puncture at the time of sacrifice using syringes containing 100 ul of citrate phosphate dextrose solution and spun at room temp for 15 min at 1000 rpm to obtain platelet rich plasma (PRP). PRP was transferred and labeled with PE-anti-mouse-CD41 and FITC-anti-mouse-CD62P (BD bioscience) antibodies following the manufacturer's protocol for "staining platelets for activation". PE-IgG1-k or FITC IgG1-λ were used as isotype control. Cells were analyzed by FACS (Guava-easy-cyte *HT) using Guava Express Pro 8.1 software, gating for CD41 positive cells (platelet marker).

Immunoprecipitation

C5a was immunoprecipitated from plasma or lung using anti-C5a antibody conjugated to protein A/G Dynal beads (Invitrogen) per the manufacturer's instructions [19].

Western blot

Tissue homogenates were separated by SDS PAGE and transferred to nitrocellulose membranes. Membranes were blocked in TBST (Tris buffered saline, 0.1% Tween 20), 5% non-fat dry milk for 30 min, followed by incubation in primary antibody. Membranes were washed in TBST before incubation for 1 h with horseradish peroxidase-conjugated secondary antibodies. Membranes were washed and developed using enhanced chemiluminescence substrate (Pierce). The intensity of the bands was quantified using Image J software (rsbweb.nih.gov/ij/).

Real time PCR

RNA was isolated after homogenization of snap frozen lungs using the RNeasy Mini Kit (Qiagen). RNA was reverse transcribed using random hexamers and reverse transcriptase enzyme (Applied Biosystems). Taqman primer/probe mix for interleukin-6, and β2 microglobulin were from Applied Biosystems. IL-6 expression was normalized to β2-microglobulin.

Statistical Analysis

Data were analyzed by Student's T-test when comparing two groups or by one-way ANOVA and Tukey's post-hoc test when comparing 3 or more groups. $P<0.05$ was considered significant.

Results

Complement deposition was assessed in lung sections of IPAH or control patients by immunofluorescent staining with anti-C3d antibody. We detected significant C3d deposition in the vascular wall of IPAH patients whereas it was nearly undetectable in control lungs (Fig. 1A–D). Likewise, C57BL/6J mice exposed to 3-weeks CH, but not normoxic controls, showed significant C3d deposition in the vascular wall (Fig. 2A–D). Quantification of C3d staining reveals that C3d deposition was increased approximately 3.5-fold in humans (Fig. 1E) and 3.9-fold in mouse (Fig. 2E).

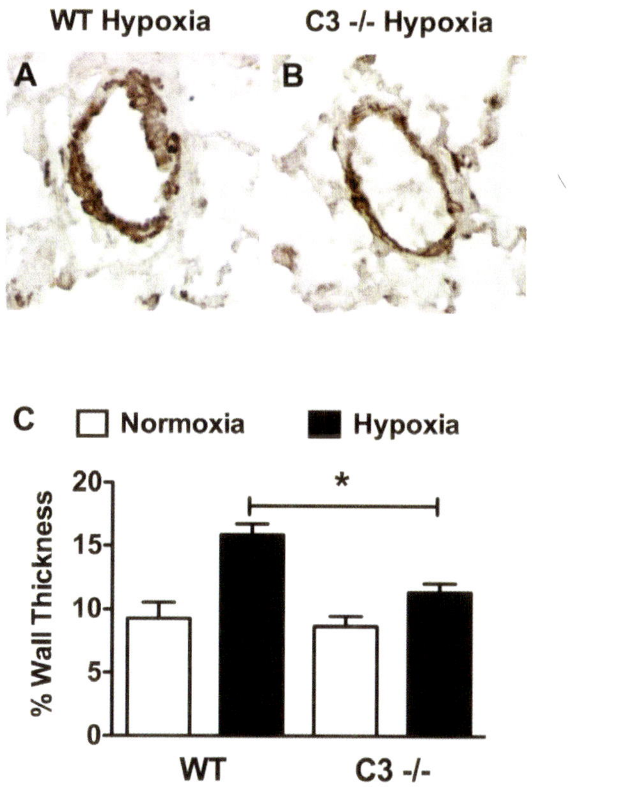

Figure 5. Loss of C3 attenuates vascular wall thickening in response to CH. (A–B) Representative photomicrographs of muscularized arterioles from (A) hypoxic WT and (B) hypoxic C3−/− mice. (C) Quantification of the % wall thickness of peripheral arterioles (<100 µm). Bars represent the mean ± SD (n = 4). *$P<0.05$.

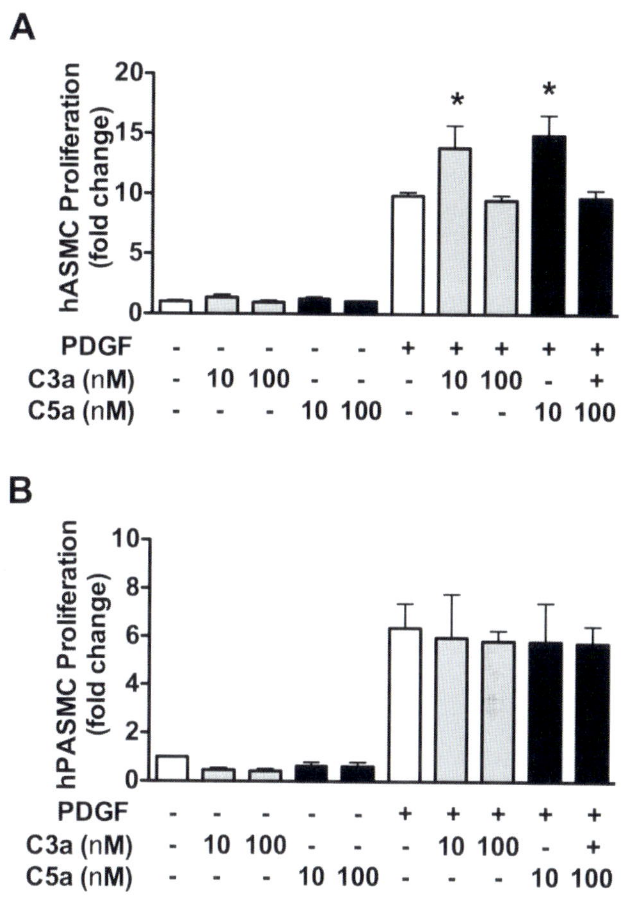

Figure 6. Complement C3a and C5a do not promote hPASMC proliferation. (**A**) **hASMC and** (**B**) hPASMC were treated with C3a or C5a with or without concurrent PDGF (10 ng/ml) stimulation and assessed for proliferation. Bars represent mean ± SD of four individual experiments. *$P<0.05$ vs. PDGF. n.s. = not significant.

Western blot analysis of lung from normoxic and hypoxic C57BL/6J mice showed a similar 3.5 fold increase in C3d in the hypoxic mouse lung (Fig. 2F–G). Immunoprecipitation of C5a from plasma or lung followed by Western blot analysis for C5a failed to detect the C5 cleavage product suggesting that activation of complement in chronic hypoxia is limited to C3 (Fig. 2H). Recombinant mouse C5a served as a positive control.

We next compared the effect of CH on WT vs. C3−/− mice. CH elicited a significant increase in RVSP in WT mice (19.9 mmHg, normoxia vs. 34.3 mmHg, hypoxia) that was attenuated in the C3−/− mice (18.3 mmHg, normoxia vs. 25.1 mm Hg, hypoxia) (Fig. 3A). Likewise, RVH, a normal sequelae of increased RVSP, was attenuated in C3−/− hypoxic mice as determined by the fulton index (0.390, WT vs. .346, C3−/−) (Fig. 3B).

Increased peripheral vascular resistance leading to elevated RVSP and RVH is in part caused by pulmonary vascular remodeling characterized by the muscularization and increased wall thickness of small (>100 µm) non-muscular arterioles. C3−/− hypoxic mice showed significantly less pulmonary vascular remodeling compared to WT hypoxic mice. SMA staining of the lung revealed significantly less muscularization of small peripheral arterioles in hypoxic C3−/− mice vs. WT mice (Fig. 4). Likewise, morphometric analysis of small peripheral arterioles revealed significantly less thickening of the vessel wall in C3−/− mice vs. WT mice (Fig. 5). Previous studies show that C3a, a cleavage product of C3, stimulates aortic smooth muscle cells [20] and genetic deletion of C3a receptor or C5a receptor attenuates neointimal hyperplasia and vascular smooth muscle cell proliferation after arterial injury. To confirm this finding we stimulated human aortic smooth muscle cells with C3a or C5a in the presence or absence of platelet-derived growth factor. In our hands C3a and C5a alone had no effect on hASMC proliferation, but enhanced PDGF-stimulated hASMC proliferation at 10 nm. Interestingly, a higher concentration of C3a or C5a (100 nM) had no effect on PDGF-stimulated hASMC (Fig. 6A). In order to determine whether C3a or C5a has a similar effect on vascular smooth muscle cells in the pulmonary vasculature, hPASMC were exposed to varying concentrations of C3a or C5a ± PDGF. Neither C3a nor C5a had any effect on hPASMC proliferation alone or in the presence of PDGF (Fig. 6B).

Endothelial dysfunction and inflammation contribute to the development of PH and are promoted by complement activation. Among inflammatory cytokines, interleukin-6 (IL-6) has recently been shown to play a prominent role in the development of pulmonary hypertension. In WT mice CH induced an approximate 2-fold increase in IL-6 mRNA at three weeks that was abrogated in C3 −/− mice (Fig. 7A). In terms of endothelial dysfunction, adhesion molecules and vasoconstrictors play important roles in PH. We observed increases in lung intracellular adhesion molecule 1 (ICAM-1) and plasma endothelin-1 (ET-1) in WT mice exposed to CH. Interestingly, while the increase in

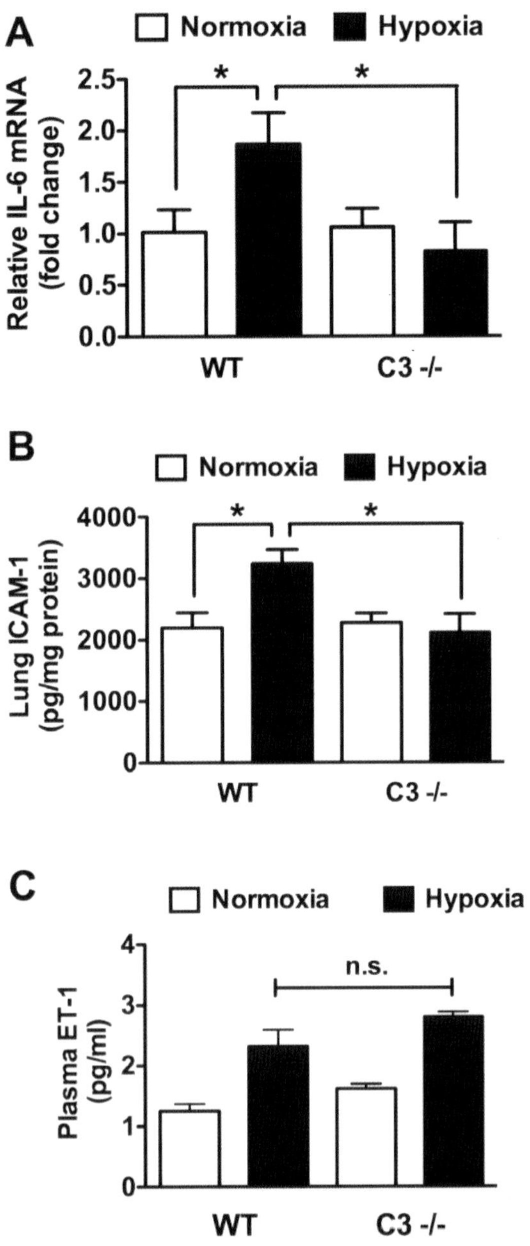

Figure 7. Markers of Inflammation and endothelial dysfunction in WT vs. C3 −/− mice. (A) IL-6 mRNA was measured by quantitative rtPCR in RNA prepared from normoxic or hypoxic WT and C3−/− lungs. IL-6 levels were normalized to the house keeping gene β2-microglobulin. (B) ICAM-1 was quantified by ELISA in lung homogenates from normoxic or hypoxic WT or C3−/− mice. (C) ET-1 was quantified by ELISA in plasma from normoxic or hypoxic WT or C3−/− mice. Bars represent mean ± SD (n = 4) for A–C. *$P<0.05$.

ICAM-1 was abrogated in C3 −/− mice the increase in ET-1 was not (Fig. 7B–C).

The complement system interacts with the coagulation cascade and C3 −/− mice exhibit abnormal platelet activation. Therefore, we were interested in determining whether the loss of C3 would protect against platelet activation caused by CH. In normoxia bleeding time, a reflection of platelet activation, was significantly prolonged in C3 −/− mice as previously described [21]. In WT mice, CH led to a significant decrease in bleeding time compared to normoxic mice (Fig. 8A). In contrast, CH had no effect on bleeding time in C3−/− mice. In concordance with decreased bleeding time, the fraction of P-selectin (a marker of activated platelets) positive platelets in hypoxic WT mice, but not C3−/− mice, was significantly increased compared to normoxic control as determined by flow cytometry (Fig. 8B–F).

Previous studies demonstrate that CH in mice results in increased TF expression and enhanced fibrin deposition [22,23]. Therefore, we further explored the interaction of the complement system with the coagulation cascade by examining TF expression and fibrin deposition in WT vs. C3−/− mice. In response to 3-weeks of CH, TF expression was significantly increased in WT but not C3 −/− mice (Fig. 9A,B). Likewise, CH increased fibrin deposition in WT mice but had no effect on fibrin deposition in C3−/− mice (Fig. 10A,B). Fibrin colocalized with vWF confirming that fibrin deposition was primarily within the vessel lumen (Fig. 10C).

Discussion

The complement system is an evolutionarily ancient and highly complex biological system playing a major role in body defense as part of the innate and adaptive immune systems. The complement system consists of three activation pathways that merge at the proteolytic cleavage of C3, the nexus of the complement system. Herein, we provide for the first time genetic evidence that the complement system contributes to the development of PAH in mice. Genetic deletion of C3 caused significant attenuation of PAH in the mouse model of CH-induced PAH. This was associated with attenuated pulmonary vascular remodeling and reversal of the pro-coagulant phenotype induced by CH exposure. Furthermore, we document the deposition of C3d, a stable C3 cleavage product, in the pulmonary vasculature of humans and mice with PAH. While genetic deficiency may lead to chronic phenotypic changes which may be the true pathogenetic factors, our data strongly support a role for C3 in the pathogenesis of PH.

Activation of C3 also leads to downstream cleavage of C5 and C5 cleavage has been shown to take place in the absence of C3 by alternative mechanisms [19]. Our results suggest that C5 does not play an active role in chronic hypoxia-induced PH since we were unable to detect the C5 cleavage product C5a in plasma or lung tissue. That being said, we can not rule out the possibility that C5 cleavage takes place at earlier time points and then dissipates by three weeks.

The loss of C3 led to decreased pulmonary vascular remodeling in response to CH. The complement component C3a stimulates the proliferation of systemic vascular smooth muscle cells [20] and genetic deletion of C3a receptor or C5a receptor attenuates neointimal hyperplasia and vascular smooth muscle cell proliferation after arterial injury [24]. Our studies confirm a role for C3a and C5a in enhancing PDGF-stimulated human aortic smooth muscle cell proliferation. In contrast, C3a or C5a had no effect on the proliferation of hPASMC. These data suggest that either different complement components are responsible for promoting hPASMC proliferation or that complement activation contributes to pulmonary vascular remodeling by indirect means. Cobra venom factor, which causes rapid activation of C3 (and then depletion), elicits acute pulmonary vasoconstriction leading to a transient increase in pulmonary arterial pressure [25]. Our data suggest more chronic complement activation, which could contribute to sustained vasoconstriction and pulmonary vascular remodeling. In addition, TF as well as chronic exposure to fibrin stimulates hPASMC proliferation [26]. Finally, ICAM-1 is a ligand for lymphocyte function-associated antigen 1 (LFA-1), a receptor found on leukocytes [27]. Activated leukocytes bind to

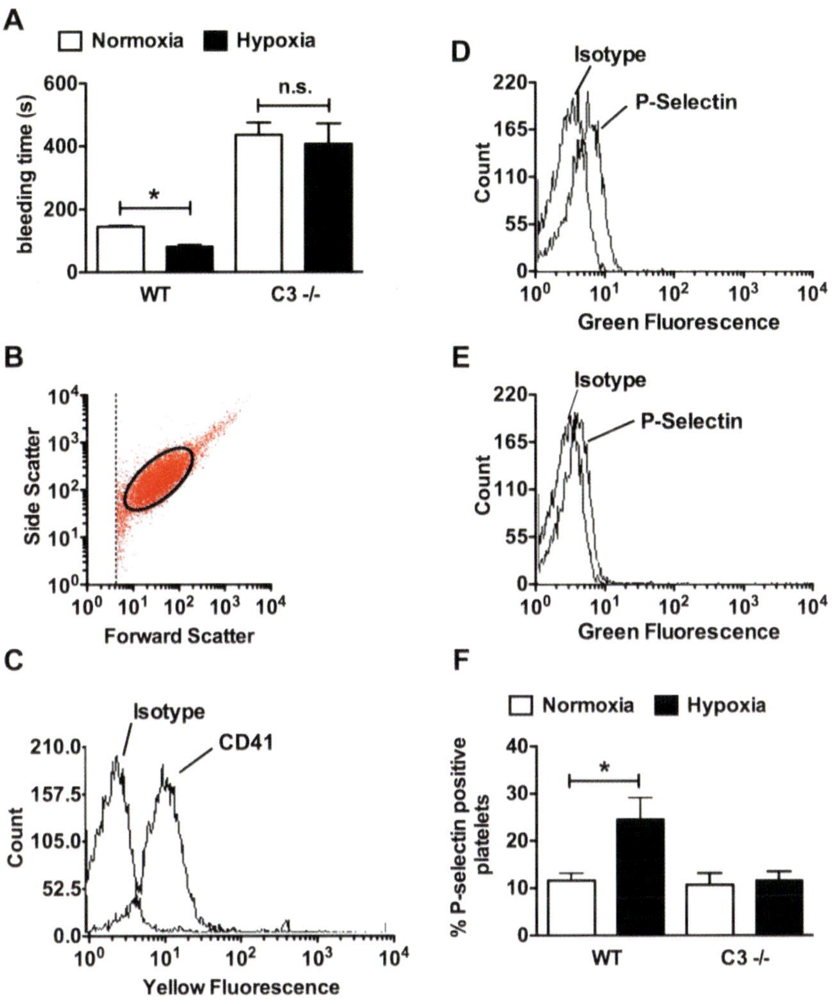

Figure 8. Loss of C3 prevents platelet activation caused by CH. (A) Bleeding time of WT and C3−/− mice exposed to normoxia or CH (n = 5–7). (B) Scatter plot showing platelet population in platelet rich plasma. All experiments were similarly gated to the area encircled. (C) Flow cytometry histogram demonstrating that the gated cell population is positive for the platelet marker CD41. (D–E) Representative flow cytometry histograms of platelets from (D) hypoxic WT or (E) hypoxic C3−/− mice stained with P-selectin antibody or isotype control. (F) Percent P-selectin positive platelets in PRP isolated from normoxic and hypoxic WT or C3−/− mice (n = 6). Bars represent mean ± SD. $^*P<0.05$; n.s. = not significant.

ECs via ICAM-1/LFA-1 allowing them to transmigrate into tissues [28]. Also C3a and C5a are potent chemoattractants promoting the recruitment of leukocytes. This suggests an additional mechanism by which complement may promote pulmonary vascular remodeling.

IL-6 has recently been shown to play a prominent role in the development of pulmonary hypertension. Overexpression of IL-6 promotes PH in mice, where as IL-6 knockout mice are protected from hypoxia-induced PH [29,30]. In addition, elevated serum IL-6 concentrations have been reported in patients with idiopathic PH or PH associated with inflammatory diseases such as scleroderma and lupus [31,32,33]. Our data suggest that complement activation may play a role in stimulating IL-6 production in pulmonary hypertension since IL-6 expression was increased in hypoxic WT mice but not in C3 −/− mice.

In contrast to IL-6 we found that the ET-1 was increased in response to CH in both WT and C3 −/− mice. ET-1 is a potent vasoconstrictor and is a well established contributor to human PAH as evidenced by the fact that the ET-1 receptor antagonist, Bosentan, is currently used to treat PAH patients [34]. Clearly more studies need to be performed to determine whether complement inhibition might be a therapeutic avenue for treating PH. However, the fact that loss of C3 attenuates PH without affecting ET-1 levels leads to the intriguing possibility that complement inhibition might make an effective combination therapy with Bosentan.

Complement contributes to coagulation by augmenting inflammation, promoting the TF coagulation pathway, activating platelets, increasing TF expression, and modifying the activity of mast cells and basophils [35]. C3 −/− mice also exhibit defective platelet activation in response to the thrombin receptor agonist PAR4 peptide, but not collagen or ADP, suggesting a role for complement in thrombin activated platelet aggregation. Interestingly, pulmonary arterial hypertensive patients have increased platelet membrane expression of PAR1 and PAR-mediated surface exposure of P-selectin which may represent increased propensity to thrombosis [36]. Experimental models have also implicated platelet abnormalities in the thrombotic tendency of PAH. In the mouse model of hypoxia-induced PAH a small number of *in situ* vascular thrombi are found in the pulmonary vasculature [37,38] and the development of monocrotaline-induced PAH in the rat is attenuated by inducing thrombocyto-

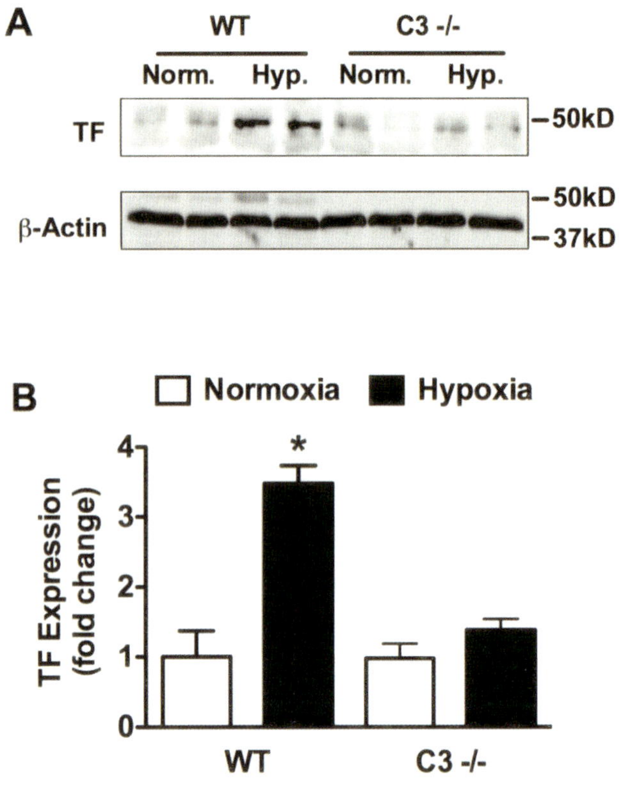

Figure 9. Loss of C3 prevents hypoxia-induced TF upregulation. (A) Representative Western blot analysis of normoxic or hypoxic WT and C3−/− lungs for TF expression. (B) Densitometric anlysis of Western blots from (A). Bars represent the mean ± SD (n = 4 animals per group). *$P<0.05$.

penia [39]. There are only a few clinical studies of platelet function and activation in patients with PAH. A case report described thrombocytosis in association with increased pulmonary vascular-specific fibrin generation and platelet activation in a patient with PAH [40]. Moreover, urinary metabolites of thromboxane A2 (TxA2) are increased in PAH vs control subjects [41]. This is consistent with significant platelet activation since TxA2 production is predominantly from platelets.

In our experiments CH led to decreased bleeding time and increased surface expression of P-selectin (CD62P) on platelets in WT mice providing evidence of platelet activation in PAH. In contrast, C3−/− mice had prolonged bleeding time in normoxia as previously described, and hypoxia had no effect on bleeding time or surface P-selectin expression in these mice. These data suggest that complement activation contributes to platelet activation in CH-induced pulmonary hypertension.

In addition to platelet activation, CH led to increased TF expression and fibrin deposition in WT mice but not C3−/− mice. TF is a procoagulant protein that triggers the extrinsic coagulation cascade leading to the generation of thrombin and conversion of fibrinogen to fibrin. Independent of its procoagulant activity TF also stimulates vascular cell migration and proliferation [42,43]. Multiple lines of evidence suggest that the TF pathway may be involved in the pathogenesis of PAH. In humans, increased pulmonary expression of TF and an increase in TF-bearing microparticles have been observed [44,45]. TF is also expressed in pulmonary plexiform lesions in humans and in a rat model of severe pulmonary hypertension [46,47]. Additionally, TF expression is strongly induced by hypoxia, promoting pulmonary fibrin deposition and pulmonary *in situ* thrombosis [22,23,48,49].

While there is little thrombosis per se in the mouse model of CH-induced PAH, increased fibrin deposition in WT but not C3 −/− mice demonstrate that, in CH, complement contributes to a pro-thrombotic environment. In addition, like TF, fibrin

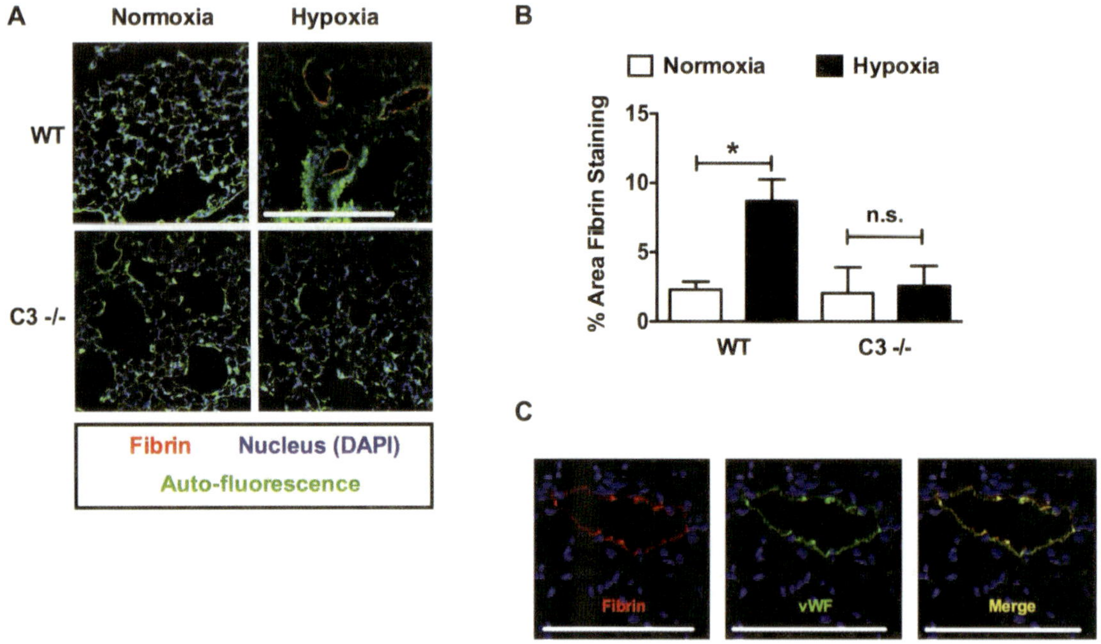

Figure 10. Decreased fibrin deposition in hypoxic C3−/− mice. (A) Representative images of lung sections from normoxic or hypoxic WT or C3 −/− mice stained for fibrin(ogen) and nuclei (DAPI). Scale bar represents 150 μm. (B) % Area fibrin staining per total lung area (n = 4) in hypoxic or normoxic WT or C3−/− mice. (C) Representative photomicrograph of WT hypoxic mouse lung showing colocalization (yellow to orange) of Fibrin (green) and vWF (red). Scale bar represents 50 μm. (A, B, E). Bars represent the mean ± SD. *$P<0.05$; n.s. = not significant.

enhances hPASMC proliferation suggesting that fibrin deposition may play a role in pulmonary vascular remodeling [26]. It is also interesting that activation of the coagulation cascade leads to activation of the complement system via cleavage of C3 and C5 [50]. This suggests the intriguing possibility that in PAH there exists a cycle of complement and coagulation system activation, each promoting the other.

In conclusion, our data provide the first evidence for a direct role of the complement system in the development of pulmonary arterial hypertension. These seminal findings have the potential to open up new areas of PAH research as well as novel therapeutic avenues in the treatment of this deadly disease.

Author Contributions

Conceived and designed the experiments: PMB EMB TRB. Performed the experiments: EMB PMB HZ. Analyzed the data: EMB PMB. Contributed reagents/materials/analysis tools: SC SE TRB. Wrote the paper: PMB EMB.

References

1. D'Alonzo GE, Barst RJ, Ayres SM, Bergofsky EH, Brundage BH, et al. (1991) Survival in patients with primary pulmonary hypertension. Results from a national prospective registry. Ann Intern Med 115: 343–349.
2. Humbert M, Morrell NW, Archer SL, Stenmark KR, MacLean MR, et al. (2004) Cellular and molecular pathobiology of pulmonary arterial hypertension. J Am Coll Cardiol 43: 13S–24S.
3. Mathew R (2010) Inflammation and pulmonary hypertension. Cardiol Rev 18: 67–72.
4. Markiewski MM, Lambris JD (2007) The role of complement in inflammatory diseases from behind the scenes into the spotlight. Am J Pathol 171: 715–727.
5. Pangburn MK, Rawal N (2002) Structure and function of complement C5 convertase enzymes. Biochem Soc Trans 30: 1006–1010.
6. Bjork J, Hugli TE, Smedegard G (1985) Microvascular effects of anaphylatoxins C3a and C5a. J Immunol 134: 1115–1119.
7. Morel DR, Zapol WM, Thomas SJ, Kitain EM, Robinson DR, et al. (1987) C5a and thromboxane generation associated with pulmonary vaso- and broncho-constriction during protamine reversal of heparin. Anesthesiology 66: 597–604.
8. Morganroth ML, Schoeneich SO, Till GO, Ward PA, Horvath SJ, et al. (1990) C3a57–77, a C-terminal peptide, causes thromboxane-dependent pulmonary vascular constriction in isolated perfused rat lungs. Am Rev Respir Dis 141: 296–300.
9. Abdul-Salam VB, Paul GA, Ali JO, Gibbs SR, Rahman D, et al. (2006) Identification of plasma protein biomarkers associated with idiopathic pulmonary arterial hypertension. Proteomics 6: 2286–2294.
10. Zhang J, Zhang Y, Li N, Liu Z, Xiong C, et al. (2009) Potential diagnostic biomarkers in serum of idiopathic pulmonary arterial hypertension. Respir Med 103: 1801–1806.
11. Aldred MA, Comhair SA, Varella-Garcia M, Asosingh K, Xu W, et al. (2010) Somatic chromosome abnormalities in the lungs of patients with pulmonary arterial hypertension. Am J Respir Crit Care Med 182: 1153–1160.
12. Fijalkowska I, Xu W, Comhair SA, Janocha AJ, Mavrakis LA, et al. (2010) Hypoxia inducible-factor1alpha regulates the metabolic shift of pulmonary hypertensive endothelial cells. Am J Pathol 176: 1130–1138.
13. Masri FA, Xu W, Comhair SA, Asosingh K, Koo M, et al. (2007) Hyperproliferative apoptosis-resistant endothelial cells in idiopathic pulmonary arterial hypertension. Am J Physiol Lung Cell Mol Physiol 293: L548–554.
14. Xu W, Kaneko FT, Zheng S, Comhair SA, Janocha AJ, et al. (2004) Increased arginase II and decreased NO synthesis in endothelial cells of patients with pulmonary arterial hypertension. FASEB J 18: 1746–1748.
15. Zuckerbraun BS, Shiva S, Ifedigbo E, Mathier MA, Mollen KP, et al. (2010) Nitrite potently inhibits hypoxic and inflammatory pulmonary arterial hypertension and smooth muscle proliferation via xanthine oxidoreductase-dependent nitric oxide generation. Circulation 121: 98–109.
16. Aytekin M, Comhair SA, de la Motte C, Bandyopadhyay SK, Farver CF, et al. (2008) High levels of hyaluronan in idiopathic pulmonary arterial hypertension. Am J Physiol Lung Cell Mol Physiol 295: L789–799.
17. Phillippi JA, Klyachko EA, Kenny JPt, Eskay MA, Gorman RC, et al. (2009) Basal and oxidative stress-induced expression of metallothionein is decreased in ascending aortic aneurysms of bicuspid aortic valve patients. Circulation 119: 2498–2506.
18. Bauer PM, Buga GM, Ignarro LJ (2001) Role of p42/p44 mitogen-activated-protein kinase and p21waf1/cip1 in the regulation of vascular smooth muscle cell proliferation by nitric oxide. Proc Natl Acad Sci U S A 98: 12802–12807.
19. Huber-Lang M, Sarma JV, Zetoune FS, Rittirsch D, Neff TA, et al. (2006) Generation of C5a in the absence of C3: a new complement activation pathway. Nat Med 12: 682–687.
20. Verdeguer F, Castro C, Kubicek M, Pla D, Vila-Caballer M, et al. (2007) Complement regulation in murine and human hypercholesterolemia and role in the control of macrophage and smooth muscle cell proliferation. Cardiovasc Res 76: 340–350.
21. Gushiken FC, Han H, Li J, Rumbaut RE, Afshar-Kharghan V (2009) Abnormal platelet function in C3-deficient mice. J Thromb Haemost 7: 865–870.
22. Lawson CA, Yan SD, Yan SF, Liao H, Zhou YS, et al. (1997) Monocytes and tissue factor promote thrombosis in a murine model of oxygen deprivation. J Clin Invest 99: 1729–1738.
23. Yan SF, Zou YS, Gao Y, Zhai C, Mackman N, et al. (1998) Tissue factor transcription driven by Egr-1 is a critical mechanism of murine pulmonary fibrin deposition in hypoxia. Proc Natl Acad Sci U S A 95: 8298–8303.
24. Sakuma M, Morooka T, Wang Y, Shi C, Croce K, et al. (2010) The intrinsic complement regulator decay-accelerating factor modulates the biological response to vascular injury. Arterioscler Thromb Vasc Biol 30: 1196–1202.
25. Cheung AK, Parker CJ, Wilcox L (1989) Effects of two types of cobra venom factor on porcine complement activation and pulmonary artery pressure. Clin Exp Immunol 78: 299–306.
26. Firth AL, Yau J, White A, Chiles PG, Marsh JJ, et al. (2009) Chronic exposure to fibrin and fibrinogen differentially regulates intracellular Ca2+ in human pulmonary arterial smooth muscle and endothelial cells. Am J Physiol Lung Cell Mol Physiol 296: L979–986.
27. Rothlein R, Springer TA (1986) The requirement for lymphocyte function-associated antigen 1 in homotypic leukocyte adhesion stimulated by phorbol ester. J Exp Med 163: 1132–1149.
28. Yang L, Froio RM, Sciuto TE, Dvorak AM, Alon R, et al. (2005) ICAM-1 regulates neutrophil adhesion and transcellular migration of TNF-alpha-activated vascular endothelium under flow. Blood 106: 584–592.
29. Steiner MK, Syrkina OL, Kolliputi N, Mark EJ, Hales CA, et al. (2009) Interleukin-6 overexpression induces pulmonary hypertension. Circ Res 104: 236–244. 228p following 244.
30. Savale L, Tu L, Rideau D, Izziki M, Maitre B, et al. (2009) Impact of interleukin-6 on hypoxia-induced pulmonary hypertension and lung inflammation in mice. Respir Res 10: 6.
31. Soon E, Holmes AM, Treacy CM, Doughty NJ, Southgate L, et al. (2010) Elevated levels of inflammatory cytokines predict survival in idiopathic and familial pulmonary arterial hypertension. Circulation 122: 920–927.
32. Pendergrass SA, Hayes E, Farina G, Lemaire R, Farber HW, et al. (2010) Limited systemic sclerosis patients with pulmonary arterial hypertension show biomarkers of inflammation and vascular injury. PLoS One 5: e12106.
33. Nishimaki T, Aotsuka S, Kondo H, Yamamoto K, Takasaki Y, et al. (1999) Immunological analysis of pulmonary hypertension in connective tissue diseases. J Rheumatol 26: 2357–2362.
34. Rubin LJ, Badesch DB, Barst RJ, Galie N, Black CM, et al. (2002) Bosentan therapy for pulmonary arterial hypertension. N Engl J Med 346: 896–903.
35. Markiewski MM, Nilsson B, Ekdahl KN, Mollnes TE, Lambris JD (2007) Complement and coagulation: strangers or partners in crime? Trends Immunol 28: 184–192.
36. Maeda NY, Carvalho JH, Otake AH, Mesquita SM, Bydlowski SP, et al. (2010) Platelet protease-activated receptor 1 and membrane expression of P-selectin in pulmonary arterial hypertension. Thromb Res 125: 38–43.
37. Cathcart MC, Tamosiuniene R, Chen G, Neilan TG, Bradford A, et al. (2008) Cyclooxygenase-2-linked attenuation of hypoxia-induced pulmonary hypertension and intravascular thrombosis. J Pharmacol Exp Ther 326: 51–58.
38. White TA, Witt TA, Pan S, Mueske CS, Kleppe LS, et al. (2009) Tissue Factor Pathway Inhibitor Overexpression Inhibits Hypoxia-induced Pulmonary Hypertension. Am J Respir Cell Mol Biol.
39. Ganey PE, Sprugel KH, White SM, Wagner JG, Roth RA (1988) Pulmonary hypertension due to monocrotaline pyrrole is reduced by moderate thrombocytopenia. Am J Physiol 255: H1165–1172.
40. Rostagno C, Prisco D, Abbate R, Poggesi L (1991) Pulmonary hypertension associated with long-standing thrombocytosis. Chest 99: 1303–1305.
41. Christman BW, McPherson CD, Newman JH, King GA, Bernard GR, et al. (1992) An imbalance between the excretion of thromboxane and prostacyclin metabolites in pulmonary hypertension. N Engl J Med 327: 70–75.
42. Cirillo P, Cali G, Golino P, Calabro P, Forte L, et al. (2004) Tissue factor binding of activated factor VII triggers smooth muscle cell proliferation via extracellular signal-regulated kinase activation. Circulation 109: 2911–2916.
43. Sato Y, Asada Y, Marutsuka K, Hatakeyama K, Sumiyoshi A (1996) Tissue factor induces migration of cultured aortic smooth muscle cells. Thromb Haemost 75: 389–392.
44. Altman R, Scazziota A, Rouvier J, Gurfinkel E, Favaloro R, et al. (1996) Coagulation and fibrinolytic parameters in patients with pulmonary hypertension. Clin Cardiol 19: 549–554.

45. Bakouboula B, Morel O, Faure A, Zobairi F, Jesel L, et al. (2008) Procoagulant membrane microparticles correlate with the severity of pulmonary arterial hypertension. Am J Respir Crit Care Med 177: 536–543.
46. White RJ, Galaria II, Harvey J, Blaxall BC, Cool CD, et al. (2005) Tissue factor is induced in a rodent model of severe pulmonary hypertension characterized by neointimal lesions typical of human disease. Chest 128: 612S–613S.
47. White RJ, Meoli DF, Swarthout RF, Kallop DY, Galaria II, et al. (2007) Plexiform-like lesions and increased tissue factor expression in a rat model of severe pulmonary arterial hypertension. Am J Physiol Lung Cell Mol Physiol 293: L583–590.
48. Yan SF, Mackman N, Kisiel W, Stern DM, Pinsky DJ (1999) Hypoxia/Hypoxemia-Induced activation of the procoagulant pathways and the pathogenesis of ischemia-associated thrombosis. Arterioscler Thromb Vasc Biol 19: 2029–2035.
49. Yan SF, Pinsky DJ, Stern DM (2000) A pathway leading to hypoxia-induced vascular fibrin deposition. Semin Thromb Hemost 26: 479–483.
50. Amara U, Flierl MA, Rittirsch D, Klos A, Chen H, et al. Molecular intercommunication between the complement and coagulation systems. J Immunol 185: 5628–5636.

Poor Agreement between Pulmonary Capillary Wedge Pressure and Left Ventricular End-Diastolic Pressure in a Veteran Population

Abbas Bitar[1], Mona Selej[2], Islam Bolad[3,4], Tim Lahm[2,4]*

1 Department of Medicine, Internal Medicine Residency Program, Krannert Institute of Cardiology, Indiana University, Indianapolis, Indiana, United States of America, **2** Department of Medicine, Division of Pulmonary, Allergy, Critical Care, Occupational and Sleep Medicine, Krannert Institute of Cardiology, Indiana University, Indianapolis, Indiana, United States of America, **3** Department of Medicine, Krannert Institute of Cardiology, Indiana University, Indianapolis, Indiana, United States of America, **4** Richard L. Roudebush Veterans Affairs Medical Center, Indianapolis, Indiana, United States of America

Abstract

Background: Accurate determination of left ventricular filling pressure is essential for differentiation of pre-capillary pulmonary hypertension (PH) from pulmonary venous hypertension (PVH). Previous data suggest only a poor correlation between left ventricular end-diastolic pressure (LVEDP) and its commonly used surrogate, the pulmonary capillary wedge pressure (PCWP). However, no data exist on the diagnostic accuracy of PCWP in veterans. Furthermore, the effects of age and comorbidities on the PCWP-LVEDP relationship remain unknown.

Methods: We investigated the PCWP-LVEDP relationship in 101 patients undergoing simultaneous right and left heart catherization at a large VA hospital. PCWP performance was evaluated using correlation and Bland-Altman analyses. Area under Receiver Operating Characteristics curves (AUROC) for PCWP were determined.

Results: PCWP-LVEDP correlation was moderate ($r = 0.57$). PCWP-LVEDP calibration was poor (Bland-Altman limits of agreement −17.2 to 11.4 mmHg; mean bias −2.87 mmHg). 59 patients (58.4%) had pulmonary hypertension; 15 (25.4%) of those met pre-capillary PH criteria based on PCWP. However, if LVEDP was used instead of PCWP, 7/15 patients (46.6%) met criteria for PVH rather than pre-capillary PH. When restricting analysis to patients with a mean pulmonary artery pressure of ≥25 mmHg and pulmonary vascular resistance of >3 Wood units ($n = 22$), 10 patients (45.4%) were classified as pre-capillary PH based on PCWP ≤15 mmHg. However, if LVEDP was used, 4/10 patients (40%) were reclassified as PVH. Among patients with any type of pulmonary hypertension, PCWP discriminated moderately between high and normal LVEDP (AUROC, 0.81; 95%CI 0.69–0.94). PCWP-LVEDP correlation was particularly poor in patients with COPD or obesity.

Conclusion: Reliance on PCWP rather than LVEDP results in misclassification of veterans as having pre-capillary PH rather than PVH in almost 50% of cases. This is clinically relevant, as misclassification may lead to inappropriate therapies and adverse events.

Editor: Antonio Abbate, Virginia Commonwealth University, United States of America

Funding: This research was funded by Indiana University and the Richard L. Roudebush Veterans Affairs Medical Center. The funders had no role in study design, data collection and analysis, decision to publish, or preparation of the manuscript.

Competing Interests: The authors have declared that no competing interests exist.

* E-mail: tlahm@iu.edu

Introduction

Pulmonary hypertension (PH) is present when the mean PA pressure (mPAP) is ≥25 mmHg [1,2]. A diagnosis of pulmonary arterial hypertension (PAH), the only PH subtype for which specific pulmonary vasodilators are FDA-approved, requires absence of left ventricular (LV) dysfunction [3]. The management of PH with elevated LV filling pressures (WHO group II PH; also referred to as "post-capillary PH", "pulmonary venous hypertension" or "PVH") differs dramatically from pre-capillary PH, which encompasses PAH and other PH forms with normal LV pressures [4,5]. In fact, the pulmonary vasodilators used for PAH worsen morbidity and mortality in PVH [4–7]. Right heart catheterization (RHC) with accurate assessment of LV filling pressures is therefore of utmost importance in making a correct diagnosis of PAH, in selecting appropriate therapies, and in differentiating PVH from pre-capillary PH.

LV filling pressures can be measured *directly* via left heart catherization (LHC) and assessment of LV end-diastolic pressure (LVEDP), or *indirectly* by measuring pulmonary capillary wedge pressure (PCWP) during RHC. However, a recent study suggested that when relying on measurement of PCWP alone, patients get misclassified (assigned to the wrong WHO PH group) in 50% of cases [8]. This is due to poor correlation and poor agreement between PCWP and the more accurate (but less frequently measured) LVEDP. Whether age and comorbidities affect PCWP-LVEDP relationship remains unknown.

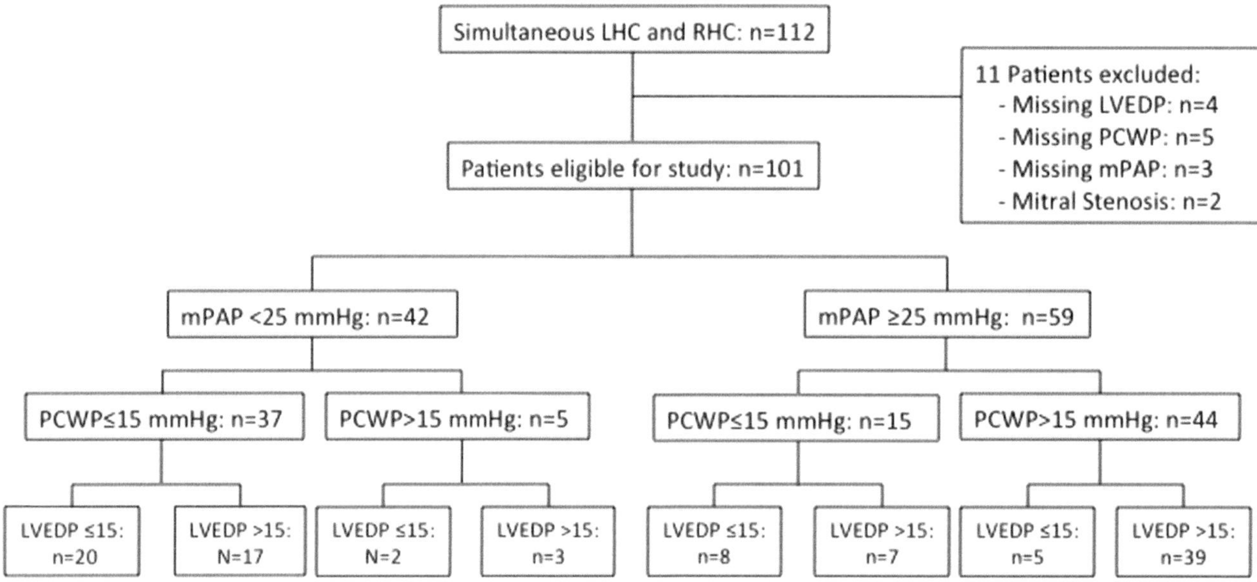

Figure 1. Patient flow chart. LHC, left heart catheterization; LVEDP, left ventricular end-diastolic pressure; mPAP, mean pulmonary artery pressure; PCWP, pulmonary capillary wedge pressure; RHC, right heart catheterization.

Furthermore, no data exist on the diagnostic accuracy of PCWP in the veteran population. The Veterans Health Administration (VHA) is the largest integrated health care system in the USA and serves 8.3 million veterans annually. Patients are characterized by male predominance, advanced age, and a large burden of chronic cardiopulmonary diseases [9]. For example, the number of veterans ≥85 years treated by the VHA has tripled from 2000 to 2011. Since cardiopulmonary hemodynamics are affected by age and gender [10–12], and since veterans are older and exhibit different male-female ratios than previously studied populations [8,13], data from other populations cannot be extrapolated to VA patients. Specific data for the veteran population are therefore needed. Furthermore, given the large prevalence and prognostic significance of PH in the veteran population [14], it is important to test whether the hemodynamic values obtained in this population are accurate.

Since misclassification of veterans with PVH as pre-capillary PH would be a particular problem in this population with poor cardiopulmonary reserve [9], we sought to determine the correlation between PCWP and LVEDP in patients undergoing combined RHC and LHC at a large VA medical center. A secondary aim was to determine how age and comorbidities affect the PCWP-LVEDP relationship.

Methods

Patient population

We retrospectively analyzed patients ≥18 years that underwent combined RHC and LHC from January 2010 until March 2012 at the Richard L. Roudebush VA Medical Center in Indianapolis, Indiana, USA, a large VA tertiary referral center affiliated with Indiana University School of Medicine. Exclusion criteria included: moderate or severe mitral stenosis, heart rate >130/minute, and missing mPAP, PCWP or LVEDP during RHC/LHC. A total of 112 patients were identified. Eleven patients met exclusion criteria (Figure 1). All information gathered was obtained during routine patient care. This work was approved and granted "exempt" status by the Indiana University Institutional Review Board (IRB; Protocol #: 1201007857). Individual patient consent was waived by the approving IRB.

Hemodynamic measurements

PH was diagnosed if the mPAP was ≥25 mmHg [1]. Group II PH was diagnosed as PH with PCWP >15 mmHg [1]. All procedures were performed under the supervision of board-certified cardiologists with specialty training in interventional cardiology. All cardiologists were faculty members of the Indiana University School of Medicine. The physicians performing the catheterizations did not follow standardized protocols for measurement of hemodynamic values; however, values from both RHC and LHC were obtained prior to the injection of contrast media for left ventriculography or coronary angiography. Catheters were connected to the transducer after placement of the tip in the right atrium. After opening the transducer to air and placing it at the mid chest position, the transducer was zeroed, and then the valve was turned to close to air and connected to the catheter tip. The cardiologist then reviewed the tracings as the catheter tip was passed to the different chambers of the right heart and the pulmonary vasculature. Measured pressures were accepted only after review of pressure tracings and confirmation of a true representation of the chamber or vascular pressure. Hemodynamic measurements were transferred directly into electronic spreadsheets and stored in an electronic database (VA CART-CL). The computer-generated values of all hemodynamic measurements were reviewed by the cardiologist and used for diagnosis and analysis if no error was detected. Digitized mean PCWP reading were used; no specific respiratory maneuvers were performed during the wedge measurements.

The pulmonary vascular resistance (PVR) was calculated as the transpulmonary gradient (TPG; mPAP minus PCWP) divided by the cardiac output (with the latter being determined by thermodilution; if that was not done, Fick cardiac output was used). PVR >3 Wood units (WU) was considered increased [1,2]. TPG was considered increased if it was >12 mmHg[1]. Diastolic pressure gradient (DPG) was determined as diastolic PAP minus PCWP, and a value ≥7 mmHg was considered abnormal [15].

Table 1. Patient characteristics of the 101 study subjects.

Age (years)		65.5±9.4
Sex	Male	94 (93.1%)
	Female	7 (6.9%)
Race	Caucasian	92 (91.1%)
	African American	8 (7.9%)
	Other	1 (1%)
Height (cm)		175±9
Weight (kg)		100.2±23.0
Tobacco use (previous or active)		78 (78.8%)
BMI	<18.5	1 (1%)
	18.5–24.9	22 (22%)
	25–29.9	21 (21%)
	30–34.9	28 (28%)
	35–39.9	15 (15%)
	>=40	13 (13%)
Comorbidities	Obstructive sleep apnea	30 (29.7%)
	COPD	21 (20.8%)
	Hypertension	78 (77.2%)
	Coronary artery disease	61 (61.6%)
	Hyperlipidemia	66 (65.3%)
	Diabetes mellitus	46 (45.5%)
	Congestive heart failure	51 (51.5%)
	• Systolic failure	38 (38.4%)
	• Diastolic failure	17 (17.2%)
Cardiac rhythm	Sinus	76 (75.2%)
	Atrial fibrillation/flutter	25 (24.8%)
h/o cardiac surgery		19 (19%)
	Coronary artery bypass grafting	16 (15.8%)
	Valve replacement	3 (3%)
Medications	Aspirin	76 (75.2%)
	ACE-inhibitor/angiotensin receptor-antagonist	61 (60.4%)
	Beta Blocker	66 (65.3%)
	Calcium channel blocker	19 (18.8%)
	Diuretic	57 (56.4%)
	Nitrate	14 (13.9%)
	Statin	67 (66.3%)
	Phosphodiesterase inhibitor	1 (1%)
	Anticoagulation	17 (16.8%)

Age, height, and weight are expressed as means±SD. All other values are expressed as absolute numbers with percent of the total study population in parenthesis.

Echocardiography

All transthoracic echocardiograms were performed for routine patient care according to current guidelines by certified technicians and interpreted by a board certified cardiologist. Echocardiograms were reviewed for the presence of mitral stenosis and other valvular heart diseases.

Clinical diagnoses were made based on standard criteria. Pulmonary function testing, laboratory testing, electrocardiography, polysomnography, and blood pressure measurements were performed according to current guidelines as part of routine patient care. Obesity was defined as a body mass index (BMI) ≥ 30.

Statistical analysis

Baseline demographic and clinical variables are descriptively summarized. Continuous variables are expressed as mean ± SD. Categorical data are presented as percent frequency. The calibration of PCWP to LVEDP was assessed using Bland-Altman analysis. The area under the receiver operating characteristic curve (AUROC) was calculated to determine the ability of PCWP to discriminate between patients with LVEDP of ≤15 mmHg and

Table 2. Hemodynamic Parameters of the 101 study subjects.

Heart rate (bpm) (n = 101)	73±11
Systolic blood pressure (mmHg) (n = 101)	121±22
Diastolic blood pressure (mmHg) (n = 101)	66±14
Left ventricular systolic pressure (mmHg) (n = 100)	135±31
Left ventricular diastolic pressure (mmHg) (n = 101)	19±8
Right atrial pressure (mmHg) (n = 101)	10±5
Mean pulmonary artery pressure (mmHg) (n = 101)	28±10
<25 mmHg	42 (41.6%)
≥25 mmHg	59 (58.4%)
Pulmonary capillary wedge pressure (mmHg) (n = 101)	16±7.4
≤15 mmHg	52 (51.5%)
>15 mmHg	49 (48.5%)
Cardiac output (L/min; thermodilution) (n = 51)	5.0±1.2
Cardiac output (L/min; Fick) (n = 97)	5.0±1.3
Cardiac index (L/min/m²; thermodilution) (n = 50)	2.3±0.54
Cardiac index (L/min/m²; Fick) (n = 95)	2.3±0.53
Pulmonary vascular resistance (Wood units) (n = 98)	2.6±2.0
Systemic vascular resistance (dynes/sec/cm⁻⁵) (n = 80)	1285±485

If a parameter was not obtained in all 101 patients, the number of patients in which this was measured is indicated in parenthesis in the left column. Values are expressed as means±SD, or as absolute numbers with percent of the total study population in parenthesis.

Table 3. Echocardiographic parameters.

Left ventricular ejection fraction (%)	48.7±15.56
Left ventricular hypertrophy	42 (50.6%)
Left atrial dilatation	48 (57.1%)
Right atrial dilatation	14 (16.5%)
Left ventricular dilatation	14 (16.5%)
Right ventricular dilatation	11 (13.4%)
Mitral stenosis	0 (0%)
Mitral Regurgitation	32 (38.1%)
• **Mild**	19 (22.6%)
• **Moderate**	7 (8.3%)
• **Severe**	6 (7.1%)
Aortic stenosis	26 (28.9%)
• **Mild**	3 (3.3%)
• **Moderate**	5 (5.6%)
• **Severe**	18 (20%)
Aortic regurgitation	14 (16.5%)
Tricuspid regurgitation	17 (19.8%)
Tricuspid stenosis	0 (0%)
Left ventricle posterior wall thickness (cm)	1.2±0.4
Interventricular septal wall thickness (cm)	1.2±0.4

Left ventricular ejection fraction, left ventricular posterior wall thickness, and interventricular septal wall thickness are expressed as means±SD. Other values are expressed as absolute numbers with percent of the total study population in parenthesis.

those with LVEDP >15 mmHg. Data collection and analysis was performed using SPSS version 17. $P<0.05$ was considered statistically significant.

Results

Patient characteristics

We analyzed data from 101 patients (Fig. 1; table 1). 93% of patients were male; mean age was 65.5±9.4 years. Comorbidities were common (table 1). 59 patients (58.4%) met PH criteria (Fig. 1). Hemodynamic and echocardiographic parameters are shown in table 2 and table 3. 95% of catheterizations were performed by one of two cardiologists.

PCWP and LVEDP relationship in entire cohort

PCWP and LVEDP correlation was moderate ($r = 0.568$, $r^2 = 0.322$; Fig. 2). Mean bias was −2.87 mmHg (95%CI −4.316 to −1.42) with 95% limits of agreement ranging from −17.21 to 11.47 mmHg (Fig. 3). This indicates that PCWP underestimates LVEDP on average by 2.87 mmHg, and that even after exclusion of the 5% of patients with the highest differences between PCWP and LVEDP, PCWP underestimated LVEDP by as much as 17.21 mmHg and overestimated it by as much as 11.47 mmHg. In 42.6% of patients the absolute difference between PCWP and LVEDP was >5 mmHg, and in 20.8% of patients >10 mmHg.

Since 18% of our patients were noted to have severe aortic stenosis on echocardiogram (table 3), we performed a sensitivity analysis without these patients. In the remaining 81 patients, the PCWP-LVEDP correlation remained moderate ($r = 0.61$; $r^2 = 0.376$; $p<0.001$), and the mean bias was −2.65 mmHg (95% CI −4.24 to −1.06), with 95% limits of agreement from −15.90 to 10.60 mmHg. Correlation coefficient and mean bias were thus grossly unchanged compared to the larger cohort that included the patients with severe aortic stenosis.

In order to determine whether there are any specific patient characteristics in those individuals with particularly large discrepancies between PCWP and LVEDP, we identified all patients in which the PCWP-LVEDP difference was >1 standard deviation (SD) from the mean bias (mean bias <−10.15 or >4.43; n = 33). When comparing this cohort with those patients in which the PCWP-LVEDP difference was within 1 SD (mean bias −10.15 to 4.43), we did not find any significant differences in age, sex, BMI, comorbidities, or medications (data not shown), suggesting that there are no particular identifiers of patients with the largest PCWP-LVEDP discrepancies.

PCWP and LVEDP relationship in patients with or without PH

Of the 59 patients with PH, 44 (74.6%) met PCWP criteria for PVH (Fig. 1; fig. 4A). On the other hand, based on PCWP ≤ 15 mmHg, 15 patients (26.4%) met criteria for pre-capillary PH (Fig. 1; fig. 4A). However, 7 of these 15 patients (46.7%) would be classified as PVH if LVEDP was used instead of PCWP (Fig. 1; shaded area in fig. 4A). On the other hand, among the 44 patients diagnosed with PVH based on elevated PCWP, only 5 individuals (11.4%) would meet pre-capillary PH criteria if LVEDP was used instead.

When limiting our correlation analysis to PH patients, a moderate correlation was confirmed ($r = 0.539$, $r^2 = 0.290$; Fig. 4A). PCWP underestimated LVEDP by 1.7 mmHg (95%CI −3.64 to 0.15); 95% limits of agreement were −15.94 to 12.54 mmHg (Fig. 4B). On the other hand, when investigating the 42 patients without PH, no significant PCWP-LVEDP

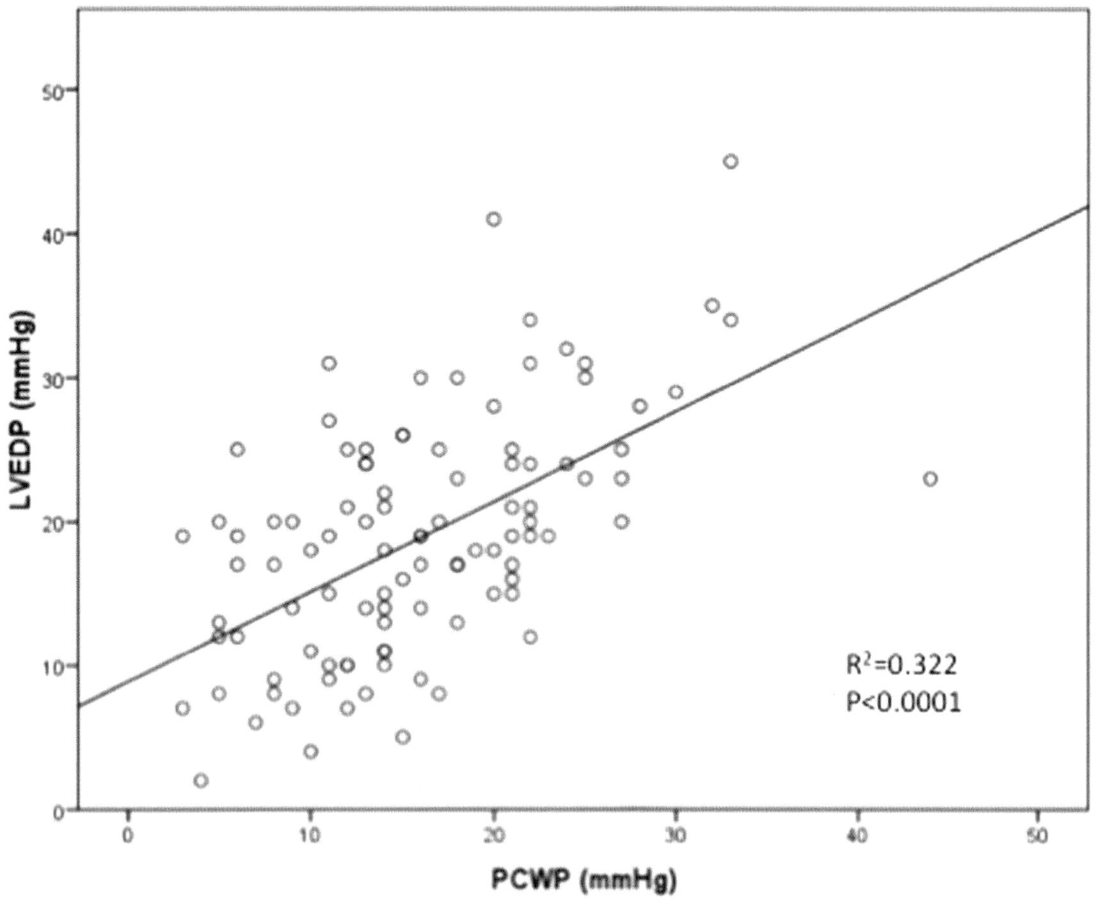

Figure 2. Correlation between PCWP and LEDP in the entire study population. Scatterplot of PCWP and LVEDP pairs for all 101 patients included in the study.

correlation was found (Fig. 4C). PCWP underestimated LVEDP by 4.4 mmHg (95%CI −6.68 to −2.21); 95% limits of agreement were −18.45 to 9.6 mmHg (Fig. 4D). These data suggest that correlation and agreement between PCWP and LVEDP are even less robust in patients without PH.

PCWP performance in patients with increased PVR, TPG or DPG

We then restricted our analysis to patients with PVR >3 WU, as this indicates significant pulmonary vascular remodeling and/or decreased CO[1,16,17]. PVR >3 WU was present in 22 patients (Fig. 5), all of which would be classified as having PH based on mPAP ≥25 mmHg. Ten patients (45.5%) would be classified as having pre-capillary PH based on PCWP ≤15 mmHg. However, if LVEDP >15 mmHg was used instead of PCWP, 4 of those 10 patients (40%) would be reclassified as having PVH. Among the 12 patients classified as having PVH based on PCWP >15 mmHg, only one (8.3%) would be reclassified as having pre-capillary PH if LVEDP was used instead.

A similar pattern was observed when analyzing the 38 patients with TPG >12 mmHg. Thirty-two of those had an mPAP ≥ 25 mmHg (Fig. 5). Fourteen (43%) of these patients would be categorized as pre-capillary PH based on PCWP ≤15 mmHg. However, 6 (42%) of those 14 patients would actually be categorized as PVH based on LVEDP >15 mmHg. Among the 18 patients categorized as PVH based on PCWP >15 mmHg, only 1 patient (5%) would be reclassified as pre-capillary PH if LVEDP was used instead.

Conversely, among the 12 PH patients with DPG ≥7 mmHg, 7 had a PCWP ≤15 mmHg, and only 1 (14%) of these patients was re-classified as PVH based on LVEDP >15 mmHg (Fig. 5). This suggests that in presence of a DPG ≥7, the diagnostic accuracy of a PCWP ≤15 mmHg may be better than in patients with increased TPG or PVR.

AUROC analyses

Among the 59 patients with PH, AUROC of PCWP against LVEDP was 0.81 (95%CI 0.69–0.94) when using a cutpoint of LVEDP ≤15 mmHg (Fig. 6A). This indicates that among all randomly selected pairs of patients in which one has an LVEDP ≤ 15 mmHg and the other has an LVEDP >15 mmHg, the patients with the higher LVEDP would have the higher PCWP in 81% of cases. If an LVEDP cutpoint of 10 or 20 mmHg was used, AUROC was 0.89 (95%CI, 0.79–0.99) and 0.75 (95%CI, 0.63–0.88) respectively (Fig. 6B+C). For the 42 patients without PH, 17 out of 37 patients with a PCWP ≤15 mmHg had an LVEDP > 15 mmHg. AUROC analysis of PCWP against LVEDP among these patients was able to discriminate patients with high or low LVEDP in 76% (95%CI, 0.67–0.86; data not shown).

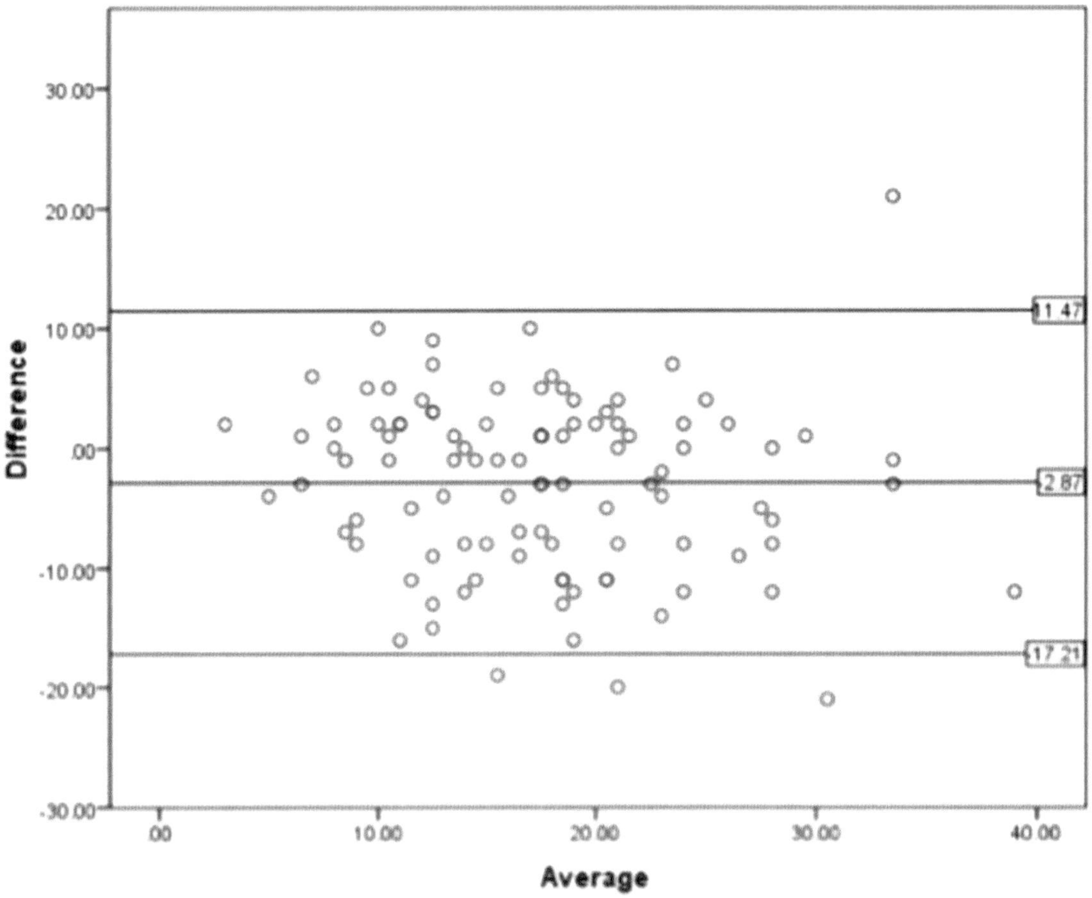

Figure 3. Agreement between PCWP and LEDP in the entire study population. Bland-Altman plot of PCWP and LVEDP pairs for all 101 patients included in the study. Difference indicates difference between PCWP and LVEDP pairs (in mmHg), with positive values indicating that PCWP is higher than corresponding LVEDP for that particular patient, and with negative values indicating that PCWP is lower. Average indicates value of corresponding PCWP and LVEDP pairs divided by 2 ([PCWP+LVEDP/2]). Upper and lower horizontal lines indicate upper and lower borders of 95% limits of agreement, respectively; horizontal line in middle represents mean bias.

PCWP and LVEDP correlations according to age, body weight, and comorbidities

Lastly, we investigated correlations between PCWP and LVEDP in presence and absence of clinically important patient characteristics (Fig. 7). We detected the strongest correlations between PCWP and LVEDP in patients with diabetes and in patients <65 years of age ($r = 0.62$, $r^2 = 0.395$, and $r = 0.63$, $r^2 = 0.4$, respectively; $p<0.0001$ for both), while no significant PCWP-LVEDP correlation was found in COPD patients ($r = 0.17$, $p = 0.46$). While a significant PCWP-LVEDP correlation was found in obese patients, this correlation was weak, and the correlation coefficient was much lower than the one in patients with a BMI <25.

Discussion

This is the first study to evaluate the PCWP-LVEDP relationship in veterans, a unique patient population with male predominance, advanced age, and multiple cardiopulmonary comorbidities [9]. Since cardiopulmonary hemodynamics are affected by age and gender [10–12], specific studies in this population are needed; results from other cohorts cannot necessarily be extrapolated to veterans.

In this cohort of veteran patients referred for RHC and LHC, PCWP and LVEDP are moderately correlated and poorly calibrated. PCWP tends to underestimate LVEDP by almost 3 mmHg, but may underestimate by as much as 17 mmHg, and overestimate by as much as 11 mmHg. Excluding patients with severe aortic stenosis did not significantly alter this relationship. Importantly, 46.7% of PH patients would be classified as having pre-capillary PH if the PCWP was used instead of LVEDP (a common clinical practice). LVEDP measurements, however, indicate that these patients have PVH rather than pre-capillary PH. This has clinical relevance, since pulmonary vasodilators indicated for pre-capillary PH may worsen heart failure and increase mortality in PVH [4–7]. This is of importance in this veteran population characterized by a high prevalence of cardiovascular and pulmonary comorbidities, and by poor cardiopulmonary reserve. These patients may not tolerate the pulmonary flooding and increased LV preload caused by pulmonary vasodilators in the setting of LV disease [4,5]. Furthermore, in light of the high cost of PAH-specific therapy, it is important that such therapy is administered to the correct patient population.

The use of PCWP as a surrogate for LVEDP is based on multiple clinical assumptions [17]. Most importantly, it assumes a static blood column between the balloon of the PA catheter and

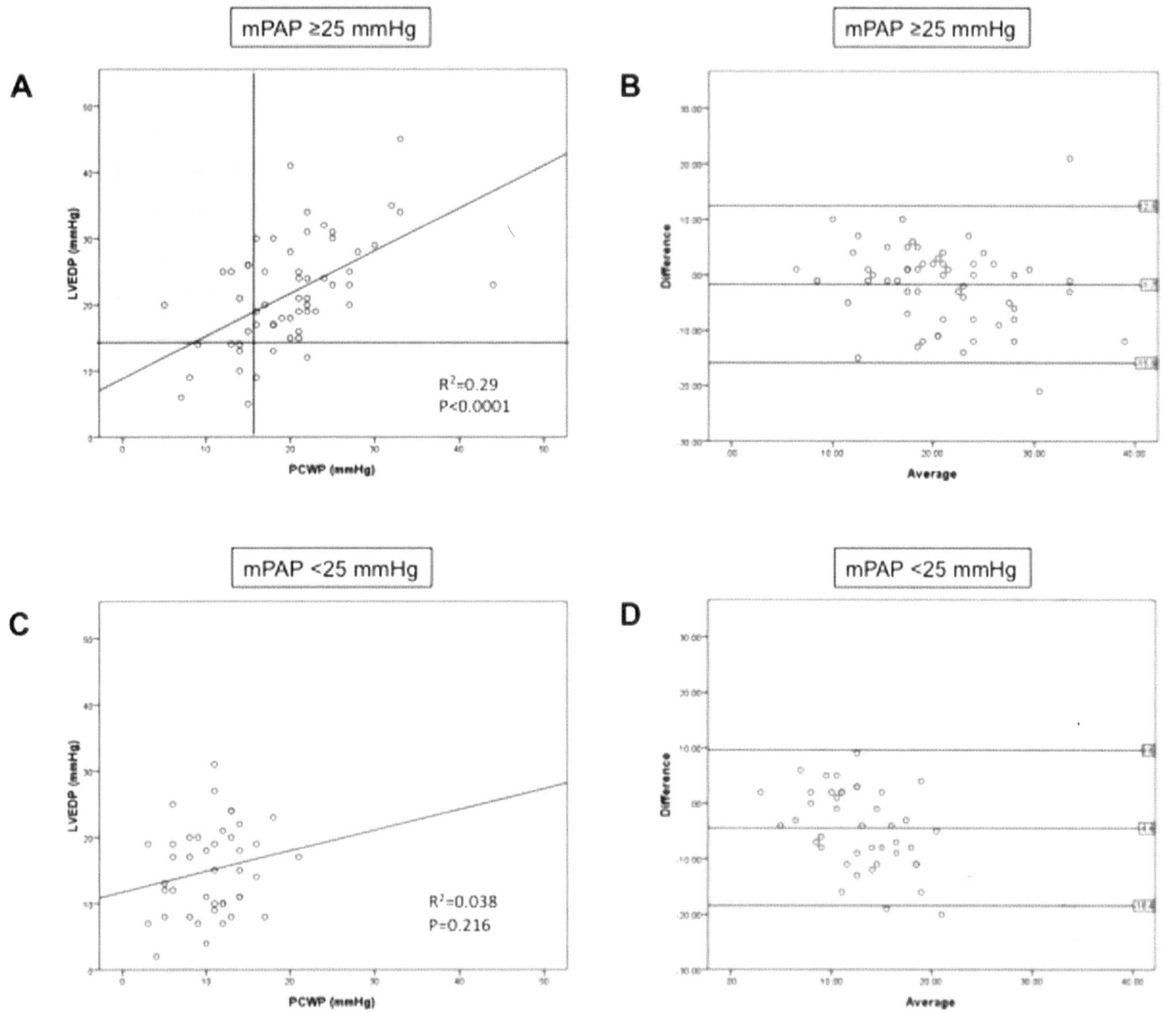

Figure 4. Correlation and agreement between PCWP and LVEDP in patients with (A, B) or without (C, D) pulmonary hypertension. Vertical line in (A) divides patients in patients with PCWP ≤15 mmHg or >15 mmHg; horizontal line divides patients in patients with LVEDP ≤ 15 mmHg or >15 mmHg. Shaded area in (A) represents the patients with PCWP ≤15 mmHg, but LVEDP >15 mmHg, thus indicating patients that would have been incorrectly classified as pre-capillary PH in absence of LVEDP measurement. See fig. 3 for explanation of Bland-Altman plot labeling.

the LV. However, this assumption may be violated in the setting of mitral valve stenosis, high alveolar pressures (as can be seen with mechanical ventilation or air trapping), significant tachycardia or hypovolemia, and if the tip of the PA catheter is not exposed to West zone 3 conditions. While mitral stenosis was an exclusion criterion in our study, it is possible that tachyarrhythmias, hypovolemia, and/or non-West zone 3 conditions may have contributed to the discrepancies between PCWP and LVEDP. Furthermore, errors in measurement and interpretation of hemodynamic values may have contributed. Lastly, use of machine-generated (digitized) mean PCWP readings instead of manually determined end-expiratory values results in underestimation of LVEDP [13]. Discrepancies are particularly pronounced in patients with increased work of breathing, a condition frequently observed in cardiopulmonary disease or obesity [16]. We used digitized mean PCWP readings, and it therefore comes as no surprise that the PCWP-LVEDP correlation was particularly poor in patients with COPD. Air trapping from COPD also may have affected the PCWP-LVEDP relationship. Along those lines, even though we found a correlation between PCWP and LVEDP in obese patients, this correlation was weak, and much less robust than the one observed in patients with a normal BMI. These data confirm that PCWP values are particularly prone to error in patients with significant respiratory excursions (as can be seen in COPD or obesity).

Almost 60% percent of our patients had PH. This is significantly higher than the 37.5% of patients with PH in the study by Halpern and Taichman [8]. Similarly, 22% of our patients had a PVR > 3 WU, compared to roughly 10% in the Halpern study. As evident from table 1, there was a high prevalence of chronic heart and lung disease, sleep-disordered breathing and obesity, all of which may cause PH [18,19]. This may explain the higher incidence of PH in our population. Despite the higher prevalence of PH in the current study, and despite differences in patient characteristics, the

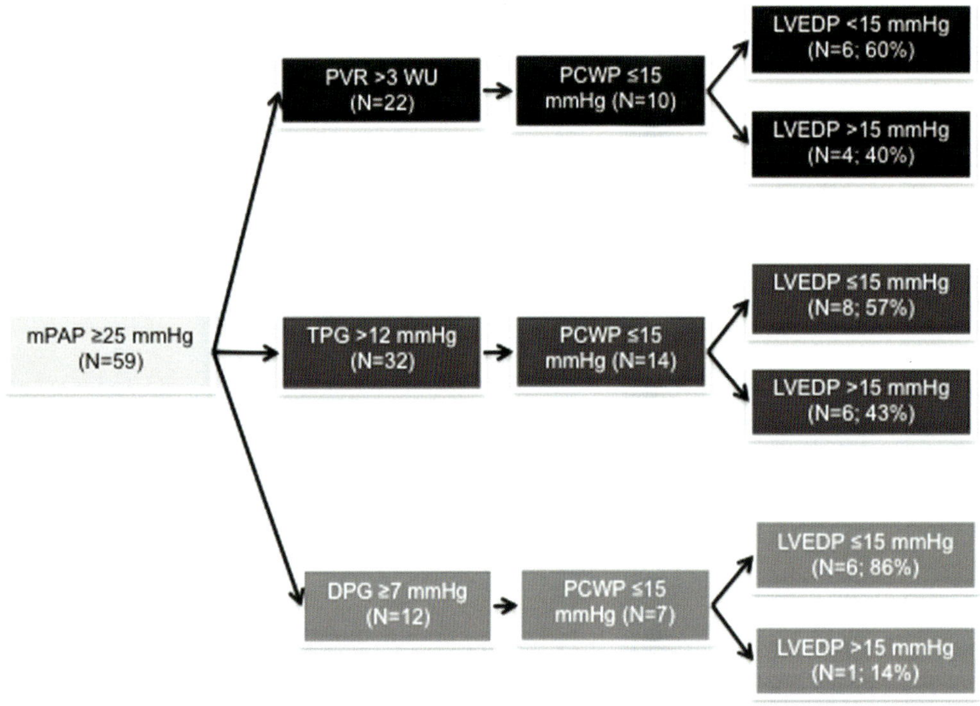

Figure 5. Distribution of patients with LVEDP ≤15 mmHg or LVEDP >15 mmHg in patients with PCWP ≤15 mmHg and PVR >3 WU (upper panel; black), TPG >12 mmHg (middle panel; dark grey), or DPG >7 mmHg (bottom panel; light grey). DPG, diastolic pressure gradient; PVR, pulmonary vascular resistance; TPG, transpulmonary gradient.

calibration of PCWP and LVEDP was identical in both studies (mean bias −2.9 mmHg). As in the Halpern/Taichman study, in the absence of LVEDP measurement almost 50% of patients would be misclassified in our study as pre-capillary PH instead of PVH. These data suggest that the PCWP-LVEDP relationship is surprisingly robust across different patient populations.

It is noteworthy that correlation and agreement between PCWP and LVEDP were worse in the group of patients without PH, where PCWP also tended to underestimate LVEDP. While less important to PH diagnosis and classification, this is of relevance to situations in which a patient's volume status or cardiac function needs to be determined. In fact, underestimation of LVEDP by PCWP also occurs in patients with acute myocardial infarction

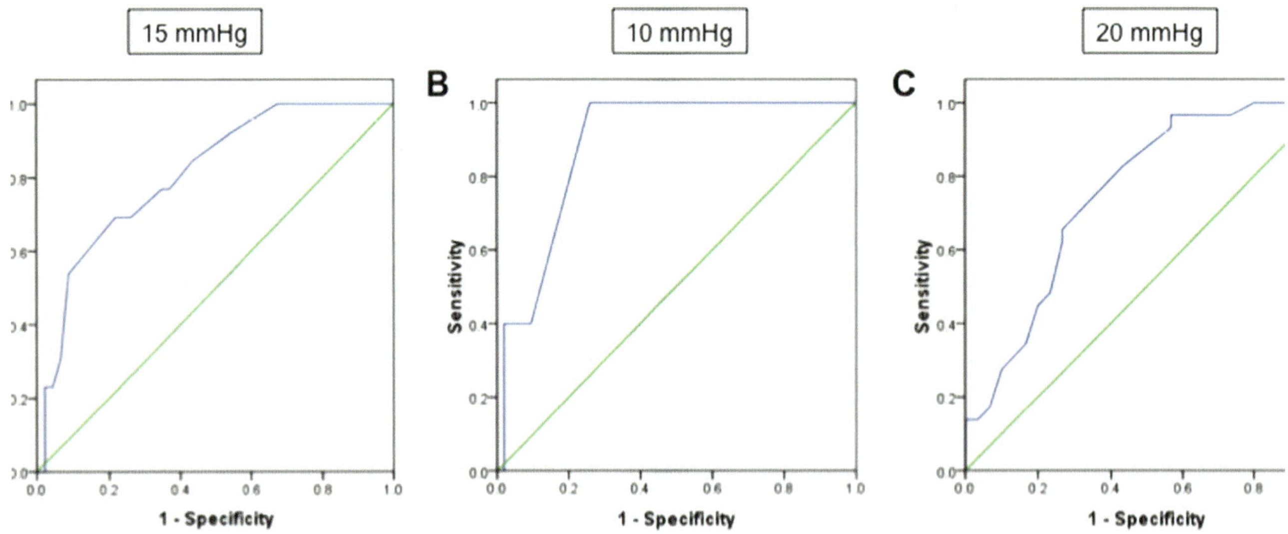

Figure 6. Area under the receiver operating characteristic curve (AUROC) of PCWP against LVEDP in the entire study population. (A) AUROC = 0.81 (95% CI, 0.69 to 0.94) using a cut point of LVEDP ≤15 mmHg to indicate pre-capillary PH. (B) If a cut point of LVEDP ≤10 mmHg was used, the AUROC would be 0.89 (95% CI, 0.79 to 0.99). (C) If a cut point of LVEDP ≤20 mmHg was used, the AUROC would be 0.75 (95% CI, 0.63 to 0.88). Sensitivity = sensitivity for the outcome of LVEDP >15 mmHg; Specificity = specificity for the outcome of LVEDP >15 mmHg.

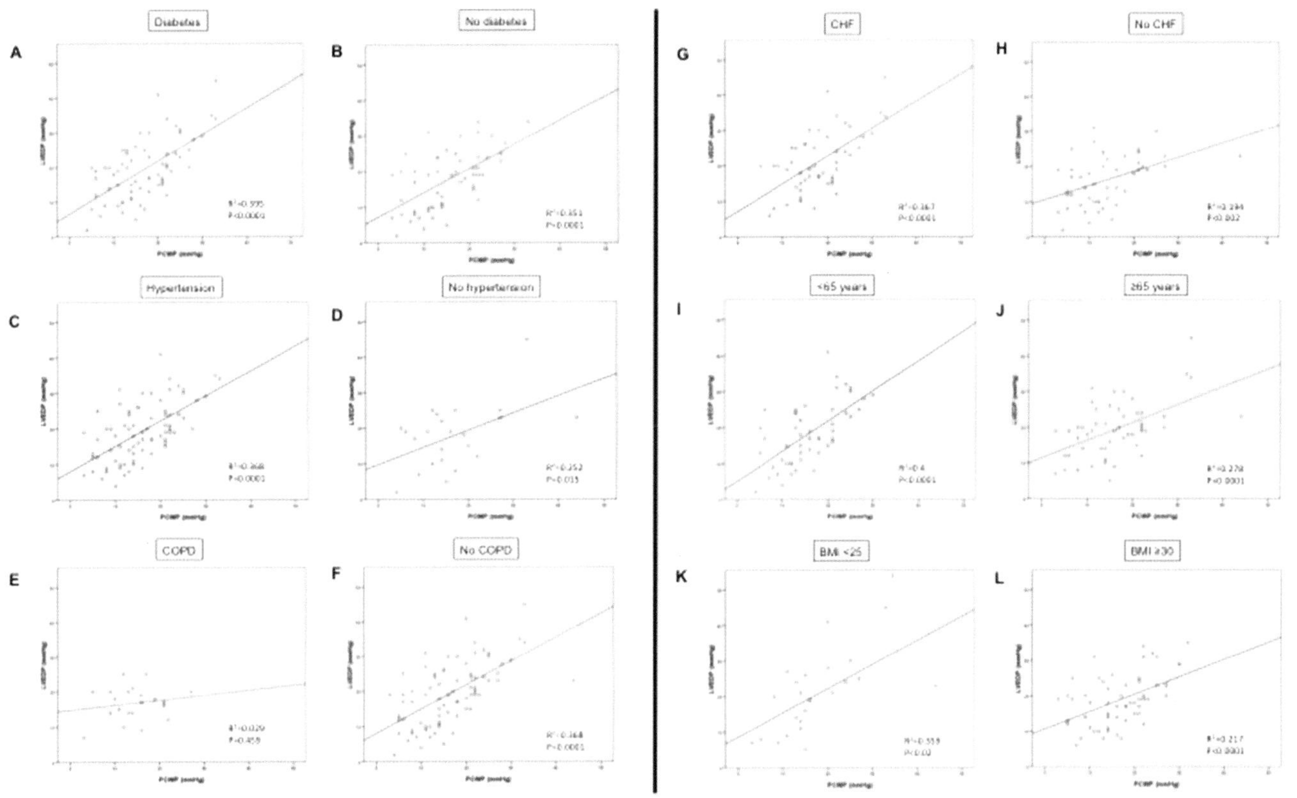

Figure 7. Correlations between PCWP and LEDP in patients with or without diabetes (A, B), hypertension (C, D), COPD (E, F) or CHF (G, H), as well as for patients < or ≥65 years of age (I, J), and for patients with a body mass index (BMI) <25 or ≥30 (K, L). Note lack of significant correlation between PCWP and LVEDP in COPD patients, and poor correlation in obese patients.

[20] and in critically ill patients [21]. This poor calibration may explain at least in part why the majority of studies of pulmonary artery catheter-guided fluid therapy have been disappointing [22,23].

As discussed by others [8], simply adding the mean bias to the PCWP is not sufficient, since the wide 95% limits of agreement demonstrate that - even though PCWP tends to underestimate LVEDP - there is a significant number of patients in which PCWP *overestimates* the latter. Systemic bias therefore is not the only explanation for the discrepancy between PCWP and LVEDP, and for any given patient it is impossible to predict whether the PCWP is higher or lower than the LVEDP. If accurate determination of cardiac filling pressures is needed, threshold for LVEDP measurement should be low.

Our results have important implications for veterans. First, PVH is common in this population (78% of all PH patients had LVEDP-confirmed PVH). This condition therefore should be aggressively looked for. We do not propose, however, aggressive treatment of PVH with PAH-specific therapy. Rather, if PVH is diagnosed, the patient should be aggressively treated with proven pharmacologic and non-pharmacologic (e.g. exercise, oxygen for hypoxemia, CPAP for obstructive sleep apnea) interventions [24].

Second, providers need to be cognizant about the potential for underdiagnosis (and, to a lesser extent, overdiagnosis) of PVH if decisions are based solely on PCWP. As previously shown [13,16], software-generated mean PCWPs frequently are inaccurate and should not be relied upon. However, even with end-expiratory PCWP there still is potential for discrepancies between PCWP and LVEDP (95% limits of agreement −5.19 to 6.93 mmHg[13]). When an accurate assessment of volume status or LV function is needed, determination of LVEDP should strongly be considered (especially if the pre-test probability for PVH is high). We consider the additional risks of LVEDP determination small as compared to the risks of inappropriate pulmonary vasodilator therapy in the setting of occult LV disease. An alternative strategy to detect occult LV disease is provocative testing during RHC (e.g. volume challenge or exercise testing) [16]. However, while promising, these provocative maneuvers still need prospective evaluation.

Misclassification of PVH as pre-capillary PH in our cohort appears to be less common in the subgroup of patients with a DPG of ≥7 mmHg. While this observation is limited by a relatively small number of patients, it is consistent with the recently reported superior ability of the DPG to recognize significant PH as compared to the TPG [15].

The major strength of our study is the investigation of a unique and clinically important patient population. Furthermore, since prior work did not investigate patient characteristics other than PH (e.g. age, BMI, co-morbidities), the investigation of these factors on the PCWP-LVEDP relationship represents another specific strength of our study.

Our study has limitations. First, this is a retrospective single center study with a limited number of patients. Our cohort is identical in age and sex distribution to other recently VA populations [9]. Similarly, the predominance of elderly Caucasian males is similar to what is observed at other large VA medical centers in the US (G. Choudhary, B. Maron; personal communication). However, despite these typical characteristics of VA cohort, our results are similar to those from a larger population [8], thus supporting their validity and generalizability. Second, selection bias may have resulted from referral of patients for combined RHC/LHC. However, most patients (>80%) were actually referred for RHC or LHC only, and the indication for combined catheterization was made later by the procedural cardiologist based on patient characteristics or intra-procedural findings in order to better understand the clinical scenario. Referral for combined RHC/LHC occurred in <20% of cases. Furthermore, previous studies demonstrated no differences in PCWP between patients undergoing combined RHC/LHC and those undergoing RHC alone. Third, hemodynamic tracings were not stored. We therefore were not able to compare the digitized with end-expiratory PCWPs. This will be the subject of further prospective study.

In conclusion, in veterans undergoing combined RHC and LHC, PCWP was poorly calibrated to LVEDP. Reliance on PCWP rather than LVEDP misclassifies veterans as having pre-capillary PH rather than PVH in almost 50% of cases. Correlations were particularly poor in patients with COPD and obesity, suggesting a significant impact of respiratory excursions on the PCWP-LVEDP relationship if automated PCWP readings are used. This is clinically relevant, as misclassification may lead to inappropriate therapies and adverse events, a particular problem in this population with high incidence of cardiovascular comorbidities and poor cardiac reserve.

Acknowledgments

We would like to acknowledge and thank our research nurse Mrs. Vicki Williams for her administrative work with this research project.

Author Contributions

Conceived and designed the experiments: TL. Performed the experiments: AB IB. Analyzed the data: AB MS TL. Contributed reagents/materials/analysis tools: IB TL. Wrote the paper: AB MS IB TL.

References

1. McLaughlin VV, Archer SL, Badesch DB, Barst RJ, Farber HW, et al. (2009) ACCF/AHA 2009 expert consensus document on pulmonary hypertension a report of the American College of Cardiology Foundation Task Force on Expert Consensus Documents and the American Heart Association developed in collaboration with the American College of Chest Physicians; American Thoracic Society, Inc.; and the Pulmonary Hypertension Association. J Am Coll Cardiol 53: 1573 1619.
2. Galie N, Hoeper MM, Humbert M, Torbicki A, Vachiery JL, et al. (2009) Guidelines for the diagnosis and treatment of pulmonary hypertension. Eur Respir J 34: 1219 1263.
3. Badesch DB, Champion HC, Sanchez MA, Hoeper MM, Loyd JE, et al. (2009) Diagnosis and assessment of pulmonary arterial hypertension. J Am Coll Cardiol 54: S55 66.
4. Hoeper MM, Barbera JA, Channick RN, Hassoun PM, Lang IM, et al. (2009) Diagnosis, assessment, and treatment of non-pulmonary arterial hypertension pulmonary hypertension. J Am Coll Cardiol 54: S85 96.
5. Guazzi M, Borlaug BA (2012) Pulmonary hypertension due to left heart disease. Circulation 126: 975 990.
6. Califf RM, Adams KF, McKenna WJ, Gheorghiade M, Uretsky BF, et al. (1997) A randomized controlled trial of epoprostenol therapy for severe congestive heart failure: The Flolan International Randomized Survival Trial (FIRST). Am Heart J 134: 44 54.
7. Packer M, McMurray J, Massie BM, Caspi A, Charlon V, et al. (2005) Clinical effects of endothelin receptor antagonism with bosentan in patients with severe chronic heart failure: results of a pilot study. J Card Fail 11: 12 20.
8. Halpern SD, Taichman DB (2009) Misclassification of pulmonary hypertension due to reliance on pulmonary capillary wedge pressure rather than left ventricular end-diastolic pressure. Chest 136: 37 43.
9. Kaboli PJ, Go JT, Hockenberry J, Glasgow JM, Johnson SR, et al. (2012) Associations between reduced hospital length of stay and 30-day readmission rate and mortality: 14-year experience in 129 Veterans Affairs hospitals. Ann Intern Med 157: 837 845.
10. Kovacs G, Berghold A, Scheidl S, Olschewski H (2009) Pulmonary arterial pressure during rest and exercise in healthy subjects: a systematic review. Eur Respir J 34: 888 894.
11. Shapiro S, Traiger GL, Turner M, McGoon MD, Wason P, et al. (2012) Sex differences in the diagnosis, treatment, and outcome of patients with pulmonary arterial hypertension enrolled in the registry to evaluate early and long-term pulmonary arterial hypertension disease management. Chest 141: 363 373.
12. Kawut SM, Lima JA, Barr RG, Chahal H, Jain A, et al. (2011) Sex and race differences in right ventricular structure and function: the multi-ethnic study of atherosclerosis-right ventricle study. Circulation 123: 2542 2551.
13. Ryan JJ, Rich JD, Thiruvoipati T, Swamy R, Kim GH, et al. (2012) Current practice for determining pulmonary capillary wedge pressure predisposes to serious errors in the classification of patients with pulmonary hypertension. Am Heart J 163: 589 594.
14. Maron BA, Choudhary G, Khan UA, Jankowich MD, McChesney H, et al. (2013) Clinical profile and underdiagnosis of pulmonary hypertension in US veteran patients. Circ Heart Fail 6: 906 912.
15. Gerges C, Gerges M, Lang MB, Zhang Y, Jakowitsch J, et al. (2013) Diastolic pulmonary vascular pressure gradient: a predictor of prognosis in "out-of-proportion" pulmonary hypertension. Chest 143: 758 766.
16. Champion HC, Michelakis ED, Hassoun PM (2009) Comprehensive invasive and noninvasive approach to the right ventricle-pulmonary circulation unit: state of the art and clinical and research implications. Circulation 120: 992 1007.
17. Sharkey SW (1997). A Guide to Interpretation of Hemodynamic Data in the Coronary Care Unit. 1st edition. Philadelphia, PA: Lippincott Williams and Wilkins.
18. Rabinovitch M (2012) Molecular pathogenesis of pulmonary arterial hypertension. J Clin Invest 122: 4306 4313.
19. Morrell NW, Adnot S, Archer SL, Dupuis J, Jones PL, et al. (2009) Cellular and molecular basis of pulmonary arterial hypertension. J Am Coll Cardiol 54: S20 31.
20. Rahimtoola SH, Loeb HS, Ehsani A, Sinno MZ, Chuquimia R, et al. (1972) Relationship of pulmonary artery to left ventricular diastolic pressures in acute myocardial infarction. Circulation 46: 283 290.
21. Calvin JE, Driedger AA, Sibbald WJ (1981) Does the pulmonary capillary wedge pressure predict left ventricular preload in critically ill patients? Crit Care Med 9: 437 443.
22. Wheeler AP, Bernard GR, Thompson BT, Schoenfeld D, Wiedemann HP, et al. (2006) Pulmonary-artery versus central venous catheter to guide treatment of acute lung injury. N Engl J Med 354: 2213 2224.
23. Shure D (2006) Pulmonary-artery catheters peace at last? N Engl J Med 354: 2273 2274.
24. Hunt SA, Abraham WT, Chin MH, Feldman AM, Francis GS, et al. (2009) 2009 focused update incorporated into the ACC/AHA 2005 Guidelines for the Diagnosis and Management of Heart Failure in Adults: a report of the American College of Cardiology Foundation/American Heart Association Task Force on Practice Guidelines: developed in collaboration with the International Society for Heart and Lung Transplantation. Circulation 119: e391 479.

18

Utility of the Physical Examination in Detecting Pulmonary Hypertension. A Mixed Methods Study

Rebecca Colman[1], Heather Whittingham[2], George Tomlinson[3], John Granton[1]*

1 Pulmonary hypertension program, Toronto General Hospital, Division of Respirology, Faculty of Medicine, University of Toronto, Toronto, Ontario, Canada, **2** Department of Critical Care Medicine, Hamilton General Hospital, McMaster University, Hamilton, Ontario, Canada, **3** Department of Medicine, Mount Sinai Hospital and University Health Network, Faculty of Medicine, University of Toronto, Toronto, Ontario, Canada

Abstract

Introduction: Patients with pulmonary hypertension (PH) often present with a variety of physical findings reflecting a volume or pressure overloaded right ventricle (RV). However, there is no consensus regarding the diagnostic utility of the physical examination in PH.

Methods: We conducted a systematic review of publications that evaluated the clinical examination and diagnosis of PH using MEDLINE (1946–2013) and EMBASE (1947–2013). We also prospectively evaluated the diagnostic utility of the physical examination findings. Patients who underwent right cardiac catheterization for any reason were recruited. After informed consent, participants were examined by 6 physicians (3 "specialists" and 3 "generalists") who were unaware of the results of the patient's hemodynamics. Each examiner independently assessed patients for the presence of a RV lift, loud P2, jugular venous distension (JVD), tricuspid insufficiency murmur and right-sided 4th heart sound at rest and during a slow inspiration. A global rating (scale of 1–5) of the likelihood that the patient had pulmonary hypertension was provided by each examiner.

Results: 31 articles that assessed the physical examination in PH were included in the final analysis. There was heterogeneity amongst the studies and many did not include control data. The sign most associated with PH in the literature was a loud pulmonic component of the second heart sound (P2). In our prospective study physical examination was performed on 52 subjects (25 met criteria for PH; mPAP ≥25 mmHg). The physical sign with the highest likelihood ratio (LR) was a loud P2 on inspiration with a LR +ve 1.9, 95% Crl [1.2, 3.1] when data from all examiners was analyzed together. Results from the specialist examiners had higher diagnostic utility; a loud P2 on inspiration was associated with a positive LR of 3.2, 95% Crl [1.5, 6.2] and a right sided S4 on inspiration had a LR +ve 4.7, 95% CI [1.0, 15.6]. No aspect of the physical exam, could consistently rule out PH (negative LRs 0.7–1.3).

Conclusions: The presence of a loud P2 or audible right-sided 4th heart sound are associated with PH. However the physical examination is unreliable for determining the presence of PH.

Editor: Harm Bogaard, VU University Medical Center, Netherlands

Funding: This study was funded through the Toronto General Hospital Foundation. The funder had no role in the design, execution or interpretation of the study results.

Competing Interests: No competing interests or conflict of interest relating to this work from any author.

* Email: John.granton@uhn.ca

Introduction

Pulmonary hypertension (PH) is defined as a mean pulmonary artery pressure (mPAP) ≥25 mmHg measured during cardiac catheterization. The World Health Organization Dana Point Classification divides pulmonary hypertension into five groups based upon similarities in therapeutic approaches, and to some extent, pathophysiologic mechanisms [1]. Although the natural history varies according to the etiology of the condition, PH is often a progressive disease characterized by increased pulmonary vascular resistance and diminished right ventricular (RV) function due to increased RV afterload [2].

Early in the disease, the symptoms of PH are often benign and non-specific but progress over time to functionally limiting dyspnea and fatigue. Patients may also experience chest pain, palpitations, pre-syncope, syncope and peripheral edema. The non-specific nature of symptoms in early disease and subtlety of clinical signs are some of the obstacles to establishing an early diagnosis. Delays in the diagnosis of PH lead to postponement of treatment and thus may have deleterious effects.

Patients with pulmonary hypertension are reported to present with a variety of physical findings reflecting a volume and/or pressure overloaded right ventricle (RV). These include a left parasternal lift, an accentuated pulmonary component of the second heart sound (P2), a pansystolic murmur of tricuspid regurgitation (TR), a diastolic murmur of pulmonary insufficiency and a third or fourth heart sound originating in the RV. In more advanced states patients may manifest jugular venous distension, hepatomegaly and peripheral edema [3]. Numerous studies have described the various findings on physical examination of PH patients but there is no consensus regarding their diagnostic utility [2,4–6].

Many early studies used phonocardiography to validate the role of the physical examination in the diagnosis pulmonary hypertension. With increased adoption of 2-dimensional and Doppler echocardiography, the phonocardiogram has fallen into disuse. Attempts to improve diagnostic accuracy of non-invasive tools other than echocardiography have included revisiting the phonocardiogram itself as well as acquisition of similar phonocardiographic data through use of electronic stethoscopes and computerized algorithms [7–11]; however the use of such tools is impractical for most clinicians, and most continue to rely on the physical examination itself, even though, to date, the diagnostic utility of the physical examination in determining the presence of PH in a symptomatic patient has not been systematically evaluated.

Our purpose was to evaluate the diagnostic utility of the physical examination in PH through literature review and empirical study. We systematically reviewed and appraised the published literature on the physical examination in PH. In addition we prospectively assessed the diagnostic utility of the various physical signs of PH described in the literature by correlation with results of right heart catheterization (RHC). (A description of physical examination techniques used to evaluate for pulmonary hypertension can be found in the appendix.) We also evaluated the potential impact of differences in observer experience (specialist vs generalist) on the detection of findings on physical examination.

Methods

Systematic review

We performed a systematic search of the published literature using MEDLINE (1946–Feb 2013) and EMBASE (1947–March 22, 2013) to identify original publications that evaluated the clinical examination and diagnosis of pulmonary hypertension. We used the following key terms or Medical Subject Headings: (EXP Hypertension, Pulmonary) AND (EXP Physical Examination OR EXP Heart Auscultation OR Heart sounds. The search was limited to English language and human studies. The titles and abstracts of articles retrieved were reviewed by two of the authors (R.C, J.G). If either reviewer chose an article as possibly useful, the article was reviewed for content. Differences between the reviewers regarding articles to be included were resolved by consensus. Reference lists from appropriate articles were carefully searched for other relevant articles. Publications were excluded if they were case reports or review articles.

Physical examination study

Six academic staff physicians, comprising three "experts" (recruited from the heart failure program (1), the division of respirology (1) and lung transplant program (1) and three "non-experts" (two from the division of general internal medicine), acted as examiners in the study. All examiners were blinded to the patients' diagnoses and none were involved in any aspect of the patients' care. All physicians participated in a common training session in which exam maneuvers were reviewed and subjects who demonstrated the findings of interest were available. Following the training session, the physicians were asked to examine a group of patients for the presence or absence of five pre-specified physical findings: a loud P2, a right ventricular heave, a right-sided S4, a murmur of tricuspid regurgitation and the height of the jugular venous distention (JVD) (Text S1). Examination was performed during quiet active breathing. Each sign was re-evaluated during a slow inspiratory maneuver followed to approximately 75% of total lung capacity to help augment right-sided auscultatory findings. The examiners documented their findings on a standardized recording sheet (Figure S1). After completing the series of maneuvers the examiners were asked to estimate the probability that the patient either did have or did not have PH by indicating the degree of certainty using a Likert scale.

The examinations occurred in a series of private examination rooms where examiners moved from one room to the next and were not permitted to discuss their findings.

Subject selection

Subjects were prospectively recruited from a list of patients who underwent right heart cardiac catheterization for any indication at a large tertiary care teaching hospital with an active PH program. Subjects were contacted by telephone and invited to participate in the study using a standardized script. Based on results of the right heart catheterization, subjects were divided into two groups: subjects with PH (those with mPAP >25 mmHg) and those with normal pulmonary artery pressures (mPAP ≤25 mmHg). Each subject was advised about the intent of the study and further advised not to discuss any aspect of their health or their diagnosis with the examining physicians. The examiners were unaware of the subjects' hemodynamics or diagnoses. Prior to the study, standardized instruction on the slow inspiratory maneuver was provided to all patients by one of the authors (JG). The study was approved by the research ethics board of the University Health Network (REB number. All participants signed written informed consent before study enrollment.

Statistical analysis

Published raw data was obtained from relevant systematic review articles whenever available and used to construct 2×2 contingency tables for clinical variables. When data for a specific variable were available from more than one source, these were combined across studies. We then used this published data to calculate sensitivity, specificity and summary positive and negative likelihood ratios (LR) along with 95% confidence intervals (CI).

For each maneuver in our prospective study, we fitted a random effects logistic regression model to account for the fact that six separate examiners assessed each subject and to allow estimation of sensitivity, specificity and the LRs for the average examiner. The probability of a patient having a positive finding on the maneuver performed by a particular examiner was related through a logit link to the patient's true PAH status and a random effect for the examiner. We also fitted a model that allowed for different average sensitivity and specificity for specialists and generalists. The models were fitted using Bayesian methods using the package rjags [12], with three parallel chains run for 10,000 burn-in iterations and 10,000 further iterations after convergence was established using the Gelman-Rubin statistic. Diffuse normal priors were used for regression parameters and uniform prior distributions on the range 0 to 1 were used for the standard deviations of the random effect. Posterior medians and 95% credible intervals (CrI) were extracted from the posterior samples [13]. For each examiner, we used the global rating to generate the non-parametric ROC curve and calculated the area under the curve and its 95% CI [14].

Results

Systematic Review

The literature search identified 1036 citations (Figure 1). Of these, 65 were determined to be duplicates and 902 were excluded after review of their titles and abstracts. Review of the references from the 69 remaining studies identified three additional studies for full text evaluation. Thus 72 studies were reviewed in detail. Of these, 31 studies were identified that assess the physical examination in pulmonary hypertension; these studies were included in the final analysis (Table S1).

There was significant heterogeneity among the studies reviewed in regard to study population, subject selection, methods/details of evaluating physical findings and results. Of the 31 studies in patients with PH, 10 [8,15–23] assessed splitting of the second heart sound (S2), but results were inconsistent. For example Bleifer *et al.* (1960) and Wood (1952) described that patients with PH exhibit narrow splitting of S2 while Xu et. al (2002) argued that as pulmonary artery pressure increases, so does the A2-P2 interval [8,16,23]. Using an intracardiac phonocardiogram at the time of right heart catheterization, Shaver *et al.* (1974) demonstrated that patients with pulmonary hypertension can have varying degrees of splitting of S2 [20].

Because the majority of papers did not include control data, the results from only six studies could be used to determine the performance characteristics of physical examination findings, and only 5 in regard to individual components of the physical examination. Several used phonocardiography to identify the characteristics of the components of the heart sounds. Ungerer *et al.* studied 49 patients with systemic sclerosis and compared the test characteristics of the physical examination, chest radiograph, EKG, echocardiogram, and pulmonary function testing (vital capacity and single breath diffusing capacity. However they defined PAH as a mean PA pressure at rest greater than 20 mmHg or an abnormal increase in PA pressure with exercise [24]. Using this unconventional definition, 16 patients met the criteria for PAH. They reported that the physical examination by two cardiologists (incorporating a prominent a-wave, parasternal heave, an increased S2, and or a right ventricular gallop was positive in 8/16 patients and in 4/33 scleroderma patients in the cohort without PAH providing a sensitivity of 50% [95% CI, 28% to 72%] and a specificity of 88% [95% CI, 73% to 95%] with a corresponding positive LR of 4.1 [95% CI, 1.5–11.7] and negative LR of 0.57 [95% CI, 0.34 to 0.94]. The details of the examination methods and relative merit of one finding over the other were not provided in this high-risk population for PAH.

In 1968, Sutton *et al.* evaluated the second heart sound in patients with pulmonary hypertension in a variety of conditions including congenital cardiac lesions, idiopathic pulmonary hypertension and chronic respiratory disease [25]. They also included a small number of "control" subjects in their analysis: patients with mitral regurgitation or intra-cardiac shunts without PH. In a second paper published in the same journal issue, the authors describe their findings regarding second heart sounds in normal subjects obtained using similar methods [26]. By combining the data from these two papers, the presence of a loud P2 (defined as the pulmonary component of the second heart sound heard louder than the aortic component (A2), assessed where both components can be heard simultaneously during splitting) has a sensitivity of 45.5% [95% CI: 36%–55%] and a specificity of 99% [95% CI: 96%–100%] with a corresponding positive LR of 56.4 [95% CI: 7.9–401.7] and negative LR of 0.5 [95% CI: 0.46–0.66] (Table 1). Another study in our review evaluated clinical predictors of PAH in 55 patients undergoing orthotopic liver transplantation and found that a loud P2 had a sensitivity of 37.5% [95% CI: 14%–69%] and a specificity of 98% [95% CI: 89%–100%] while an RV heave had a sensitivity of 37.5% [95% CI: 14%–69%] and a specificity of 96% [95% CI: 86%–99%](Table 1) [27]. However, only eight patients in this study had pulmonary arterial hypertension (PAH), limiting the precision of the estimates of sensitivity. In 1980 Stein and Sabbah reported intracardiac sound and pressure recordings in 24 subjects in an attempt to determine whether RV failure modified the intensity of P2 in pulmonary hypertension. Eight subjects had pulmonary hypertension with normal RV function, 8 had pulmonary hypertension with evidence of RV dysfunction and 8 were controls with normal PAP [28]. They found that the amplitude of P2 was significantly higher in the pulmonary hypertension subjects compared to controls. There was no significant difference in amplitude of P2 in subjects with PH and evidence of right heart failure compared to those with PH and

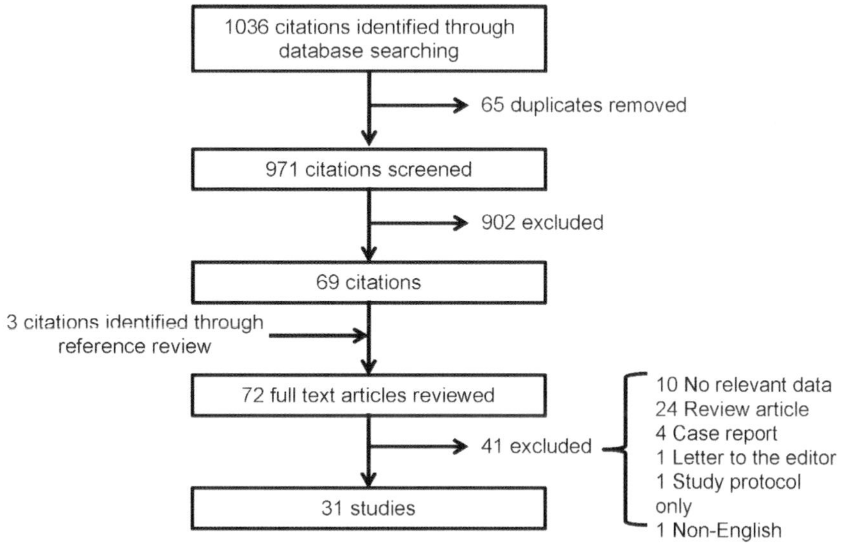

Figure 1. Summary of literature search and identification of publications.

Table 1. 2×2 contingency tables and derived test characteristics from relevant studies.

Study	Finding	PH	No PH	Sn	Sp	LR+ve	LR −ve
Sutton, Harris & Leatham [25] AND Harris & Sutton [26] (1968)	P2>A2			45.5%	99%	56.36 [7.91–401.72]	0.55 [0.46–0.66]
	Finding +ve	45	1				
	Finding −ve	54	123				
Sutton, Harris & Leatham [25] (1968)	P2>A2			45.5%	98.6%	31.85 [2.02–503.37]	0.55 [0.46–0.66]
	Finding +ve	45	0				
	Finding −ve	54	34				
Sutton, Harris & Leatham [25] (1968)	P2≥A2			72.7%	70.6%	2.47 [1.45–4.22]	0.39 [0.26–0.57]
	Finding +ve	72	10				
	Finding −ve	27	24				
Pilatis [27]. (2000)	'loud P2'			37.5%	97.9%	17.63 [2.08–149.12]	0.64 [0.37–1.09]
	Finding +ve	3	1				
	Finding −ve	5	46				
Pilatis [27]. (2000)	RV heave			37.5%	95.7%	8.81 [1.74–44.74]	0.65 [0.38–1.12]
	Finding +ve	3	2				
	Finding −ve	5	45				
Ungerer [15]. (1983)	"Physical exam			50%	95.2%	4.12 [1.46–11.68]	0.57 [0.34–0.94]
	Finding +ve	8	4				
	Finding -ve	8	29				

Sn: sensitivity, SP: specificity, LR +ve: positive likelihood ratio, LR−ve: negative likelihood ratio, RV: right ventricle.

Table 2. Baseline characteristics of study population.

Variable	Mean PAP ≤25 mmHg (N = 27)	Mean PAP >25 mmHg (N = 25)
Mean/Median PA pressure	**17/16 mmHg**	**35.9/32 mmHg**
Range of PA pressure	**10–25 mmHg**	**26–61 mmHg**
Age (median, range)	64 (33–83)	65.5 (28–82)
Female	10	10
Diagnosis		
Mitral valve disease	**6**	**5**
Aortic valve disease	**7**	**0**
Cardiomyopathy	**2**	**6**
Ischaemic heart disease	**0**	**5**
Lung disease	**4**	0
Connective tissue disease	**2**	0
PAH*	**0**	6
Other	**6**	3
Wedge pressure or left ventricular end-diastolic pressure >15 mmHg	**0**	**17**

normal RV function. Because the results of the study are provided as average sound pressure measurements for an entire group, data to assess the performance characteristics of a loud P2 in a given patient are not available in the publication.

Recently, Chan *et al.* investigated the quantitative relationship between acoustic characteristics of S1 and S2 in patients with PAH compared to controls using phonocardiography [7]. They demonstrated that the normal acoustic profile observed in controls, of increased S1 complexity and intensity compared to S2, was altered in subjects with PAH; the PAH subjects were found to have increased S2 complexity compared to S1. Additionally, the mPAP was found to be an independent predictor of S2 complexity in patients with PAH [7]. Similar to the Stein study described above, the results are provided as average sound intensity and complexity measurements for the entire group therefore making it difficult to determine performance characteristics of the loud P2.

Physical examination study

In our empiric study, physical examination was performed on 52 subjects. Of these, 25 had mPAP >25 mmHg. Baseline characteristics of study participants are provided in Table 2. The two groups were similar with respect to age and sex. There were slightly more patients with a diagnosis of connective tissue disease in the normal PAP group.

As shown in Table 3, when data from all examiners were analyzed together no sign reliably predicted nor excluded the presence of pulmonary hypertension. While many of the signs had high specificities (88% for an S4 on inspiration, 85% for a loud P2 on inspiration, 84% for an RV lift on inspiration), the sensitivities were low (12%, 29% and 21% respectively). The physical sign with the highest positive LR was a loud P2 on inspiration (LR +ve 1.9, 95% CrI [1.2, 3.1]) and all negative LRs were approximated 1.0.

However, when results from examination by the specialist group were analyzed separately from those from the "generalist group", a loud P2 on inspiration (specificity 87%, sensitivity 37%, positive LR 3.2, 95% CrI [1.5, 6.2]) and a right sided S4 on inspiration (specificity 96%, sensitivity 13%, positive LR 4.7, 95% CrI [1.0, 15.6]) were the best predictors of pulmonary hypertension. The same maneuvers are not predictive when performed by the generalist physicians (positive LR 1.2, 95% CrI [0.58, 2.4] and 0.6, 95% CI [0.24, 1.2] respectively). Although the differences between LRs in specialists and generalists were not large for these two maneuvers, the probabilities that the specialists had larger LRs were 96% and 97%. We found no aspect of the physical exam, alone or used in combination in a global rating, could consistently rule out pulmonary hypertension, with estimates of negative LRs ranging from 0.7 to 1.3. (Table 3).

When examiners were asked to estimate their confidence as to whether or not a patient had pulmonary hypertension at the end of the assessment (presumably based on a gestault of their findings and clinical biases), the accuracy of diagnosis was quite low. The areas under the ROC curves for specialists ranged from 0.57–0.62 while for generalists they ranged from 0.41–0.56 (Table 4).

Discussion

In this study, we sought to validate the physical examination for pulmonary hypertension through review of the literature and empirical study. Although the accurate diagnosis of PH is important, there are very few prior studies evaluating the role of the clinical examination. The results of the available studies are often not applicable to present practice, especially because phonocardiography is no longer generally available. As well, although most of the papers derive from an era in which there was heavier reliance on physical examination for diagnosis that was also an era when less emphasis was placed on study design, especially noted in the absence of control groups. Consequently historical studies have methodological limitations relating to cohort assembly, lack of controls and uncertain blinding. Our review found that the literature is dominated by heterogeneous, small, cross-sectional and retrospective studies. Consequently, it is not possible to form evidence-based conclusions from the existing published data.

A common theme in the limited studies available is investigator interest in the characteristics of the second heart sound in pulmonary hypertension. In that regard, the utility of the duration

Table 3. Summary of test characteristics for each component of the physical examination that was performed, with comparisons between specialists and generalists.

Sign	All Examiners				Specialists				Generalists			
	Sn	Sp	LR+	LR−	Sn	Sp	LR+	LR−	Sn	Sp	LR+	LR−
RV Lift	32	72	1.1 [0.78,1.6]	1.0 [0.81,1.1]	34	73	1.3 [0.74,2.1]	0.9 [0.72,1.1]	31	70	1.0 [0.58,1.7]	1.0 [0.78,1.3]
RV Lift (insp)	21	84	1.3 [0.78,2.1]	1.0 [0.82,1.1]	32	76	1.4 [0.79,2.5]	0.9 [0.68,1.1]	13	88	1.2 [0.42,2.8]	1.0 [0.85,1.1]
Loud P2	43	74	1.6 [1.2,2.4]	0.8 [0.63,0.92]	52	70	1.8 [1.2,2.8]	0.7 [0.48,0.90]	34	77	1.5 [0.84,2.6]	0.9 [0.67,1.1]
Loud P2 (insp)	29	85	1.9 [1.2,3.1]	0.8 [0.71,0.96]	37	87	3.2 [1.5,6.2]	0.7 [0.51,0.90]	22	81	1.2 [0.58,2.4]	1.0 [0.78,1.2]
S4	20	83	1.2 [0.73,2.0]	1.0 [0.84,1.1]	16	94	3.0 [0.94,8.3]	0.9 [0.77,1.0]	28	69	0.94 [0.52,1.6]	1.0 [0.82,1.3]
S4 (insp)	12	88	1.0 [0.51,1.9]	1.0 [0.9[illegible],1.1]	13	96	4.7 [1.0,15.6]	0.9 [0.79,1.0]	13	77	0.6 [0.24,1.2]	1.1 [0.96,1.4]
TR	28	69	0.9 [0.62,1.3]	1.0 [0.89,1.2]	30	82	1.8 [0.9,3.2]	0.9 [0.67,1.0]	26	56	0.6 [0.33,0.95]	1.3 [1.0,1.8]
TR (insp)	22	81	1.1 [0.71,1.8]	1.0 [0.85,1.1]	22	86	1.7 [0.77,3.4]	0.9 [0.75,1.1]	22	75	0.93 [0.46,1.6]	1.0 [0.86,1.3]

of the A2 to P2 interval (S2 splitting) for estimation of pulmonary pressure is questionable. In our study, we did not formally evaluate duration of S2 splitting given the inconsistent literature and the difficulty in accurately assessing and documenting the finding with tools available in routine clinical practice. The literature does support that the presence of a loud P2 is associated with an increased likelihood of pulmonary hypertension while its absence may make the diagnosis less likely. However, different authors provide varying definitions of "loud" thus compromising the generalizability of the finding.

The results of our clinical evaluation do support the notion derived from prior studies, limited though they may be, that a loud P2 is a physical sign predictive of pulmonary hypertension. We found, however, that meaningful value was only achieved when the assessment was made by a specialist (with experience in examining patients with PH) during a slow inspiratory maneuver. Even so, in our evaluation, the maximum LR +ve associated with this finding was only 3.2, much lower than the LR+ve of >56 calculated from the data of Sutton *et al.* This difference may be explained by differences in study design and subject selection. The high testing characteristics obtained by Sutton *et al.* are likely an overestimation stemming from a study of a cohort of patients with a known diagnosis of pulmonary hypertension. In addition, they used phonocardiography, rather than auscultation, to evaluate the heart sounds. In our study, we evaluated patients referred for right heart catheterization, without prior knowledge of pulmonary pressures. Nevertheless the population of patients that we studied likely has a higher prevalence of PH than the general population, because they had some indication for measurement of right ventricular/pulmonary hemodynamics. Consequently, our test characteristics may overestimate utility of the manoeuvres that we evaluated if they were applied to the general population. Furthermore the physical examination, used because we felt that our findings would be more applicable to everyday practice, is likely to be less precise than phonocardiography in assessing the absolute and relative loudness of heart sounds. This may also explain why in contrast to the literature the absence of a loud P2 cannot not be used to rule out PH.

In our study the finding that was most predictive of PH (LR +ve 4.7) was a right-sided S4. There are claims in the literature that the presence of a right-sided S3 or S4 supports PH but published data in the literature to support such claims is lacking.

In our study, "specialists" performed slightly better than "generalists". This is not surprising when one considers the subtlety of the positive findings. An individual with a trained ear would presumably have less difficulty recognizing a loud P2 compared to someone with less experience. Similarly, a clinician who is unaccustomed to assessing for right-sided heart sounds may not easily appreciate sounds that are louder, or only noticeable, on inspiration, such as a right-sided S4.

Consistent with published data, we found that physical examination is more reliable at ruling disease in, based on the higher specificity and positive likelihood ratios. In contrast, low sensitivity and negative likelihood ratios close to 1.0 preclude reliance on negative findings on physical examination to exclude presence of pulmonary hypertension.

In conclusion, although we demonstrate that the physical findings of a right-sided S4 and a loud P2 are associated with PH, the physical examination is unreliable overall for the diagnosis of PH. Positive findings are only modestly predictive when their presence is noted by "specialists" and they are not predictive when noted by "generalists". Absence of findings is of no use to exclude the diagnosis of PH. Previously published literature manifests weaknesses in subject selection and study design that has led to

Table 4. ROC curves for each physician's estimate of the probability that the patient either did have or did not have PH.

Examiner	Area under ROC curve (95% C.I.)
Specialist 1	0.61 (0.45–0.77)
Specialist 2	0.57 (0.39–0.75)
Specialist 3	0.62 (0.44–0.80)
Generalist 1	0.43 (0.25–0.61)
Generalist 2	0.56 (0.38–0.74)
Generalist 3	0.41 (0.21–0.61)

The degree of certainty was estimated for each patient at the end of the examination using a Likert scale.

overestimation of the utility of physical examination findings to support or exclude the diagnosis of pulmonary hypertension.

Supporting Information

Figure S1 Standardized recording sheet used by examiners to record their findings for each patient. A Likert scale was used to estimate the examiner's impression regarding the likelihood of pulmonary hypertension at the end of each examination.

Table S1 Summary of the 31 studies were identified that assess the physical examination in pulmonary hypertension and were included in the final analysis.

Text S1 Details of the physical examination maneuvers provided to each examiner who participated in the study.

Checklist S1 PRISMA Checklist.

Author Contributions

Conceived and designed the experiments: JG HW RC. Performed the experiments: JG HW RC. Analyzed the data: JG HW RC GT. Contributed reagents/materials/analysis tools: JG HW RC GT. Wrote the paper: JG RC HW GT. Review of studies included in systematic review: JG RC.

References

1. Simonneau G, Robbins IM, Beghetti M, Channick RN, Delcroix M, et al. (2009) Updated clinical classification of pulmonary hypertension. J Am Coll Cardiol 54: S43–54.
2. Gaine SP, Rubin LJ (1998) Primary pulmonary hypertension. Lancet 352: 719–725.
3. Galie N, Hoeper MM, Humbert M, Torbicki A, Vachiery JL, et al. (2009) Guidelines for the diagnosis and treatment of pulmonary hypertension: the Task Force for the Diagnosis and Treatment of Pulmonary Hypertension of the European Society of Cardiology (ESC) and the European Respiratory Society (ERS), endorsed by the International Society of Heart and Lung Transplantation (ISHLT). Eur Heart J 30: 2493–2537.
4. Galie N, Hoeper MM, Humbert M, Torbicki A, Vachiery JL, et al. (2009) Guidelines for the diagnosis and treatment of pulmonary hypertension. Eur Respir J 34: 1219–1263.
5. Gaine S (2000) Pulmonary hypertension. JAMA 284: 3160–3168.
6. McGoon M, Gutterman D, Steen V, Barst R, McCrory DC, et al. (2004) Screening, early detection, and diagnosis of pulmonary arterial hypertension: ACCP evidence-based clinical practice guidelines. Chest 126 (1 SUPPL.): 14S–34S.
7. Chan W, Woldeyohannes M, Colman R, Arand P, Michaels AD, et al. (2013) Haemodynamic and structural correlates of the first and second heart sounds in pulmonary arterial hypertension: an acoustic cardiography cohort study. BMJ Open 3.
8. Xu J, Durand LG, Pibarot P (2002) A new, simple, and accurate method for non-invasive estimation of pulmonary arterial pressure. Heart 88 (1): 76–80.
9. Nigam V, Priemer R (2006) A dynamic method to estimate the time split between the A2 and P2 components of the S2 heart sound. Physiological Measurement 27: 553–567.
10. Javed F, Venkatachalam PA, Hani AFM (2007) Knowledge based system with embedded intelligent heart sound analyser for diagnosing cardiovascular disorders. Journal of Medical Engineering and Technology 31 (5): 341–350.
11. Dennis A, Michaels AD, Arand P, Ventura D (2010) Noninvasive diagnosis of pulmonary hypertension using heart sound analysis. Computers in Biology and Medicine 40 (9): 758–764.
12. Plummer M (2013) Plummer, Martyn. riags: Bayesian graphical models using MCMC. R package version 3-10, Available: http://CRAN.R-project.org/package=rjags.
13. Sung L, Hayden J, Greenberg ML, Koren G, Feldman BM, et al. (2005) Seven items were identified for inclusion when reporting a Bayesian analysis of a clinical study. J Clin Epidemiol 58: 261–268.
14. Hanley JA, McNeil BJ (1982) The meaning and use of the area under a receiver operating characteristic (ROC) curve. Radiology 143: 29–36.
15. Craige E (1960) Phonocardiography in interventricular septal defects. American Heart Journal 60 (1): 51–60.
16. Bleifer S, Donoso E, Grishman A (1960) The auscultatory and phonocardiographic signs of ventricular septal defects. American Journal of Cardiology 5 (2): 191–198.
17. Karnegis JN, Wang Y (1964) The Phonocardiogram in Idiopathic Dilatation of the Pulmonary Artery. American Journal of Cardiology 14: 75–78.
18. Goryanina NK (1964) THE SIGNIFICANCE of the SECOND CARDIAC SOUND in THE DIAGNOSIS of PULMONARY HYPERTENSION (Russian). Terapevticheskii Arkhiv 36 (4): 85–89.
19. Slodki SJ, Shah PM (1965) The Q-II interval. II. A study of the second heart sound in pulmonary hypertension. Chic Med Sch Quart 25 (3): 108–113.
20. Shaver JA, Nadolny RA, O'Toole JD, Thompson ME, Reddy PS, et al. (1974) Sound pressure correlates of the second heart sound. An intracardiac sound study. Circulation 49: 316–325.
21. Harris A (1970) The second heart sound in health and in pulmonary hypertension. American Heart Journal 79 (2): 145–148.
22. Leatham A, Gray I (1956) Auscultatory and phonocardiographic signs of atrial septal defect. Brit Heart T 18 (2): 193–208.
23. Wood P (1952) Pulmonary hypertension. Br Med Bull 8: 348–353.
24. Ungerer RG, Tashkin DP, Furst D, Clements PJ, Gong H Jr, et al. (1983) Prevalence and clinical correlates of pulmonary arterial hypertension in progressive systemic sclerosis. American Journal of Medicine 75: 65–74.
25. Sutton G, Harris A, Leatham A (1968) Second heart sound in pulmonary hypertension. British Heart Journal 30 (6): 743–756.
26. Harris A, Sutton G (1968) Second heart sound in normal subjects. Br Heart J 30: 739–742.
27. Pilatis ND, Jacobs LE, Rerkpattanapipat P, Kotler MN, Owen A, et al. (2000) Clinical predictors of pulmonary hypertension in patients undergoing liver transplant evaluation. Liver Transplantation 6 (1): 85–91.
28. Stein PD, Sabbah H (1980) Intensity of the second heart sound. Relation of physical, physiological and anatomic factors to auscultatory evaluation. Henry Ford Hospital Medical Journal 28: 205–209.

Comparative Analyses of Lung Transcriptomes in Patients with Alveolar Capillary Dysplasia with Misalignment of Pulmonary Veins and in *Foxf1* Heterozygous Knockout Mice

Partha Sen[1*¶], Avinash V. Dharmadhikari[2,3¶], Tadeusz Majewski[4], Mahmoud A. Mohammad[1], Tanya V. Kalin[5], Joanna Zabielska[6], Xiaomeng Ren[5], Molly Bray[7], Hannah M. Brown[2,8], Stephen Welty[1], Sundararajah Thevananther[1,3], Claire Langston[9], Przemyslaw Szafranski[2], Monica J. Justice[2,3], Vladimir V. Kalinichenko[5], Anna Gambin[6,10], John Belmont[1,2], Pawel Stankiewicz[2,3*]

1 Department of Pediatrics, Baylor College of Medicine, Houston, Texas, United States of America, **2** Department of Molecular & Human Genetics, Baylor College of Medicine, Houston, Texas, United States of America, **3** Interdepartmental Program in Translational Biology and Molecular Medicine, Baylor College of Medicine, Houston, Texas, United States of America, **4** Department of Pathology, University of Texas MD Anderson Cancer Center, Houston, Texas, United States of America, **5** Division of Pulmonary Biology, Cincinnati Children's Hospital Research Foundation, Cincinnati, Ohio, United States of America, **6** Institute of Informatics, University of Warsaw, Warsaw, Poland, **7** Department of Epidemiology, University of Alabama at Birmingham, Birmingham, Alabama, United States of America, **8** Robinson Research Institute, School of Pediatrics and Reproductive Health, University of Adelaide, Adelaide, Australia, **9** Department of Pathology, Baylor College of Medicine, Houston, Texas, United States of America, **10** Mossakowski Medical Research Center, Polish Academy of Sciences, Warsaw, Poland

Abstract

Alveolar Capillary Dysplasia with Misalignment of Pulmonary Veins (ACDMPV) is a developmental disorder of the lungs, primarily affecting their vasculature. *FOXF1* haploinsufficiency due to heterozygous genomic deletions and point mutations have been reported in most patients with ACDMPV. The majority of mice with heterozygous loss-of-function of *Foxf1* exhibit neonatal lethality with evidence of pulmonary hemorrhage in some of them. By comparing transcriptomes of human ACDMPV lungs with control lungs using expression arrays, we found that several genes and pathways involved in lung development, angiogenesis, and in pulmonary hypertension development, were deregulated. Similar transcriptional changes were found in lungs of the postnatal day 0.5 *Foxf1*$^{+/-}$ mice when compared to their wildtype littermate controls; 14 genes, *COL15A1, COL18A1, COL6A2, ESM1, FSCN1, GRINA, IGFBP3, IL1B, MALL, NOS3, RASL11B, MATN2, PRKCDBP,* and *SIRPA,* were found common to both ACDMPV and *Foxf1* heterozygous lungs. Our results advance knowledge toward understanding of the molecular mechanism of ACDMPV, lung development, and its vasculature pathology. These data may also be useful for understanding etiologies of other lung disorders, e.g. pulmonary hypertension, bronchopulmonary dysplasia, or cancer.

Editor: Michael Koval, Emory University School of Medicine, United States of America

Funding: Part of this work was supported by a NORD grant and Pilot Project Award from the Texas Children's Hospital, Houston TX to P. Sen, and NIH grant 1RO1HL101975-01 to P. Stankiewicz. The funders had no role in study design, data collection and analysis, decision to publish, or preparation of the manuscript.

* E-mail: psen@msn.com (P. Sen); pawels@bcm.edu (P. Stankiewicz)

¶ These authors contributed equally to this work.

Introduction

Alveolar Capillary Dysplasia with Misalignment of Pulmonary Veins (ACDMPV; MIM# 265380) is a rare developmental disorder of the lung [1]. ACDMPV was first described by McMahon [2] and its genetic basis emerged as more patients [3] and familial cases were reported [4]. The primary diagnostic features of ACDMPV include misalignment (malposition) of pulmonary veins, medial thickening of smooth muscles in pulmonary arteries, hyperplasia of alveolar epithelium, and drastically decreased number of capillaries and lobular underdevelopment [5]. Approximately one third of the patients also have lymphangiectasis. The disease usually presents within a few hours after birth although late presentations have been reported [6,7]. Treatment, including high pressure oxygen, nitric oxide, extra corporeal membrane oxygenation (ECMO) [8–11], and more recently Sildenafil [12], only provide temporary relief as the disease is uniformly lethal. Most patients die within the first few weeks of life although some prolonged survivals have been described [13]. The majority of the patients with ACDMPV also have extra-pulmonary anomalies, including gastrointestinal, cardiovascular, and genitourinary systems [14].

We have shown that ACDMPV results from haploinsufficiency of *FOXF1* [15]. To date 42 point mutations and 18 genomic deletions involving *FOXF1* or its upstream regulatory region have been identified in patients with ACDMPV [15–17]. Interestingly, our recent work has indicated that *FOXF1* is incompletely paternally imprinted in human lungs [17,18]. *Foxf1*$^{+/-}$ mice exhibit neonatal mortality similar to human infants with ACDMPV and die due to defects in vasculogenesis and alveolarization [19]. They also demonstrate other foregut malformations such as narrowing of the esophagus and trachea, esophageal atresia and trachea-esophageal fistula [20]. Unlike in humans, *Foxf1* was not found to be imprinted in mice (data not shown).

To better understand the molecular bases of ACDMPV and to identify major genes and pathways involved in lung development, we performed comparative analyses of lung transcriptomes in patients with ACDMPV and in *Foxf1*$^{+/-}$ mice using Human Ref-8 v3 and Mouse WG-6 v2 Expression BeadChip Illumina microarrays, respectively.

Materials and Methods

Ethics Statement

Patients with histopathologically-verified ACDMPV were recruited after signing consent for the study, Institutional Review Board (IRB) protocol # H-8712 "Molecular genetics of Alveolar capillary dysplasia with misalignment of pulmonary veins (ACDMPV)" approved by the IRB for Baylor College of Medicine (BCM) and Affiliated Hospitals. All mouse experiments were carried out under the approval of the Institutional Animal Care and Use Committee (IACUC) at BCM. Mice were housed in the Transgenic Mouse Facility (barrier level 3) under the care of the Center for Comparative Medicine (CCM), which is accredited by the Association for Assessment and Accreditation of Laboratory Animal Care (AAALAC).

Patients

The clinical descriptions are shown in Table 1. Patients 3 and 6 were of Hispanic ethnicity and the remainder were Caucasians. Patients 2–8 had sporadic ACDMPV and patient 1 represents a familial case with neither point mutation in *FOXF1* nor deletion in the 16q24.1 region identified. Patients 3 & 4 and 2, 5, & 6 were reported by Stankiewicz et al (2009) (pts D4 and M4) and by Sen et al (2013) (pts 15, 1, and 2), respectively. Patients 2 and 5 had missense mutations, patient 4 had a no stop mutation, patient 6 had a nonsense mutation and patient 3 had an approximately 1 Mb deletion involving *FOXF1* as well its upstream regulatory region. Patients 2–6 had associated anomalies of the gastrointestinal system. Butterfly vertebrae were identified in the patients 3 and 6. In patient 1, autopsy was limited to heart and lung. No clinical or molecular information about patients 7 and 8 was available.

Animals

Foxf1$^{+/-}$ mice with one *Foxf1* allele disrupted by deletion of the forkhead binding domain were generated (Figure S1) and maintained on a mixed 129-C57BL6/J background. The midday of vaginal plug identification was considered as embryonic day 0.5 and the mid-day when pups were born was considered as postnatal day (P) 0.5.

RNA isolation

Total RNA was isolated from approximately 10 mg frozen lung samples from patients and normal control humans using TRIzol (Invitrogen). Controls C1-C4 are age-matched lung samples from individuals that had no lung problems and died of other reasons. Control samples C1-C3 are from females and control sample C4 is a male sample. Control sample C5 is a commercially available human total lung RNA (Life Technologies Cat. No# AM7968). The tissue was homogenized in microfuge tubes with a hand held homogenizer in the presence of 200 µl of TRIzol. The aqueous phase was collected after spinning at 10,000 rpm for 5 min. This step was repeated and the pooled aqueous phase was loaded onto an RNeasy column (Qiagen). RNA was eluted from the columns following the manufacturer's instruction. The RNA was quantified using Nanodrop and its quality was assessed on a BioRad Bioanalyzer. In spite of the differences in their process of collection and preservation, the RNA isolated from the lung tissues of patients with ACDMPV were of good quality.

Mouse RNA was extracted from frozen whole lungs of P0.5 *Foxf1*$^{+/-}$ mice and their wildtype littermate controls. Whole lungs were homogenized using TissueLyser LT (Qiagen) in QIAzol lysis reagent (Qiagen) according to manufacturer's instructions. Total RNA was isolated from lung homogenates using the miRNeasy mini kit (Qiagen). RNAs were tested for quality on the Agilent 2100 bioanalyzer and quantified on the Nanodrop Spectrophotometer by the Genomic and RNA Profiling Core (GARP) facility at BCM.

Microarray analysis

500 ng of total human RNA was converted into cDNA and then cRNA following the manufacturer's instructions. The cRNA was biotinylated and hybridized to the Human Ref8.V3 microarray (Illumina) contains probes representing ~22,000 curated genes and ESTs conjugated with streptavidin-Cy3. Quality standards for hybridization, labeling, staining, background signal, and basal level of housekeeping gene expression for each chip were verified. The scanned images of the chip were analyzed using GenomeStudio software (Illumina). Gene expression analyses of RNA from patients' lungs ($n = 8$) was compared to those from the control lungs ($n = 5$).

Transcriptomes of six *Foxf1*$^{+/-}$ and six wildtype littermate samples were assessed in two separate microarray experiments using MouseWG-6 v2.0 Expression BeadChip kit (Illumina) containing probes for over 45,200 transcripts. 500 ng of total RNA was labeled using Illumina TotalPrep RNA Amplification Kit (Ambion) and hybridized as per manufacturer's instructions. The array data were analyzed using the lumi bioconductor package [21], normalized by robust spline normalization (RST), and transformed using variance stabilization transformation (VST) [22]. ComBAT batch correction [23] was applied to correct for differences in expression values between the two separate microarray experiments. Two-sample t-test was applied to determine differentially expressed genes between *Foxf1*$^{+/-}$ and wild type lung groups. Differential expression *p*-values were adjusted for false discovery rates (FDR). Fold changes were calculated using reverse VST.

Database for Annotation, Visualization, and Integrated Discovery (DAVID), Ingenuity pathway analysis (IPA), and Gene set enrichment analysis (GSEA) softwares were used for gene ontology, pathway, and network analyses.

The ACDMPV and *Foxf1*$^{+/-}$ lung microarray data sets can be accessed through the NCBI Gene Expression Omnibus (GEO) (http://www.ncbi.nih.gov/geo/) under accession numbers GSE54780 and GSE54128, respectively.

qRT-PCR

Confirmation of the differential gene expression was done by qRT-PCR using an ABI 7900HT Fast real time PCR System. Universal probe library and Fast start probe master mix from

Table 1. ACDMPV patient sample information.

Patient	Gender	Ethnicity	Inheritance	Life span (days)	*FOXF1* molecular defect	Associated anomalies
P1	M	Caucasian	Familial	48	None	Limited autopsy
P2	M	Caucasian	Sporadic	7	Missense mutation (c.286G> A;p.V96M)	Malrotation of the intestine, atrial septal defect, thick distended bladder with muscular hypertrophy, mild bilateral hydroureter and hydronephrosis
P3	F	Hispanic	Sporadic	21	Deletion (chr16: 84,402,571–85,435,712) (hg18)	Imperforate anus, suspected malrotation of the intestine, bicornuate uterus, multiple butterfly vertebrae
P4	M	Caucasian	Sporadic	46	No stop mutation (c.1138T> C;*380Rext*73)	Malrotation of the colon, Meckel's diverticulum
P5	M	Caucasian	Sporadic	28	Missense mutation (c.145C> T;p.P49S)	Incomplete rotation of bowel, right colon unfixed
P6	F	Hispanic	Sporadic	18	Nonsense mutation (c.89C> A;p.S30*	Malrotation of the intestine, imperforate anus, butterfly vertebrae, ventricular septal defect

No clinical or genetic information is available for patients 7 and 8.

Roche Applied Science was used following manufacturer's instructions.

For the mouse microarray analysis validation, RNA was reverse transcribed to cDNA using the SuperScript III First-Strand Synthesis System (Life Technologies) and amplified using the Power SYBR Green PCR Master Mix (Life Technologies). Primers used for qRT-PCR validation of the mouse microarray are listed in table S5.

Immunohistochemistry

Antibody against COL1A1 was obtained from Sigma-Aldrich. The respective dilutions of antibodies and other experimental conditions used were following manufacturer's instructions.

Results

ACDMPV lung gene expression analysis

Statistical analysis revealed 337 genes deregulated in ACDMPV lungs compared to control lungs (adjusted p-value <0.05, fold-change approximately $>/=2$ or $</=-2$), of which 205 (60.83%) were down-regulated and 132 (39.17%) were up-regulated (Figure 1A, Table S1). DAVID analysis revealed gene ontologies (GO) related to inflammation and immune responses, vasculature development, cell adhesion and chemotaxis associated with the deregulated genes (Figure 1B). The microarray data were validated using qRT-PCR for eight differentially expressed genes: *IL8*, *SPP1*, *IGFBP3*, *COL1A1*, *SOD2*, *GLI2*, *ANGPTL4*, and *HES4* (data not shown). Further, differences in protein quantity were assessed by immunohistochemistry (IHC) using antibodies against a significantly differentially expressed (*COL1A1*) product (Figure 1C). The amount of COL1A1 was significantly higher in the patient samples as compared to the control lung.

GSEA and DAVID analyses showed enrichment of pathways related to signaling in the immune system, hemostasis, cell surface interactions at the vascular wall, and the lysosome (Table S2). Further analyses by GSEA allowed determining gene sets associated with chemical and genetic perturbations enriched in the 337 genes deregulated in the ACDMPV lungs (Table S3). Genes up-regulated in vascular smooth muscle cells by MAPK8, and genes up-regulated in the Kras2LA lung cancer mouse model, are enriched in the list of down-regulated genes. Genes up-regulated by E-cadherin, and genes down-regulated in the Kras2LA lung cancer mouse model are enriched in the list of up-regulated genes. IPA pathway analysis was used to build networks and demonstrate interactions among the deregulated genes (Figure 2). Top networks involve cellular movement, cellular proliferation, inflammatory response, cardiovascular disease, hematological system development, and carbohydrate and lipid metabolism.

Foxf1$^{+/-}$ mouse lung gene expression analysis

Statistical analysis showed 789 deregulated genes in *Foxf1*$^{+/-}$ lungs compared to control lungs (FDR$<$ 0.05, fold-change $>/=1.5$ and $</=-1.5$) (Figure 3A). 394 genes of them (49.93%) were down-regulated and 395 (50.06%) were up-regulated (Table S4). GSEA and DAVID analyses revealed GO terms related to response to cytokine stimulus, cell division, blood circulation, regulation of cell proliferation and cell adhesion associated with deregulated genes (Figure 3B).

The microarray data were confirmed using qRT-PCR for five differentially expressed genes: *Dll4*, *Hgf*, *Sema3C*, *Cma1*, and *Ren1* (Figure 3C). Canonical pathways affected include genes involved in focal adhesion, homeostasis, p53 signaling, as well as in Vegf, Endothelin, and Notch signaling (Table S6). Additional GSEA analysis identified genes down-regulated by E-cadherin and genes up-regulated in vascular smooth muscle cells by MAPK8 to be enriched in the list of down-regulated genes. Genes regulated by hypoxia were found to be enriched in the list of up-regulated genes (Table S7). Network analysis by IPA identified interactions amongst genes involved in cellular movement, inflammatory response, and hematological and cardiovascular system development (Figure 4).

Gene expression alterations common to both ACDMPV and *Foxf1*$^{+/-}$ lung transcriptomes

To identify genes regulated by both *FOXF1* and *Foxf1* in human and mouse lungs, respectively, we compared genes with similarly altered expression in both ACDMPV patients and P0.5 *Foxf1*$^{+/-}$ pups and identified fourteen intersecting genes (Figure 5; Table S8). Ten genes: *COL15A1*, *COL18A1*, *COL6A2*, *FSCN1*, *IGFBP3*, *MALL*, *MATN2*, *NOS3*, *PRKCDBP*, and *RASL11B* upregulated in ACDMPV patients were also upregulated in *Foxf1*$^{+/-}$ pups. Four

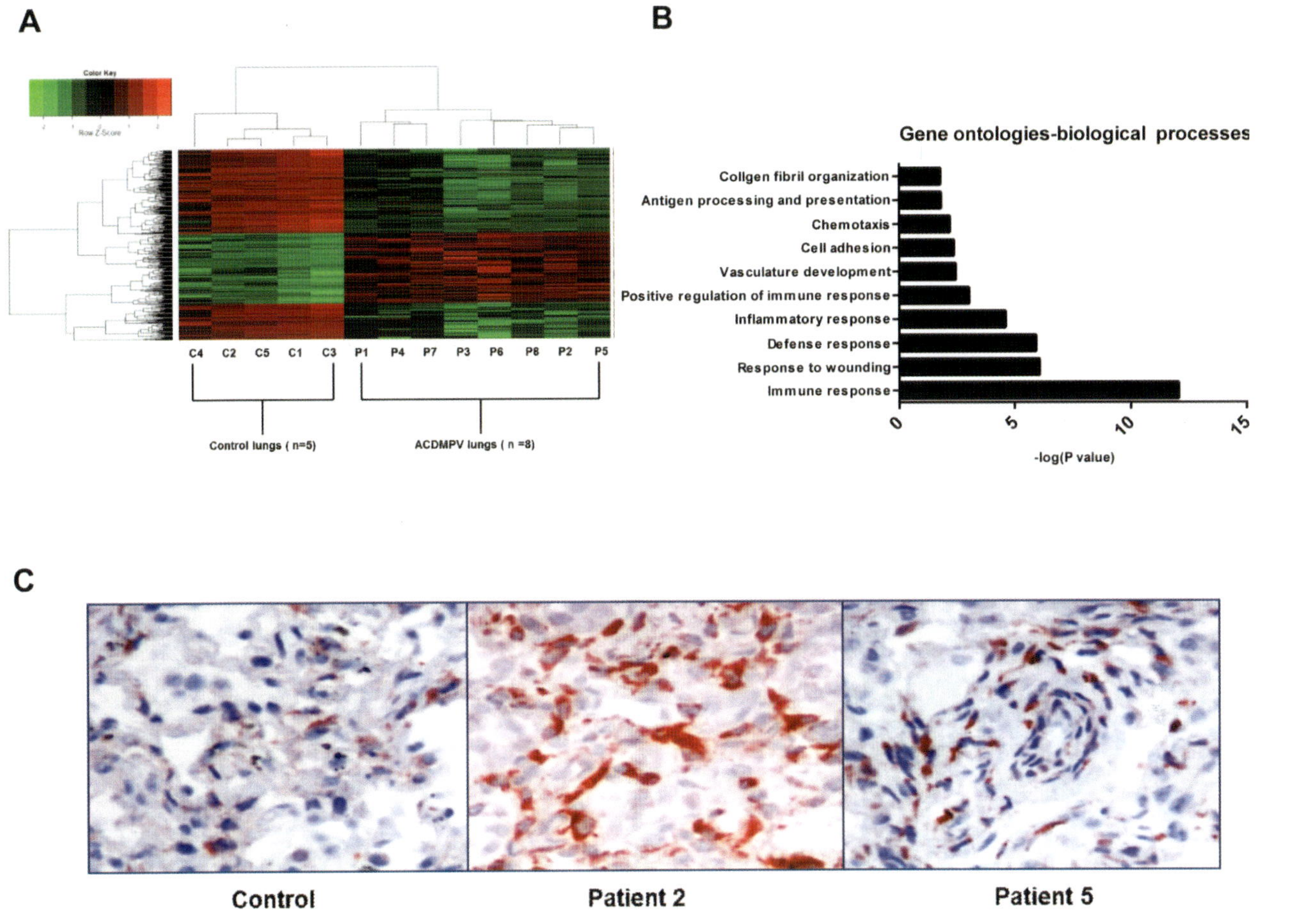

Figure 1. ACDMPV lung microarray analysis: heat map, clustering, DAVID analysis, and IHC validation. (A) Heat map for genes differentially expressed (adjusted p-value <0.05, fold change approximately $>/= 2$ or $</= -2$) between ACDMPV lungs ($n = 8$) and control lungs ($n = 5$); Decreased gene expression is shown in green and increased gene expression is shown in red. (B) Top significant gene ontology (biological processes) terms associated with deregulated genes identified by DAVID analysis. (C) IHC validation for COL1A1; Representative slides from two patients' and one control sample at 20× magnification. A commercial control lung sample C5 clustered with the age-matched control lung samples C1-4. A lung sample from a patient who died from a different congenital diffuse lung developmental disorder was also included in the analysis. The deregulated genes in this sample clustered differently than those in ACDMPV lung samples (data not shown), confirming the validity of our approach.

genes: *ESM1*, *GRINA*, *IL1B*, and *SIRPA* were downregulated in ACDMPV patients and also *Foxf1*$^{+/-}$ pups. However, five genes *ORM1*, *FGG*, *KLF4*, *IGFBP5*, and *GAMT* were found to be differentially altered in the human vs mouse microarray datasets.

Discussion

To date, we have recruited greater than 100 families with children affected with ACDMPV. This is the largest collection of ACDMPV samples worldwide. To identify transcriptional changes in the neonate ACDMPV lungs, we compared the whole genome expression in the lungs of eight patients with ACDMPV with transcriptional changes in P0.5 *Foxf1*$^{+/-}$ mouse lungs, and appropriate control lungs. This approach enabled us to identify gene ontologies and pathways associated with ACDMPV and gain a better understanding of the disease.

The *Foxf1*$^{+/-}$ mouse lungs showed down-regulation of Notch signaling genes *Dll4* and *Notch1* and slightly lower but significant (fold change: −1.46) down-regulation of the Notch target gene *Hey1* (data not shown). Notch signaling has been reported to be affected in *Foxf1*$^{+/-}$ lungs [24]. Genes involved in pulmonary vasculature development, *Sema3c* and lung branching morphogenesis, *Hgf* and *Lama1*, were also down-regulated. *Sema3c*, a semaphorin gene expressed in the lung endothelium, interacts with neuropillin-1 during vasculature development; loss of semaphorin-neuropilin-1 signaling showed lung pathology reminiscent of ACDMPV [25]. *Sema3c* was down-regulated in our study and *Foxf1* was down-regulated in lungs of *Nrp1*$^{Sema-}$ mice, suggesting a possible interaction between *Foxf1* and *Sema3C* in murine lung pathology. These transcriptional changes potentially lead to underdeveloped lungs causing respiratory distress at birth.

Transcriptional changes found in *Foxf1*$^{+/-}$ lungs, potentially resulting from the respiratory distress, include deregulation of pathways associated with hypoxia-induced vascular remodeling. There is increased expression of α-smooth muscle actin *Acta2*, indicating greater muscularization of pulmonary vessels and possible pulmonary hypertension. Greater expression of *Acta2* could also be due to endothelium-to-mesenchyme transition that is found to accompany vascular remodeling in pulmonary hypertension [26]. Additionally, members of the Endothelin-1 signaling pathway were deregulated. Endothelin-1 (ET-1) is a potent vasoconstrictor regulating vascular tone and is implicated in pulmonary hypertension. *Edn1* over-expression in mice leads to

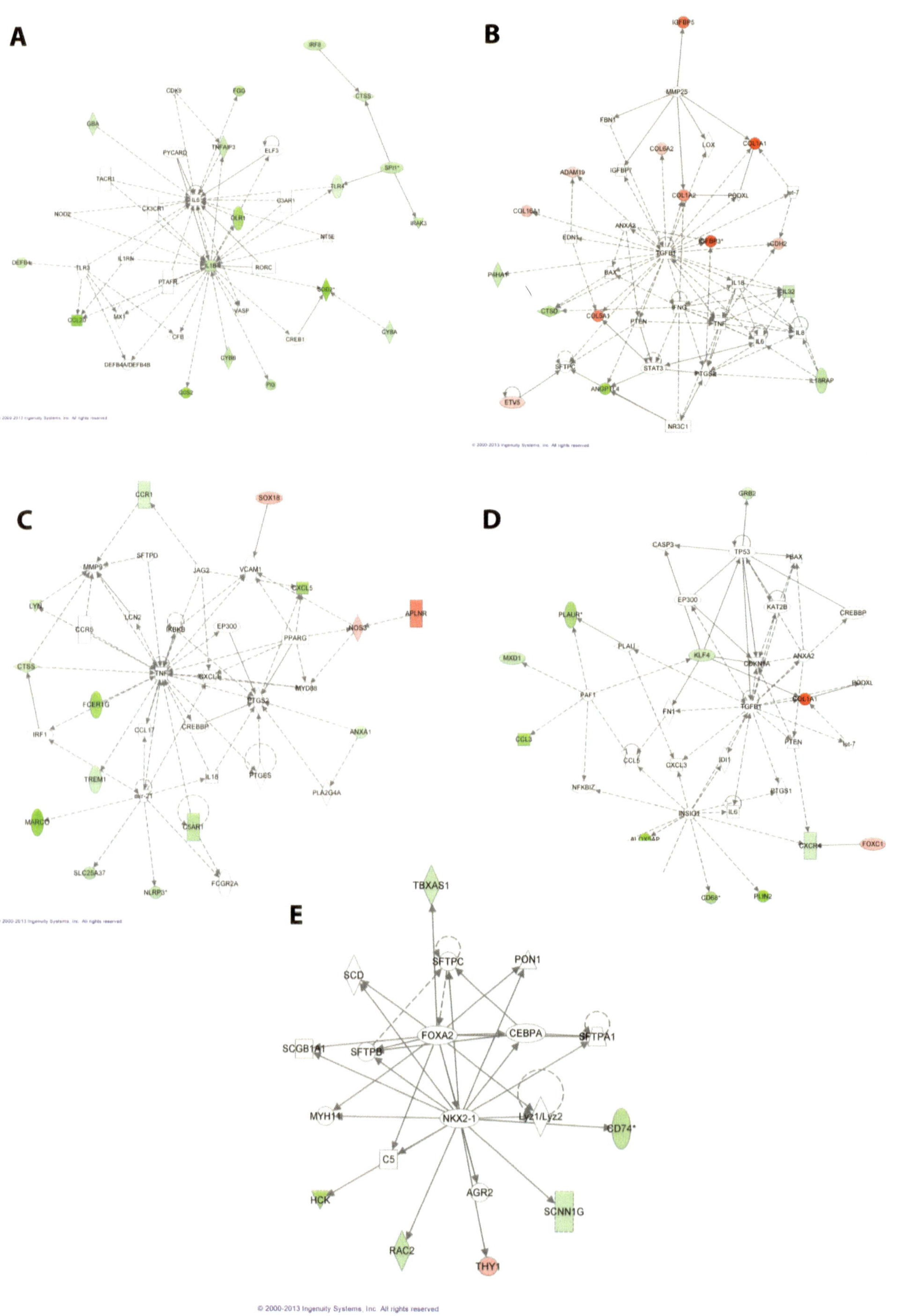
A
B
C
D
E
TBXAS1
SFTPC
PON1
SCD
FOXA2
CEBPA
SCGB1A1
SFTPB
SFTPA1
MYH11
NKX2-1
Lyz1/Lyz2
CD74*
C5
HCK
AGR2
SCNN1G
RAC2
THY1
© 2000-2013 Ingenuity Systems, Inc. All rights reserved

Figure 2. Networks involving deregulated genes in ACDMPV lungs identified using IPA; down-regulated genes are shown in green and up-regulated genes are shown in red. Deregulated genes involved in (A) Cellular movement, immune cell trafficking, inflammatory response; (B) Cellular development, cellular growth and proliferation, tumor morphology; (C) Cellular development, hematological system development and function, immune cell trafficking; (D) Cardiovascular disease, inflammatory response and cellular movement; (E) Carbohydrate metabolism, lipid metabolism and molecular transport.

development of systemic hypertension with altered vascular reactivity [27].

Fibronectin and several members of the collagen gene family are also found to be up-regulated, likely leading to increased production of extracellular matrix (ECM) proteins. Accumulation of ECM proteins such as collagen, elastin, and fibronectin leads to thickening of pulmonary blood vessels, likely contributing to pulmonary hypertension. Interestingly, endothelin induced collagen remodeling has been reported in a mouse model of pulmonary hypertension [28], indicating that the increased endothelin-1 signaling in *Foxf1*$^{+/-}$ lungs may be causing an increase in collagen production. Integrins involved in cell surface interactions at the vascular wall were also found to be down-regulated. Similar transcriptional changes have been observed to be associated with matrix and vasculature remodeling in TGF-α induced pulmonary fibrosis [29]. *Foxf1* was shown to play an essential role in mesenchymal migration by transcriptionally regulating integrin-β3 (Itgβ3) [30]. Integrin-ECM interactions also contribute to vascular remodeling. Altered integrin-ECM interactions have been documented in chronic hypoxia and monocrotaline-induced pulmonary hypertension [31].

Mast cell chymase and tryptase genes (*Mcpt4*, *Mcpt6*, *Cma1*, and *Cpa3*) are highly up-regulated i n *Foxf1*$^{+/-}$ lungs, showing evidence of pulmonary mastocytosis. Pulmonary mastocytosis and enhanced lung inflammation in *Foxf1*$^{+/-}$ mice after chemically induced or allergen-mediated lung injury was reported [32]. These inflammatory molecules could contribute to the vascular remodeling through their effects on vascular cell wall permeability, matrix protein production, and by inducing recruitment of mesenchymal precursor cells [33]. Similar accumulation of mast cell mediators was found in lungs of *Fgfr3/4* mutant mice that exhibit Bronchopulmonary Dysplasia (BPD) like pathology and in lungs

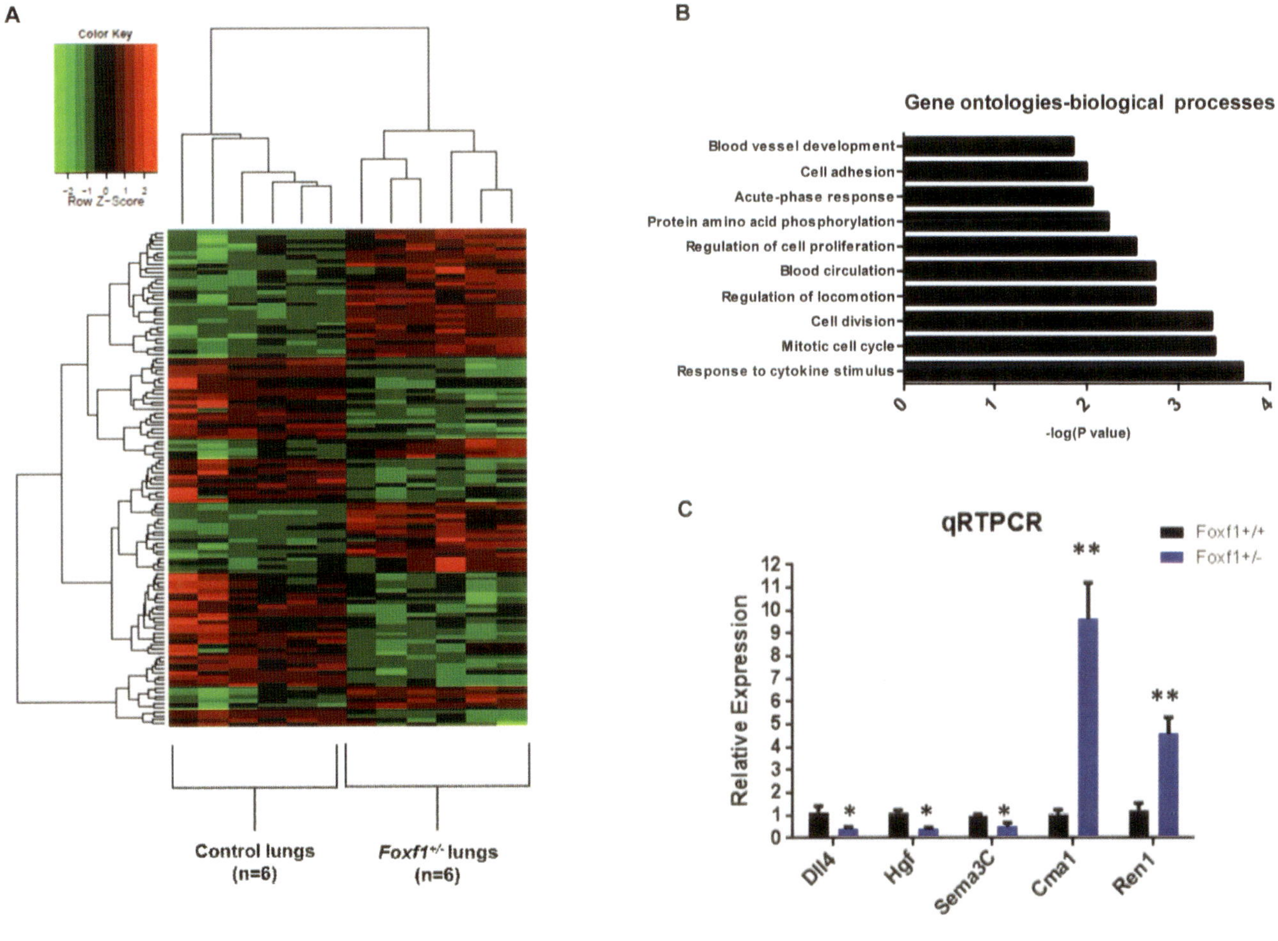

Figure 3. *Foxf1*$^{+/-}$ mouse lung microarray analysis: heat map, clustering, DAVID analysis, and qRT-PCR validation. (A) Heat map for genes differentially expressed (fdr <0.05, fold change >/= 2 or </= − 2) between *Foxf1*$^{+/-}$ lungs (n = 6) and littermate control lungs (n = 6); Decreased gene expression is shown in green and increased gene expression is shown in red; *Foxf1*$^{+/-}$ lung samples and wildtype lung samples cluster as two separate groups. (B) Top significant gene ontology (biological processes) terms associated with deregulated genes from DAVID analysis. (C) qRT-PCR validation for down-regulated genes (*Sema3C*, *Dll4*, and *Hgf*) and up-regulated genes (*Cma1* and *Ren1*); n = 6 for each group; * = p value <0.05; ** = p value <0.001.

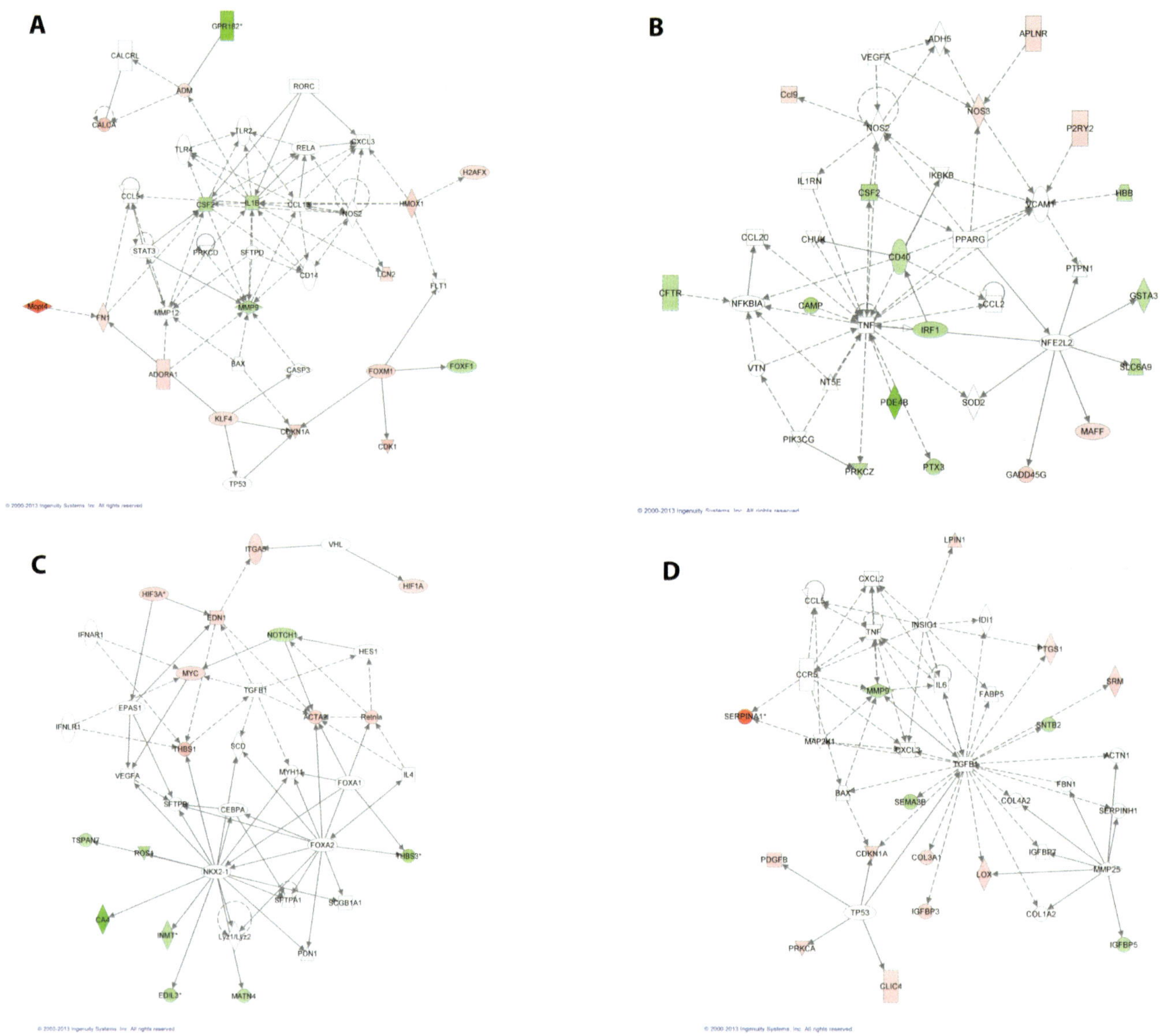

Figure 4. Networks involving deregulated genes in *Foxf1*$^{+/-}$ lungs identified using IPA. Deregulated genes involved in (A) Inflammatory response, cellular movement, cardiovascular disease; (B) Cell-to-cell signaling and interaction, cellular movement, hematological system development and function; (C) Embryonic development, organ development; (D) Cardiovascular system development and function, organ development, cellular movement; down-regulated genes are shown in green and up-regulated gens are shown in red.

of children with BPD [34], suggesting that pulmonary mastocytosis could be a common feature found in diffuse lung developmental conditions. *Ren1* which along with *Cma1* and *Cpa3* is a component of the blood pressure regulating renin angiotensin system is also up-regulated.

Other transcriptional changes include up-regulation of *Mki67*, *Ccnd1*, and *Foxm1*, showing an increase in proliferation in the lung. *Foxf1* has been reported to be down-regulated in mice with endothelial cell-specific deletion of *Foxm1* [35], indicating a reciprocal feedback loop between *Foxf1* and *Foxm1*. Finally, up-regulation of *Hif3α* and *Nos3* is also observed, suggesting a compensatory mechanism to counteract the effects of hypoxia-induced pulmonary hypertension.

Microarray analysis of ACDMPV human lung transcriptomes primarily identified deregulation of genes involved in inflammation and cell surface interactions at the vascular wall. Members of the collagen gene family are highly up-regulated similar to the up-regulation seen in *Foxf1*$^{+/-}$ lungs, potentially leading to increased ECM collagen production, causing thickening of pulmonary blood vessels, and resulting in pulmonary hypertension, a typical feature found in neonates with ACDMPV.

IHC for COL1A1 confirmed the increased protein levels of COL1A1 in ACDMPV patient lungs (Figure 1C). Structural changes in ACDMPV lungs that could be attributed to hypoxia-induced vascular remodeling include medial thickening of smooth muscles in pulmonary arteries. Transcriptional changes which could be described as compensatory mechanisms to counteract the pulmonary hypertension include down-regulation of genes involved in TREM1 signaling (*TREM1, TLR4, IL1B,* and *ITGAX*) and up-regulation of *NOS3*. Pulmonary inflammatory responses play an important role in hypoxia-induced vascular remodeling [33] and down-regulation of TREM1 signaling could be a

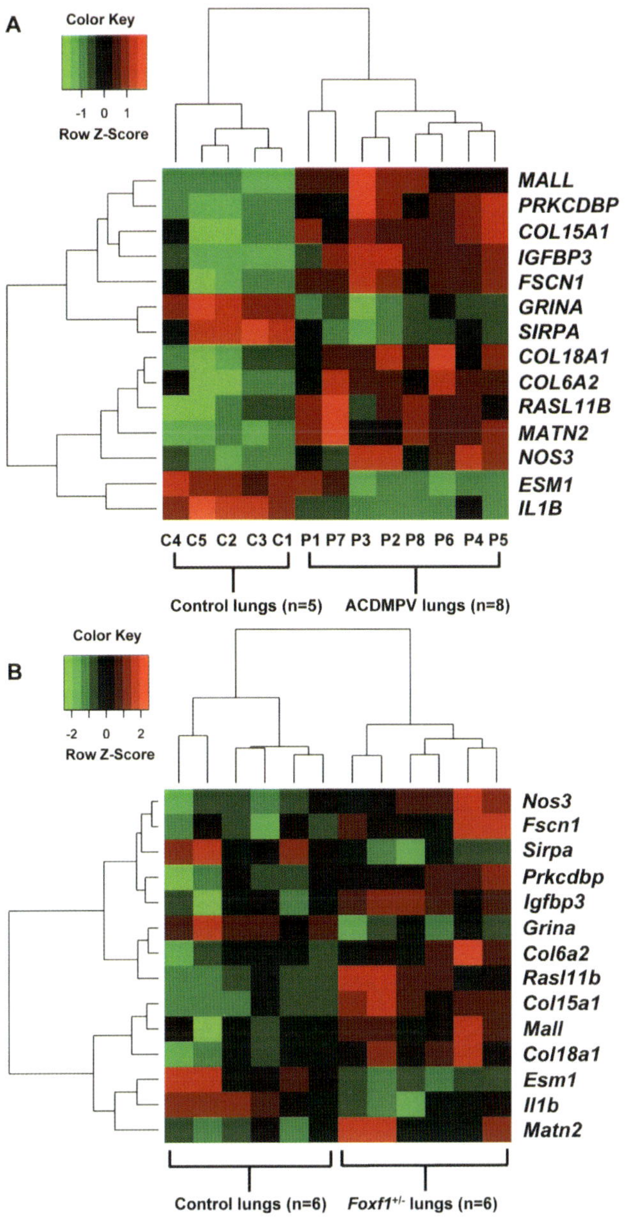

Figure 5. Deregulated genes common to both ACDMPV lungs and P0.5 *Foxf1*$^{+/-}$ lungs. (A) Heat map comparing expression of 14 overlapping genes in ACDMPV lung samples and control lung samples; (B) Heat map comparing expression of 14 overlapping genes in *Foxf1*$^{+/-}$ lung samples and control lung samples.

compensatory response to attenuate pulmonary inflammatory responses. *Tlr-4* deficient mice were shown to be resistant to chronic hypoxia-induced pulmonary hypertension by attenuating the pulmonary vascular inflammatory response to hypoxia [36]. Up-regulation of *NOS3* also could be a compensatory response to counteract the hypertension.

Other affected pathways include signaling related to the lysosome function, carbohydrate metabolism, cell cycle, and axon guidance which are also deregulated in *Foxf1*$^{+/-}$ lungs. Interestingly, we found targets of E-cadherin enriched in the deregulated genes. Recently, E-cadherin has been shown to be a target of FOXF1, which in turn has been shown to be a target of p53, regulating cancer cell migration and invasiveness [37]. Additionally, *FOXF1* expression has been shown to be changed in numerous human malignancies [38–45].

Comparison of the deregulated genes in both experiments enabled identification of 14 genes, *COL15A1, COL18A1, COL6A2, ESM1, FSCN1, GRINA, IGFBP3, IL1B, MALL, NOS3, RASL11B, MATN2, PRKCDBP,* and *SIRPA,* similarly altered in both ACDMPV and *Foxf1* heterozygous lung transcriptomes. *ESM1* is mainly expressed in endothelial cells and its expression is upregulated by cytokines like TNFα and IL-1β suggesting that it plays a role in endothelium-dependent pathological disorders [46]. *ESM1* as well as *IL1B* are downregulated in both the microarray datasets. *ESM1* has also been computationally predicted to have a FOX: ETS binding motif in its vicinity suggesting that it could be a direct target of *FOXF1* in endothelial cells [47]. Another common downregulated gene in both datasets, *SIRPA* has been shown to interact with surfactant proteins A & D in the absence of inflammation to suppress alveolar macrophage phagocytosis [48]. Whereas there is greater variation for *Sirpa* in the mouse data, the average fold change difference for this gene correlates with the human data.

In aggregate, we present the results of genome-wide analyses of transcriptional changes in lungs from patients with ACDMPV due to point mutations or genomic deletions in *FOXF1* and in mice heterozygous for *Foxf1* loss. The transcriptional changes should help better define the molecular mechanisms involved in the pathogenesis of ACDMPV and may also be a valuable source for future research on lung vasculature development and pulmonary disease conditions such as pulmonary hypertension, bronchopulmonary dysplasia, and lung cancer.

Supporting Information

Figure S1 Generation of the *Foxf1*$^{+/-}$ mouse line. Single allele deletion of the *Foxf1* gene was achieved by breeding of *Foxf1*-floxed heterozygous females with EIIa-Cre male mice. *Foxf1*-floxed allele possesses two LoxP sites (white arrowhead) and one Frt site that surround exon 1, encoding the Forkhead DNA-binding domain of the *Foxf1* protein. Cre-mediated recombination occurs in a wide range of tissues, including the germ cells that transmit *Foxf1*-null allele to offspring. Exon 1 and part of the promoter of *Foxf1* are deleted. The GRCm38/mm10 coordinates of the deleted region are chr8:121,083,499-121,085,436 (1938 bp). *Fendrr* is a long non coding RNA gene located upstream to *Foxf1*, and negatively regulates it. Primer sequences used to genotype mice with heterozygous loss of *Foxf1* are: F: 5′-TTCAGATCTGAGAGTGGCAGCTTC-3′; R1:5′-GCTTTGTCTCCAAGCGCTGC-3′; and R2:5′GAAGGAACCCAGATGTTCCCTG-3′.
(TIF)

Table S1 ACDMPV lung microarray analysis: List of deregulated genes (adjusted p value <0.05, fold change> / = 2 or </ = - 2).
(XLSX)

Table S2 Pathways enriched in ACDMPV lung transcriptomes: GSEA and DAVID analyses (p-value <0.05).
(XLSX)

Table S3 Chemical and genetic perturbation gene sets enriched in ACDMPV lungs: GSEA analysis (fdr <0.05).
(XLSX)

Table S4 *Foxf1*$^{+/-}$ mouse lung microarray analysis: List of deregulated genes (fdr <0.05, fold change > / = 1.5 or </ = − 1.5).
(XLSX)

Table S5 List of primer sequences used for qRT-PCR validation using SYBR.
(XLSX)

Table S6 Pathways enriched in *Foxf1*$^{+/-}$ lung transcriptomes: GSEA and DAVID analyses (p-value <0.05).
(XLSX)

Table S7 Chemical and genetic perturbation gene sets enriched in *Foxf1*$^{+/-}$ lungs: GSEA analysis (fdr <0.05).
(XLSX)

Table S8 GO terms associated with genes similarly altered in both ACDMPV lungs and *Foxf1*$^{+/-}$ lungs.
(XLSX)

Acknowledgments

We thank J. Crowe and M. Hill for technical assistance and Drs. W.Y. Wan, K.M. Aagaard, and I.B. Van den Veyver for helpful discussion and assistance with microarray analysis.

Author Contributions

Conceived and designed the experiments: P. Sen AVD HB P. Stankiewicz. Performed the experiments: P. Sen AVD TM MM MB ST P. Szafranski. Analyzed the data: P. Sen AVD JZ AG JB CL. Contributed reagents/materials/analysis tools: TVK XR VVK MJJ SW. Wrote the paper: P. Sen AVD P. Stankiewicz.

References

1. Bishop NB, Stankiewicz P, Steinhorn RH (2011) Alveolar capillary dysplasia. Am J Respir Crit Care Med 184: 172–179.
2. MacMahon HE (1948) Congenital alveolar dysplasia; a developmental anomaly involving pulmonary alveoli. Pediatrics 2: 43–57.
3. Janney CG, Askin FB, Kuhn C 3rd (1981) Congenital alveolar capillary dysplasia–an unusual cause of respiratory distress in the newborn. Am J Clin Pathol 76: 722–727.
4. I, Reichman B, Schibi G, Brish M (1984) Familial persistent pulmonary hypertension. Arch Dis Child 59: 783–785.
5. Langston C (1991) Misalignment of pulmonary veins and alveolar capillary dysplasia. Pediatr Pathol 11: 163–170.
6. Abdallah HI, Karmazin N, Marks LA (1993) Late presentation of misalignment of lung vessels with alveolar capillary dysplasia. Crit Care Med 21: 628–630.
7. Shankar V, Haque A, Johnson J, Pietsch J (2006) Late presentation of alveolar capillary dysplasia in an infant. Pediatr Crit Care Med 7: 177–179.
8. Thibeault DW, Garola RE, Kilbride HW (1999) Alveolar capillary dysplasia: an emerging syndrome. J Pediatr 134: 661–662.
9. Kitayama Y, Kamata S, Okuyama H, Usui N, Sawai T, et al. (1997) Nitric oxide inhalation therapy for an infant with persistent pulmonary hypertension caused by misalignment of pulmonary veins with alveolar capillary dysplasia. J Pediatr Surg 32: 99–100.
10. Alameh J, Bachiri A, Devisme L, Truffert P, Rakza T, et al. (2002) Alveolar capillary dysplasia: a cause of persistent pulmonary hypertension of the newborn. Eur J Pediatr 161: 262–266.
11. Al-Hathlol K, Philips S, Seshia MK, Casiro O, Alvaro RE, et al. (2000) Alveolar capillary dysplasia. Report of a case of prolonged life without extracorporeal membrane oxygenation (ECMO) and review of the literature. Early Hum Dev 57: 85–94.
12. Plat G, Rouquette I, Marcoux MO, Bloom MC, Acar P, et al. (2007) Alveolar capillary dysplasia and persistent pulmonary hypertension of the newborn Arch Mal Coeur Vaiss 100: 458–461.
13. Licht C, Schickendantz S, Sreeram N, Arnold G, Rossi R, et al. (2004) Prolonged survival in alveolar capillary dysplasia syndrome. Eur J Pediatr 163: 181–182.
14. Sen P, Thakur N, Stockton DW, Langston C, Bejjani BA (2004) Expanding the phenotype of alveolar capillary dysplasia (ACD). J Pediatr 145: 646–651.
15. Stankiewicz P, Sen P, Bhatt SS, Storer M, Xia Z, et al. (2009) Genomic and genic deletions of the FOX gene cluster on 16q24.1 and inactivating mutations of *FOXF1* cause alveolar capillary dysplasia and other malformations. Am J Hum Genet 84: 780–791.
16. Sen P, Yang Y, Navarro C, Silva I, Szafranski P, et al. (2013) Novel *FOXF1* Mutations in Sporadic and Familial Cases of Alveolar Capillary Dysplasia with Misaligned Pulmonary Veins Imply a Role for its DNA Binding Domain. Hum Mutat 34: 801–811.
17. Szafranski P, Dharmadhikari AV, Brosens E, Gurha P, Kolodziejska KE, et al. (2013) Small noncoding differentially methylated copy-number variants, including lncRNA genes, cause a lethal lung developmental disorder. Genome Res 23: 23–33.
18. Sen P, Gerychova R, Janku P, Jezova M, Valaskova I, et al. (2013) A familial case of alveolar capillary dysplasia with misalignment of pulmonary veins supports paternal imprinting of *FOXF1* in human. Eur J Hum Genet 21: 474–477.
19. Kalinichenko VV, Lim L, Stolz DB, Shin B, Rausa FM, et al. (2001) Defects in Pulmonary Vasculature and Perinatal Lung Hemorrhage in Mice Heterozygous Null for the Forkhead Box f1 Transcription Factor. Dev Biol 235: 489–506.
20. Mahlapuu M, Enerbäck S, Carlsson P (2001) Haploinsufficiency of the forkhead gene *Foxf1*, a target for sonic hedgehog signaling, causes lung and foregut malformations. Development 128: 2397–2406.
21. Du P, Kibbe WA, Lin SM (2008) lumi: a pipeline for processing Illumina microarray. Bioinformatics 24: 1547–1548.
22. Lin SM, Du P, Huber W, Kibbe WA (2008) Model-based variance-stabilizing transformation for Illumina microarray data. Nucleic Acids Res 36: e11.
23. Johnson WE, Rabinovic A, Li C (2007) Adjusting batch effects in microarray expression data using empirical Bayes methods. Biostatistics 8: 118–127.
24. Kalinichenko VV, Gusarova GA, Kim IM, Shin B, Yoder HM, et al. (2004) *Foxf1* haploinsufficiency reduces Notch-2 signaling during mouse lung development. Am J Physiol Lung Cell Mol Physiol 286: 521–530.
25. Joza S, Wang J, Fox E, Hillman V, Ackerley C, et al. (2012) Loss of semaphorin-neuropilin-1 signaling causes dysmorphic vascularization reminiscent of alveolar capillary dysplasia. Am J Pathol 181: 2003–20017.
26. Arciniegas E, Frid MG, Douglas IS, Stenmark KR (2007) Perspectives on endothelial-to-mesenchymal transition: potential contribution to vascular remodeling in chronic pulmonary hypertension. Am J Physiol Lung Cell Mol Physiol 293: 1–8.
27. Leung JW, Wong WT, Koon HW, Mo FM, Tam S, et al. (2011) Transgenic mice over-expressing ET-1 in the endothelial cells develop systemic hypertension with altered vascular reactivity. PLoS One 6: e26994.
28. Mansoor AM, Honda M, Saida K, Ishinaga Y, Kuramochi T, et al. (1995) Endothelin induced collagen remodeling in experimental pulmonary hypertension. Biochem Biophys Res Commun 215: 981–986.
29. Hardie WD, Korfhagen TR, Sartor MA, Prestridge A, Medvedovic M, et al. (2007) Genomic profile of matrix and vasculature remodeling in TGF-alpha induced pulmonary fibrosis. Am J Respir Cell Mol Biol 37: 309–321.
30. Malin D, Kim IM, Boetticher E, Kalin TV, Ramakrishna S, et al. (2007) Forkhead box F1 is essential for migration of mesenchymal cells and directly induces integrin-beta3 expression. Mol Cell Biol 27: 2486–2498.
31. Umesh A, Paudel O, Cao YN, Myers AC, Sham JS (2011) Alteration of pulmonary artery integrin levels in chronic hypoxia and monocrotaline-induced pulmonary hypertension. J Vasc Res 48: 525–537.
32. Kalin TV, Meliton L, Meliton AY, Zhu X, Whitsett JA, et al. (2008) Pulmonary mastocytosis and enhanced lung inflammation in mice heterozygous null for the *Foxf1* gene. Am J Respir Cell Mol Biol 39: 390–399.
33. Stenmark KR, Fagan KA, Frid MG (2006) Hypoxia-induced pulmonary vascular remodeling: cellular and molecular mechanisms. Circ Res 99: 675–691.
34. Bhattacharya S, Go D, Krenitsky DL, Huyck HL, Solleti SK, et al. (2012) Genome-wide transcriptional profiling reveals connective tissue mast cell accumulation in bronchopulmonary dysplasia. Am J Respir Crit Care Med 186: 349–358.
35. Balli D, Zhang Y, Snyder J, Kalinichenko VV, Kalin TV (2011) Endothelial cell-specific deletion of transcription factor *FoxM1* increases urethane-induced lung carcinogenesis. Cancer Res 71: 40–50.
36. Young KC, Hussein SM, Dadiz R, deMello D, Devia C, et al. (2010) Toll-like receptor 4-deficient mice are resistant to chronic hypoxia-induced pulmonary hypertension. Exp Lung Res 36: 111–119.
37. Tamura M, Sasaki Y, Koyama R, Takeda K, Idogawa M, et al. (2013) Forkhead transcription factor *FOXF1* is a novel target gene of the p53 family and regulates cancer cell migration and invasiveness. Oncogene doi: 10.1038/onc.2013.427.
38. Lo PK, Lee JS, Liang X, Han L, Mori T, et al. (2010) Epigenetic inactivation of the potential tumor suppressor gene *FOXF1* in breast cancer. Cancer Res 70: 6047–6058.
39. Su Z, Gay LJ, Strange A, Palles C, Band G, et al. (2012) Common variants at the MHC locus and at chromosome 16q24.1 predispose to Barrett's esophagus. Nat Genet 44: 1131–1136.
40. Levine DM, Ek WE, Zhang R, Liu X, Onstad L, et al. (2013) A genome-wide association study identifies new susceptibility loci for esophageal adenocarcinoma and Barrett's esophagus. Nat Genet 45: 1487–1493.
41. van der Heul-Nieuwenhuijsen L, Dits NF, Jenster G (2009) Gene expression of forkhead transcription factors in the normal and diseased human prostate. BJU Int 103: 1574–1580.
42. Armeanu-Ebinger S, Bonin M, Häbig K, Poremba C, Koscielniak E, et al. (2011) Differential expression of invasion promoting genes in childhood rhabdomyosarcoma. Int J Oncol 38: 993–1000.
43. Lo PK, Lee JS, Chen H, Reisman D, Berger FG, et al. (2013) Cytoplasmic mislocalization of overexpressed *FOXF1* is associated with the malignancy and metastasis of colorectal adenocarcinomas. Exp Mol Pathol 94: 262–269.

44. Wendling DS, Luck C, von Schweinitz D, Kappler R (2008) Characteristic overexpression of the forkhead box transcription factor *Foxf1* in Patched-associated tumors. Int J Mol Med 22: 787–792.
45. Saito RA, Micke P, Paulsson J, Augsten M, Peña C, et al. (2010) Forkhead box F1 regulates tumor-promoting properties of cancer-associated fibroblasts in lung cancer. Cancer Res 70: 2644–2654.
46. Lassalle P, Molet S, Janin A, Heyden JV, Tavernier J, et al. (1996) ESM-1 is a novel human endothelial cell-specific molecule expressed in lung and regulated by cytokines. J Biol Chem 271: 20458–20464.
47. De Val S, Chi NC, Meadows SM, Minovitsky S, Anderson JP, et al. (2008) Combinatorial regulation of endothelial gene expression by Ets and Forkhead transcription factors. Cell 135: 1053–1064.
48. Janssen WJ, McPhillips KA, Dickinson MG, Linderman DJ, Morimoto K, et al. (2008) Surfactant proteins A and D suppress alveolar macrophage phagocytosis via interaction with SIRP alpha. Am J Respir Crit Care Med 178: 158–167.

20

Muscle RING Finger-1 Promotes a Maladaptive Phenotype in Chronic Hypoxia-Induced Right Ventricular Remodeling

Matthew J. Campen[1]*, Michael L. Paffett[1], E. Sage Colombo[1], Selita N. Lucas[1], Tamara Anderson[2], Monique Nysus[2], Jeffrey P. Norenberg[2], Ben Gershman[3], Jacob Hesterman[3], Jack Hoppin[3], Monte Willis[4]

1 Department of Pharmaceutical Sciences, College of Pharmacy, University of New Mexico Health Sciences Center, Albuquerque, New Mexico, United States of America, **2** Radiopharmaceutical Sciences Program, College of Pharmacy, University of New Mexico Health Sciences Center, Albuquerque, New Mexico, United States of America, **3** inviCRO, LLC., Boston, Massachusetts, United States of America, **4** McAllister Heart Institute and Department of Pathology and Laboratory Medicine, University of North Carolina, Chapel Hill, North Carolina, United States of America

Abstract

Exposure to chronic hypoxia (CH) induces elevated pulmonary artery pressure/resistance, leading to an eventual maladaptive right ventricular hypertrophy (RVH). Muscle RING finger-1 (MuRF1) is a muscle-specific ubiquitin ligase that mediates myocyte atrophy and has been shown to play a role in left ventricular hypertrophy and altered cardiac bioenergetics in pressure overloaded hearts. However, little is known about the contribution of MuRF1 impacting RVH in the setting of CH. Therefore, we hypothesized that MuRF1 deletion would enhance RVH compared to their wild-type littermates, while cardiac-specific overexpression would reduce hypertrophy following CH-induced pulmonary hypertension. We assessed right ventricular systolic pressure (RVSP), right ventricle to left ventricle plus septal weight ratio (RV/LV+S) and hematocrit (Hct) following a 3-wk isobaric CH exposure. Additionally, we conducted dual-isotope SPECT/CT imaging with cardiac function agent ^{201}Tl-chloride and cell death agent ^{99m}Tc-annexin V. Predictably, CH induced pulmonary hypertension, measured by increased RVSP, RV/LV+S and Hct in WT mice compared to normoxic WT mice. Normoxic WT and MuRF1-null mice exhibited no significant differences in RVSP, RV/LV+S or Hct. CH-induced increases in RVSP were also similar between WT and MuRF1-null mice; however, RV/LV+S and Hct were significantly elevated in CH-exposed MuRF1-null mice compared to WT. In cardiac-specific MuRF1 overexpressing mice, RV/LV+S increased significantly due to CH exposure, even greater than in WT mice. This remodeling appeared eccentric, maladaptive and led to reduced systemic perfusion. In conclusion, these results are consistent with an atrophic role for MuRF1 regulating the magnitude of right ventricular hypertrophy following CH-induction of pulmonary hypertension.

Editor: Sudhiranjan Gupta, Texas A & M, Division of Cardiology, United States of America

Funding: This work is supported by the National Institutes of Health (NIH ES014639 to MJC and R01HL104129 to MW), the University of New Mexico Cancer Center (NIH P30 CA118100-06), the W.M. KECK Foundation, and the Leducq Foundation (MW). inviCRO, LLC provided support in the form of salaries for authors JH, JH, and BG, but did not have any additional role in the study design, data collection and analysis, decision to publish, or preparation of the manuscript. The specific roles of these authors are articulated in the author contributions section.

Competing Interests: Jack Hoppin, Jacob Hesterman, and Ben Gershman are employees of inviCRO, LLC. There are no patents, products in development or marketed products to declare.

* E-mail: mcampen@salud.unm.edu

Introduction

Right ventricular hypertrophy (RVH) occurs in the setting of primary pulmonary arterial hypertension (PAH) and frequently precipitates mortality in this disease [1], with recent estimates of 44% of PAH patients dying from right ventricular failure or sudden cardiac death [2]. The manifestation of a dilated hypertrophic phenotype, characterized by a large RV volume and reduced stroke volume, correlates with an even worse prognosis [3]. RVH also contributes to mortality as a comorbid condition in a number of other syndromes, such as chronic obstructive pulmonary disease and scleroderma [4] [5]. Even without progressing to frank failure, progressive remodeling of the RV may generate a substrate for electrocardiographic abnormalities [6], which may contribute to the incidence of sudden cardiac death [7]. As such, improved understanding of molecular pathways that contribute to or modify RVH phenotypes may provide important clues towards novel therapies for PAH treatment.

Muscle RING finger 1 (MuRF1) is a ubiquitin ligase that regulates atrophy processes in striated muscle [8–10]. A critical component to the regulation of muscle mass is the turnover over and degradation of sarcomere proteins, which MuRF1 has been reported to ubiquitinate and target for proteasome-mediated degradation, including cardiac troponin I and beta-Myosin heavy chain [11,12]. MuRF1 also interacts with a number of other sarcomere-associated proteins, including myosin light chain 2, titin, myotilin, and TnT, and may be responsible for the turnover of these and other yet to be identified proteins [13,14]. However, the ability of MuRF1 to regulate signal transduction through its interaction with transcription factors may play a more prominent role in its regulation of cardiac hypertrophy. For example, in ischemia-reperfusion injury, MuRF1 regulates JNK-mediated apoptosis through its interaction, poly-ubiquitination, and degradation of phosphorylated c-Jun activated by reperfusion [15]. In pathological cardiac hypertrophy, MuRF1-/- mice undergo an exaggerated hypertrophy in vivo, suggesting an anti-hypertrophic activity of MuRF1 [8]. One possible mechanism by which MuRF1 exerts this activity is through its direct interaction with the transcription factor SRF, which it inhibits without affecting its protein level [8]. Using MuRF1 Tg mice with increased cardiac MuRF1 expression, it was shown that MuRF1 acts through the regulation of creatine kinase activity to alter cellular metabolism [10]. In models of cardiac atrophy and left ventricular cardiac hypertrophy reversal, MuRF1 is a critical mediator, as demonstrated in MuRF1-/- mice, resistant to both processes [9].

In contrast to the left ventricle, the right functions with low-pressure working conditions and a complex geometry different from the left ventricle. Despite the more passive role the RV may appear to play, it is important in the interdependence between left and right systolic and diastolic function. Pulmonary hypertension, for example, causes a leftward shift of the interventricular septum that can negatively affect LV function [16] [17]. Recent studies have investigated the role of the ubiquitin proteasome system in a right ventricular hypertrophy model [18]. After induction of PAH and the development of right ventricular hypertrophy, increased poly-ubiquitination and free ubiquitin was detected in the hearts [18]. Given MuRF1's presence in both the left and right ventricles and MuRF1's regulation of LV cardiomyocyte hypertrophy by multiple mechanisms, we hypothesized that MuRF1 would regulate right ventricular hypertrophy *in vivo*. To test this, we challenged MuRF1-/- and MuRF1 Tg+ mice to hypoxia-induced pulmonary hypertension to detect the role of MuRF1 in the compensatory mechanisms of a model of pulmonary artery hypertension.

Methods

Animal Model

Mice were obtained from colonies whose derivation has been previously described [8,10] or from a commercial vendor (C57BL/6 mice from Taconic; Oxnard, CA) and shipped to the University of New Mexico. Following a week-long quarantine, mice were moved to a control chamber or normobaric hypoxia chamber, but maintained in standard shoebox cages with food and water available ad libitum throughout. The hypoxia chamber was set at 10.0% oxygen (partial pressure of oxygen roughly 65 mmHg in Albuquerque) and monitored both by the digital feedback-control system (Biospherix, Colorado) as well as by a secondary O_2/CO_2 monitor (O2Cap, OxiGraf, Inc.; Mountain View, CA). The hypoxia exposure lasted 3 weeks with twice-weekly cage changes and standard 12 h light:dark cycle. Procedures were conducted under full isoflurane anesthesia to minimize or eliminate risk of pain and discomfort. All procedures were conducted with full approval by the University of New Mexico Institutional Animal Care and Use Committee and carried out in compliance with the National Institutes of Health Guide for the Care and Use of Laboratory Animals.

Single-Photon Emission Computed Tomography

On the final day of hypoxia or normoxia exposures, mice were slowly injected via a bolus tail vein injection of approximately 0.75 mCi of ^{201}TlCl in 0.9% NaCl, USP for ECG-gated SPECT/CT assessments of cardiac perfusion, volume and function. Imaging was conducted at approximately 30 minutes post injection as previously described [17]. As in this previous work, RV imaging in normoxic mice was occasionally sub-optimal due to a large signal from the left ventricle that overwhelmed our ability to discriminate the RV. For this reason, data for normoxic mice are frequently pooled to facilitate statistical comparisons. In hypoxic mice, RV hypertrophy was sufficient to mitigate this challenge.

Volume and radioactivity concentration were estimated from 3D regions-of-interest (ROIs), including left & right ventricle, left & right myocardium, entire heart, and fixed-volume lung and muscle sub-regions, generated using VivoQuant (inviCRO) image processing software. A flow quantification software FlowQuant (University of Ottawa, Heart Institute) was used to estimate cardiac ejection fraction.

Right Ventricular Pressure, Hypertrophy, and Hematocrit

Immediately following the SPECT/CT assessments, mice were rapidly intubated and artificially ventilated with 2% isoflurane/balance O_2. Under anesthesia, a thoracotomy was performed and a saline-filled catheter was inserted into the right ventricle. Stable pressure measurements were obtained for >30 seconds from which right ventricular systolic, mean, and diastolic pressures were obtained. Next, blood was rapidly withdrawn into capillary tubes and spun for hematocrit readings, while the heart was excised and carefully dissected into right ventricle and left ventricle + septum to obtain separate weights for derivation of RV/LVS ratios, as previously described [19].

Quantitative Polymerase Chain Reaction

qPCR was conducted as previously described [20] [21] using a Roche 480 LightCycler instrument. Primers were obtained from a commercial vendor (Life Technologies) and shown in Table 1.

Statistics

Considerations for pooling of data were given for normoxia and WT groups in all scenarios. Where either variation or means were statistically different, pooling was not conducted. However, for most endpoints, no differences were observed between WT KO and WT Tg+ in hypoxic groups or between any strain in normoxia. A clear exception to this was overall heart weights, where the Normoxic MuRF1-/- mice had evident cardiac enlargement compared to most other strains. All data were examined for assumptions of normal distribution. Data were routinely compared by 2-factor Analysis of Variance, considering the roles of hypoxia and genotype, and using a Bonferroni post-hoc test to explore specific group effects. Probability values of less than 0.05 were considered significant.

Results

Right ventricular MuRF1 mRNA expression decreases in response pulmonary hypertension

C57BL/6 mice challenged to chronic hypoxia exhibited increased right ventricular hypertrophy. Exposure to 10% O_2 for 3 weeks resulted in significantly increased right ventricular systolic pressure, resulting in an increase in right ventricular mass measured by the Fulton index (RV/LVS; Fig. 1, A and B). BNP expression was significantly increased in the right ventricle, consistent with the hypertrophic response observed (Fig. 1C). The expression of the RV MuRF1 mRNA decreased compared to normoxic control mice (Fig. 1D).

Table 1. Primers used for quantitative PCR.

Gene Name	Gene Symbol	Primer ID
TATA Box Protein	TBP	Mm00446971_m1
Muscle RING finger 1 (MuRF1)	Trim63	Mm01185221_m1
B-type Natriuretic Peptide (BNP)	Nppb	Mm01255770_g1
Beta Myosin Heavy Chain (bMHC)	Myh7b	Mm01249941_m1
Alpha Smooth Muscle Actin	Acta2	Mm01546133_m1
NADH-Ubiquinone Oxidoreductase Chain 2	MtND2	Mm04225288_s1

Chronic Hypoxia Increases Right Ventricular Pressure and Hematocrit

Both MuRF1-/-, MuRF1 Tg+, and their respective strain-matched wild type controls exhibited a statistically equivalent increase in RV systolic pressure 3 weeks of hypoxia (35.5–40.7 mm Hg) (Figure 2A, right). The systolic pressure in parallel normoxia treated mice did not differ between the pooled strain-matched WT controls, MuRF1 -/-, and MuRF1 Tg+ mice with mean values of 26.8, 25.6, and 28.5 mmHg, respectively (Figure 2A, left).

Hematocrit in normoxia-challenged controls was statistically similar across strains (Figure 2B, left). Hypoxia exposure induced a predictable increase in hematocrit, with values of 74.3, 77.7 and 80.1 for WT (pooled), MuRF1-/- and MuRF1 Tg+ strains, respectively, all significantly elevated over normoxic controls. Interestingly, in response to hypoxia, the MuRF1 Tg+ mice developed a significantly greater polycythemia than WT hypoxic mice ($P<0.05$, 2-way ANOVA with Bonferroni posthoc test). It should also be noted that we observed two lethalities in the MuRF Tg+ hypoxia group, one after two weeks and one just prior to imaging at 3 weeks. Lethality in the 10% O_2 exposure is highly unusual in our experience.

Weight Loss due to hypoxia is attenuated in MuRF1 -/- mice

Normoxic control mice increased body weight over the 3 week experimental period, with no differences observed between the genotypes (Figure 3). WT, MuRF1-/- and MuRF1 Tg+ mice challenged with hypoxia in parallel underwent significant body weight, owing to reductions in food and water intake, of roughly 6 g over the first week (Figure 3A). MuRF -/- mice displayed a significant attenuation in this response compared to wildtype mice (Figure 3A), while MuRF1 Tg+ tracked consistently with their respective WT strain (Figure 3B). After one week, both MuRF1-/- and MuRF1 Tg+ mice undergoing hypoxia treatment stabilized body weight and consistently increased over the remaining 2 weeks.

Right Ventricular Growth is Enhanced by MuRF1 Deletion, Unaltered by Overexpression

Gravimetric and SPECT/CT assessment of the hearts from MuRF1 -/- and MuRF1 Tg+ mice challenged with hypoxia for 3 weeks demonstrated a significant right ventricular hypertrophy compared to all normoxic control groups (Figure 4). As predicted, hypoxia treatment induced a significant elevation in RV/LVS in the WT strains (0.37; pooled). MuRF1-/- mice after hypoxia treated exhibited an exaggerated cardiac hypertrophy, illustrated by a RV/LVS mean value of 0.48 that was significantly greater

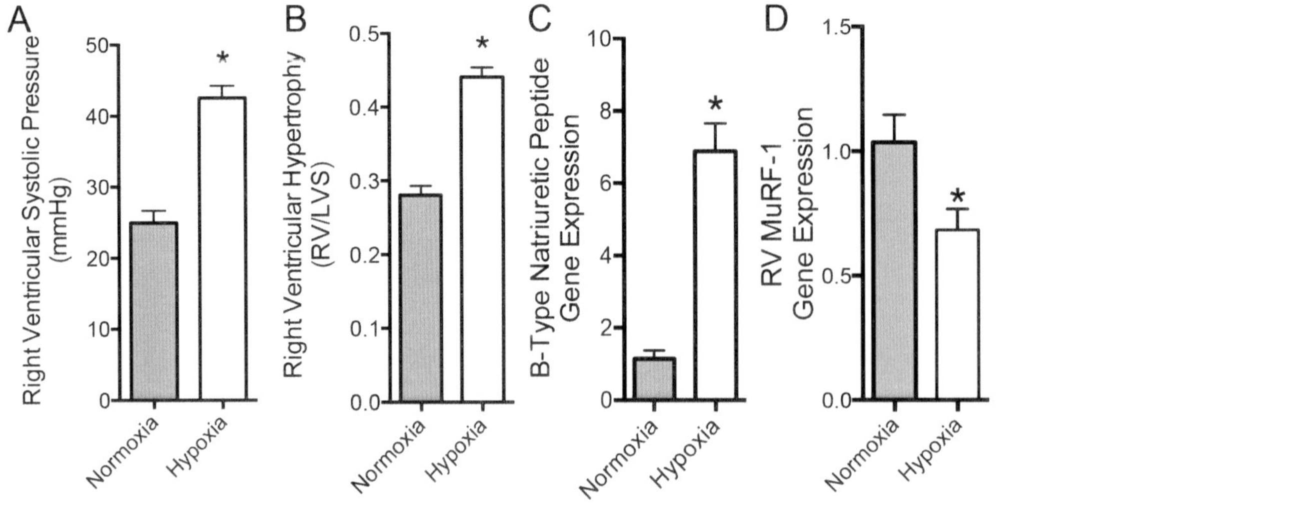

Figure 1. WT C57BL/6 mouse response to hypoxia in terms of right ventricular systolic pressure (A), right ventricular hypertrophy (B), right ventricular expression of B-type natriuretic peptide mRNA (C) and right MuRF1 mRNA (D). Asterisks denote significant difference from normoxic controls ($p<0.05$) by two-tailed t-test (N = 7-8 per group).

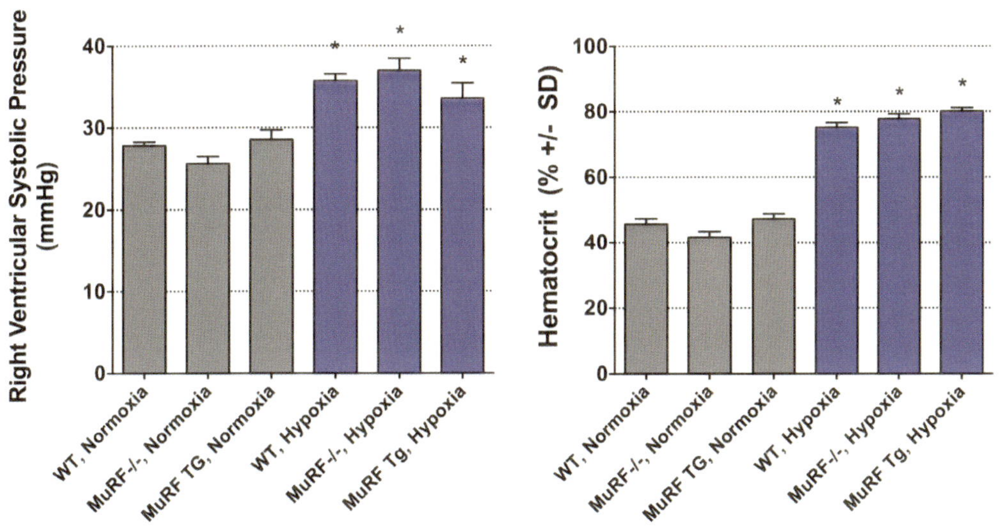

Figure 2. Hemodynamic and Hematologic Responses to Hypoxia in MuRF1 -/- and MuRF1 cardiac Tg+ mice. Chronic normobaric hypoxia ($FiO_2 = 0.10$) led to predictable increase in right ventricular systolic pressure and hematocrit in WT and $MuRF^{-/-}$ mice, as measured at 21 days (*left*). Asterisks denote significant difference from normoxia control groups ($P < 0.05$; N = 5–11 per group). All strains exhibited increases in hematocrit (N = 5–11 per group, *$p < 0.001$; *right*).

than both WT and MuRF1 Tg+ exposed to hypoxic conditions. Interestingly, mice with increased cardiac-specific MuRF1 expression and challenged with hypoxia for 3 weeks had increased right ventricular growth, rather than inhibited growth, as was expected. In fact, the MuRF1 Tg+ RV/LVS values (0.42) were significantly greater than WT, although significantly less than MuRF1-/- mice. SPECT/CT imaging revealed a pattern of RV growth in MuRF1 Tg+ mice that appeared more dilated than that of WT or MuRF1-/- mice (Figure 4B).

To quantify the degree of dilation observed in the SPECT/CT assessment, we compared the gravimetrically-determined mass of the RV free wall with the SPECT/CT-derived RV[1] chamber volume, which showed a significant reduction in hypoxia exposed MuRF1 Tg+ mice relative to all other groups, confirming a dilated phenotype (Figure 4C). Ejection fractions were also determined on those subjects for whom adequate ECG-gated images were collected; notably normoxic mice had smaller RV mass compared to LV mass, which was a limitation in this study, necessitating pooling of data for all strains in the normoxia treatment (Figure 4D). Not only did MuRF1 Tg+ hearts appear dilated after 3 weeks of hypoxia treatment, they exhibited a significant decrease in RV ejection fraction compared to normoxic controls ($P < 0.05$), in contrast to wild type and MuRF1-/- mice, which were generally unaffected (Figure 4D). Overall systolic and diastolic volumes in the MuRF1 Tg+ hearts also appeared dilated compared to MuRF-/- mice (Fig. 4E).

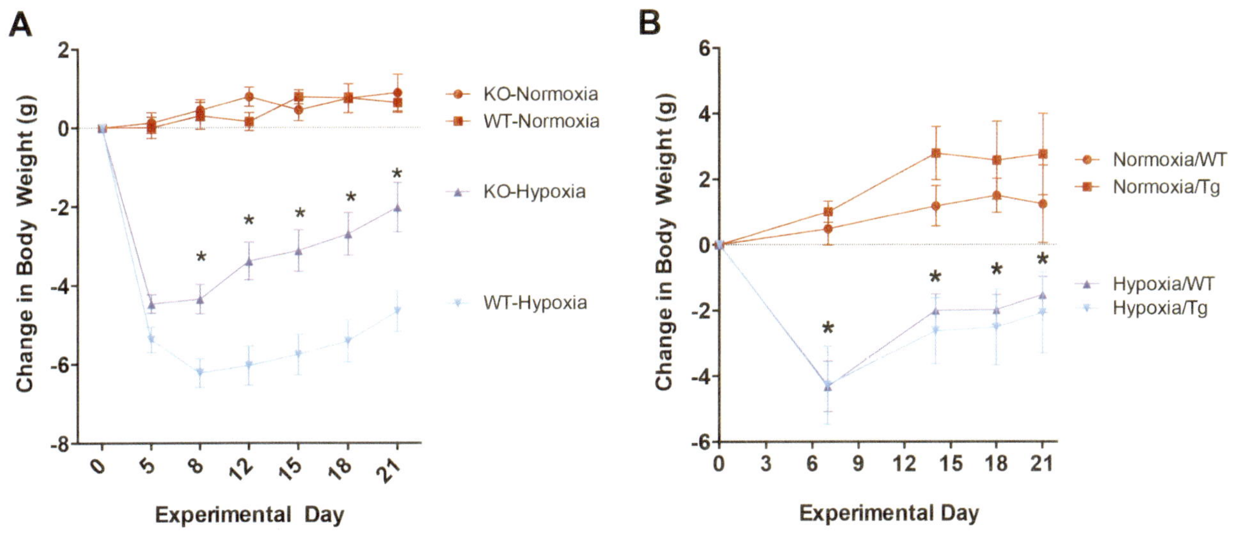

Figure 3. Body weight response to CH is evident in global *MuRF1 -/-* mice compared to cardiac-specific MuRF1 Tg^+ mice. Longitudinal weight change profile during chronic hypoxia exposure illustrates global MuRF1 deletion attenuates weight loss with similar gain to WT *(A)*, whereas MuRF1 Tg^+ mice have similar weight loss and gain compared to WT *(B)*. N = 5-6 per group, *$p < 0.05$ from WT.

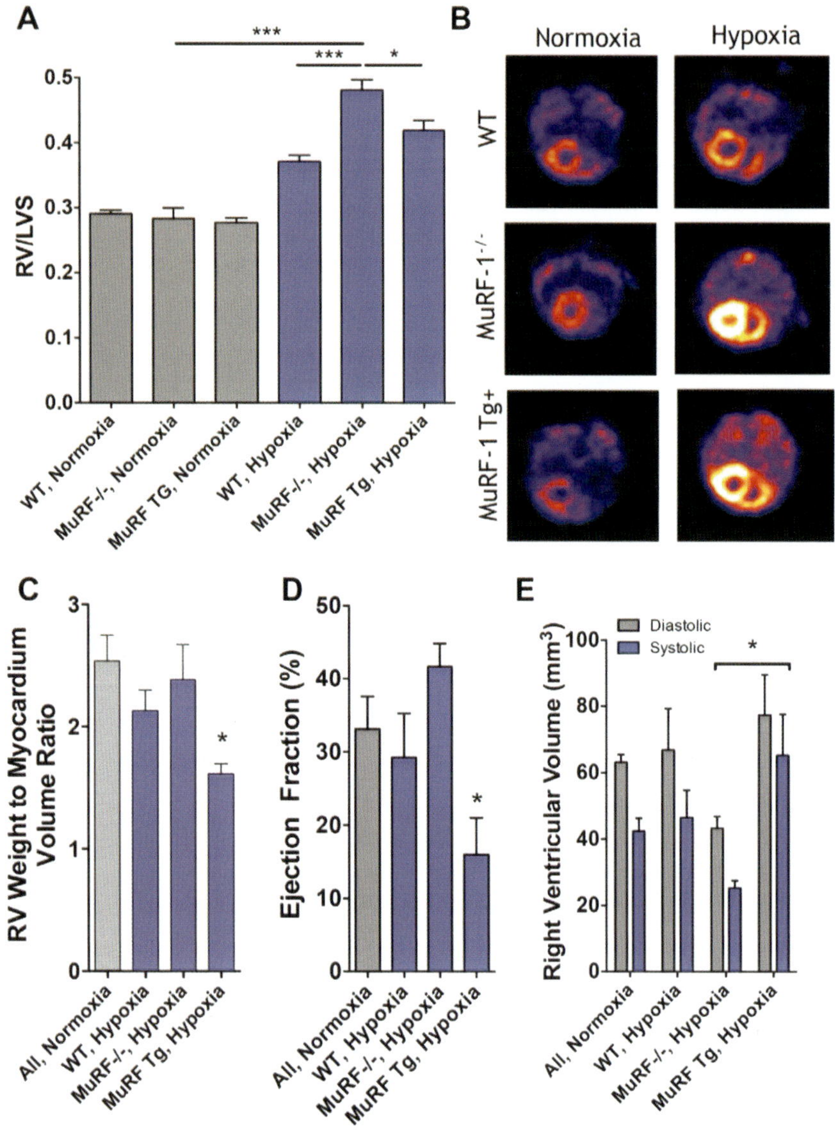

Figure 4. Hypoxia-induced right ventricular remodeling is enhanced by MuRF1 deletion, while cardiac-specific MuRF1 overexpression leads to a maladaptive dilated phenotype. (A) Chronic hypoxia induced predictable increases in RV/LVS, more so in the *MuRF1 -/-* mice than in WT. Interestingly, cardiac-specific overexpression of this atrophy-mediating ubiquitin ligase had no protective effect in terms of net hypertrophy of the right ventricle and in fact led to exacerbation of hypoxia-induced RVH relative to WT (*significantly greater than all control groups, $p<0.01$; **significantly greater than all control groups and WT hypoxia, $p<0.01$; ***significantly greater than all other groups, $p<0.01$). (B) Axial SPECT/CT cross-section images obtained at diastole reveal marked hypertrophy of the RV in hypoxia-exposed mice, with the appearance of dilation in the MuRF1 Tg+ mice. (C) Right ventricular weight to chamber volume ratio (D) ejection fraction and (E) RV systolic and diastolic volumes determined from ECG-gated SPECT/CT images are shown. As RV wall motion was difficult to image in normoxia mice, all genotypes are pooled. (N = 3-6 per group; *significantly lower than KO, Hypoxia mice, $p<0.05$).

MuRF1 and RV expression of pathologic cardiac hypertrophy markers in response to hypoxia

The expression of mRNA normally found in the fetal heart, but not adult heart, were identified in mice challenged to hypoxia. Smooth muscle alpha-actin, myosin heavy chain beta, and BNP were measured in after 2 weeks of hypoxia challenge (Figure 5). Cardiac markers of pathologic hypertrophy demonstrated mixed outcomes related to the hypoxia and genetic factors. Hypoxia consistently induced RV expression of SM a-actin mRNA, with no major differences apparent among the strains (Fig. 5A). βMyHC mRNA did not show a substantial increase in most strains, despite the hypertrophic findings, but was significantly elevated in MuRF1 Tg+ mice. BNP mRNA was not significantly altered by chronic hypoxia in the MuRF1-/- mice or their genetic background strain, but both MuRF1 Tg+ and their background strain showed significant increases. Lastly, we assessed a marker of mitochondrial density, MtND2 DNA, which was significantly reduced by chronic hypoxia in both MuRF1 Tg+ mice and their background strain, but not in the MuRF1-/- mice or their background strain.

Cardiac and Skeletal Muscle Perfusion

SPECT/CT imaging of ^{201}TlCl was used to assess overall perfusion of cardiac tissue and a region of skeletal muscle in a small cohort of exposed mice (Fig. 6A). Again, because the normal

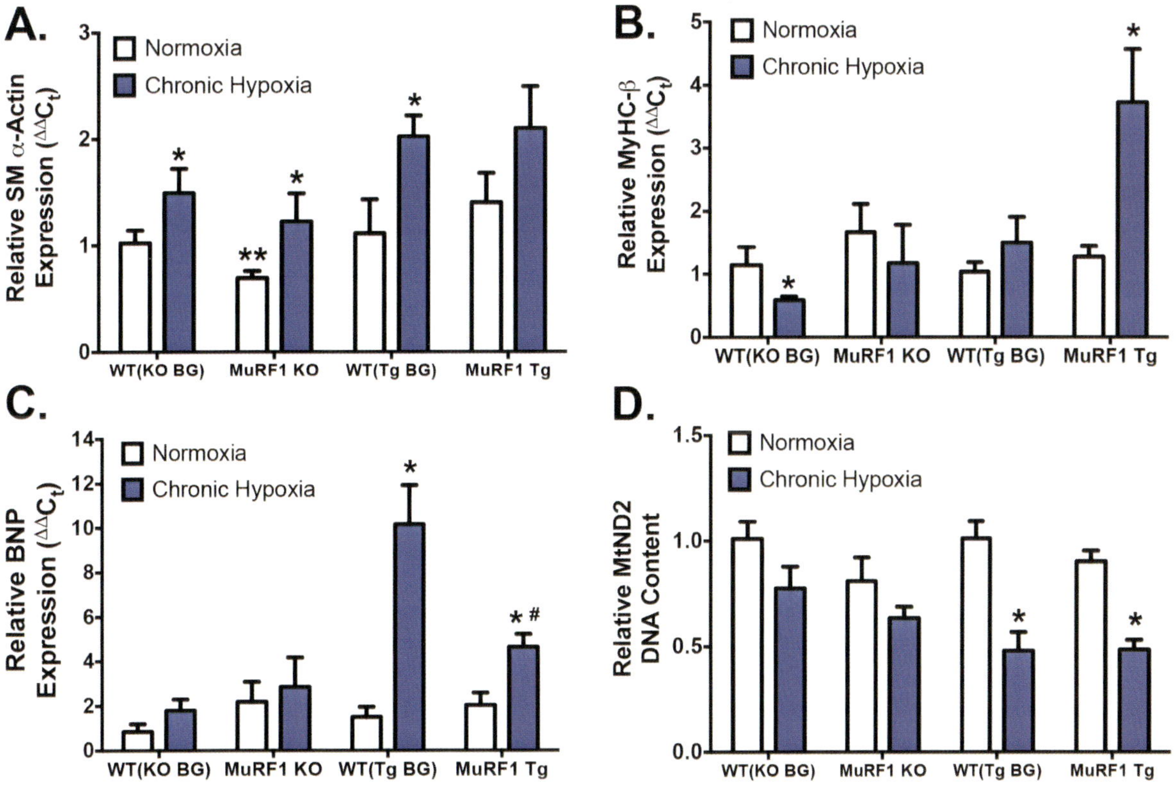

Figure 5. Differential Induction of Cardiac Hypertrophy/Failure Transcripts in MuRF$^{-/-}$ & *MuRF1 Tg+* Mice Following CH. Effects of CH-induced PH on relative RV transcript expression of *(A)* SM a-actin, *(B)* MyHC-b, *(C)* BNP and *(D)* mtND2 DNA content from *MuRF1 -/-* and MuRF1 Tg+ mice. BNP, MyHC-b and SM a-actin expression normalized to TATA binding protein. MtND2 DNA content normalized to 18S DNA. N = 5 per group, *p<0.05 vs respective normoxic control; #p<0.05 vs chronic hypoxia Tg^{+}; **p<0.05 vs respective WT.

RV is small in comparison to the LV, the normoxic RV was often difficult to reliably assess. For this reason, data for RV total perfusion in normoxic mice were pooled across strains in mice that could be assessed. RV perfusion was significantly elevated in hypoxia-exposed MuRF1-/- and MuRF1 Tg+ mice compared to normoxic controls (Fig. 6B). A modest, but non-significant perfusion increase was seen in hypoxia-exposed WT mice; a restricted group subanalysis of the hypoxia effect in WT mice by Student's *t*-test revealed a likely effect compared to normoxia-exposed mice (P = 0.035). When ^{201}TlCl uptake for the whole heart was calculated, hypoxia as an independent treatment factor caused a significant increase in perfusion, most pronounced in the MuRF1-/- and MuRF1 Tg+ mice (Fig. 6C). However, when skeletal muscle perfusion was analyzed, MuRF1-/- and MuRF1 Tg+ mice trended in opposite directions, with greater skeletal muscle perfusion seen in MuRF1-/- mice and reduced perfusion in MuRF1 Tg+ hearts.

Discussion

MuRF1 regulates atrophy of cardiac muscle through the degradation of structural and regulatory proteins [22]. In the setting of hypoxia-induced PAH, RV MuRF1 mRNA expression was downregulated, potentially to permit cellular hypertrophic responses. The deletion of MuRF1 expectedly led to exaggerated growth of the right ventricle relative to the left in response to hypoxia-induced PAH. However, cardiac-specific overexpression of MuRF1 did not have the opposite effect (*i.e.*, preventing growth), but rather led to a maladaptive phenotype associated with wall thinning, lower ejection fraction, and reduced perfusion. We speculate that selective overexpression of MuRF1 may enhance degradation and therefore reduce abundance of sarcomeric proteins, with minimal impact on growth-related signaling for other cellular components, thus allowing for enlargement of cells with reduced contractile force. On the other hand, inhibition (or deletion) of MuRF1 may permit an enhanced contractile phenotype. The short time frame (3 weeks) of the hypoxia model limits the conclusions as to the potential positive or negative implications of the enhanced growth in MuRF1-/- mice, but increased growth in the presence of adequately compensated perfusion suggests a beneficial adaptation.

Right ventricular failure is a common and defining outcome in many forms of pulmonary hypertension [4] [5]. Little research has been conducted on ride-sided cardiac hypertrophy and failure in terms of proteolysis and ubiquitin ligase involvement. However, a great deal is known about left-sided hypertrophy and failure and the role of MuRF1, specifically. In LV pathologic cardiac hypertrophy, MuRF1 inhibits pathologic cardiac hypertrophy in a transaortic constriction (TAC) model without affecting function [8,10]. However, cardiac-specific overexpression of MuRF1 in the TAC mode led to eccentric remodeling similar to that seen in the present study with hypoxia-induced right ventricular remodeling [9]. MuRF1 regulates the creatine kinase activity in MuRF1 Tg+ hearts and increases susceptibility to TAC-induced heart failure, while doing little to inhibit cardiac hypertrophy. While much of this is consistent with the influence of MuRF1 overexpression on hypoxia-induced right ventricular changes, in the TAC model mitochondrial numbers were significantly increased in MuRF1

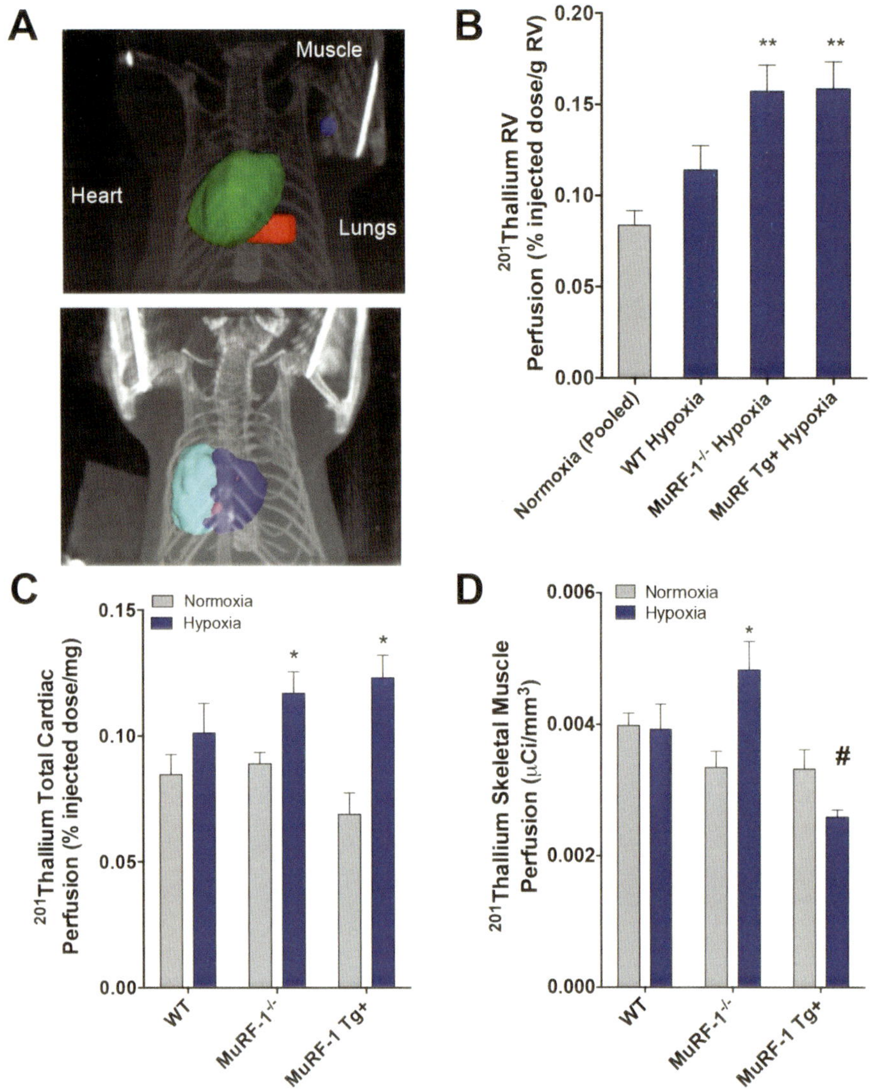

Figure 6. Relative perfusion of right ventricular myocardium, total heart, and skeletal muscle as a reference, as determined by SPECT/CT using ^{201}TlCl uptake. Region of interest phantoms are depicted in (A). Hypoxia caused a significant increase in perfusion in the RV (B) of both *MuRF1 -/-* and *MuRF1 Tg+* mice relative to RV mass (N = 5–8 per group; ** denotes $p<0.01$ compared to normoxia mice by ANOVA). The RV perfusion was not consistently observable in controls, so results are pooled for all mouse models. The total heart uptake also showed an effect of hypoxia that was predominant in the *MuRF1 -/-* and *MuRF1 Tg+* mice relative to WT (C). Skeletal muscle perfusion (C) was elevated in hypoxia-exposed MuRF1 -/-mice but reduced in hypoxia-exposed *MuRF1 Tg+* mice. (B,C: N = 5–8 per group; * indicates $p<0.05$ compared to normoxic conditions for the same strain; † indicates $P<0.05$ compared to WT).

Tg+ mice, while we observed a reduction in cardiac MtDNA levels due to hypoxia that was unaffected by MuRF1.

We had previously investigated the roles of MuRF1 and a related ubiquitin ligase, atrogin-1 or MAFbx, in pulmonary vascular smooth muscle hypertrophy stemming from pulmonary hypertension [23]. In the monocrotaline (MCT) model, rat pulmonary arteries demonstrated significant reductions in atrogin-1 expression that tightly followed the timecourse of vascular hypertrophy and hemodynamic changes. We then used resveratrol to specifically upregulate atrogin-1, both in whole animal and vascular smooth muscle cell culture studies, which led to a reversal of the hypertrophic/hyperplastic phenotype. While off-target pleiotropic effects of resveratrol cannot be discounted, these findings motivated further inquiry into the role of ubiquitin ligases in aspects of PAH. Subsequent studies of MCT found atrogin-1 to be downregulated in the right ventricle, as well [21]. Interestingly, MuRF1 is not highly expressed in smooth muscle cells, despite its prominent role in skeletal and cardiac muscle growth.

Resveratrol was initially used in the MCT model due to our hypothesis that inducing a caloric restriction phenotype in myocytes would reduce growth pathways. In cardiac muscle this might reduce the size of the myocytes, while in smooth muscle it may also reduce hyperplasia. Pathways upregulated by caloric restriction, related to AMP kinase and sirtuin signaling, oppose IGF-1/Akt signaling in cardiomyocytes. AMPK, activated via caloric restriction or pharmacologically (AICAR), induces MuRF1 and atrogin-1 in cardiomyocytes [24]. Caloric restriction also maintains elevated levels of skeletal muscle MuRF1 and atrogin-1 [25]. These studies highlight a key involvement of MuRF1 in energy-saving benefits in scenarios of reduced energy bioavailability or increased metabolic demand, such as in the case of elevated pulmonary vascular resistance. However, for cardiomyocytes, activating MuRF1 and impeding the matched growth of contractile components compared to other cellular components may lead to maladaptive stretching of the myocytes and eccentric remodeling. Therapeutic interventions that antagonize MuRF-1, on the other hand, may permit the increased abundance of contractile proteins and enhance force generation, with the caveat that failure to remove aging sarcomeric components would soon lead to negative outcomes.

One interesting observation in this study was that MuRF1-/- mice were partially protected against the weight loss that occurred during the mid-to-late phases of the hypoxic exposure (Figure 3). The present hypoxia model incorporates a weight loss phase that is a combination of hypoxia and starvation, as the mice decrease activity and ingest less food and water in the first week of treatment. Weight loss in this model results in ~6 g decrease in body weight in wild-type mice. Our findings suggest that MuRF-1 did not affect the initial magnitude of weight loss, which is consistent with the literature defining this initial period as a lack of food consumption. In comparable studies, hypoxia-induced weight loss is directly related to early deficits in food and water consumption; supplementing hypoxic rats with erythrocytes to offset reduced oxygen availability did not reduce the initial weight loss phase [26]. On the other hand, in the later phases of the hypoxia model the mice are chronically hypoxic and the absence of MuRF-1 led to a faster recovery of body weight, presumably muscular weight. Mice deficient in erythropoietin exhibit significant reductions in hematocrit and muscle oxygenation, which induces skeletal muscle proteolysis [27]. Rats in a 5-week hypobaric hypoxia model exhibited increased skeletal muscle expression of a related ubiquitin ligase, atrogin-1[28]. It may also be that hypoxia-related inactivity plays an important role, and it has been documented that MURF1 -/- mice are resistant to skeletal muscle atrophy in response to a denervation model [29].

It is unknown to what extent these factors (anorexia, hypoxia, inactivity) may also contribute to the cardiac muscle mass changes and MuRF1 activity beyond the obvious mechanical stress incurred by the hemodynamic changes in this PAH model. While more detailed histopathology and complementary functional assessments would be ideal, the data from this study strongly suggests that functionality of the whole heart is better preserved when MuRF1 is absent and impaired when it is overexpressed (Figure 6). In human heart failure, skeletal muscle undergoes a number of atrophic changes, including reduced Akt phosphorylation [30], mitochondrial density [31], and cross-bridge kinetics [32]. In MuRF1-/- mice, systemic perfusion was preserved, possibly even increased over controls, while the cardiac-specific MuRF1 overexpression led to reduced skeletal muscle perfusion, as assessed by SPECT/CT. The recovery of body weight in the MuRF1-/- mice may relate in part to this preserved cardiac function, but more detailed studies are needed to define this phenomenon.

One clear limitation to the present study is the lack of assessment of pulmonary vascular remodeling and resistance. Because we did not see clear differences in RVSP or HCT that would drive the pattern of RV/LVS phenotypes, we believe it is unlikely that a substantial load-dependent differential was incurred by the genetic manipulations in this study. MuRF1, unlike its relative ubiquitin ligase Atrogin-1 (paffet, that uterus study) [21] [33], does not appear to have an important role in smooth muscle regulation. Alternatively, one might consider a role for MuRF1 in response to hypoxia globally. This may in part explain the modest, significant increase in HCT in the hypoxic MuRF1 Tg+ mice compared to WT and MuRF1-/- mice, but postulating how a cardiac-specific overexpression of MuRF1 drives an increased erythropoeitic response would be challenging. Perhaps more compelling argument relates to the reduced perfusion in the failing heart of hypoxic MuRF1 Tg+ mice, which leads to reduced perfusion of kidneys and increased erythropoeitic signaling.

In summary, MuRF1 plays an important role in modulating the degree and quality of hypertrophic manifestations resulting from the hypoxia-induced PAH model. The overexpression of MuRF1 led to an eccentric and maladaptive hypertrophy, while deletion of MuRF1 permitted greater hypertrophy without a loss of function. While we foresee a limited and biphasic benefit, there may be a strategic therapeutic opportunity to antagonize MuRF1 to allow for improved growth of the RV to match elevated pulmonary arterial resistance. A better understanding of MuRF1 and overall proteasomal function in cardiac hypertrophic may enable interventions for modifying chronic hypertrophic remodeling towards a more benign outcome.

Author Contributions

Conceived and designed the experiments: MJC MLP JPN MSW. Performed the experiments: MJC MLP SNL TA MVN ESC. Analyzed the data: MJC J.Hoppin BG J.Hesterman MLP. Contributed reagents/materials/analysis tools: MSW J.Hesterman. Wrote the paper: MJC JPN J.Hesterman MSW.

References

1. Vonk Noordegraaf A, Galie N (2011) The role of the right ventricle in pulmonary arterial hypertension. Eur Respir Rev 20: 243–253.
2. Tonelli AR, Arelli V, Minai OA, Newman J, Bair N, et al. (2013) Causes and circumstances of death in pulmonary arterial hypertension. Am J Respir Crit Care Med 188: 365–369.
3. van Wolferen SA, Marcus JT, Boonstra A, Marques KM, Bronzwaer JG, et al. (2007) Prognostic value of right ventricular mass, volume, and function in idiopathic pulmonary arterial hypertension. Eur Heart J 28: 1250–1257.
4. Minai OA, Chaouat A, Adnot S (2010) Pulmonary hypertension in COPD: epidemiology, significance, and management: pulmonary vascular disease: the global perspective. Chest 137: 39S–51S.
5. Tyndall AJ, Bannert B, Vonk M, Airo P, Cozzi F, et al. (2010) Causes and risk factors for death in systemic sclerosis: a study from the EULAR Scleroderma Trials and Research (EUSTAR) database. Ann Rheum Dis 69: 1809–1815.
6. Tverskaya MS, Sukhoparova VV, Karpova VV, Kadyrova M, Klyuchikov VY (2011) Pathomorphology of the heart conduction system: comparative study during increase in left or right ventricular afterload. Bull Exp Biol Med 151: 634–637.
7. Patel AR, Hurst JR (2011) Extrapulmonary comorbidities in chronic obstructive pulmonary disease: state of the art. Expert Rev Respir Med 5: 647–662.
8. Willis MS, Ike C, Li L, Wang DZ, Glass DJ, et al. (2007) Muscle ring finger 1, but not muscle ring finger 2, regulates cardiac hypertrophy in vivo. Circ Res 100: 456–459.
9. Willis MS, Rojas M, Li L, Selzman CH, Tang RH, et al. (2009) Muscle ring finger 1 mediates cardiac atrophy in vivo. Am J Physiol Heart Circ Physiol 296: H997–H1006.
10. Willis MS, Schisler JC, Li L, Rodriguez JE, Hilliard EG, et al. (2009) Cardiac muscle ring finger-1 increases susceptibility to heart failure in vivo. Circ Res 105: 80–88.
11. Kedar V, McDonough H, Arya R, Li HH, Rockman HA, et al. (2004) Muscle-specific RING finger 1 is a bona fide ubiquitin ligase that degrades cardiac troponin I. Proc Natl Acad Sci U S A 101: 18135–18140.
12. Fielitz J, Kim MS, Shelton JM, Latif S, Spencer JA, et al. (2007) Myosin accumulation and striated muscle myopathy result from the loss of muscle RING finger 1 and 3. J Clin Invest 117: 2486–2495.
13. Witt CC, Witt SH, Lerche S, Labeit D, Back W, et al. (2008) Cooperative control of striated muscle mass and metabolism by MuRF1 and MuRF2. EMBO J 27: 350–360.
14. Witt SH, Granzier H, Witt CC, Labeit S (2005) MURF-1 and MURF-2 target a specific subset of myofibrillar proteins redundantly: towards understanding MURF-dependent muscle ubiquitination. J Mol Biol 350: 713–722.

15. Li HH, Du J, Fan YN, Zhang ML, Liu DP, et al. (2011) The ubiquitin ligase MuRF1 protects against cardiac ischemia/reperfusion injury by its proteasome-dependent degradation of phospho-c-Jun. Am J Pathol 178: 1043–1058.
16. Forfia PR, Vaidya A, Wiegers SE (2013) Pulmonary heart disease: The heart-lung interaction and its impact on patient phenotypes. Pulm Circ 3: 5–19.
17. Paffett ML, Hesterman J, Candelaria G, Lucas S, Anderson T, et al. (2012) Longitudinal in vivo SPECT/CT imaging reveals morphological changes and cardiopulmonary apoptosis in a rodent model of pulmonary arterial hypertension. PLoS One 7: e40910.
18. Rajagopalan V, Zhao M, Reddy S, Fajardo GA, Wang X, et al. (2013) Altered Ubiquitin-Proteasome Signaling in Right Ventricular Hypertrophy and Failure. Am J Physiol Heart Circ Physiol.
19. Campen MJ, Shimoda LA, O'Donnell CP (2005) Acute and chronic cardiovascular effects of intermittent hypoxia in C57BL/6J mice. J Appl Physiol 99: 2028–2035.
20. Paffett ML, Lucas SN, Campen MJ (2012) Resveratrol reverses monocrotaline-induced pulmonary vascular and cardiac dysfunction: a potential role for atrogin-1 in smooth muscle. Vascul Pharmacol 56: 64–73.
21. Paffett ML, Channell MM, Naik JS, Lucas SN, Campen MJ (2012) Cardiac and vascular atrogin-1 mRNA expression is not associated with dexamethasone efficacy in the monocrotaline model of pulmonary hypertension. Cardiovasc Toxicol 12: 226–234.
22. Willis MS, Schisler JC, Patterson C (2008) Appetite for destruction: E3 ubiquitin-ligase protection in cardiac disease. Future Cardiol 4: 65–75.
23. Paffett ML, Lucas SN, Campen MJ (2011) Resveratrol reverses monocrotaline-induced pulmonary vascular and cardiac dysfunction: A potential role for atrogin-1 in smooth muscle. Vascul Pharmacol.
24. Baskin KK, Taegtmeyer H (2011) AMP-Activated Protein Kinase Regulates E3 Ligases in Rodent Heart. Circ Res.
25. Hepple RT, Qin M, Nakamoto H, Goto S (2008) Caloric Restriction Optimizes the Proteasome Pathway with Aging in Rat Plantaris Muscle: Implications for Sarcopenia. Am J Physiol Regul Integr Comp Physiol.
26. Norese MF, Lezon CE, Alippi RM, Martinez MP, Conti MI, et al. (2002) Failure of polycythemia-induced increase in arterial oxygen content to suppress the anorexic effect of simulated high altitude in the adult rat. High Alt Med Biol 3: 49–57.
27. Mille-Hamard L, Billat VL, Henry E, Bonnamy B, Joly F, et al. (2012) Skeletal muscle alterations and exercise performance decrease in erythropoietin-deficient mice: a comparative study. BMC Med Genomics 5: 29.
28. Hayot M, Rodriguez J, Vernus B, Carnac G, Jean E, et al. (2011) Myostatin up-regulation is associated with the skeletal muscle response to hypoxic stimuli. Mol Cell Endocrinol 332: 38–47.
29. Bodine SC, Latres E, Baumhueter S, Lai VK, Nunez L, et al. (2001) Identification of ubiquitin ligases required for skeletal muscle atrophy. Science 294: 1704–1708.
30. Toth MJ, Ward K, van der Velden J, Miller MS, Vanburen P, et al. (2011) Chronic heart failure reduces Akt phosphorylation in human skeletal muscle: relationship to muscle size and function. J Appl Physiol 110: 892–900.
31. Toth MJ, Miller MS, Ward KA, Ades PA (2012) Skeletal muscle mitochondrial density, gene expression, and enzyme activities in human heart failure: minimal effects of the disease and resistance training. J Appl Physiol 112: 1864–1874.
32. Miller MS, VanBuren P, LeWinter MM, Braddock JM, Ades PA, et al. (2010) Chronic heart failure decreases cross-bridge kinetics in single skeletal muscle fibres from humans. J Physiol 588: 4039–4053.
33. Bdolah Y, Segal A, Tanksale P, Karumanchi SA, Lecker SH (2007) Atrophy-related ubiquitin ligases atrogin-1 and MuRF-1 are associated with uterine smooth muscle involution in the postpartum period. Am J Physiol Regul Integr Comp Physiol 292: R971–976.

Local and Systemic RAGE Axis Changes in Pulmonary Hypertension: CTEPH and iPAH

Bernhard Moser[1]*, Anna Megerle[1], Christine Bekos[1,2], Stefan Janik[1], Tamás Szerafin[3], Peter Birner[4], Ana-Iris Schiefer[4], Michael Mildner[5], Irene Lang[6], Nika Skoro-Sajer[6], Roela Sadushi-Kolici[6], Shahrokh Taghavi[1], Walter Klepetko[1], Hendrik Jan Ankersmit[1,2]

1 Department of Thoracic Surgery, Division of Surgery, Medical University Vienna, Vienna, Austria, **2** Christian Doppler Laboratory for the Diagnosis and Regeneration of Cardiac and Thoracic Diseases, Medical University Vienna, Vienna, Austria, **3** Department of Cardiac Surgery, University of Debrecen, Debrecen, Hungary, **4** Department of Pathology, Medical University Vienna, Vienna, Austria, **5** Department of Dermatology, Medical University Vienna, Vienna, Austria, **6** Department of Internal Medicine II, Division of Cardiology, Medical University Vienna, Vienna, Austria

Abstract

Objective: The molecular determinants of chronic thromboembolic pulmonary hypertension (CTEPH) and idiopathic pulmonary arterial hypertension (iPAH) remain poorly understood. The receptor for advanced glycation endproducts (RAGE) and its ligands: HMGB1 and S100A9 are involved in inflammatory disorders. We sought to investigate the role of the RAGE axis in patients with CTEPH undergoing pulmonary endarterectomy (PEA), iPAH undergoing lung transplantation (LuTX). The high pulmonary vascular resistance in CTEPH/iPAH results in pressure overload of the right ventricle. We compared sRAGE measurements to that of patients with aortic valve stenosis (AVS) – pressure overload of the left ventricle.

Methods: We enrolled patients with CTEPH(26), iPAH(15), AVS(15) and volunteers(33). Immunohistochemistry with antibodies to RAGE and HMGB1 was performed on PEA specimens and lung tissues. We employed enzyme-linked immunosorbent assays to determine the concentrations of sRAGE, esRAGE, HMGB1 and S100A9 in serum of volunteers and patients with CTEPH, iPAH, AVS before and after PEA, LuTX and aortic valve replacement (AVR).

Results: In endarterectomised tissues from patients with CTEPH RAGE and HMGB1 were identified in myofibroblasts (α-SMA^{+}vimentin^{+}CD34^{-}), recanalizing vessel-like structures of distal myofibrotic tissues and endothelium of neointima. RAGE was differentially expressed in prototypical Heath Edwards lesions in iPAH. We found significantly increased serum concentrations of sRAGE, esRAGE and HMGB1 in CTEPH. In iPAH, sRAGE and esRAGE were significantly higher than in controls. Serum concentrations of sRAGE were significantly elevated in iPAH($p<0.001$) and CTEPH($p=0.001$) compared to AVS. Serum sRAGE was significantly higher in iPAH compared to CTEPH($p=0.042$) and significantly reduced in AVS compared to controls($p=0.001$). There were no significant differences in sRAGE serum concentrations before and after surgical therapy for CTEPH, iPAH or AVS.

Conclusions: Our data suggest a role for the RAGE pathway in the pathophysiology of CTEPH and iPAH. PEA improves the local control of disease but may not influence the systemic inflammatory mechanisms in CTEPH patients through the RAGE pathway.

Editor: James West, Vanderbilt University Medical Center, United States of America

Funding: The study was funded by the Research laboratories of the Department of Surgery (FOLAB ARGE Moser) of the Medical University Vienna and the Christian Doppler laboratory for the Diagnosis and Regeneration of Cardiac and Thoracic Diseases. The funders had no role in study design, data collection and analysis, decision to publish, or preparation of the manuscript.

Competing Interests: The authors have declared that no competing interests exist.

* Email: bernhard.moser@meduniwien.ac.at

Introduction

Pulmonary hypertension (PH) is currently defined as a hemodynamic and pathophysiological condition with a mean pulmonary artery pressure (PAP*mean*) of ≥25 mmHg at rest. The European Society of Cardiology (ESC) and European Respiratory Society (ERS) have classified these conditions into six groups. Pulmonary arterial hypertension (PAH, group 1) can be the result of a wide array of underlying diseases. The entity idiopathic pulmonary arterial hypertension (iPAH, group 1.1) is used if no underlying causative disease can be diagnosed. The increase in pulmonary vascular resistance (PVR) is related to different mechanisms, including vasoconstriction, proliferative and obstructive remodeling of the pulmonary vessel wall, inflammation and thrombosis. The pathology of idiopathic pulmonary arterial hypertension affects the small distal pulmonary arteries (PAs) with a diameter less than 500 µm. Typical findings are hypertrophy of the media, intimal proliferative and fibrotic changes, thickening of the adventitia with perivascular inflammatory infiltrates, complex

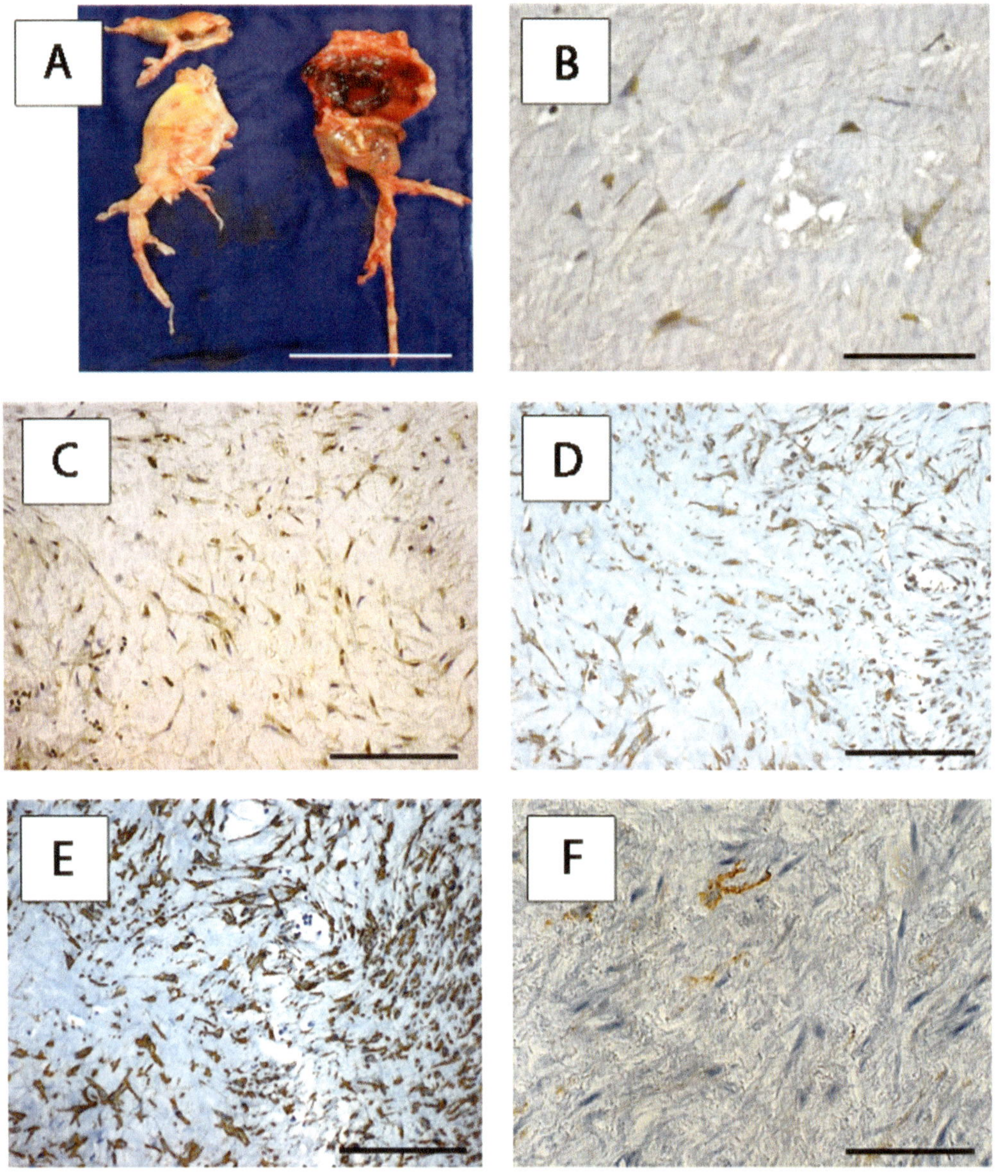

Figure 1. RAGE and HMGB1 are expressed in myofibroblasts of endarterectomised chronic thromboembolic tissues of CTEPH patients. One representative patient is shown (12 out of 15 patients (80%) displayed analogous staining patterns. Photograph showing the macroscopic aspect of a representative PEA specimen (A). Scale bar: 6 cm. Immunohistochemical expression of RAGE (B, scale bar: 20 μm), HMGB1 (C), vimentin (D), alpha-smooth muscle actin (E) and CD34 (F) on adjacent tissue sections of the PEA specimen shown in (A). Scale bar: 40 μm. *RAGE* receptor for advanced glycation endproducts, *HMGB1* high mobility group box 1, *CTEPH chronic thromboembolic pulmonary hypertension, PEA* pulmonary endarterectomy.

and thrombotic lesions [1]. A widely used pathological grading system for pulmonary arterial changes in hypertensive pulmonary vascular disease was published by Heath and Edwards in 1958 [2,3].

In stark contrast to iPAH, the characteristic pathology of chronic thromboembolic pulmonary hypertension (CTEPH, group 4) is remodeled central and proximal PAs. Organized thrombotic formations build the luminal lining of the PA vessel wall replacing physiological intima [1]. Endarterectomized tissues from patients with CTEPH show vessel-like structures in material obtained from distal areas, whereas proximal material is characterized by lower cell density and sometimes the accumulation of fresh thrombotic material [4].

As described above, iPAH and CTEPH are progressive diseases of the distal (iPAH) and proximal (CTEPH) pulmonary vessels leading to increased PVR and PAP. In the further course of these diseases right ventricular dysfunction and ultimately right ventricular failure is the leading cause of death. The prognosis of patients is associated to right ventricular performance measures, such as cardiac index and right atrial pressure. Right heart failure is caused by pressure overload of the right ventricle. The increase in wall stress leads to increased wall thickness by muscular hypertrophy (increase in cell size by addition of sarcomeres).

Table 1. The basic characteristics of patients with CTEPH and controls (healthy volunteers) are listed.

	CTEPH (n = 26)	Controls (n = 33)	*p* value
Age *in years*	51.9 (56.2) ±14.7 (2.9), [31–75]	54.2 (54.0) ±15.2 (2.6), [30–83]	0.828
F:M ratio *n (%)*	9:17 (34.6:65.4)	12:21 (36.4:63.6)	0.985
PAP_{mean} *[mmHg]*	52.9 (52.0) ±14.6 (2.9), [32–90]		
PVR *[dynes·s^{-1}·cm^{-5}]*	787.2 (757.0) ±386.6 (75.8), [281–1646]		
CI *[l/min/m^2]*	4.4 (4.5) ±0.99 (0.19), [2.2–5.4]		
sRAGE *[pg/ml]*	467.2 (331.8) ±370.4 (72.6), [105.0–1461.6]	198.6 (142.8) ±162.9 (28.3), [6.4–807.6]	0.001
esRAGE *[pg/ml]*	703.7 (610.8) ±309.3 (63.1), [170.0–1370.0]	414.5 (378.8) ±177.1 (31.8), [180.0–790.0]	<0.001
S100A9 *[μg/ml]*	2.1 (0.7) ±3.9 (0.8), [0.3–18.2]	0.7 (0.6) ±0.5 (0.09), [0.2–2.1]	0.064
HMGB1 *[pg/ml]*	1141.1 (865.8) ±865.6 (173.1), [226.5–3584.8]	464.3 (411.3) ±371.1 (66.6), [0–1818.4]	0.001

Reported is mean (median) ± standard deviation (standard error mean), [range].
CTEPH chronic thromboembolic pulmonary hypertension, *n* number of patients, *F:M* ratio female to male ratio, *PAP_{mean}* mean pulmonary artery pressure, *PVR* pulmonary vascular resistance; *CI* cardiac index, *sRAGE* soluble receptor for advanced glycation endproducts, *esRAGE* endogenous secretory receptor for advanced glycation endproducts, *S100A9* member of S100 family of Ca^{+} binding proteins, *HMGB1* high mobility group box1.

However, the chronic exposure to high RV pressures results in RV dilation with a decrease in contractile forces. Pathological inflammatory responses, oxidative stress and humoral responses may further promote right heart failure [5]. The consequences of RV failure are intractable ascites, renal impairment, malnutrition and immobility [5,6]. Pharmacological therapy effective in PAH did not prove to benefit patients with CTEPH [7]. Surgical therapy for selected patients with CTEPH is pulmonary endarterectomy (PEA) [8]. Patients with CTEPH who are not amenable to PEA and patients with iPAH are possible candidates for lung transplantation (LuTX).

The overexpression of cytokine cascades may contribute to the progression of heart failure - "cytokine hypothesis" for heart failure [9]. Most of our knowledge on neurohormonal and cytokine signaling, oxidative stress, inflammation, ischemia, and cell death which may contribute to RV dilatation and failure is inferred from research on left sided heart failure [10]. In patients with chronic left-sided heart failure increased serum concentrations of proinflammatory cytokines, such as tumor necrosis factor-alpha (TNF-alpha), interleukin(IL)-1, and IL-6 correlate with clinical and hemodynamic parameters of disease severity [11,12]. A S100 protein family member, S100A8/A9, has recently been shown to activate cardiac fibroblasts to initiate angiotensin II-induced hypertension cardiac injury [13]. Recently, increased left ventricular hypertrophy (LVH) and diastolic dysfunction was demonstrated in chronic uremic mice with transgenic expression of the human S100/Calgranulin gene cluster containing the genes and regulatory elements for S100A8, S100A9, and S100A12. S100/calgranulin-mediated inflammation induced fibroblast growth factor 23 (FGF23) in cardiac fibroblasts which in a paracrine manner may mediate LVH and diastolic dysfunction [14]. The role of biomarkers in pulmonary hypertension has been reviewed recently [15].

The Receptor for Advanced Glycation Endproducts (RAGE), a transmembrane receptor, is a member of the immunoglobulin superfamily of receptors that interacts with different ligands. Since its first characterization in 1992 where a high basal expression in the lung was shown [16] a vast literature around this receptor, its lung and vascular biology and pathology has evolved [17,18,19,20]. First, advanced glycation endproducts (AGEs) were identified as ligands [16]. Next, RAGE was identified as a cell surface receptor for S100/Calgranulins amplifying chronic cellular activation and tissue injury [21]. Further ligands were detected later: high-mobility group box 1 (HMGB1) - also known as amphoterin [22], Mac-1 and others. The current view that RAGE - RAGE-ligand interaction augments pro-inflammatory pathways is supported by the detection of RAGE and RAGE ligands in tissues of various disease processes, such as arteriosclerosis [18], diabetes [23], glomerulosclerosis [24], periodontal disease [25], arthritis [26], transplantation [27] and other chronic inflammatory disorders.

The extracellular soluble form of the receptor (sRAGE) can be detected in serum of patients [28]. Proteolytic shedding of RAGE by metalloproteinases has been described [29,30]. It functions to bind ligands and thereby blocks interaction with and activation of cell surface RAGE. An increased concentration of RAGE-ligands leads to the formation of circulating sRAGE-ligand complexes. An increasing occupation of sRAGE leads to lower concentration of free sRAGE in serum and therefore directs to increased surface RAGE-ligand interaction and possibly to a boost in inflammation. Nevertheless, it is currently unknown if high plasma/serum concentrations of sRAGE can be interpreted as protection against chronic inflammation or correlated with high levels of ongoing inflammation [29]. Currently available tools to measure sRAGE don't separate between sRAGE-ligand complexes and free sRAGE. There is an alternative splice variant of the RAGE gene, called endogenous secretory RAGE (esRAGE) that is actively secreted. [31,32]. In conclusion, neither the function nor the source of sRAGE in human physiology is known. Expression profiling for esRAGE in multiple human organs and RAGE in human thymus has recently been performed [33,34]. Plasma/serum concentrations of sRAGE in diabetes mellitus type 2 and coronary artery disease have been studied with conflicting findings [35,36].

The RAGE ligand HMGB1 is a non-histone chromosomal protein which functions as a DNA chaperone. The molecule is composed of two homologous DNA binding domains and an acidic tail. Different binding domains for its receptors: RAGE, Toll-like receptor 4 (TLR4) and a p53 transactivation domain have been identified. Once HMGB1 is released from the cell it acts as a signaling molecule, namely a damage-associated molecular pattern molecule (DAMP) [37,38].

There is a myriad of studies (mostly animal models) implicating a role for RAGE and its ligands in the pathogenesis of vascular disease. Most of these studies have investigated the systemic vessels. Studies in mice with diabetic atherosclerosis showed that

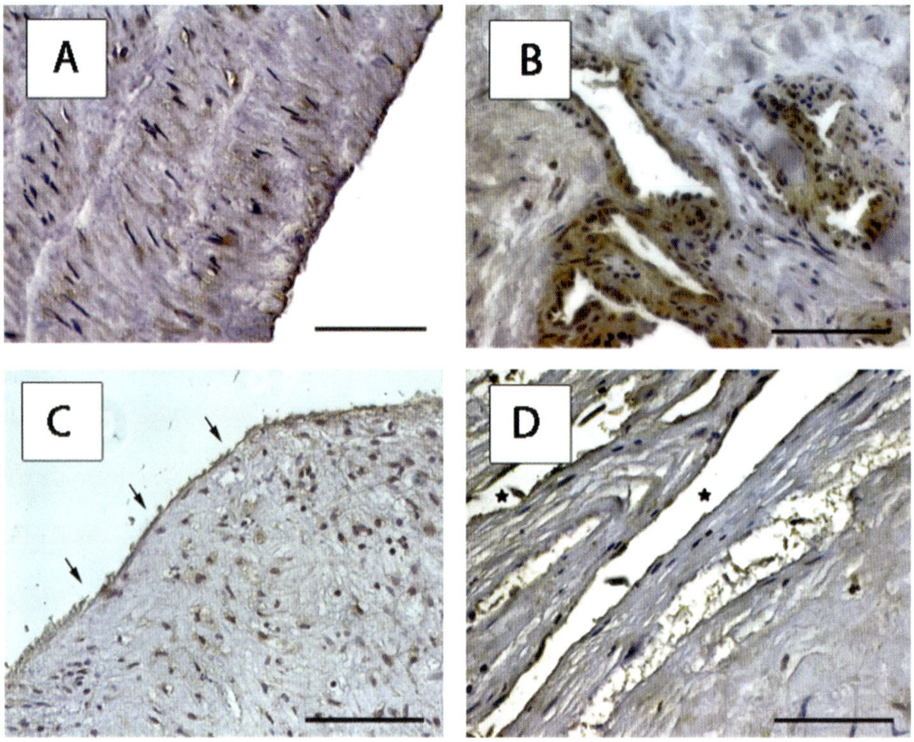

Figure 2. RAGE and HMGB1 expression on endothelial cells of regular PA and endarterectomised tissues. Representative examples of 12 examined patients are shown. Immunohistochemical analysis of regular main pulmonary artery with RAGE expression on endothelium and smooth muscle cells is shown (A). Scale bar: 40 µm. RAGE expressing endothelial cells in vessel-like structures recanalizing the matrix of distal PEA material (B). Endothelial cells expressing RAGE in proximal PEA tissue (arrows point at neointima, C) and HMGB1 (* in recanalizing vessel-like structures, D) in distal PEA specimen are displayed. Scale bar: 20 µm. *RAGE* receptor for advanced glycation endproducts, *HMGB1* high mobility group box 1, *PA* pulmonary artery, *PEA* pulmonary endarterectomy.

treatment with murine sRAGE suppressed the development of accelerated diabetic atherosclerosis in a dose-dependent manner [39,40].

The hypothesis that RAGE could be a key player in pulmonary hypertension was inferred from evidenced based reviews of the scientific literature [41]. The RAGE – RAGE-ligand axis might drive the inflammatory changes in the walls of pulmonary vessels (macro- and microangiopathy) in a similar way as has been shown for the systemic vasculature. A role for RAGE in human pulmonary artery smooth muscle cells (hPASMCs) of patients with idiopathic pulmonary arterial hypertension (iPAH) and in *in vivo* animal models of monocrotaline- and Sugen-induced PAH was recently described [42]. Further, HMGB1 was shown to contribute to PH via a Toll-like receptor 4 (TLR4)-dependent mechanism in a murine model of chronic hypoxia (CH)-induced PH [43].

In a mouse model of hypobaric hypoxia (10% O_2)-induced PH treatment with sRAGE was protective against increases in RV pressure but did not affect distal pulmonary vascular remodeling. In vitro the administration of sRAGE modulated vasoreactivity of intralobar pulmonary arteries from hypobaric hypoxic mice and further enhanced hypoxia-induced proliferation of Chinese hamster lung fibroblasts [44].

We sought to investigate a possible role of RAGE and HMGB1 in diseased main to segmental pulmonary arteries of patients with CTEPH undergoing PEA and small PAs (<500 µm) in iPAH patients undergoing lung transplantation. Moreover, we hypothesized that systemic inflammatory changes pertaining to RAGE and RAGE ligands (HMGB1, S100A9) can be measured in patients with CTEPH and iPAH. We compared systemic measurements of CTEPH and iPAH patients to those of patients with aortic valve stenosis (AVS). We aimed to filter out changes specific to PH, a disease characterized by pressure overload of the right ventricle in comparison to a disease that inflicts pressure overload on the left ventricle, such as AVS. Lastly, we sought to investigate the effects of surgical therapy, such as PEA, LuTX and AVR on systemic inflammation.

Materials and Methods

Ethics Statement

Ethical approval was obtained from the Medical University Vienna review board on human research. Written informed consent was obtained from all patients and volunteers participating in this study.

Definitions

PH is defined as an increase in mean pulmonary arterial pressure (PAP) ≥25 mmHg at rest as assessed by right heart catheterization [1]. CTEPH is defined by the following observations after ≥3 months of effective anticoagulation: (1) mean PAP≥ 25 mmHg with a pulmonary capillary wedge pressure (PCWP) ≤ 15 mmHg; and (2) at least one (segmental) perfusion defect detected by lung scanning, multi-detector computed tomography angiography or pulmonary angiography [45].

iPAH is a clinical condition characterized by the presence of precapillary PH in the absence of other causes of precapillary PH [1].

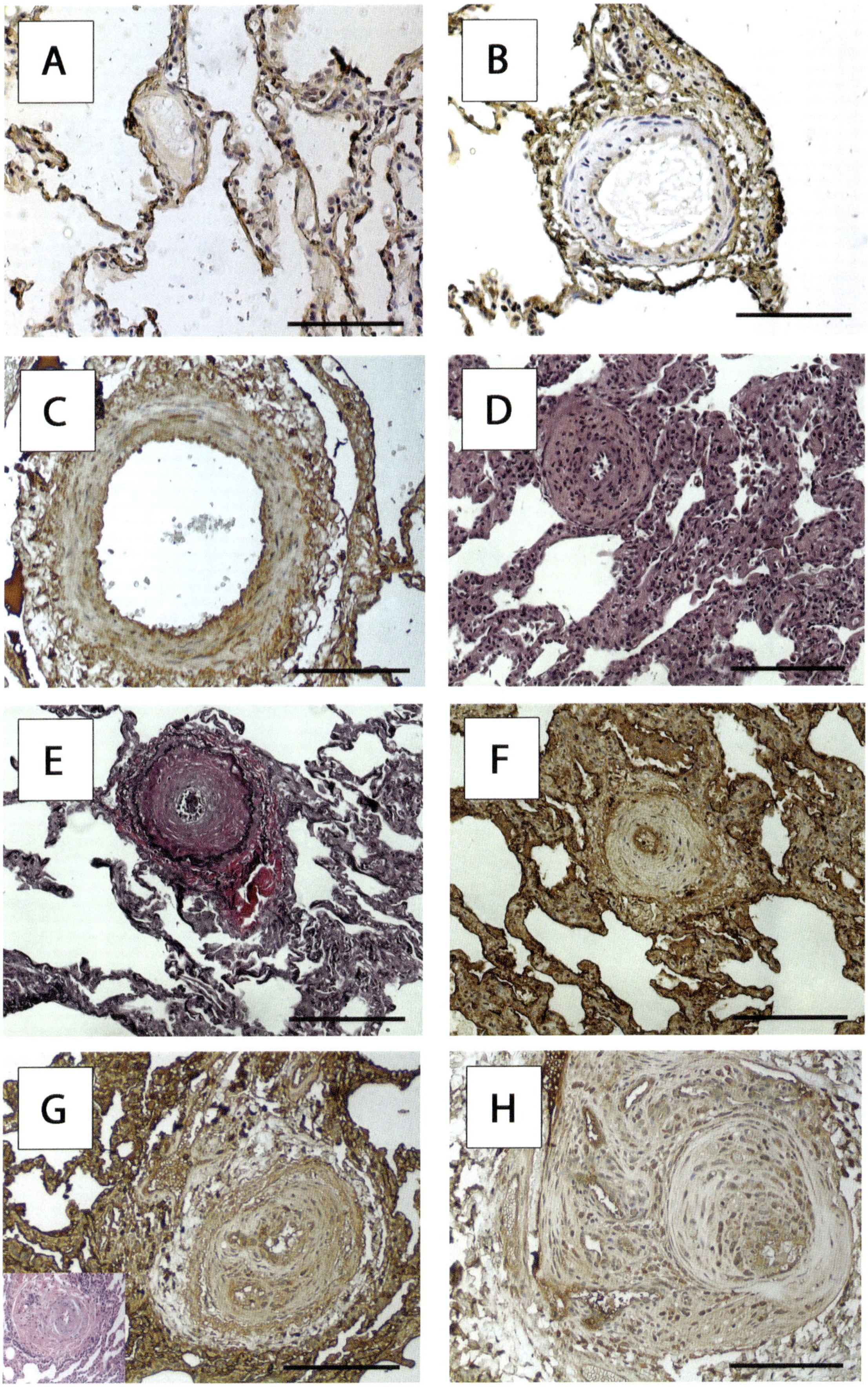
A
B
C
D
E
F
G
H

Figure 3. RAGE expression in pulmonary vascular changes of patients with iPAH. Representative examples of immunohistochemical analyses of pathognomonic lesions in lung of patients with iPAH according to the modified Heath Edwards classification in PA vessels smaller than 500 µm in diameter are shown (3 patients per every Heath Edwards group were analysed). RAGE expression in (A) a morphologically regular small PA - stage 0 and (B) a stage 1 histological change in lung of a patient operated for pneumothorax (COPD 0, centriacinar emphysematous changes). RAGE expression in characteristic stage 2 changes in a lung of a patient with iPAH (C). Scale bar in A, B and C: 80 µm. Adjacent sections of H&E (D) and EvG (E) and RAGE staining (F) for stage 3 changes in iPAH. Scale bar in D, E and F: 40 µm. Stage 4, angiomatoid (insert with adjacent H&E section, G), and stage 5, plexiform (H) PA vessel changes are shown. Scale bar in G and H: 80 µm. *iPAH* idiopathic pulmonary arterial hypertension, *PA* pulmonary artery, *RAGE* receptor for advanced glycation endproducts, *COPD* chronic obstructive pulmonary disease, *H&E* hematoxylin and eosin staining, *EvG* Elastica van Gieson staining.

Subjects

We prospectively enrolled 26 patients with CTEPH undergoing PEA, 15 patients with iPAH undergoing lung transplantation, 15 patients with severe aortic stenosis undergoing aortic valve replacement and 33 healthy control subjects between 2010 and 2014. PEA and LuTX surgery were carried out at the department of thoracic surgery, Medical University Vienna, aortic valve replacement (AVR) surgery at the department of cardiac surgery, University Debrecen. The diagnosis of CTEPH and indication for PEA surgery was established by teams of specialists in the diagnosis and treatment of patients with pulmonary hypertension, CTEPH and lung transplantation in every case. All patients with CTEPH were classified to have type 2 disease, intimal thickening and fibrosis proximal to the segmental arteries, according to the intraoperative classification system [8]. The diagnosis of AVS and indication for AVR surgery was established by teams of specialists in cardiology and cardiac surgery in every case. Patient characteristics are given in Tables 1–3.

None of the control subjects studied had any evidence or suspicion of any form of pulmonary hypertension, autoimmune disease, malignancies or infectious conditions at the time of entry into this study. None of the volunteers received anticoagulants,

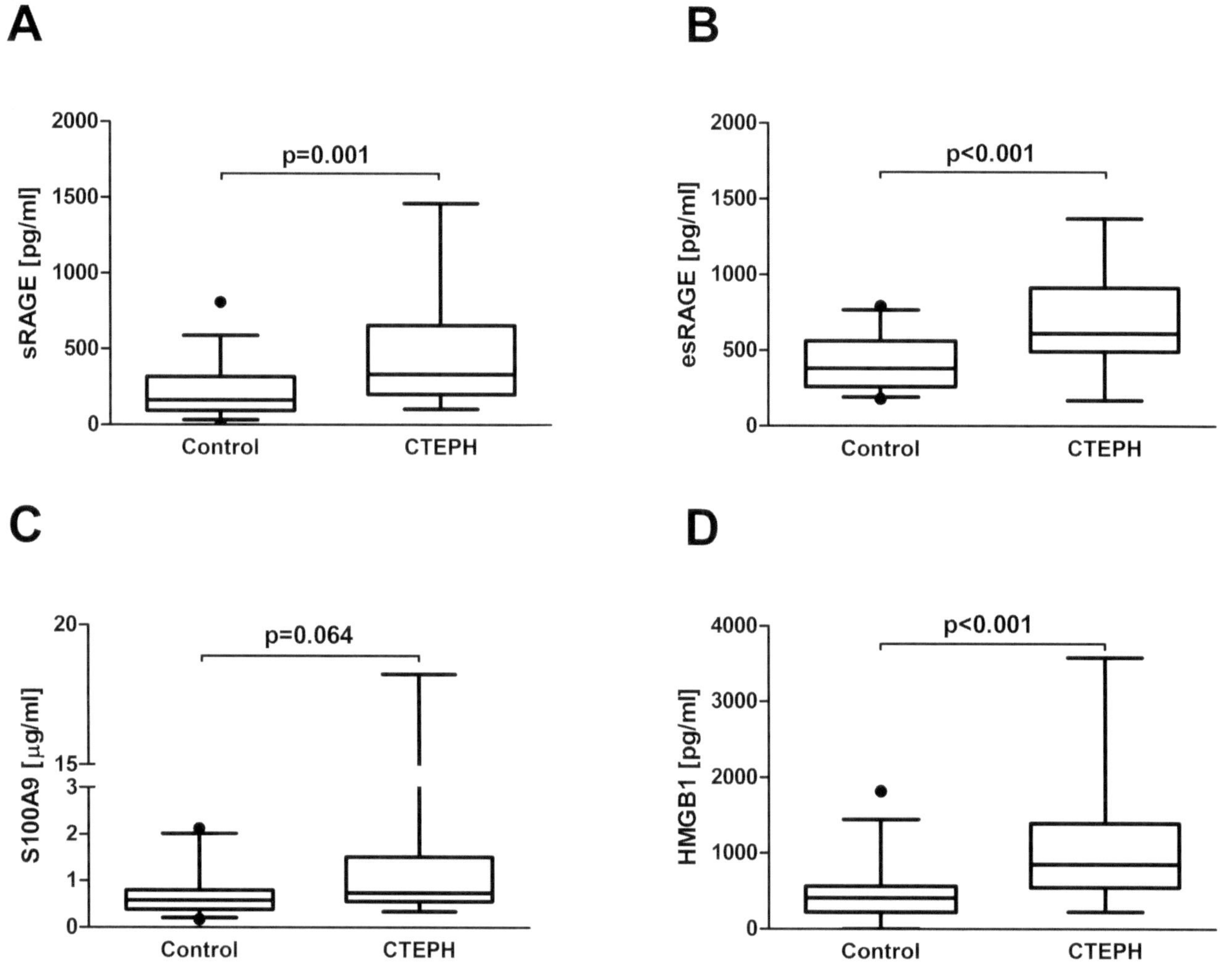

Figure 4. Serum concentrations of RAGE axis molecules in patients with CTEPH. Box plot analysis of serum concentrations of sRAGE (A), esRAGE (B), S100A9 (C) and HMGB1 (D) in patients with CTEPH (n = 26) and controls (n = 33). Independent Student's t-test was used to compare groups. *RAGE* receptor for advanced glycation endproducts, *sRAGE* soluble RAGE, *esRAGE* endogenous secretory RAGE, *S100A9* member of S100 family of Ca+ binding proteins, *HMGB1* high mobility group box1, *CTEPH* chronic thromboembolic pulmonary hypertension.

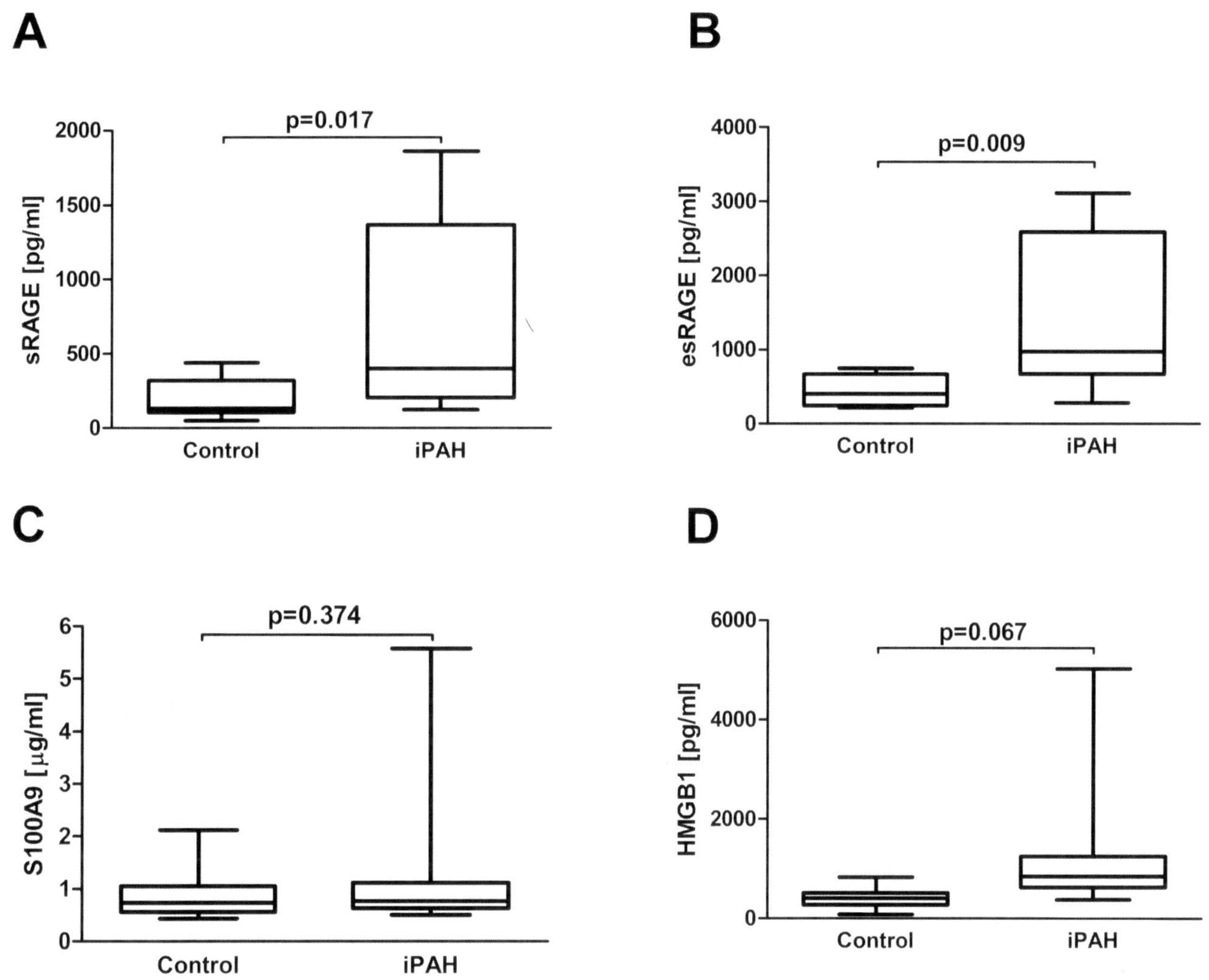

Figure 5. Serum concentrations of RAGE axis molecules in patients with iPAH. Box plot analysis of serum concentrations of sRAGE (A), esRAGE (B), S100A9 (C) and HMGB1 (D) in patients with iPAH (n = 8) and controls (n = 11). Independent Student's t-test was used to compare groups. *RAGE* receptor for advanced glycation endproducts, *sRAGE* soluble RAGE, *esRAGE* endogenous secretory RAGE, *S100A9* member of S100 family of Ca+ binding proteins, *HMGB1* high mobility group box1, *iPAH* idiopathic pulmonary arterial hypertension.

Table 2. The basic characteristics of patients with iPAH and controls (healthy volunteers) are listed.

	iPAH (n = 8)	Controls (n = 11)	*p* value
Age *in years*	36.6 (37.4) ±9.9 (3.5), [21–50]	36. 4(33.0) ±12.3 (3.7), [22–62]	0.963
F:M ratio *n (%)*	8:0 (100:0)	10:1 (90.9:9.1)	0.381
PAP_{mean} *[mmHg]*	54.5 (57.5) ±20.0 (10.0), [28–75]		
PVR *[$dynes \cdot s^{-1} \cdot cm^{-5}$]*	1425.0 (1505.0) ±582.1 (291.0), [706–1984]		
CI *[$l/min/m^2$]*	3.7 (3.8) ±0.4 (0.1)		
sRAGE *[pg/ml]*	743.7 (401.9) ±672.9 (254.3), [123.9–1861.7]	195.5 (130.8) ±130.9 (39.5), [51.0–441.1]	0.017
esRAGE *[pg/ml]*	1391.1 (972.9) ±1073.2 (379.4), [280.0–3110.0]	423.2 (399.4) ±197.1 (59.4), [210.0–750.0]	0.009
S100A9 *[µg/ml]*	1.4 (0.8) ±1.7 (0.6), [0.5–5.6]	0.9 (0.7) ±0.5 (0.1), [0.4–2.1]	0.374
HMGB1 *[pg/ml]*	1419.4 (845.2) ±1614 (610.1), [381.5–5020.9]	415.1 (410.6) ±207.0 (65.5), [80.6–833.3]	0.067

Reported is mean (median) ± standard deviation (standard error mean), [range].
iPAH idiopathic pulmonary arterial hypertension, *n* number of patients, *F:M* ratio female to male ratio, *PAP_{mean}* mean pulmonary artery pressure, *PVR* pulmonary vascular resistance; *CI* cardiac index, *sRAGE* soluble receptor for advanced glycation endproducts, *esRAGE* endogenous secretory receptor for advanced glycation endproducts, *S100A9* member of S100 family of Ca^+ binding proteins, *HMGB1* high mobility group box1.

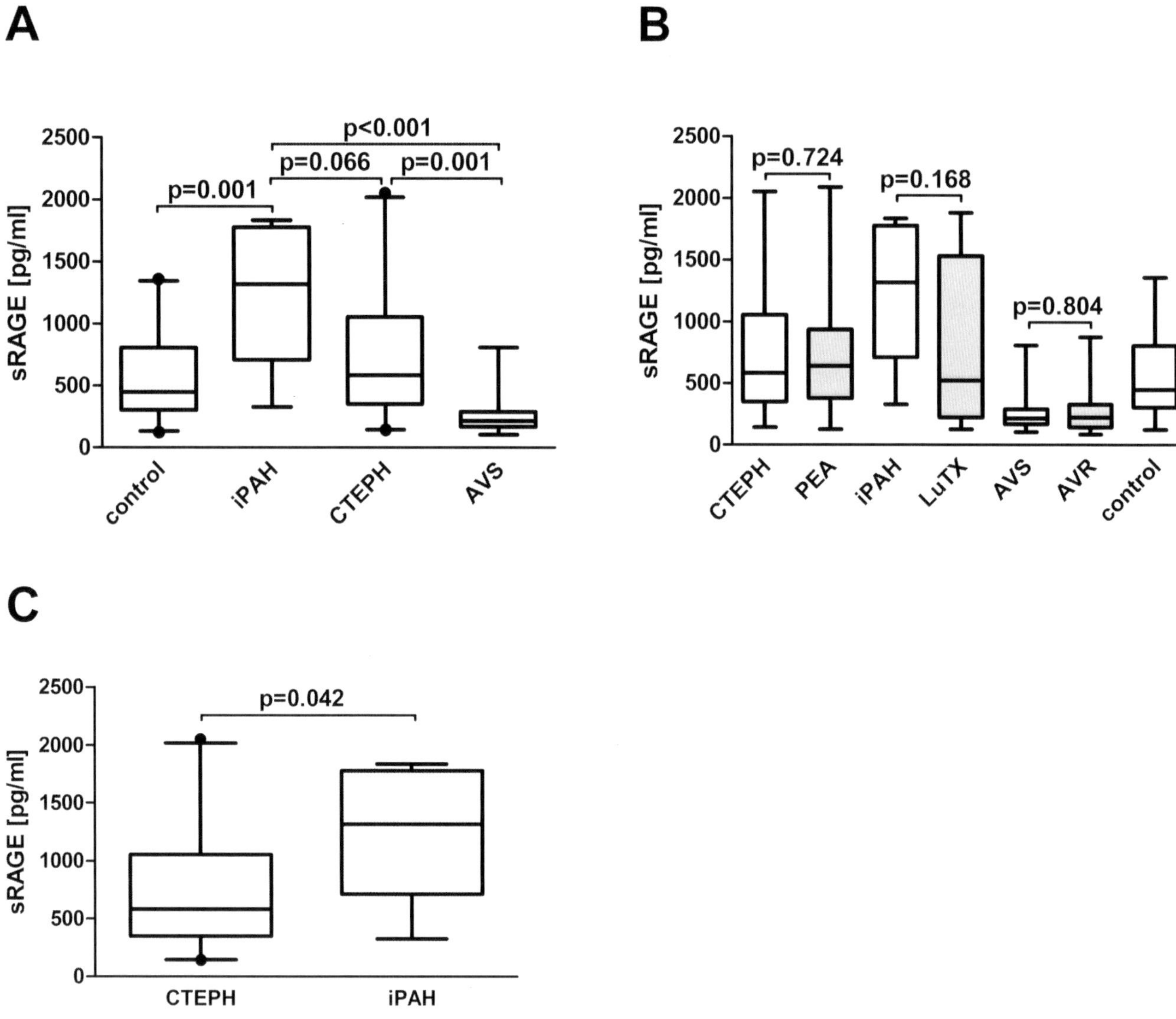

Figure 6. Serum concentrations of sRAGE in patients before and after surgery for CTEPH, iPAH and AVS. Box plot analysis of serum concentrations of sRAGE in patients with CTEPH (n = 20), iPAH (n = 7), AVS (n = 15) and controls (n = 28, A). Box plot analysis of sRAGE in serum of patients with CTEPH before and after PEA, in patients with iPAH before and after double lung transplantation and in patients with AVS before and after AVR (B). Box plot analysis of serum concentrations of sRAGE in patients with CTEPH and iPAH (C). One-way ANOVA was used to compare groups. Post hoc comparisons were computed with the Tukey correction. *RAGE* receptor for advanced glycation endproducts, *sRAGE* soluble RAGE, *CTEPH* chronic thromboembolic pulmonary hypertension, *PEA* pulmonary endarterectomy, *iPAH* idiopathic pulmonary arterial hypertension, *AVS* aortic valve stenosis, *AVR* aortic valve replacement.

prostaglandins, immunosuppressant therapy or any other type of prescribed medication.

Human tissue and serum sample collection

Fresh tissues (PEA specimens, pulmonary arteries and lung tissues) were harvested at the time of PEA (from patients with CTEPH), lung transplantation (from patients with iPAH, CF and COPD) and video-assisted thoracoscopic surgery for recurrent primary spontaneous pneumothorax (otherwise healthy individuals). Histological diagnoses and classification of iPAH in this study was routinely performed at the clinical institute of pathology at the Medical University Vienna.

Serum samples were centrifuged within 60 minutes of collection and stored at −80°C until analysis. In CTEPH the first results from serum analysis were obtained in 26 patients compared to 33 controls (table 1). For the next step we collected serum samples 10 days after (12 patients) and 1 year after PEA (9 different patients; summarized in table 3). Similarly, in iPAH the first result was obtained in serum of 8 patients compared to controls (table 2). In the next step we collected serum samples of 7 different patients with iPAH before and 3 weeks after lung transplantation (table 3). A total of 15 patients with iPAH were included in the study. Age- and sex-matched controls used for subset analysis are part of the whole control pool. Serum samples were collected before and 10 days after AVR (table 3). All postoperatively collected serum samples stem from patients with an uneventful postoperative course.

Table 3. Clinical characteristics of patients with CTEPH before and after PEA, iPAH before and LuTX, AVS before and after AVR.

CTEPH (n = 20)	**Before PEA**	**After PEA**	**p value**
sRAGE *[pg/ml]*	743.29 (582.90) ±117.62 (26.98), [125.33–2085.55]	688.70 (609.14) ±396.60 (88.68), [141.84–1712.88]	0.724
Age *in years*	60.24 (63.99) ±12.99 (2.91), [31–78]		
F:M ratio *n (%)*	5:15		
PAP_{mean} *[mmHg]*	53.53 (53.00) ±15.26 (3.50), [28.00–90.00]	27.42 (27.00) ±6.05 (1.39), [18.00–39.00]	<0.001
PVR *[$dynes \cdot s^{-1} \cdot cm^{-5}$]*	701.27 (690.00) ±277.95 (67.41), [329.00–1257.00]	265.37 (248.00) ±117.62 (26.98), [88.00–539.00]	<0.001
CI *[$l/min/m^2$]*	1.92 (2.12) ±1.13 (0.25), [0.00–4.20]	2.08 (2.20) ±1.42 (0.33), [0.00–3.86]	0.542
iPAH (n = 7)	**Before LuTX**	**After LuTX**	
sRAGE *[pg/ml]*	1216.05 (1315.27) ±564.95 (213.53), [326.47–1835.31]	772.83 (519.91) ±694.85 (262.63), [125.95–1880.66]	0.168
Age *in years*	33.43 (34.00) ±6.23 (2.35), [21–40]		
F:M ratio *n (%)*	5:2		
PAP_{mean} *[mmHg]*	82.57 (77.00) ±17.63 (6.66), [54.00–103.00]	22.57 (22.00) ±3.41 (1.29), [19.00–29.00]	<0.001
PVR *[$dynes \cdot s^{-1} \cdot cm^{-5}$]*	1733.60 (1800.00) ±200.71 (89.76), [1452.00–1984.00]		
CI *[$l/min/m^2$]*	1.99 (2.00) ±0.27 (0.11), [1.70–2.30]	4.27 (4.50) ±0.59 (0.34), [3.60–4.70]	0.074
AVS (n = 15)	**Before AVR**	**After AVR**	
sRAGE *[pg/ml]*	260.26 (216.04) ±171.40 (44.26), [104.01–808.26]	274.45 (221.26) ±199.24 (51.44), [83.91–874.58]	0.804
Age *in years*	65.23 (64.50) ±10.31 (2.66), [44–86]		
F:M ratio *n (%)*	6:9		
PAP_{mean} *[mmHg]*	18.87 (19.00) ±4.94 (1.28), [9.00–28.00)		
Mean grad	47.47 (43.00) ±16.22 (4.19), [29.00–84.00]		
Vmax *m/s*	4.47 (4.30) ±0.73 (0.19), [3.80–6.20]		
AVA	0.76 (0.80) ±0.21 (0.06), [0.30–1.00]		
Controls (n = 28)			
sRAGE *[pg/ml]*	567.80 (446.78) ±329.09 (62.19) [122.48–1355.13]		
Age *in years*	58.50 (62.00) ±20.72 (3.92) [30–91]		
F:M ratio *n (%)*	12:16		

Reported is mean (median) ± standard deviation (standard error mean), [range].
CTEPH chronic thromboembolic pulmonary hypertension *PEA* pulmonary endarterectomy, *iPAH* idiopathic pulmonary arterial hypertension, *LuTX* double lung transplantation, *AVS* aortic valve stenosis; *AVR* aortic valve replacement, *Mean grad* mean transvalvular pressure gradient, *Vmax* maximum aortic stenosis jet velocity, *AVA* aortic valve area, *F:M* ratio female to male ratio, PAP_{mean} mean pulmonary artery pressure, *PVR* pulmonary vascular resistance; *CI* cardiac index, *sRAGE* soluble receptor for advanced glycation endproducts, *n* number of patients.

Immunohistochemistry

Formaldehyde-fixed and paraffin-embedded human PEA specimens, lung tissues and PAs were prepared according to routine protocols of the clinical institute of pathology. Briefly, sections 2 µm in thickness, were baked for 1 hour at 55°C, deparaffinized in three xylenes and rehydrated in ethanol as follows: 2×100%, 1×95%, 1×90%, and 1×70%, followed by PBS. Antigen retrieval was performed by boiling slides at 600 watt (3×5 min) in a microwave oven using citrate buffer at pH 6.0 (Target Retrieval Solution, Dako, USA). Endogenous peroxidase activity was blocked by applying hydrogen peroxide 0.3%. Sections were incubated with 2% bovine serum albumin or blocking serum of the same species as the biotinylated secondary antibody to deplete unspecific protein-protein interactions. Sections were stained using affinity-purified polyclonal goat anti-human RAGE IgG (R&D Systems, Minneapolis, MN, USA) or monoclonal mouse anti-human HMGB1 IgG2b (R&D Systems) and biotinylated anti-goat IgG or anti-mouse IgG secondary antibodies (Vector Laboratories, Burlingame, CA, USA). Immunoreactivity was amplified using biotin-avidin peroxidase conjugates (Vectastain ABC kit, Vector Laboratories). 3,3′-diaminobenzidine was used as chromogen (DAB Peroxidase substrate kit, Vector Laboratories). Counterstaining was performed using Mayer's hematoxylin. Slides were dehydrated with ethanol: 1×95% for 1 min, 1×100% for 6 min and cleared in n-Butanol before mounting (Pertex Mounting Media, Leica Microsystems, Germany).

Immunohistochemistry for representative markers of hematopoietic precursor cells CD34, the intermediate filament vimentin and smooth muscle α-actin (α-SMA) were performed on adjacent sections of PEA specimens using the automated Ventana Benchmark platform (Ventana Medical Systems, Tucson, AZ, USA) according to routine protocols of the clinical institute of pathology. Sections were stained with monoclonal mouse anti-human α-SMA (Clone1A4; Dako, Denmark, Europe), monoclonal mouse anti-human CD34 IgG_1 (Clone QBEnd/10; Novocastra, Leica Biosystems Newcastle, UK, Europe) and monoclonal rabbit anti-human vimentin IgG (clone SP20; Thermo Fisher Scientific, Fremont, USA). Heat pre-treatment was conducted in Ultra cell conditioner number 1 buffer (Ultra CC1; pH 6). Color was developed with Ultraview Universal Detection DAB-kit (Ventana Medical Systems). Immunohistochemical staining for RAGE and HMGB1 was reproduced with the described automated system.

Omission of primary antibody served as negative control. Hematoxylin and eosin (H&E) staining was performed according to routine protocols. Analysis and image documentation was done with Axio Imager 2 microscope and AxioVision software (Carl Zeiss International, Germany).

Grading of pulmonary vascular lesions

Specimens of explanted lungs from patients undergoing lung transplantation for iPAH were harvested at the time of transplantation. Sections were stained for hematoxylin and eosin (H&E) and Elastica van Gieson (EvG) to visualize elastin and analyzed according to a modified Heath Edwards classification system changes in small pulmonary arteries. Grade 1 is characterized by extension of muscle cells into distal arterioles and thickening of the media of muscular arteries. Grade 2 is defined as hypertrophy of the media with intimal proliferation in small muscular arteries. Grade 3 shows progressive fibrous vascular occlusion and concentric intimal fibrosis. Grade 4 is characterized by progressive arterial dilatation with plexiform lesions, grade 5 by chronic dilatation with fibrosis of intima and media, prominent plexiform and angiomatoid lesions and pulmonary hemosiderosis.

Evaluation of immunoreactivity

Analysis of immunoreactivity was performed by two observers blinded to the type of antibodies used for staining. Two to four slides per patient were assessed. We assigned a score from 0 to 3 to assess staining intensity for RAGE or HMGB1 cytoplasmic or nuclear expression in PEA specimens, PA and small PA in lungs of patients with pneumothorax, iPAH and COPD (0, no staining; 1, weak; 2, moderate; 3, strong).

Detection of serum proteins

To test the hypothesis that RAGE and HMGB1 are involved systemically in patients with pulmonary hypertension, we employed enzyme-linked immunosorbent assays (ELISA) for the detection of sRAGE, esRAGE, S100A9 and HMGB1 in serum of patients with CTEPH, iPAH, AVS and healthy volunteers. All ELISA tests were performed according to the manufacturers' instructions: sRAGE (RAGE Duoset Elisa, RnD Systems, Minneapolis, MN, USA), esRAGE (B-Bridge International Inc., CA, USA), S100A9 (Abnova, Taipei City, Taiwan) and HMGB1 (IBL International GmbH, Hamburg, Germany). Researchers performing the assays and data analyses were blinded to the groups associated with each sample.

Statistical methods

We performed an observational study with longitudinal (cohort study, measurements before and after PEA, LuTX and AVR) and cross-sectional design (e.g. serum sRAGE concentration in CTEPH/iPAH compared to controls). Statistical analysis of data was performed using SPSS software (version 20; IBM SPSS Inc., IL, USA). Data were reported as mean (median) ± standard deviation (and standard error mean) in tables and as mean ± standard error mean in the abstract and results section. The concentrations of proteins in serum of patients with CTEPH, iPAH and AVS were compared to those of healthy volunteers using independent Student's t test or One-way ANOVA for normal (Gaussian) distributions. Kruskal-Wallis rank test or Mann-Whitney U test was used to evaluate non-normal distributions. Post hoc comparisons were computed with the Tukey correction. The paired t-test was applied to before and after measurements made on the same group of subjects, such as sRAGE serum concentrations before and after PEA. Pearson's $\chi 2$ test for independence was used for analysis of categorical data, such as sex differences. Spearman's rank correlation test was used to assess possible correlations of sRAGE and mean pulmonary artery pressure. The level of statistical significance was set at < 0.05 (two-tailed p-values).

Results

Expression of RAGE and HMGB1 in endarterectomized tissue from CTEPH patients, regular PA morphology and diseased small PAs in patients with iPAH

Expression of RAGE and HMGB1 in endarterectomized tissues of patients with CTEPH. Diseased central, lobar and segmental PAs in CTEPH patients undergoing PEA showed thromboembolic material incorporated into the remodeled vessel wall in the form of intimal thickening and formation of neointima. The macroscopic aspect of a representative PEA specimen is shown (Fig. 1A). Hematoxylin and eosin stained sections revealed the prototypic morphology of fibroblasts/fibrocytes forming a honeycomb-like network. To test the hypothesis that RAGE and HMGB1 are involved in CTEPH, we employed immunohistochemical analysis for the detection of RAGE and HMGB1 in PEA specimens (fig. 1B+C). We found cytoplasmic staining for RAGE and cytoplasmic and nuclear staining for HMGB1 in the majority of patients examined (12 out of 15 patients, 80.0%). The specimens of the same 12 patients stained for RAGE and HMGB1. Nuclear staining for RAGE was not detected. In positive specimens 70.9±4.2% of cells showed RAGE and 72.8±4.6% showed HMGB1 expression.

Identification of RAGE and HMGB1 expressing cells as myofibroblasts. We performed analysis on adjacent sections to further characterize $RAGE^+$ and $HMGB1^+$ cells in endarterectomized tissues. We found that $RAGE^+$ and $HMGB1^+$ cells were also expressing the intermediate filament vimentin and α-SMA. CD34, a representative marker of hematopoietic precursor cells, did not correlate with the expression pattern seen for $RAGE^+$ $HMGB1^+$ $vimentin^+$ $\alpha\text{-SMA}^+$ cells. The expression of CD34 expressing cells can rather be described as sporadic nests in 30.0% of tissues, a homogeneous distribution throughout any of the specimens was not found (fig. 1).

RAGE and HMGB1 expression in neointima and small vessel-like structures recanalizing distal "myofibrotic" clots. RAGE cytoplasmic staining was detected in endothelium of the intimal vessel wall (100% of endothelial cells) and smooth muscle cells of the media (64.8%) of regular main PAs. Vessel-like structures in distal areas of endarterectomized tissues showed RAGE and HMGB1 expression. Neointima (cell layer outlining the luminal surface) covering the organized thromboembolic material of diseased PAs displayed RAGE and HMGB1 expression (fig. 2). These staining patterns were analogous in all 12 patients examined.

Differentiated expression of RAGE in small PAs (<500 μm in diameter). In order to quantify the expression of RAGE in PA changes prototypical for PH we employed immunohistochemical analysis for the detection of RAGE in lung tissue specimens of patients with iPAH, COPD and pneumothorax (fig. 3). Prototypical Heath Edwards lesions were identified by H&E and EvG staining. We investigated lesions from three patients for every Heath Edwards group. Cytoplasmic RAGE expression was found in endothelium of Heath Edwards stages 0–5. The staining intensity in endothelial cells was as follows: stages 0–1: weak, stages 2–5: moderate. In smooth muscle cells of small muscular PAs RAGE was detectable with the following staining intensities: stages 0–1 (absent to weak), stages 2–5 (weak to moderate). Nuclear staining for RAGE was not detected. The described staining patterns and intensities were uniform throughout all patients examined.

Systemic measurements: Concentration of sRAGE, esRAGE and RAGE ligands: HMGB1 and S100A9 in serum of patients with PH and AVS

Increased levels of sRAGE, esRAGE and HMGB1 in serum of patients with CTEPH. Basic demographic and hemodynamic data of patients with CTEPH and volunteers are detailed in table 1. There was no statistically significant difference in age ($p = 0.828$) and sex ($p = 0.985$) between patients with CTEPH ($n = 26$) and controls ($n = 33$). We found significantly elevated serum concentrations of sRAGE in patients with CTEPH compared to controls (sRAGE [pg/ml] 467.2±72.6 vs.198.6±28.3; $p = 0.001$). Similarly, serum concentrations of the splice variant esRAGE were significantly higher than those of controls (esRAGE [pg/ml] 703.7±63.1 vs. 414.5±31.8; $p < 0.001$). The RAGE ligand S100A9 was not significantly different (S100A9 [μg/ml] 2.1±0.8 vs. 0.7±0.09; $p = 0.064$) whereas HMGB1 was significantly elevated in serum of patients with CTEPH (HMGB1 [pg/ml] 1141.1±173.1 vs. 464.3±66.6; $p = 0.001$; fig. 4, table 1). There was no significant correlation of serum sRAGE concentrations with mean pulmonary artery pressure in patients with CTEPH (correlation coefficient 0.116, $p = 0.646$).

Higher concentrations of sRAGE and esRAGE, but not HMGB1 and S100A9 in patients with iPAH. Basic demographic and hemodynamic data of patients with iPAH and volunteers are detailed in table 2. There was no significant difference in age ($p = 0.963$) and sex ($p = 0.381$) between patients with iPAH and controls. We found significantly elevated concentrations of sRAGE and esRAGE in patients with iPAH (sRAGE [pg/ml]: 743.7±254.3 vs. 195.5±39.5; $p = 0.017$; esRAGE [pg/ml] 1391.1±379.4 vs. 423.2±59.4; $p = 0.009$). Conversely, the measured RAGE ligands: serum S100A9 and HMGB1 in patients with iPAH did not differ from controls (S100A9 [μg/ml] 1.4±0.6 vs. 0.9±0.1, $p = 0.374$; and HMGB1 [pg/ml] 1419.4±610.1 vs. 415.1±65.5, $p = 0.067$; fig. 5, table 2). There was no significant correlation of serum sRAGE concentrations with mean pulmonary artery pressure in patients with iPAH (correlation coefficient −0.144, $p = 0.734$).

Serum concentrations of sRAGE were significantly higher in iPAH and CTEPH (iPAH>CTEPH) in relation to reduced concentrations in AVS patients. We wanted to test the hypothesis that sRAGE serum concentrations are only elevated in diseases of the pulmonary circulation leading to pressure overload of the right ventricle compared to disease leading to pressure overload of the left ventricle, such as AVS. Basic demographic and hemodynamic data of patients with CTEPH undergoing PEA, iPAH undergoing lung transplantation, AVS undergoing AVR and volunteers are detailed in table 3.

ANOVA analysis of sRAGE concentrations from patients with CTEPH, iPAH, AVS and healthy volunteers revealed significant differences ($p < 0.001$). *Post-hoc* comparisons showed significantly higher serum concentrations of sRAGE in patients with iPAH ($p < 0.001$) and CTEPH ($p = 0.001$) compared to AVS (fig. 6). Further *post-hoc* comparisons revealed no difference in serum sRAGE concentration between patients with CTEPH and iPAH ($p = 0.066$). Separate analysis of patients with CTEPH and iPAH showed significantly higher serum sRAGE concentrations in patients with iPAH compared to CTEPH (independent samples t-test: $p = 0.042$). Serum sRAGE concentrations were significantly reduced in patients with AVS compared to controls ($p = 0.001$).

Influence of surgical therapy on serum sRAGE concentrations. There were no significant differences in sRAGE serum concentrations before and after surgical therapy for CTEPH, iPAH or AVS. Basic demographic and hemodynamic data are detailed in table 3. The results were as follows: CTEPH patients before and after PEA (sRAGE [pg/ml] 743.29±26.98 vs. 688.70±88.68, $p = 0.724$), iPAH patients before and after lung transplantation (sRAGE [pg/ml] 1216.0±213.5 vs. 772.8±262.6, $p = 0.168$) and patients with AVS before and after AVR (sRAGE [pg/ml] 260.2±44.2 vs. 274.4±51.4, $p = 0.804$; table 3, fig. 6).

For patients undergoing PEA, early (10 days after PEA) and late (one year after PEA) postoperative serum samples were available: There was no difference in sRAGE concentrations when measurements were stratified between early and late: before and early after PEA ($n = 12$): (sRAGE [pg/ml]: 692.8±168.3 vs. 534.1±59.8, $p = 0.451$; before and one year after PEA ($n = 9$): 804.9±214.7 vs. 877.6±167.1, $p = 0.767$; in comparison to all patients ($n = 21$) together: as above: $p = 0.724$.

Discussion

The results of this study describe for the first time the expression of RAGE and HMGB1 in myofibroblasts of patients with CTEPH. Prior studies have shown the majority of cells in endarterectomised tissues from patients with CTEPH to be myofibroblasts [46,47]. The presence of multipotent mesenchymal progenitor cells (capable of adipogenic and osteogenic differentiation) was described [46]. Further, endothelial progenitor cells ($CD34^+CD133^+Flk\text{-}1^+$) were identified in neointima of proximal thromboembolic material as well as distal regions (downstream of the thromboembolic material) [47]. Myofibroblast-like cells were described as hyperproliferative, anchorage-independent, invasive and serum-independent [48]. These myofibroblast-like cells were later termed sarcoma-like cells as the injection into the tail veins of C.B-17/Icr-scid/scidJcl mice led to the development of tumors growing along the intimal surface of the pulmonary vessels (a mouse model for pulmonary artery intimal sarcoma) [49]. A possible functional role of RAGE and HMGB1 in myofibroblasts of remodeled PA vessels in patients with CTEPH may be inferred from recent studies describing a role for RAGE in iPAH. In PASMCs of patients with PAH, RAGE was 6-fold upregulated, induced STAT3 activation and decreased the expression of BMPR2 and PPARγ. The described cell phenotype could be induced by RAGE agonist 100A4 in control PASMCs and reversed by RAGE blockade with RAGE small interfering RNA (siRNA) in both cell types. RAGE blockade reduced PA pressures and right ventricular remodeling associated with improved lung perfusion and vascular remodeling in *in vivo* animal models of monocrotaline- and Sugen-induced PAH. Immunofluorescence staining revealed a correlation of RAGE protein expression with disease severity in patients with PAH [42]. Disease severity was classified as mild, moderate and severe. As increased sRAGE concentrations in our study did not correlate with PAP*mean*, we chose to investigate RAGE expression in prototypical vessel changes according to the modified Heath and Edwards classification that was routinely applied during the diagnostic workup of lungs with iPAH at our institution. We found a greater staining intensity in endothelial cells as well as smooth muscle cells of higher Heath Edwards grades.

Recently, a role of the damage-associated molecular pattern molecule (DAMP) HMGB1 was shown to contribute to PH via a TLR4-dependent mechanism in a mouse model of CH-induced PH. In patients with iPAH extra-nuclear HMGB1 in pulmonary vascular lesions was identified. Increased concentrations of serum HMGB1 correlated with PAP*mean*. In C57BL6/J mice exposed to CH-induced PH a statistically not significant nearly two-fold increase in RAGE mRNA was observed. Also of interest are the observations in RAGE knockout ($RAGE^{-/-}$) compared to wild-type mice exposed to CH: there was the same increase in right ventricular (RV) systolic pressure, but decreased RV hypertrophy in $RAGE^{-/-}$ mice. In the same model $RAGE^{-/-}$ mice neither showed significantly different vascular changes nor did the levels of mouse endothelin −1 (ET-1) or mouse soluble intracellular adhesion molecule 1 (sICAM-1) differ [43]. Our data on human patients support a role of the RAGE axis, namely RAGE and HMGB1, in iPAH. The lack of significant differences in pulmonary vascular changes and circulating cytokines in $RAGE^{-/-}$ mice is puzzling and does not parallel our data – stronger expression of RAGE in higher Heath Edwards stages - or the above described data by Meloche et al - 6-fold upregulation of RAGE in PASMCs of patients with PAH [42]. With the current limited evidence we can only attribute the differences between mice and men to intrinsic mechanisms of the mouse model of CH-induced PH.

The migration of human pulmonary artery endothelial cells (huPAEC) in vitro could be inhibited by HMGB1 via TLR4 and IRF3-dependent mechanisms [50]. If this HMGB1 effect can also be reversed by blockade of RAGE still has to be tested. In our study we demonstrated RAGE expression in endothelial cells of large and small (<500 μm) regular PAs, neointima of proximal remodeled PAs and recanalizing vessel-like structures of distal endarterectomised tissue of patients with CTEPH, as well as prototypical Heath Edwards lesions in patients with PH. Endothelial RAGE was present in health and disease. The behavior of endothelial cells from diseased and healthy tissues could reveal further information.

In patients with chronic heart failure and impaired left ventricular function activation of the immune system as measured by increased levels of proinflammatory cytokines is associated with poor prognosis [51,52]. No differences in serum concentrations of the measured cytokines: TNF-alpha, its soluble receptors 1 and 2 (sTNFR1 and 2), IL-10, high sensitivity C-reactive protein (hsCRP) and N-terminal-pro-B-type natriuretic peptide (NT-proBNP was measured in plasma) were found when right ventricular dysfunction due to CTEPH and left ventricular dysfunction due to chronic heart failure were compared [51]. In order to help untangle the possible sources by which sRAGE serum concentrations increased in patients with CTEPH and iPAH we compared serum measurements in patients with CTEPH before and after PEA and in patients with iPAH before and after lung transplantation to those of patients with AVS before and after AVR. In this experiment right ventricular remodeling with pressure overload resulting from pulmonary vascular disease (CTEPH and iPAH) is compared to left ventricular remodeling as a consequence of the pressure-overloaded left ventricle observed in patients with aortic stenosis. The results of our experiment point to a pulmonary source of sRAGE as there was no elevation in serum of patients with AVS. A normalization of sRAGE in serum after PEA or lung transplantation can probably not be expected regarding the neurohumoral and immunological disturbances occurring in these patients [10]. Possible pitfalls of our model are two emerging conceptual differences between right and left ventricular adaptation and remodeling: (1) right ventricular enlargement occurs earlier in the course of PAH when compared to pressure-overloaded left ventricles, probably because of the smaller thickness of the right ventricle that will experience greater wall stress for comparable increases in pressure. And second, there is much less myocardial fibrosis in patients with RV pressure overload compared to patients with AVS which explains the high rate of recovery of right ventricular function after lung transplantation, even when right ventricular ejection fraction was severely reduced at the time of transplantation [53,54,55]. Regarding these differences, we cannot exclude the possibility that sRAGE is derived (in part) from a myocardial source. Concerning the myocardium, the intra-coronary administration of sRAGE attenuated cardiac remodeling and fibrosis in minipigs with ischemia-reperfusion injury [56].

Our results on patients with AVS are in line with a previous study that showed that plasma sRAGE levels were significantly lower in patients with AVS than in controls and independently associated with the risk for AVS. In that study there was an inverse correlation with age, cholesterol levels and coronary calcification [57].

In lung transplant recipients elevated plasma sRAGE concentrations measured four hours after reperfusion of the lung allograft were associated with longer duration of mechanical ventilation and longer intensive care unit length of stay [58]. Increased plasma levels of sRAGE were associated with primary graft dysfunction at six and 24 hours after lung transplantation [59]. Elevated plasma sRAGE measured 24 hours postoperatively was associated with the development of bronchiolitis obliterans syndrome [60]. No data exist on RAGE and lung transplantation for iPAH. In our study there was a non-significant reduction in serum sRAGE concentrations in stable lung transplant recipients 3 weeks post transplantation.

Multivariate logistic regression analysis revealed plasma sRAGE concentrations immediately after cardiopulmonary bypass surgery to be an independent predictor for postoperative acute lung injury after cardiac surgery in children [61]. Similarly, S100A12 and sRAGE were associated with increased length of hospitalization after non-urgent coronary artery bypass grafting surgery [62]. The comparison of early (ten days) and late (one year) sRAGE measurement in our study did not show significant differences which infers that the high serum concentrations also after surgery may not only be influenced by the trauma of the surgical intervention alone but also by disease specific alterations in the RAGE axis that may not be influenced by current treatment modalities.

Current standard preoperative evaluation of PEA candidates is unreliable in predicting patients at risk for persistent pulmonary hypertension because of surgically inaccessible thromboembolic material or coexistent small vessel disease which are major reasons for poor outcome [63]. Attempts to identify high risk patients are currently investigated. In a recent study, the preoperative assessment of upstream resistance correlated with postoperative pulmonary resistance index and PAP*mean* [64]. In our study, preoperative sRAGE serum concentrations were significantly higher in patients with iPAH compared to CTEPH and did not correlate with the height of pulmonary artery pressures. This could have implications on the decision to perform pulmonary endarterectomy on patients with CTEPH. The question that has to be answered in future studies is: can high serum concentrations of sRAGE, such as measured in iPAH in this study, unmask distal disease that is not accessible to PEA and thus be of value in preoperative decision making regarding operability of CTEPH patients with high pulmonary vascular resistance (PVR>1200 $dynes.cm/s^5$) [65]?

As sRAGE serum concentrations did not correlate with their corresponding pulmonary artery pressures in this study we can only hypothesize about an on/off-phenomenon of chronic inflammation in iPAH and CTEPH patients. The current information raises new questions. What pathophysiologic threshold has to be reached to turn on chronic inflammation through the RAGE axis? Is the RAGE axis involved in the primary events of remodeling of the thromboembolic material into the PA vessel wall or is it turned on at later stages of CTEPH and iPAH? Could

RAGE blockade terminate chronic inflammation in these diseases and be of clinical value in patients as an adjunct to current therapies?

We are not suggesting that our absolute concentration values can be used to make any judgments about the diagnosis of, for example CTEPH. While comparative results (e.g. control vs. CTEPH) gained during one experiment could be repeated in separate ELISA experiments, the absolute values for the individual serum samples vary in our experienced hands with the recommended additional reagents from the manufacturer. So we never compare absolute values from samples measured with the RAGE Duoset from different experiments. The intraassay coefficient of variation was 2.3%. We run control serum samples on each ELISA. The RAGE Duoset has quite some interassay variability. The commercially available ELISA is sold for research use only and not for diagnostic purposes. We don't see this interassay variability with the other ELISA assays used in this manuscript.

Soluble RAGE was measured in serum/plasma of other pulmonary diseases with different methods. In stable COPD patients plasma sRAGE was significantly lower compared to healthy control subjects: 400.2 pg/ml vs. 783.3 pg/ml, $p<0.001$; measured by ELISA, R&D systems, Minneapolis, MN, USA [66]. Another study used two different multiplex platforms (Luminex multi-analyte profiling at Rules Based Medicine, RBM, Austin, TX and Searchlight at Aushon Biosystems, Bellaria, MA) to find significant differences in serum sRAGE concentrations in non-smokers, smokers, COPD I/II and COPD III/IV: median sRAGE values [ng/ml] 4.2, 3.2, 2.7 and 2.2, $p = 0.003$ [67]. A study using Quanitkine human RAGE ELISA kit (R&D systems, Minneapolis, MN, USA) found significantly different lower sRAGE concentrations in patients with COPD compared to smoking and nonsmoking controls subjects: sRAGE values [pg/ml]: 1351.1 vs. 1736.6 and 1797.3, $p<0.001$ [68]. There are 2.8- to 10.5-fold differences between the controls or COPD patients when the three studies with different analytical methods and different population samples are compared. Regarding the different absolute concentrations reported for sRAGE as exemplified with three studies for COPD as another pulmonary disease, it is too vague for us to draw conclusions from the comparison of absolute sRAGE measurements between our and other studies.

In summary, we have shown the expression of RAGE and HMGB1 in myofibroblasts of endarterectomised tissues from patients with CTEPH and increased expression of RAGE in prototypical lesions in lung of patients with iPAH. Our immunohistochemical results were corroborated by alterations in the serum concentration of soluble RAGE variants and HMGB1. The results may have substantial implications for diagnosis and/or treatment of patients with pulmonary hypertension. PEA improves the local control of disease with the resultant decrease in pulmonary artery pressure but may not influence the systemic inflammatory mechanisms in CTEPH patients through the RAGE pathway. A more detailed understanding of the RAGE-HMGB1 axis and related molecules in diseases associated with pulmonary hypertension is needed and warrants future study.

Acknowledgments

We thank Andrea Alvarez Hernandez for technical help with immunohistochemical techniques.

Author Contributions

Conceived and designed the experiments: BM. Performed the experiments: BM AM SJ TS CB PB AIS MM. Analyzed the data: BM AM CB SJ TS PB AIS MM IL RSK NSS ST WK HJA. Contributed reagents/materials/analysis tools: BM TS PB AIS IL NSS ST WK HJA. Contributed to the writing of the manuscript: BM AM CB SJ HJA.

References

1. Galiè N, Hoeper MM, Humbert M, Torbicki A, Vachiery JL, et al. (2009) Guidelines for the diagnosis and treatment of pulmonary hypertension. Eur Respir J 34(6): 1219–63.
2. Heath D, Edwards JE (1958) The pathology of hypertensive pulmonary vascular disease; a description of six grades of structural changes in the pulmonary arteries with special reference to congenital cardiac septal defects. Circulation 18(4 Part 1): 533–47.
3. Carlsen J, Hasseriis Andersen K, Boesgaard S, Iversen M, Steinbrüchel D, et al. (2013) Pulmonary arterial lesions in explanted lungs after transplantation correlate with severity of pulmonary hypertension in chronic obstructive pulmonary disease. J Heart Lung Transplant 32(3): 347–54.
4. Zabini D, Nagaraj C, Stacher E, Lang IM, Nierlich P, et al. (2012) Angiostatic factors in the pulmonary endarterectomy material from chronic thromboembolic pulmonary hypertension patients cause endothelial dysfunction. PLoS One 7(8): e43793. doi: 10.1371/journal.pone.0043793.
5. Delcroix M, Vonk Noordegraaf A, Fadel E, Lang I, Simonneau G, et al. (2013) Vascular and right ventricular remodelling in chronic thromboembolic pulmonary hypertension. Eur Respir J 41(1): 224–32.
6. van de Veerdonk MC, Kind T, Marcus JT, Mauritz GJ, Heymans MW, et al. (2011) Progressive right ventricular dysfunction in patients with pulmonary arterial hypertension responding to therapy. J Am Coll Cardiol 58(24): 2511–9.
7. Kim NH, Lang IM (2012) Risk factors for chronic thromboembolic pulmonary hypertension. Eur Respir Rev 21(123): 27–31.
8. Thistlethwaite PA, Mo M, Madani MM, Deutsch R, Blanchard D, et al. (2002) Operative classification of thromboembolic disease determines outcome after pulmonary endarterectomy. J Thorac Cardiovasc Surg 124(6): 1203–11.
9. Seta Y, Shan K, Bozkurt B, Oral H, Mann DL (1996) Basic mechanisms in heart failure: the cytokine hypothesis. J Card Fail 2(3): 243–9. Review.
10. Bogaard HJ, Abe K, Vonk Noordegraaf A, Voelkel NF (2009) The right ventricle under pressure: cellular and molecular mechanisms of right-heart failure in pulmonary hypertension. Chest 135(3): 794–804.
11. Mann DL (2002) Inflammatory mediators and the failing heart: past, present, and the foreseeable future. Circ Res 91(11): 988–98. Review.
12. Hartupee J, Mann DL (2013) Positioning of inflammatory biomarkers in the heart failure landscape. J Cardiovasc Transl Res 6(4): 485–92. Review.
13. Wu Y, Li Y, Zhang C, A X, Wang Y, et al. (2014) S100a8/a9 Released by CD11b+Gr1+ Neutrophils Activates Cardiac Fibroblasts to Initiate Angiotensin II-Induced Cardiac Inflammation and Injury. Hypertension. 2014 Apr 7. [Epub ahead of print] PMID: 24711518.
14. Yan L, Mathew L, Chellan B, Gardner B, Earley J, et al. (2014) S100/Calgranulin-mediated inflammation accelerates left ventricular hypertrophy and aortic valve sclerosis in chronic kidney disease in a receptor for advanced glycation end products-dependent manner. Arterioscler Thromb Vasc Biol 34(7): 1399–411.
15. Foris V, Kovacs G, Tscherner M, Olschewski A, Olschewski H (2013) Biomarkers in pulmonary hypertension: what do we know? Chest 144(1): 274–83. Review.
16. Neeper M, Schmidt AM, Brett J, Yan SD, Wang F, et al. (1992) Cloning and expression of a cell surface receptor for advanced glycosylation end products of proteins. J Biol Chem 267(21): 14998–5004.
17. Morbini P, Villa C, Campo I, Zorzetto M, Inghilleri S, et al. (2006) The receptor for advanced glycation end products and its ligands: a new inflammatory pathway in lung disease? Mod Pathol 19(11): 1437–45.
18. Bucciarelli LG, Wendt T, Qu W, Lu Y, Lalla E, et al. (2002) RAGE blockade stabilizes established atherosclerosis in diabetic apolipoprotein E-null mice. Circulation 106(22): 2827–35.
19. Ramasamy R, Yan SF, Herold K, Clynes R, Schmidt AM (2008) Receptor for advanced glycation end products: fundamental roles in the inflammatory response: winding the way to the pathogenesis of endothelial dysfunction and atherosclerosis. Ann N Y Acad Sci 1126: 7–13.
20. Yan SF, Ramasamy R, Naka Y, Schmidt AM (2003) Glycation, Inflammation, and RAGE: A Scaffold for the Macrovascular Complications of Diabetes and Beyond. Circ. Res 93;1159–1169.
21. Hofmann MA, Drury S, Fu C, Qu W, Taguchi A, et al. (1999) RAGE mediates a novel proinflammatory axis: a central cell surface receptor for S100/calgranulin polypeptides. Cell 97(7): 889–901.
22. Hori O, Brett J, Slattery T, Cao R, Zhang J, et al. (1995) The receptor for advanced glycation end products (RAGE) is a cellular binding site for amphoterin. Mediation of neurite outgrowth and co-expression of rage and amphoterin in the developing nervous system. J Biol Chem 270(43): 25752–61.
23. Yan SF, Ramasamy R, Bucciarelli LG, Wendt T, Lee LK, et al. (2004) RAGE and its ligands: a lasting memory in diabetic complications? Diab Vasc Dis Res. 1(1): 10–20.

24. Wendt TM, Tanji N, Guo J, Kislinger TR, Qu W, et al. (2003) RAGE drives the development of glomerulosclerosis and impli-cates podocyte activation in the pathogenesis of diabetic nephropathy. Am J Pathol 162(4): 1123–37.
25. Lalla E, Lamster IB, Stern DM, Schmidt AM (2001) Receptor for advanced glycation end products, inflammation, and accelerated periodontal disease in diabetes: mechanisms and insights into therapeutic modalities. Ann Periodontol 6(1): 113–8. Review.
26. Hofmann MA, Drury S, Hudson BI, Gleason MR, Qu W, et al. (2002) RAGE and arthritis: the G82S polymorphism amplifies the inflammatory response. Genes Immun 3(3): 123–35.
27. Moser B, Szabolcs MJ, Ankersmit HJ, Lu Y, Qu W, et al. (2007) Blockade of RAGE suppresses alloimmune reactions in vitro and delays allograft rejection in murine heart transplantation. Am J Transplant 7(2): 293–302.
28. Maillard-Lefebvre H, Boulanger E, Daroux M, Gaxatte C, Hudson BI, et al. (2009) Soluble receptor for advanced glycation end products: a new biomarker in diagnosis and prognosis of chronic inflammatory diseases. Rheumatology (Oxford) 48(10): 1190–6.
29. Raucci A, Cugusi S, Antonelli A, Barabino SM, Monti L, et al. (2008) A soluble form of the receptor for advanced glycation endproducts (RAGE) is produced by proteolytic cleavage of the membrane-bound form by the sheddase a disintegrin and metalloprotease 10 (ADAM10). FASEB J 22(10): 3716–27.
30. Zhang L, Bukulin M, Kojro E, Roth A, Metz VV, et al. (2008) Receptor for advanced glycation end products is subjected to protein ectodomain shedding by metalloproteinases. J Biol Chem 283(51): 35507–16.
31. Kalea AZ, Schmidt AM, Hudson BI (2011) Alternative splicing of RAGE: roles in biology and disease. Front Biosci 1(17): 2756–2770.
32. Hudson BI, Carter AM, Harja E, Kalea AZ, Arriero M, et al. (2008) Identification, classification, and expression of RAGE gene splice variants. FASEB J 22(5): 1572–80.
33. Cheng C, Tsuneyama K, Kominami R, Shinohara H, Sakurai S, et al. (2005) Expression profiling of endogenous secretory receptor for advanced glycation end products in human organs. Mod Pathol 18(10): 1385–96.
34. Moser B, Janik S, Schiefer AI, Müllauer L, Bekos C, et al. (2014) Expression of RAGE and HMGB1 in thymic epithelial tumors, thymic hyperplasia and regular thymic morphology. PLoS One 9(4): e94118. doi: 10.1371/journal.-pone.0094118. eCollection 2014.
35. Prasad K (2014) Low levels of serum soluble receptors for advanced glycation end products, biomarkers for disease state: myth or reality. Int J Angiol 23(1): 11–6.
36. Koyama H, Yamamoto H, Nishizawa Y (2007) Endogenous Secretory RAGE as a Novel Biomarker for Metabolic Syndrome and Cardiovascular Diseases. Biomark Insights 2: 331–9.
37. Kang R, Zhang Q, Zeh HJ 3rd, Lotze MT, Tang D (2013) HMGB1 in Cancer: Good, Bad, or Both? Clin Cancer Res 19(15): 4046–57.
38. Sims GP, Rowe DC, Rietdijk ST, Herbst R, Coyle AJ (2010) HMGB1 and RAGE in inflammation and cancer. Annu Rev Immunol 28: 367–88. Review.
39. Park HY, Yun KH, Park DS (2009) Levels of Soluble Receptor for Advanced Glycation End Products in Acute Ischemic Stroke without a Source of Cardioembolism. J Clin Neurol 5(3): 126–32.
40. Naka Y, Bucciarelli LG, Wendt T, Lee LK, Rong LL, et al. (2004) RAGE axis: Animal models and novel insights into the vascular complications of diabe-tes. Arterioscler Thromb Vasc Biol 24(8): 1342–9.
41. Farmer DG, Kennedy S (2009) RAGE, vascular tone and vascular disease. Pharmacol Ther 124(2): 185–94. Review.
42. Meloche J, Courchesne A, Barrier M, Carter S, Bisserier M, et al. (2013) Critical role for the advanced glycation end-products receptor in pulmonary arterial hypertension etiology. J Am Heart Assoc 16;2(1): e005157.
43. Bauer EM, Shapiro R, Zheng H, Ahmad F, Ishizawar D, et al. (2013) High Mobility Group Box 1 Contributes to the Pathogenesis of Experimental Pulmonary Hypertension via Activation of Toll-like Receptor 4. Mol Med 18: 1509–18.
44. Farmer DG, Ewart MA, Mair KM, Kennedy S (2014) Soluble receptor for advanced glycation end products (sRAGE) attenuates haemodynamic changes to chronic hypoxia in the mouse. Pulm Pharmacol Ther 2014 Jan 10. pii: S1094-5539(14)00003–0. doi: 10.1016/j.pupt.2014.01.002. [Epub ahead of print].
45. Lang IM, Pesavento R, Bonderman D, Yuan JX (2013) Risk factors and basic mechanisms of chronic thromboembolic pulmonary hypertension: a current understanding. Eur Respir J 41(2): 462–8.
46. Firth AL, Yao W, Ogawa A, Madani MM, Lin GY, et al. (2010) Multipotent mesenchymal progenitor cells are present in endarterectomized tissues from patients with chronic thromboembolic pulmonary hypertension. Am J Physiol Cell Physiol 298(5): C1217–25.
47. Yao W, Firth AL, Sacks RS, Ogawa A, Auger WR, et al. (2009) Identification of putative endothelial progenitor cells (CD34+CD133+Flk-1+) in endarterectomized tissue of patients with chronic thromboembolic pulmonary hypertension. Am J Physiol Lung Cell Mol Physiol 296(6): L870–8.
48. Maruoka M, Sakao S, Kantake M, Tanabe N, Kasahara Y, et al. (2012) Characterization of myofibroblasts in chronic thromboembolic pulmonary hypertension. Int J Cardiol 159(2): 119–27.
49. Jujo T, Sakao S, Kantake M, Maruoka M, Tanabe N, et al. (2012) Characterization of sarcoma-like cells derived from endarterectomized tissues from patients with CTEPH and establishment of a mouse model of pulmonary artery intimal sarcoma. Int J Oncol 41(2): 701–11.
50. Bauer EM, Shapiro R, Billiar TR, Bauer PM (2013) High mobility group Box 1 inhibits human pulmonary artery endothelial cell migration via a Toll-like receptor 4- and interferon response factor 3-dependent mechanism(s). J Biol Chem 288(2): 1365–73.
51. von Haehling S, von Bardeleben RS, Kramm T, Thiermann Y, Niethammer M, et al. (2010) Inflammation in right ventricular dysfunction due to thromboembolic pulmonary hypertension. Int J Cardiol 144(2): 206–11.
52. Anker SD, von Haehling S (2004) Inflammatory mediators in chronic heart failure: an overview. Heart 90(4): 464–70.
53. Vonk-Noordegraaf A, Haddad F, Chin KM, Forfia PR, Kawut SM, et al. (2013) Right heart adaptation to pulmonary arterial hypertension: physiology and pathobiology. J Am Coll Cardiol 62(25 Suppl): D22–33.
54. Sanz J, Dellegrottaglie S, Kariisa M, Sulica R, Poon M, et al. (2007) Prevalence and correlates of septal delayed contrast enhancement in patients with pulmonary hypertension. Am J Cardiol 100(4): 731–5.
55. Kasimir MT, Seebacher G, Jaksch P, Winkler G, Schmid K, et al. (2004) Reverse cardiac remodelling in patients with primary pulmonary hypertension after isolated lung transplantation. Eur J Cardiothorac Surg 26(4): 776–81.
56. Lu L, Zhang Q, Xu Y, Zhu ZB, Geng L, et al. (2010) Intra-coronary administration of soluble receptor for advanced glycation endproducts attenuates cardiac remodeling with decreased myocardial transforming growth factor-beta1 expression and fibrosis in minipigs with ischemia-reperfusion injury. Chin Med J (Engl) 123(5): 594–8.
57. Basta G, Corciu AI, Vianello A, Del Turco S, Foffa I, et al. (2010) Circulating soluble receptor for advanced glycation endproduct levels are decreased in patients with calcific aortic valve stenosis. Atherosclerosis 210(2): 614–8.
58. Calfee CS, Budev MM, Matthay MA, Church G, Brady S, et al. (2007) Plasma receptor for advanced glycation end-products predicts duration of ICU stay and mechanical ventilation in patients after lung transplantation. J Heart Lung Transplant 26(7): 675–80.
59. Christie JD, Shah CV, Kawut SM, Mangalmurti N, Lederer DJ, et al. (2009) Plasma levels of receptor for advanced glycation end products, blood transfusion, and risk of primary graft dysfunction. Am J Respir Crit Care Med. 2009 Nov 15;180(10): 1010–5.
60. Shah RJ, Bellamy SL, Lee JC, Cantu E, Diamond JM, et al. (2013) Early plasma soluble receptor for advanced glycation end-product levels are associated with bronchiolitis obliterans syndrome. Am J Transplant 13(3): 754–9.
61. Liu X, Chen Q, Shi S, Shi Z, Lin R, et al. (2012) Plasma sRAGE enables prediction of acute lung injury after cardiac surgery in children. Crit Care 16(3): R91.
62. Scheiber-Camoretti R, Mehrotra A, Yan L, Raman J, Beshai JF, et al. (2013) Elevated S100A12 and sRAGE are associated with increased length of hospitalization after non-urgent coronary artery bypass grafting surgery. Am J Cardiovasc Dis 3(2): 85–90.
63. Moser KM, Bloor CM (1993) Pulmonary vascular lesions occurring in patients with chronic major vessel thromboembolic pulmonary hypertension. Chest 103(3): 685–92.
64. Kim NH, Fesler P, Channick RN, Knowlton KU, Ben-Yehuda O, et al. (2004) Preoperative partitioning of pulmonary vascular resistance correlates with early outcome after thromboendarterectomy for chronic thromboembolic pulmonary hypertension. Circulation 109(1): 18–22.
65. Lang IM, Klepetko W (2008) Chronic thromboembolic pulmonary hypertension: an updated review. Curr Opin Cardiol. 2008 Nov;23(6): 555–9.
66. Smith DJ, Yerkovich ST, Towers MA, Carroll ML, Thomas R, et al. (2011) Reduced soluble receptor for advanced glycation end-products in COPD. Eur Respir J 37(3): 516–22.
67. Cockayne DA, Cheng DT, Waschki B, Sridhar S, Ravindran P, et al. (2012) Systemic biomarkers of neutrophilic inflammation, tissue injury and repair in COPD patients with differing levels of disease severity. PLoS One 7(6): e38629. doi: 10.1371/journal.pone.0038629.
68. Cheng DT, Kim DK, Cockayne DA, Belousov A, Bitter H, et al. (2013) Systemic soluble receptor for advanced glycation endproducts is a biomarker of emphysema and associated with AGER genetic variants in patients with chronic obstructive pulmonary disease. Am J Respir Crit Care Med 188(8): 948–57.

22

Upregulated Copper Transporters in Hypoxia-Induced Pulmonary Hypertension

Adriana M. Zimnicka[1], Haiyang Tang[1], Qiang Guo[1], Frank K. Kuhr[1], Myung-Jin Oh[1,2], Jun Wan[1], Jiwang Chen[1], Kimberly A. Smith[1], Dustin R. Fraidenburg[1], Moumita S. R. Choudhury[1], Irena Levitan[1,2], Roberto F. Machado[1], Jack H. Kaplan[3], Jason X.-J. Yuan[1,2,4]*

1 Department of Medicine, Section of Pulmonary, Critical Care, Sleep and Allergy Medicine, University of Illinois at Chicago, Chicago, Illinois, United States of America, **2** Department of Pharmacology, University of Illinois at Chicago, Chicago, Illinois, United States of America, **3** Department of Biochemistry and Molecular Genetics, University of Illinois at Chicago, Chicago, Illinois, United States of America, **4** Center for Cardiovascular Research, University of Illinois at Chicago, Chicago, Illinois, United States of America

Abstract

Pulmonary vascular remodeling and increased arterial wall stiffness are two major causes for the elevated pulmonary vascular resistance and pulmonary arterial pressure in patients and animals with pulmonary hypertension. Cellular copper (Cu) plays an important role in angiogenesis and extracellular matrix remodeling; increased Cu in vascular smooth muscle cells has been demonstrated to be associated with atherosclerosis and hypertension in animal experiments. In this study, we show that the Cu-uptake transporter 1, CTR1, and the Cu-efflux pump, ATP7A, were both upregulated in the lung tissues and pulmonary arteries of mice with hypoxia-induced pulmonary hypertension. Hypoxia also significantly increased expression and activity of lysyl oxidase (LOX), a Cu-dependent enzyme that causes crosslinks of collagen and elastin in the extracellular matrix. In vitro experiments show that exposure to hypoxia or treatment with cobalt ($CoCl_2$) also increased protein expression of CTR1, ATP7A, and LOX in pulmonary arterial smooth muscle cells (PASMC). In PASMC exposed to hypoxia or treated with $CoCl_2$, we also confirmed that the Cu transport is increased using ^{64}Cu uptake assays. Furthermore, hypoxia increased both cell migration and proliferation in a Cu-dependent manner. Downregulation of hypoxia-inducible factor 1α (HIF-1α) with siRNA significantly attenuated hypoxia-mediated upregulation of CTR1 mRNA. In summary, the data from this study indicate that increased Cu transportation due to upregulated CTR1 and ATP7A in pulmonary arteries and PASMC contributes to the development of hypoxia-induced pulmonary hypertension. The increased Cu uptake and elevated ATP7A also facilitate the increase in LOX activity and thus the increase in crosslink of extracellular matrix, and eventually leading to the increase in pulmonary arterial stiffness.

Editor: Philip Michael Bauer, University of Pittsburgh School of Medicine, United States of America

Funding: This work was supported by grants from the National Heart, Lung, and Blood Institute of the National Institutes of Health [HL114014 (JXY), HL066012 (JXY), HL098053 (JXY), and HL072742 (AMZ)]. The funders had no role in study design, data collection and analysis, decision to publish, or preparation of the manuscript.

Competing Interests: The authors have declared that no competing interests exist.

* E-mail: jxyuan@uic.edu

Introduction

Pulmonary arterial hypertension (PAH) is a severe, progressive disease of the pulmonary circulation manifested by increased pulmonary arterial pressure (PAP) and elevated pulmonary vascular resistance (PVR) that can lead to right ventricular failure and death [1,2]. The pathogenic mechanism responsible for the elevated of PAP and PVR results from sustained pulmonary vasoconstriction and progressive pulmonary vascular remodeling [3]. The latter involves pulmonary arterial medial hypertrophy due to a combination of excessive proliferation ("muscularization"), decreased apoptosis of smooth muscle cells, adventitial thickening from excessive deposition of collagen and elastin [4,5,6,7,8], endothelial dysfunction leading to the plexiform arteriopathy [9], and luminal obliteration. Despite our growing knowledge of the pathogenic mechanisms and new targeted therapies for PAH, there are still many questions that remain [10]. A more thorough understanding of PAH development and progression will hopefully lead to novel cellular and molecular mechanisms that can be targeted therapeutically in order to change the course of this life-threatening disease.

Cu is an essential micronutrient; its importance in angiogenesis, wound healing, and anti-oxidant defense has been appreciated for many years. More recently, Cu transporters, ATP7A/B and CTR1, have been identified to be the major membrane proteins that mediate cellular Cu transport. Cu ions have an ability to shift readily between reduced (Cu^{+}) and oxidized (Cu^{2+}) states, which makes Cu an ideal cofactor in biochemical processes relying on electron transfer, such as respiration (cytochrome c oxidase), anti-oxidation (Cu,Zn-superoxide dismutase (SOD) or SOD1), Fe transport (ceruloplasmin and hephaestin), connective tissue integrity (LOX), among others [11,12]. At the same time, the propensity of Cu to easily donate and accept electrons makes it potentially toxic through generation of hydroxyl free radicals via Fenton chemistry [13]. For these reasons, it is important that the intracellular Cu concentration is tightly regulated [14].

At the molecular level, Cu has many effects on the pulmonary vasculature that potentially could lead to physiological and pathophysiological variations. Cu,Zn-SOD and eSOD modulate ROS signaling, which has been implicated in vasoreactivity and vascular remodeling [15,16]. Cu-dependent lysyl oxidase (LOX) is an important contributor to crosslinking of collagen and elastin fibers in the extracellular matrix (ECM) which may promote vascular stiffening/remodeling. LOX is being increasingly recognized as a significant factor contributing to vascular stability and function. Patients with Menkes disease, a disorder where Cu deficiencies (due to mutations in ATP7A) result in inactive LOX, are characterized by a structurally weak, convoluted vasculature leading to aortic aneurysm [17]. LOX is initially synthesized as a 46–48 kDa pro-LOX peptide, and it is then further processed by glycosylation. Incorporation of Cu occurs when passing through the trans-Golgi network. Pro-LOX is secreted from the cell and cleaved by extracellular metalloproteinases, such as BMP-1, into ~30 kD mature active LOX enzyme [18]. Incorporation of Cu as a cofactor is crucial for activity of the expressed LOX protein, and its activity was shown to be modified in rats by manipulating nutritional Cu levels [18].

Cu enters the cell through the high affinity Cu transporter CTR1 [19], and once inside the cell, it is handled by acceptor-specific Cu-chaperones including Cu chaperone for SOD1 (CCS)

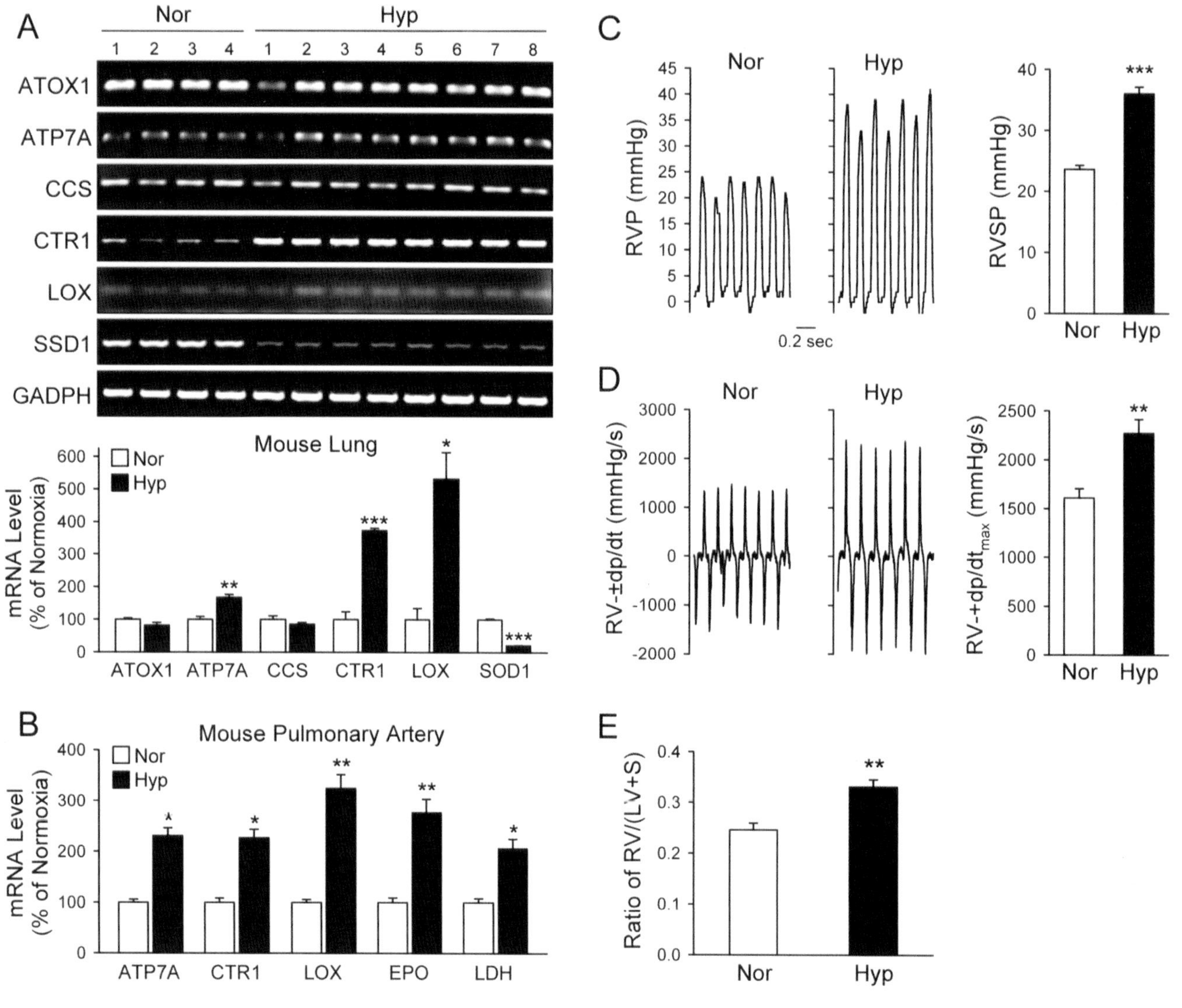

Figure 1. The mRNA expression level of Cu transporters (CTR1 and ATP7A) and lysyl oxidase (LOX) is increased in whole-lung and pulmonary artery (PA) tissues of mice with chronically hypoxia-induced pulmonary hypertension (HPH). Whole lung tissues and isolated PA tissue from normoxic (Nor, 21% O_2) and hypoxic (Hyp, 10% O_2 for 5 weeks) mice were homogenized and their mRNA transcripts evaluated by RT-PCR utilizing primers specific for ATOX1, ATP7A, CCS, CTR1, LOX, GAPDH or 18s rRNA (internal controls). A: RT-PCR products from whole-lung tissues were separated on 2% agarose gels (upper panel) and the band intensities quantitated by ImageJ, normalized to intensity of GAPDH, and graphed relative to Nor (n = 4 Nor mouse lungs; n = 8 Hyp mouse lungs). B: PA dissected from Nor and Hyp mice were used for RNA extraction (n = 5) and analyzed by quantitative PCR. Real-time PCR reaction was set with primers specific for the indicated genes. The cycle threshold C(t) values were normalized to 18s rRNA to obtain ΔC(t), quantified relative to normoxic control for each of the indicated genes (ΔΔC(t)), and graphed as % of normoxic control. C: Representative records of right ventricular pressure (RVP, left panel) and summarized data (mean ± SE) showing RV systolic pressure (RVSP) in Nor (n = 6) and Hyp (n = 13) mice. D: Representative records (left panel) and summarized data (right panel, mean ± SE) of right ventricular contractility (RV-±dp/dt_{max}) in Nor and Hyp mice. E: Summarized data (mean ± SE) showing the ratio of right ventricle (RV) weight to left ventricle (LV) and septum (S) weight [RV/(LV+S)] in Nor (n = 7) and Hyp (n = 7) mice. *$P<0.05$, **$P<0.01$, ***$P<0.001$ vs. Nor.

that delivers Cu to cytosolic SOD1, COX17 that transfers Cu to mitochondrial cytochrome, and ATOX1 that delivers Cu to ATPases, ATP7A and ATP7B, also known as Menkes and Wilson disease proteins, respectively [20]. Cu-dependent ATPases reside in the Golgi apparatus, transporting Cu inside to be incorporated into newly synthesized proteins (such as pro-LOX, or erythropoietin) bound for secretion [21]. During Cu overload, ATP7A translocates from the Golgi to the plasma membrane to mediate Cu efflux [22,23]. Recently, White et al. reported that hypoxia is a stimulus for enhanced intracellular Cu transport in murine macrophages [24], while Bogaard et al. described an intriguing link between Cu availability and pulmonary plexiform arteriopathy [25]. Using a rat Sugen5416+hypoxia (SuHx) model of severe PH, the authors were able to prevent the formation of plexiform lesions by restricting dietary Cu content, as well as reverse plexiform lesions and pulmonary hypertension by treating the animals with a Cu chelator, tetrathiomolybdate (TTM) [25]. Hypoxia has also been shown to induce expression of Cu-dependent LOX in metastatic cancer [26]. The goal of this investigation was to examine the role of Cu transport and its downstream effects on LOX in the pathogenesis of chronic hypoxia-induced pulmonary hypertension (HPH).

Materials and Methods

Ethics Statement

All animal experiments were conducted according a protocol approved by the University of Illinois at Chicago Institutional Animal Care and Use Committee (Protocol Number 13-086). For hemodynamic measurements, mice were anesthetized with ketamine/xylazine and all efforts were made to minimize suffering.

Cell culture

Human pulmonary arterial smooth muscle cells (PASMC) obtained from Lonza (Walkersville, MD) were used between passages 7–9. Cells were cultured in M199 medium (CellGro) supplemented with 10% fetal bovine serum (FBS), 20 μg/ml cell growth supplement (BD Biosciences), 25 mg/l of D-valine, 100 IU/ml penicillin and 100 μg/ml streptomycin, in a humidified atmosphere at 37°C and 5% CO_2. For normobaric hypoxia treatments, cells were incubated for 48–72 hrs in a humidified chamber at 37°C and 5% CO_2, with 100% N_2 displacing room air (21% O_2) down to 3% O_2, as indicated by an oxygen sensor and controlled by an oxygen pressure control system.

Chronic hypoxia mouse model of pulmonary hypertension

8-week-old male C57BL/6 mice were exposed to normobaric chronic hypoxia (10% O_2) or room air (21% O_2, normoxic control) in a ventilated chamber for 28–35 days according to a protocol approved by the University of Illinois at Chicago Institutional Animal Care and Use Committee (Protocol Number 13-086).

Hemodynamic measurement and right ventricular hypertrophy

Pulmonary hemodynamic and right ventricular hypertrophy (RVH) measurements were determined as previously described [27]. Briefly, right ventricular pressure (RVP) was measured by a catheter (Millar, Houston, TX) inserted into the right ventricle (RV) via the external right jugular vein. To determine RV hypertrophy, the RV was dissected away from the left ventricle (LV) and septum (S). The Fulton index or the ratio of RV weight to LV+S weight [RV/(LV+S)] was determined and calculated as a measurement for RVH.

Western blotting

Protein samples were prepared based on the type of protein being analyzed: for cytosol-soluble proteins, cells were lysed in 1×RIPA buffer (BioRad); for integral membrane proteins, cells or tissues were homogenized in HB buffer (150 mM NaCl, 10 mM Tri-HCl saline buffer, pH 7.5, 1 mM EDTA) and spun down at 500 g for 5 min to remove nuclei and unbroken cells, followed by ultracentrifugation at 100,000 g. The supernatant (post-nuclear fraction) was isolated to yield total membranes by ultracentrifugation at 100,000 g. The resulting membrane pellet was resuspended in 1× RIPA buffer. For analysis of HIF-1α, cells or tissues were processed as for total membranes, but the low speed centrifugation step (to remove nuclei) was omitted. Protein concentration was determined and samples were run on SDS gels and transferred to nitrocellulose membranes according to a standard WB protocol. Primary antibodies used: CTR1, ATOX1 (Abcam, ab54865) and LOX (Thermo Scientific, PA 1–16955), HIF-1α (Abcam, ab113642), β-tubulin (Santa Cruz Biotechnology, Inc., sc-9104), and β-actin (Santa Cruz Biotechnology, Inc., sc-81178).

RT-PCR and Real-time RT-PCR

RNA from cell lysates or tissue homogenates was isolated with TRIzol reagent and quantitated by NanoDrop (Thermo Scientific). 0.5–1 μg of total cellular RNA was taken for reverse transcription with Taq Man Reverse Transcription Reagents (Applied Biosystems), and the resulting first-strand cDNA was used as a template for PCR reaction with High Fidelity Master Mix (New England Biolabs). PCR primers designed to recognize 200–500 bp sequences specific to CTR1, ATP7A, LOX, Cu/Zn-SOD, CCS, and ATOX1 genes were designed at the Invitrogen.com site and subsequently purchased. RT-PCR results were analyzed using 2% agarose gels and ethidium bromide staining. For quantitative Real-Time PCR experiments, SYBER green supermix (Applied Biosciences) was used and results analyzed by the CFX-Manager software (BioRad).

^{64}Cu uptake

For Cu uptake experiments, PASMC cells were plated in 6-well plates, at 70% confluence. After attaching overnight, cells were divided into two groups, that were either treated, or not, with $CoCl_2$ (100 μM $CoCl_2$ in M199/10% FBS growth medium) for 48 hrs, or were incubated in a normoxic or hypoxic incubator for 48 hrs prior to the assay. Before initiating the assay, cells were washed twice with PBS and 2 ml of fresh M199 growth medium supplemented with 10% FBS was added to each well and cells were equilibrated with the fresh media for 30 min at 37°C. Cu uptake was initiated by adding 200 μl of 10× [$CuCl_2$] labeled with trace amounts of ^{64}Cu (MIR radiological sciences, Washington University Medical School). Cells were incubated for the desired times (5 min or 60 min) at 37°C and Cu uptake was terminated by addition of ice-cold stop buffer (150 mM NaCl, 5 mM KCl, 2.5 mM $MgCl_2$, 25 mM HEPES, pH 7.4, and 10 mM Na_2-EDTA), after which cells were washed three additional times with ice-cold stop buffer. Cells were lysed with 1 ml of 1N NaOH and 700 μl of lysates were taken for scintillation counting (Beckman-Coulter LS6500) with Eco-Lume scintillation liquid (ICN Biomedicals #882470). The remaining portion of cell lysates was left until radioactivity decayed, for the determination of total protein concentration in each sample, Bio-Rad Protein Assay (BioRad #500-0006). ^{64}Cu transport measurements were carried

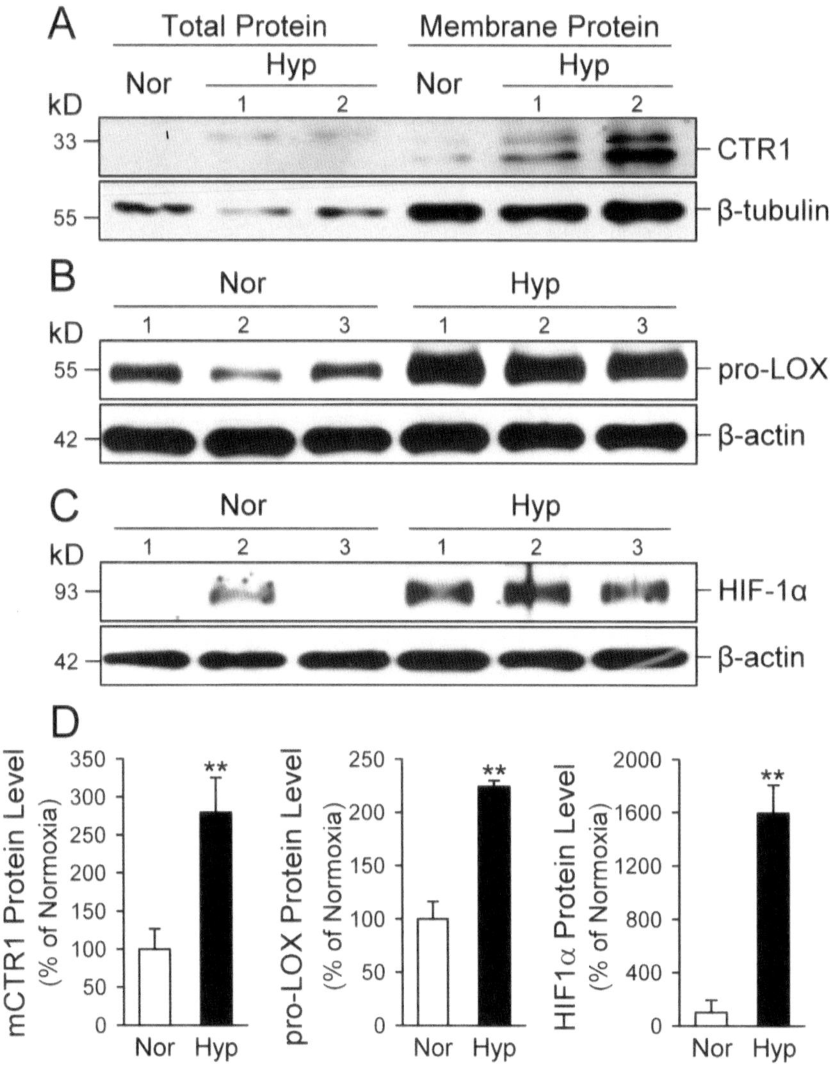

Figure 2. The protein expression level of CTR1, pro-LOX and HIF-1α is increased in whole-lung tissues of mice with HPH. A–C: Western blot analysis of mouse CTR1 (A), pro-LOX (B) and HIF-1α (C) in total and membrane proteins extracted from whole-lung lung tissues of normoxic control mice (Nor, n = 5) and chronically hypoxic (Nor, n = 5) mice. Proteins from Nor and Hyp mouse lungs were solubilized in 3% DDM/1× RIPA buffer and utilized for Western blot analysis using antibodies specific for mouse CTR1, pro-LOX, and HIF-1α. β-actin or β-tubulin was used as a loading control. D: Summarized data (mean±SE) showing protein expression levels of CTR1, pro-LOX and HIF-1α in lungs tissues isolated from Nor and Hyp mice. The band intensity was quantitated with ImageJ software, normalized with respect to the loading control, and then shown relative to control (% of Nor). $^{**}P<0.01$ vs. Nor.

out in triplicates. ^{64}Cu content of the initial tracer-containing buffer was determined for the calculation of specific activity and, following determination of the protein content, Cu uptake was then expressed as picomoles of Cu taken up by the cells per milligram of total cellular protein per minute.

LOX activity

Activity in the conditioned media and the cell extracts was measured using the Fluorimetric Lysyl Oxidase Assay Kit (AAT Bioquest, Inc., prod. no. 15255). Conditioned media was obtained by culturing PASMC cells for 48–72 hours in phenol red-free M199 medium supplemented with PDGF, under hypoxic or normoxic conditions, and then collecting the growth medium after the incubation period ended. Phenol red-free M199 medium not incubated with the cells was used as a blank. Conditioned media were further concentrated for the LOX assays by centrifugation in commercial protein concentrators (SpinX UF20, Corning, prod. No. 431488). LOX activity was measured according to the manufacturer's instructions, by monitoring LOX-catalyzed H_2O_2 release from the fluorescent substrate in an HRP-coupled reaction. To calculate value of Cu-dependent LOX activity, fluorescence of the samples treated with BCS was subtracted from the values of the untreated samples.

Cell Migration

For a scratch wound assay, PASMC cells were counted and cultured until confluent. A day before the assay, cells were serum starved overnight, washed with PBS, scraped with a sterilized pipet tip, and stimulated with 50 ng/ml of PDGF in M199 medium. Wound closure was monitored for 24 hrs by photographing the same spot (marked with pen) at 0 hr, and then every 6 hrs thereafter, using AM Scope 3.0 camera attached to a light

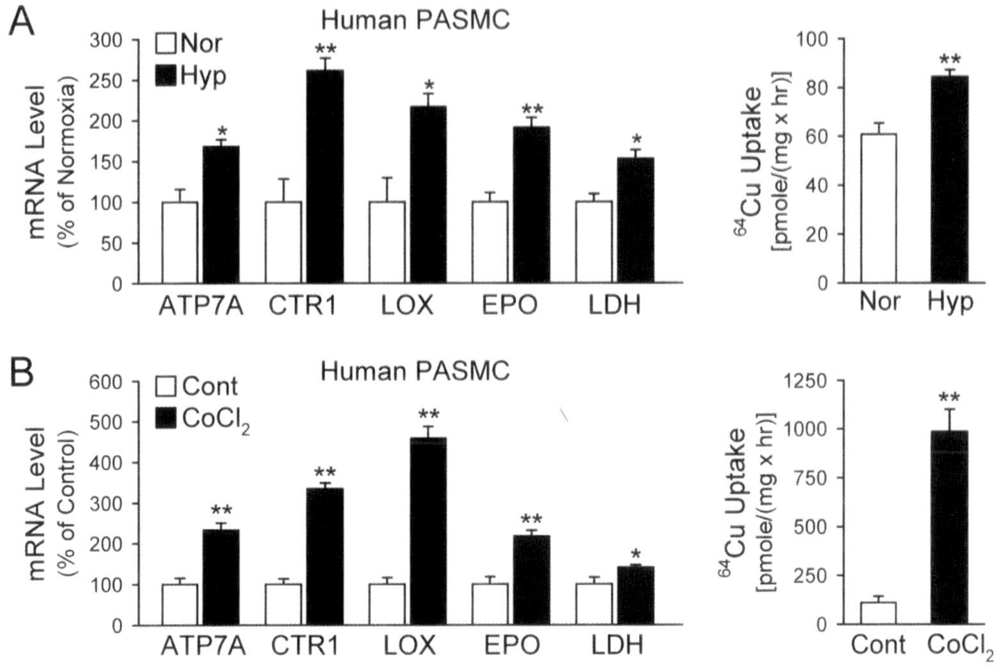

Figure 3. Hypoxia-mediated upregulation of mRNA expression of Cu transporters (CTR1, ATP7A) and lysyl oxidase (LOX) is associated with an increase in Cu transportation in human pulmonary arterial smooth muscle cells (PASMC). A: Real-time RT-PCR analysis on ATP7A, CTR1, and LOX (left panel) and ^{64}Cu uptake (mean±SE) in human PASMC exposed to normoxia (Nor) and hypoxia (Hyp, 3% O_2 for 48 hrs, n = 3; right panel). B: Real-time RT-PCR analysis on ATP7A, CTR1, and LOX (left panel) and ^{64}Cu uptake (mean±SE, right panel) in human PASMC treated with vehicle (Cont) and $CoCl_2$ (100 μM for 48 hrs, n = 3; right pane). Lactate dehydrogenase (LDH) and erythropoietin (EPO) were used as positive controls. *$P<0.05$, **$P<0.01$, ***$P<0.001$ vs. Hyp or $CoCl_2$.

microscope. For the experiment, cells were split into four groups, either treated with or without LOX inhibitor βAPN (Sigma Aldrich, prod. no. M27603), and grown in either a hypoxic or normoxic incubator.

In addition, cell migration was quantitated in Boyden chamber assay, using 24-well Transwells with 8 μm-pores (Corning, Inc., prod. no. 3422). PASMC cell suspensions (5×10^4 cells), untransfected or transfected with CTR1 siRNA (or scrambled siRNA), were plated on top of the porous membrane, and fresh M199 medium with 0.3% FBS was added to the top and bottom Transwell compartments, supplemented with 200 μM BCS, as indicated. The chamber was incubated at 37°C for 8 hrs. The membrane was fixed and stained using Diff-Quick, and random fields at 200× magnifications were counted.

Cell proliferation

Bromodeoxyuridine (BrdU) incorporation assay (Calbiochem, prod. no. QIA58) was used to determine cell proliferation. Cells were serum starved overnight, then fresh M199/10% FBS medium was added, and cells were either left untreated (control), or treated with aphidicolin (3 μM), TTM, βAPN, or low serum (0.3%) for the total of 48 hrs. For the last 12 hrs of incubation, BrdU was added to be incorporated into actively dividing cells. Cells were fixed/denatured in ice cold ethanol/0.1N NaOH, and probed with anti-BrdU antibody, followed by HRP-conjugated secondary antibody, and tetramethylbenzidine (TMB) substrate to detect horseradish peroxidase activity. Alternatively, cell proliferation was determined by the degree of expression of proliferating cells nuclear antigen (PCNA), using the Western blot analysis (Santa Cruz, Inc. prod. no. FL-261).

siRNA treatment

siRNA oligos for HIF-1α, HIF-2α, and CTR1 knockdowns were purchased from Ambion (prod. nos. s6539, s4700, and s3377), and used at final concentration of 100 pmol per 6 well-plate for 48–72 hrs. siRNA was introduced into the cells using RNA Max Lipofectamine reagent (Invitrogen). For the HIF-1α and HIF-2α knockdowns, cells were grown under hypoxic conditions.

Microaspiration

Micropipette aspiration of attached PASMC was performed as previously described [28]. Briefly, plasma membranes were visualized with a fluorescent membrane dye, carbocyanide DiIC18 (Molecular Probes, Eugene, OR), and then aspirated using micropipettes with 6–9 μm outer diameter pulled from borosilicate glass capillaries (SG10 glass; Richland Glass, Richland, NJ). Zeiss microscopy (Axiovert 200 M) was used for capturing the membrane deformation at multiple time points. Negative pressure was applied to a pipette by a pneumatic transducer tester (BioTek Instruments,Winooski, VT).

Statistical analysis

Sigma Plot software was used for Student's *t*-test to calculate significance between two groups, and One Way ANOVA for many groups. Composite data are shown as the mean ± S.E. and significant difference is expressed as *$P<0.05$, **$P<0.01$, and ***$P<0.001$.

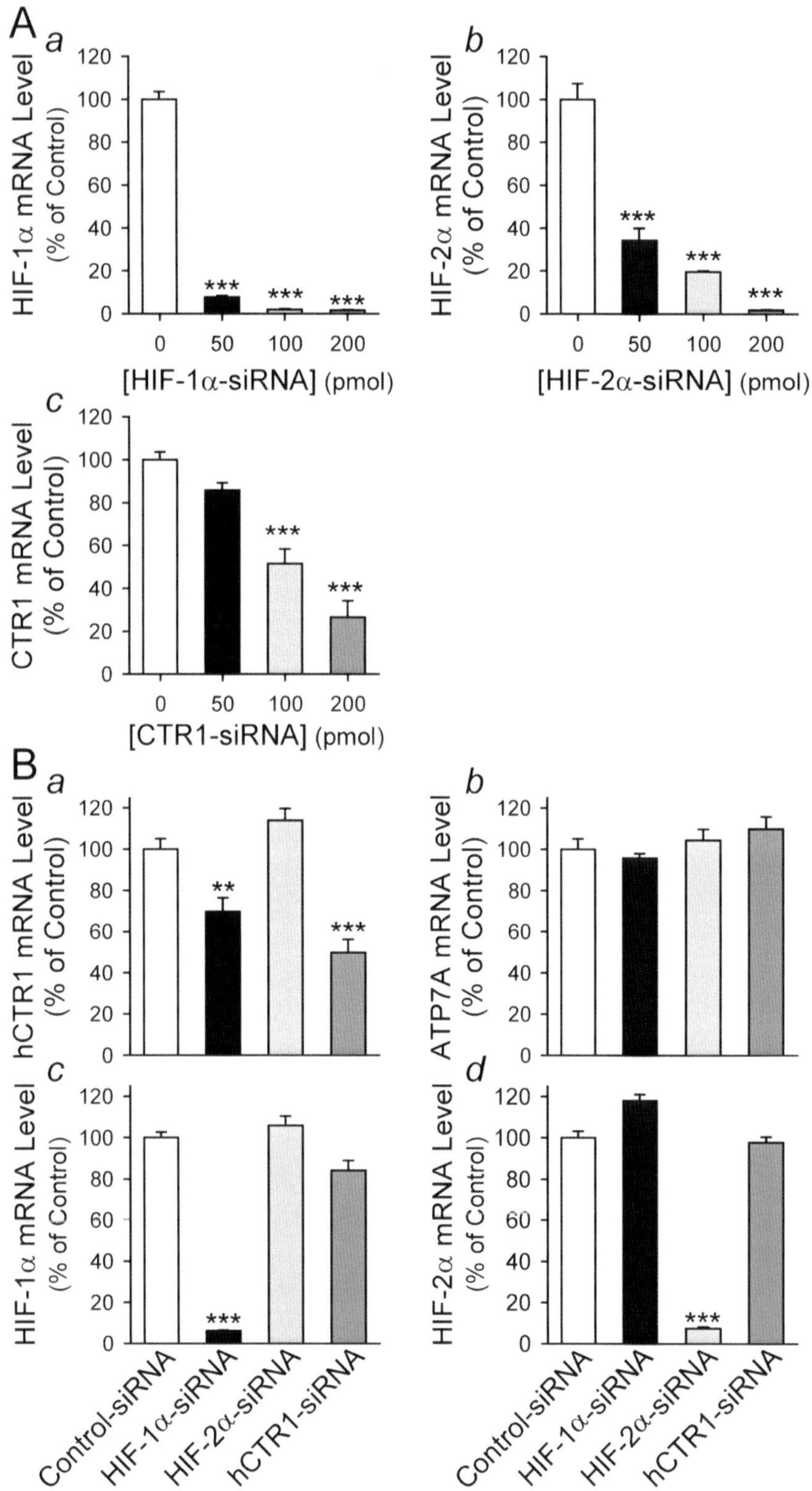

Figure 4. Downregulation of HIF-1α by siRNA significantly attenuates mRNA expression of CTR1 in hypoxic PASMC. A: Real-time RT-PCR analysis on HIF-1α (*a*), HIF-2α (*b*) and CTR1 (*c*) in hypoxic PASMC treated with (50–200 pmol) or without (0 pmol) siRNA specifically targeting HIF-1α, HIF-2α and CTR1, respectively. Data are shown in mean±SE. ****P*<0.01 vs. control hypoxic cells (0-pmol siRNA). B: Real-time RT-PCR analysis on human CTR1 (*a*), ATP7A (*b*), HIF-1α (*c*) and HIF-2α (*d*) in hypoxic PASMC treated with 100-pmol scrambled siRNA (Control-siRNA, open bars), HIF-1α-siRNA (solid bars), HIF-2α-siRNA (light grey bars), and CTR1-siRNA (dark grey bars), respectively. ****P*<0.01 vs. hypoxic cells treated with scrambled siRNA (Control-siRNA).

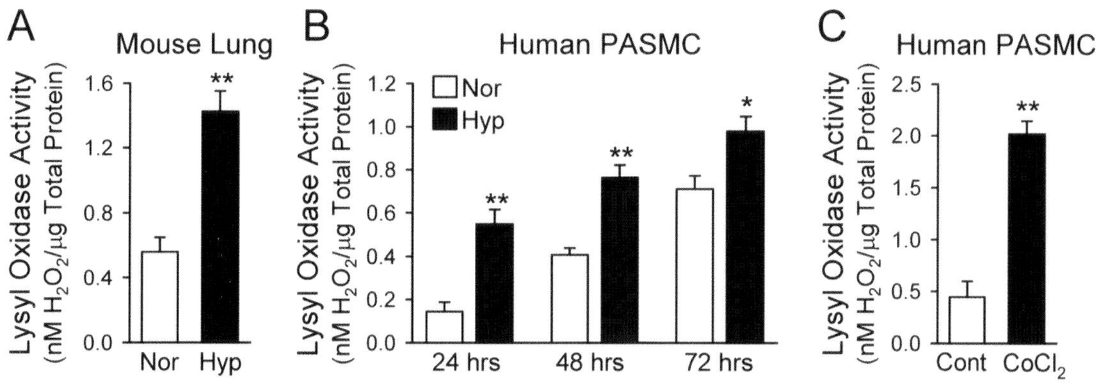

Figure 5. Activity of lysyl oxidase (LOX) is increased in whole-lung tissues of chronically hypoxic mice and in culture media from human PASMC exposed to hypoxia or treated with $CoCl_2$. Enzymatic activity of LOX was determined using Fluorimetric Lysyl Oxidase Assay Kit by monitoring LOX-catalyzed H_2O_2 release from the fluorescent substrate in HRP-coupled reaction. A: LOX activity in lung tissue homogenates from normoxic (Nor, room air for 5 weeks, n = 5) and hypoxic (Hyp, 10% O_2 for 5 weeks, n = 5) mice. $^{**}P<0.01$ vs. Nor. B: LOX activity in culture media collected from human PASMC after 24, 48 and 72 hrs of exposure to normoxia (Nor, 21% O_2) or hypoxia (Hyp, 3% O_2). $^{*}P<0.05$, $^{**}P<0.01$ vs. Nor. C: LOX activity in culture media collected from PASMC treated with vehicle (Cont) or $CoCl_2$ (100 μM for 48 hrs). $^{**}P<0.01$ vs. Cont. Each bar graph displays the Cu-dependent activity of LOX determined by subtracting values obtained in the presence of BCS (a Cu chelator) from values in the absence of BCS. LOX activity is expressed in nanomoles of H_2O_2 released from the cells and normalized to the amount of total protein in each sample. Data are shown as mean±SE.

Results

Upregulated mRNA and protein expression of Cu transporters in lung and pulmonary artery tissues isolated from mice with HPH

To examine whether Cu transportation is involved in the development of HPH, we first measured and compared mRNA and protein levels of the Cu transporters (CTR1 and ATP7A), Cu chaperones (ATOX1 and CCS) and Cu-dependent enzymes (LOX) in lung tissues from normoxic and hypoxic mice. As shown in Figure 1, the mRNA expression level of CTR1, ATP7A and LOX in lung tissues was significantly upregulated in chronically hypoxic mice (10% O_2, for 4 weeks) in comparison to control mice (21% O_2, for 4 weeks). The mRNA levels of the Cu chaperones, ATOX1 and CCS, however, remained unchanged in lung tissues isolated from mice chronically exposed to hypoxia (Fig. 1A upper and lower panels). The real-time RT-PCR experiments indicated that the mRNA expression levels of CTR1, ATP7A and LOX in isolated pulmonary arteries were all significantly higher in hypoxic (Hyp) mice than in normoxic (Nor) mice (Fig. 1B). Lactase dehydrogenase (Ldh) and erythropoietin (Epo) were used as control genes known to be upregulated by hypoxia (Fig. 1B) [29].

Chronically hypoxic mice exhibited significantly higher right ventricular systolic pressure (RVSP, 36.01±1.09 vs. 23.59±0.66 mmHg; $P<0.001$, Fig. 1C), greater right ventricular contractility (RV-dp/dt_{max}, 1609.46±305.52 vs. 2268.78±322.54 mmHg/s; $P<0.01$, Fig. 1D) and greater Fulton index (0.330±0.014 vs. 0.246±0.013; $P<0.01$, Fig. 1E) than normoxic controls. These data indicate that the upregulated mRNA expression of CTR1, ATP7A and LOX in whole-lung tissues and isolated pulmonary arteries is associated with HPH.

Western blot analysis of whole lung tissues was then used to determine whether increased mRNA expression of CTR1 and LOX resulted in a corresponding increase in CTR1 and LOX protein expression level. CTR1 is an integral membrane protein with a relatively low basal expression. To determine the protein expression level of CTR1 in the plasma membrane, we concentrated lung tissue homogenates by spinning down total membranes and then solubilizing membrane proteins for the Western blot experiments. Using a previously characterized c-terminal CTR1 antibody [30] and a commercially available LOX antibody (Sigma), we recognized a glycosylated and non-cleaved form of LOX (pro-LOX ~58 kD) and a processed LOX (~35 kD).

As shown in Figure 2, the protein expression levels of CTR1 and pro-LOX in whole lung tissues from mice with HPH were significantly higher than in lung tissues from normoxic control mice (Fig. 2A, 2B and 2D, left panels). The upregulated expression of CTR1 and pro-LOX was associated with a significantly upregulated expression of HIF-1α (Fig. 2C and 2D, right panel). The protein level of HIF-1α in lung tissues of hypoxic animals was approximately 14 times the level in lung tissues of normoxic control animals (Fig. 2C and 2D, right panel), while the intensity of CTR1 band (at 33 kD) in hypoxic mice was approximately 2.2 times higher than in normoxic mice (Fig. 2D, left panel). Lysyl oxidase (LOX) was detected mostly as a 58-kD pro-LOX band which was approximately 2.1 fold higher in hypoxic mouse lungs than in normoxic control lungs (Fig. 2D, middle panel). These results indicate that both mRNA and protein expression levels of CTR1 and pro-LOX were significantly increased in lung tissues of mice with HPH.

Hypoxia and $CoCl_2$ upregulate mRNA expression of Cu transporters and increases Cu uptake in human PASMC

In addition to the in vivo experiments shown above, we conducted in vitro experiments to examine whether hypoxic exposure of human PASMC exerts the same effect on the Cu transporters and chaperones. Our real-time RT-PCR experiments showed that incubation of PASMC under hypoxic conditions (3% O_2 for 48 hrs), or treatment of PASMC with $CoCl_2$, which can also increase HIF-1α level to activate the HIF-1α-dependent signaling cascades [31], significantly increased the mRNA expression level of ATP7A, CTR1 and LOX in PASMC (Fig. 3A and 3B, left panels). We used lactase dehydrogenase (Ldh) and erythropoietin (Epo) as control genes known to be upregulated by hypoxia (Fig. 3, left panels) [29].

To determine whether the hypoxia-induced increase in CTR1 expression in PASMC results in an increase in transportation of

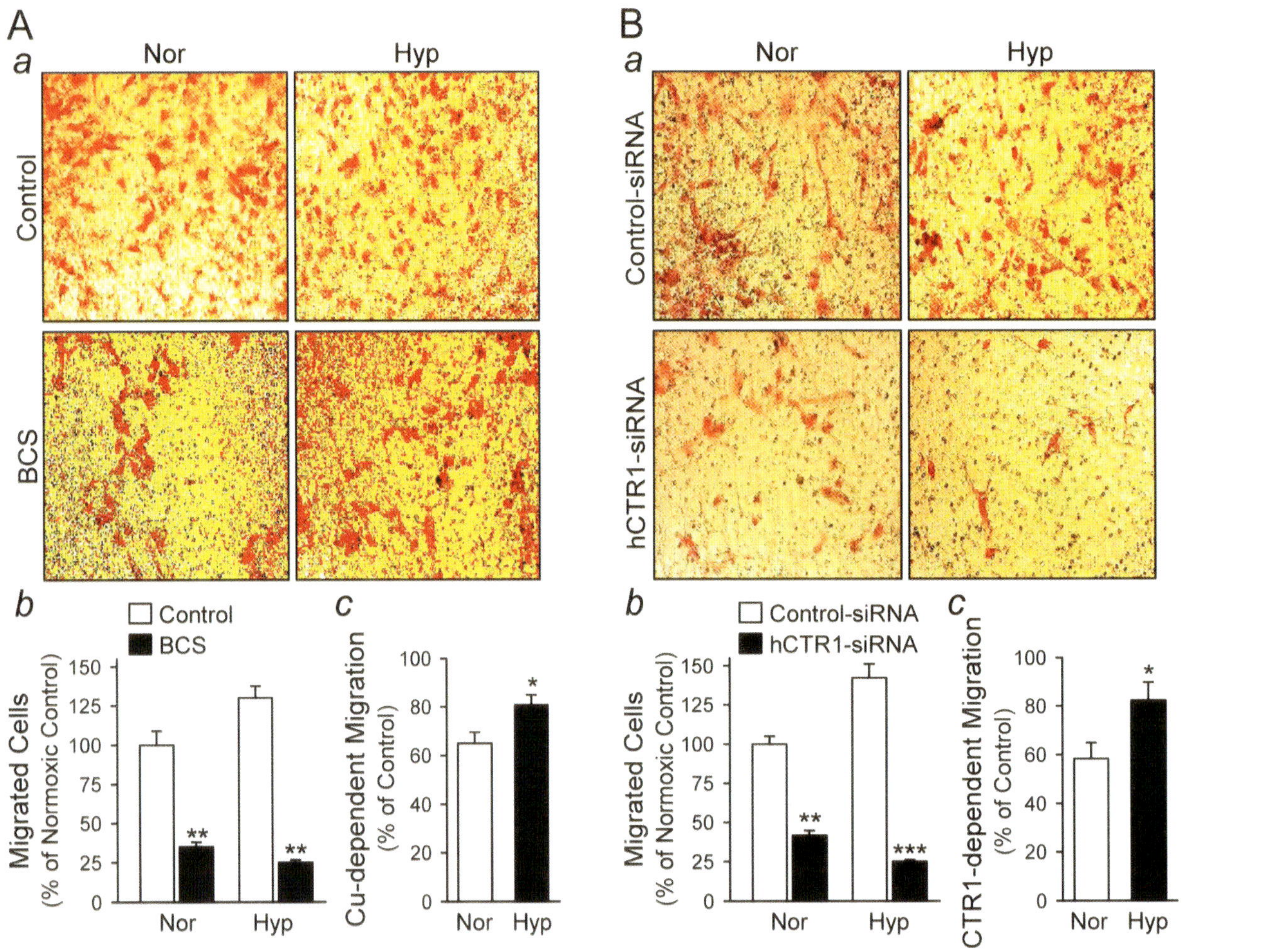

Figure 6. PASMC migration is dependent on Cu and inhibited by knockdown of CTR1. Cell migration was determined by the modified Boyden chamber assay. Cells were plated on top of the porous (8-μm pore) membrane. After 48 hrs, the membrane was fixed and stained using Diff-Quick and the migrated cells in randomly chosen fields were counted at 200× magnification. A: Representative images (*a*) showing human PASMC cultured under normoxic (Nor) or hypoxic (Hyp) conditions in the absence (Control) or presence (BCS) of 200 μM BCS (a Cu chelator). Summarized data (mean±SE) showing migrated cell counts (*b*) in normoxic (Nor) and hypoxic (Hyp) PASMC treated with (BCS) or without (Control) BCS. ***P*<0.01 vs. Control. The Cu-dependent cell migration (*c*) was determined by the percent changes in migrated cell counts between Control and BCS-treated cells in Nor and Hyp. Data are shown as mean±SE. **P*<0.05 vs. Nor. B: Representative images (*a*) showing human PASMC treated with scrambled siRNA (Control-siRNA) or CTR1-siRNA under Nor or Hyp conditions. Summarized data (mean±SE) showing migrated cell counts (*b*) in Nor and Hyp PASMC treated with Control-siRNA (solid bars) or CTR1-siRNA (open bars). ***P*<0.01 vs. Control. The Cu-dependent cell migration (*c*) was determined by the percent changes in migrated cell counts between PASMC treated with Control-siRNA and CTR1-siRNA in normoxia (Nor) and hypoxia (Hyp). Data are shown as mean±SE. **P*<0.05 vs. Nor.

Cu, we measured and compared ^{64}Cu uptake in PASMC under normoxic and hypoxic conditions. Incubation of PASMC under hypoxic condition (3% O_2 for 48 hrs) significantly enhanced ^{64}Cu uptake by approximately 30% (Fig. 3A, right panel). Treatment of PASMC with 100-μM $CoCl_2$ (for 48 hrs) led to a dramatic increase in the uptake of ^{64}Cu (by approximately 16 fold) (Fig. 3B, right panel). These observations indicate that the upregulated expression of CTR1 was associated with a significantly increased Cu uptake in PASMC. The hypoxia- (or $CoCl_2$-) induced increase in CTR1 expression and Cu uptake results in a significant increase in the amount of Cu in PASMC.

HIF-1α is involved in hypoxia-mediated upregulation of CTR1 mRNA expression in PASMC

Recently, HIF-2α was found to be important for transcription of the Cu-ATPase, ATP7A [32]. To examine whether HIF-1α or HIF-2α is necessary for hypoxia-mediated upregulation of CTR1 and ATP7A, we compared mRNA expression levels of CTR1 and ATP7A in PASMC during hypoxia (and in PASMC treated with $CoCl_2$) [31]. To optimize the experimental condition, we first conducted a dose-response experiment for two specific siRNA we used to knockdown HIF-1α and HIF-2α. As shown in Figure 4A, the siRNA (at the doses of 50, 100 and 200 pmol) for HIF-1α (Hif-1α-siRNA) efficiently decreased mRNA level of Hif-1α (Fig. 4A*a*), while the siRNA (at the doses of 50, 100 and 200 pmol) for HIF-2α (Hif-2α-siRNA) significantly decreased Hif-2α mRNA level (Fig. 4A*b*) in PASMC incubated under hypoxic condition. The inhibitory effect of the siRNA for CTR1 (CTR1-siRNA) on CTR1 mRNA level was dose-dependent; 50 pmol of CTR1-siRNA seemed to be insufficient to knockdown CTR1, while 100 and 200 pmol of CTR1-siRNA significantly decreased CTR1 mRNA level (Fig. 4A*c*) in PASMC. Interestingly, we found that downregulation of HIF-1α with Hif-1α-siRNA only significantly

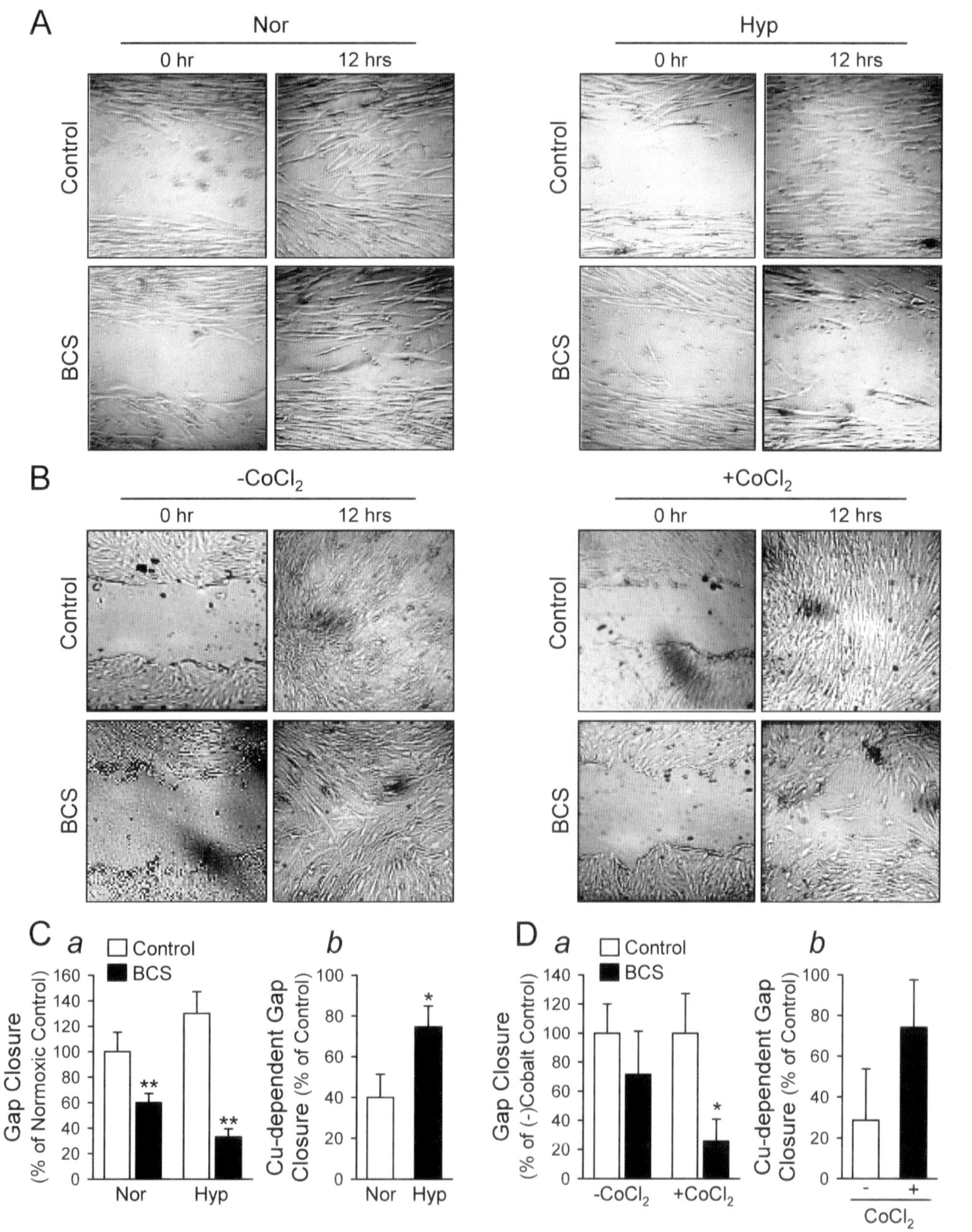

Figure 7. PASMC motility is dependent on Cu and the Cu-dependent PASMC motility is augmented by hypoxia. Cell motility was determined by a scratch wound assay over a period of 12 hours. A: Representative images showing normoxic (Nor) and hypoxic (Hyp) PASMC immediately (0 hr) or 12 hrs after scratch with a sterile pipette in the absence (Control) or presence (BCS) of 200 μM BCS (a Cu chelator). B: Representative images showing control (-$CoCl_2$) and 100-μm $CoCl_2$-treated PASMC immediately (0 hr) or 12 hrs after scratch in the absence (Control) or presence (BCS) of BCS. C: Summarized data (mean±SE) showing gap closure (*a*) measured at 12 hr in Nor and Hyp PASMC treated with (BCS) or

without (Control) BCS. **$P<0.01$ vs. Control. The Cu-dependent cell motility (*b*) was determined by the percent changes in gap closure between Control and BCS-treated PASMC under Nor and Hyp conditions. *$P<0.05$ vs. Nor. D: Summarized data (mean±SE) showing gap closure (*a*) measured at 12 hr in PASMC treated with (+$CoCl_2$) or without (-$CoCl_2$) $CoCl_2$ in the absence (Control) or presence (BCS) of BCS. *$P<0.05$ vs. Control. The Cu-dependent cell motility (*b*) was determined by the percent changes in gap closure between Control and BCS-treated PASMC in the absence (-) or presence (+) of $CoCl_2$.

decreased mRNA level of CTR1 in hypoxic PASMC, but not ATP7A mRNA level (Fig. 4B*a-d*). Knockdown of HIF-2α with Hif-2α-siRNA, however, had no effect on either CTR1 or ATP7A (Fig. 4B*a–d*). These results indicate that HIF-1α is potentially a transcription factor involved in hypoxia-mediated upregulation of CTR1 in PASMC, whereas hypoxia-mediated upregulation of ATP7A may be due to a HIF-1α/2α-independent mechanism.

Hypoxia increases lysyl oxidase activity

As described above, hypoxia upregulates CTR1, enhances Cu uptake and leads to an increase in the amount of Cu in PASMC. A fraction of the increased cellular Cu would be delivered to ATP7A at the Golgi membrane and then incorporated into newly synthesized pro-LOX protein, which traffics through the trans-Golgi network to be secreted out of the cell. To examine whether upregulated CTR1 and augmented Cu uptake lead to increased LOX secretion, we measured the activity of LOX protein secreted from PASMC under hypoxic conditions by collecting and concentrating the conditioned culture medium. Values for each sample were normalized to the total protein concentration in the conditioned medium, and an irreversible LOX inhibitor, β-aminopropionitrile (βAPN), was used as negative control. The amount of Cu-dependent LOX activity was calculated by subtracting LOX activity of the samples in the presence of a Cu chelator, bathocuproine disulphonate (BCS), from the total LOX activity.

As shown in Figure 5A, there was an approximately 2.3 fold increase in LOX activity in supernatants of lung tissue homogenates isolated from hypoxic mice in comparison to normoxic control mice. Similarly, the in vitro experiments also indicated that enzymatic activity of LOX in conditioned media collected from PASMC incubated under hypoxic condition (Fig. 5B) or treated with $CoCl_2$ (Fig. 5C) was significantly higher than in normoxic PASMC and cells treated with vehicle.

Hypoxia significantly increases Cu-dependent PASMC migration

The next set of experiments was designed to define the role of Cu in PASMC migration. Boyden chamber migration and scratch wound assays were utilized to examine whether CTR1-dependent Cu affects PASMC migration incubated under hypoxic condition. Typical smooth muscle cell culture medium (e.g., M199) contains approximately 1 μM Cu [33]. To examine the effect of this basal amount of Cu on cell migration, we treated cells with or without a Cu chelator, BCS, under normoxic and hypoxic conditions. In the Boyden chamber migration assay, Cu chelation dramatically inhibited PASMC migration under both normoxic (Nor) and hypoxic (Hyp) conditions (Fig. 6A*a* and *b*); Cu-dependent migration (Control minus BCS treatment) was significantly greater in PASMC exposed to hypoxia in comparison to PASMC exposed to normoxia (Fig. 6A*c*, $P<0.05$). Consistent with the inhibitory effect of Cu chelation by BCS, knockdown of CTR1 with siRNA led to a comparable decrease in cell migration (Fig. 6B*a* and B*b*), which was again significantly greater in hypoxic compared to normoxic PASMC (Fig. 6B*c*, $P<0.05$). These data indicate that hypoxia-mediated increase in the Cu uptake via CTR1 contributes to enhanced PASMC migration.

In addition, our results obtained for the scratch wound assay also show a significant decrease in PASMC motility when cells were treated with BCS (Fig. 7). Chelation of Cu with BCS significantly decreased PASMC motility (determined by gap closure) in both normoxic and hypoxic PASMC (Fig. 7A and 7C*a*); an effect that was more pronounced under hypoxic conditions (Fig. 7C*b*). PASMC motility was also assessed with and without $CoCl_2$ treatment and a significant decrease in motility was observed with Cu chelation after treatment with $CoCl_2$ (Fig. 7B and 7D*a*). There was a trend toward decreased migration without the addition of $CoCl_2$ and though $CoCl_2$ treatment does appear to show greater Cu-dependent migration, no statistical differences were observed due to a wide variability in outcomes (Fig. 7D*b*).

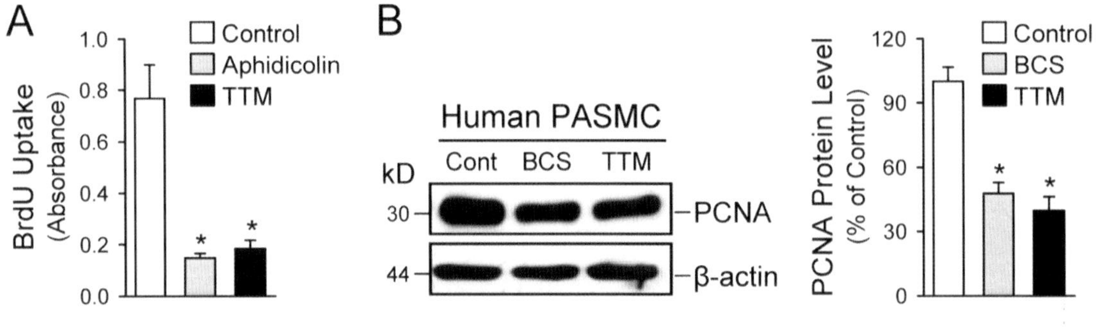

Figure 8. Chelation of Cu diminishes human PASMC proliferation. A: BrdU incorporation (mean±SE) in control PASMC and PASMC treated with aphidcolin (a DNA-replication inhibitor, 48 hrs) and 100 μM tetrathiomolybadate (TTM, a Cu chelator, 48 hrs). *$P<0.05$ vs. Control. Cells treated with aphidicolin were used as a negative control. B: Western blot analysis (left panel) on PCNA (a proliferating cell nuclear antigen) in control (Cont) PASMC and PASMC treated with the Cu chelators, BCS and TTM. Summarized data (right panel, mean±SE) showing PCNA protein levels in control cells, BCS-treated cells and TTM-treated cells. *$P<0.05$ vs. Control.

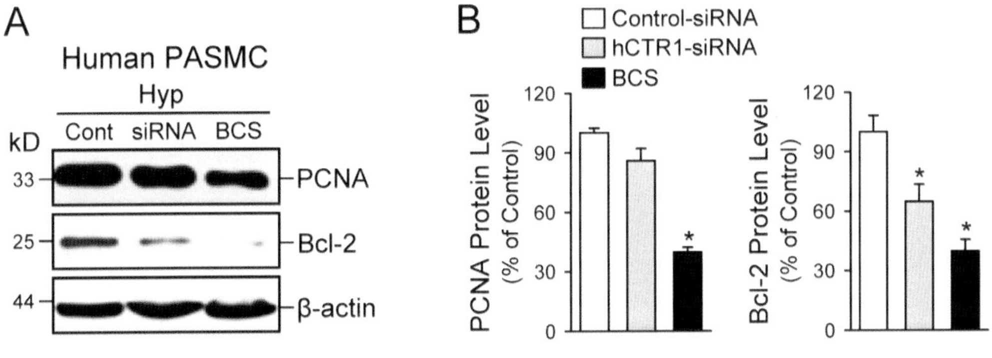

Figure 9. Chelation of Cu and knockdown of CTR1 both decrease Bcl-2 expression in human PASMC during hypoxia. A: Western blot analysis on PCNA (a marker for cell proliferation) and Bcl-2 (an anti-apoptotic protein) in PASMC transfected with scrambled siRNA (Cont) or human CTR1-siRNA (siRNA) and PASMC treated with the Cu chelator BCS. B: Summarized data (mean±SE) showing PCNA (left panel) and Bcl-2 (right panel) protein levels in PASMC transfected with Control-siRNA or hCTR1-siRNA and PASMC treated with BCS. *$P<0.05$ vs. Control-siRNA.

Cu chelation attenuates proliferation of PASMC and decreases expression of the anti-apoptotic protein Bcl-2

Next, the effect of Cu and CTR1 on the proliferation of PASMC cells was evaluated by the bromodeoxyuridine (BrdU) incorporation assay, as well as by the Western blot analysis with anti-proliferating cell nuclear antigen (PCNA) antibody. Figure 8A indicates that the treatment of PASMC with 100 μM tetrathiomolybdate (TTM), a cell permeable Cu chelator, results in a dramatic decrease of BrdU incorporation, comparable to the aphidicolin treatment (an inhibitor of DNA replication, used as the negative control here). Similar to the case of BrdU assay, the expression of PCNA was decreased in cells treated with either BCS or TTM, indicating that Cu is required for cell proliferation (Fig. 8B, left and right panels). We anticipated that TTM would have a greater inhibitory effect on proliferation than BCS because TTM can cross the plasma membrane [34], and should chelate the intra- and extra-cellular Cu and BCS is a membrane-impermeable compound [34], and therefore should only bind the extracellular Cu. Both compounds (BCS and TTM) had a similar inhibitory effect on the PCNA expression (Fig. 8B). It is likely that TTM does not further inhibit proliferation because it is not able to out-compete the Cu-chaperones and glutathione for Cu binding [35], as all of the intracellular Cu is either protein- or glutathione-bound [36,37].

In addition to the level of PCNA, we examined the effect of BCS on the expression of Bcl-2, an anti-apoptotic protein, during hypoxia (Fig. 9A). We found that Cu-chelation (by BCS), not only downregulated protein expression level of PCNA (Fig. 9A), but also significantly decreased levels of Bcl-2 protein by ~60% (Fig. 9B). These data indicate that Cu ions, or inward transportation of Cu ions, are important for activation of cell survival or anti-apoptotic signals (determined by Bcl-2 expression level) and for cellular proliferation (determined by PCNA expression level).

Knockdown of CTR1 exerts apoptotic effect on PASMC

To investigate whether inward transportation of Cu ions through CTR1 is involved in PASMC proliferation and survival, we also measured and compared the expression levels of PCNA (a marker for cell proliferation) and Bcl–2 (an anti-apoptotic protein) in human PASMC treated with control siRNA (Cont) and siRNA specifically targeting human CTR1 (hCTR1-siRNA). The real-time RT-PCR experiments showed that 100 μM of hCTR1-siRNA treatment decreased CTR1 mRNA level by 45–55% in PASMC (data not shown). As shown in Figure 9, knockdown of CTR1 with siRNA (hCTR1-siRNA) in PASMC during hypoxia negligibly affected the protein expression level of PCNA, but significantly decreased the protein expression level of Bcl–2 (by approximately 36%, $P<0.05$ vs. cells treated with control siRNA). Chelation of Cu with BCS, a membrane impermeable Cu chelator, significantly decreased the protein expression level of both PCNA and Bcl–2 in PASMC during hypoxia (Fig. 9). These data indicate that, while Cu ions are required for or involved in

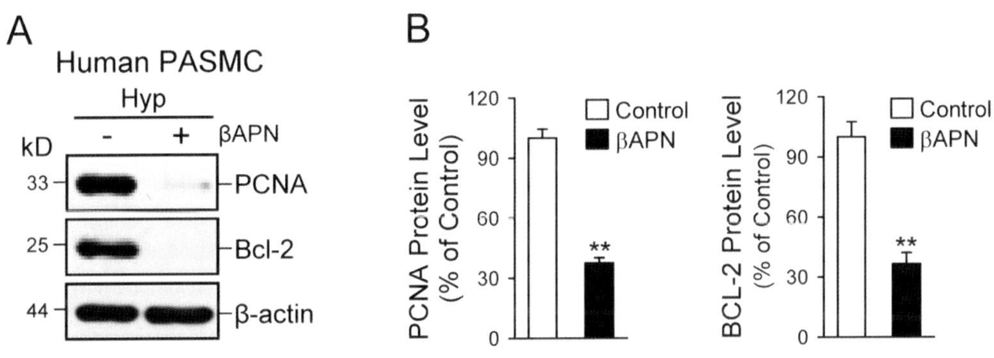

Figure 10. Inhibition of LOX downregulates PCNA (a marker for cell proliferation) and Bcl–2 (an anti-apoptotic protein) in human PASMC during hypoxia. A: Western blot analysis on PCNA and Bcl–2 in hypoxic PASMC treated with (+) or without (-) the irreversible LOX inhibitor βAPN (for 48 hrs). B: Summarized data (mean±SE) showing PCNA (left panel) and Bcl–2 (right panel) protein levels in control PASMC (open bars) and PASMC treated with βAPN (solid bars). **$P<0.01$ vs. Control.

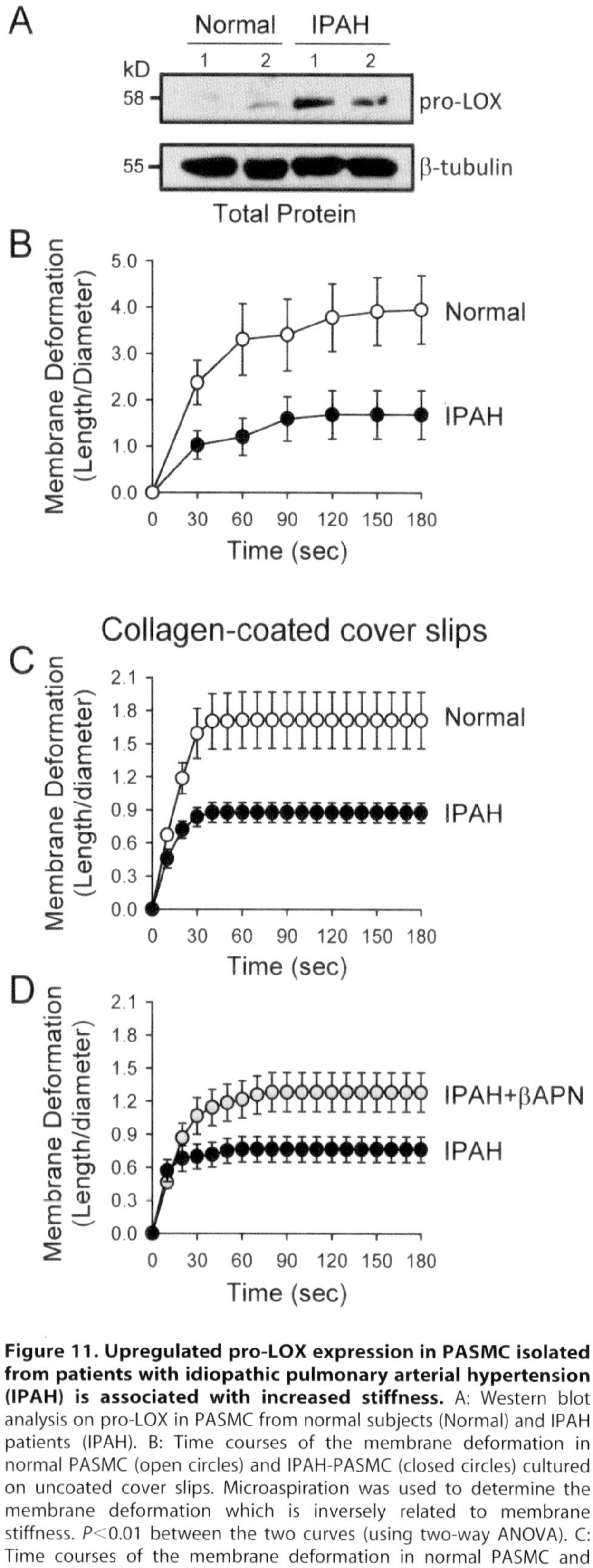

Figure 11. Upregulated pro-LOX expression in PASMC isolated from patients with idiopathic pulmonary arterial hypertension (IPAH) is associated with increased stiffness. A: Western blot analysis on pro-LOX in PASMC from normal subjects (Normal) and IPAH patients (IPAH). B: Time courses of the membrane deformation in normal PASMC (open circles) and IPAH-PASMC (closed circles) cultured on uncoated cover slips. Microaspiration was used to determine the membrane deformation which is inversely related to membrane stiffness. $P<0.01$ between the two curves (using two-way ANOVA). C: Time courses of the membrane deformation in normal PASMC and IPAH-PASMC cultured on collagen-coated cover slips. $P<0.01$ between the two curves (using two-way ANOVA). D: Time courses of the membrane deformation in IPAH-PASMC treated with (IPAH+βAPN) or without (IPAH) the LOX inhibitor βAPN. $P<0.01$ between the two curves (using two-way ANOVA).

exerting pro-proliferative (determined by PCNA expression level) and anti-apoptotic (determined by Bcl-2 expression level) effects on PASMC, transportation of Cu ions through CTR1 seems to be involved only in upregulation of Bcl-2 in PASMC (or the anti-apoptotic effect on PASMC) based on the downregulating effect of BCS on Bcl-2 as shown in Figure 9. The results further imply that CTR1 plays a predominant role in cell survival (potentially via its upregulating effect on the anti-apoptotic protein Bcl-2 since downregulation of CTR1 with siRNA only decreased Bcl–2 level but negligibly affected PCNA level, as shown in Figure 9B) while its role in cell proliferation can be compensated, possibly by an alternative mechanism of cellular Cu uptake.

Inhibition of lysyl oxidase inhibits proliferation and enhances apoptosis in PASMC

Lysyl oxidase (LOX) regulates extracellular matrix organization by crosslinking collagen and elastin, and increased activity (and/or secretion) of LOX increases ECM rigidity or stiffness [38]. The next set of experiments was designed to examine whether blockade of LOX affects PASMC proliferation and migration. As shown in Figure 10, treatment of human PASMC during hypoxia with β-aminopropionitrile (βAPN, for 48–72 hrs) significantly decreased the protein expression level of PCNA (a marker for cell proliferation) and Bcl–2 (an anti-apoptotic protein). These results imply that LOX is involved in regulating PASMC proliferation and survival by affecting extracellular matrix and cellular stiffness.

IPAH-PASMC have increased pro-LOX and show increased cellular stiffness

As shown above, hypoxia-induced pulmonary vascular remodeling is, at least in part, associated with *a*) HIF-1α-dependent upregulation of CTR1 and pro-LOX in PASMC, and *b*) LOX-mediated extracellular matrix and cellular stiffness. To confirm that LOX-mediated cellular stiffness is not only a mechanism partially involved in the development of hypoxia-mediated pulmonary hypertension, but also a potential mechanism for idiopathic pulmonary arterial hypertension (IPAH), we measured and compared deformability or stiffness of PASMC isolated from normal subjects and IPAH patients using micropipette aspiration or microaspiration.

Microaspiration is a simple method to estimate cell stiffness by measuring the degree of membrane deformation in response to negative pressure applied by a glass micropipette to the cell surface. Using microaspiration, investigators have shown previously that plasma membrane composition, such as the cholesterol content [39], the level of oxidized oxLDL [40,41], and sub-membrane cytoskeleton [28,42] all affect the degree of cellular stiffness and membrane deformation [43]. Here, we show that PASMC derived from IPAH patients (IPAH-PASMC) exhibited significantly higher expression of pro-LOX than normal PASMC (Fig. 11A). Deformation of cells measured by microaspiration was significantly decreased in IPAH-PASMC compared to normal PASMC, implying a greater overall stiffness of IPAH-PASMC cultured on glass cover slips (Fig. 11B) or collagen-coated cover slips (Fig. 11C). Inhibition of LOX activity with β-aminopropionitrate (βAPN) significantly increased the degree of membrane deformation (i.e., significantly decreased the stiffness) of IPAH-PASMC cultured on collagen-coated cover slips, implying that LOX may contribute to the increased cell stiffness in IPAH-PASMC (Fig 11D).

Discussion

Pulmonary vascular remodeling and increased stiffness of pulmonary arteries both contribute to the development and progression of pulmonary hypertension. In this study, we identified a novel mechanism in which chronic hypoxia caused increased Cu transport and LOX activity that promoted the development of pulmonary hypertension in a murine model. In lung tissues and isolated pulmonary arteries from animals with HPH and in PASMC exposed to hypoxia, our data indicated that mRNA and protein expression level of the high affinity Cu transporter CTR1 was significantly upregulated in comparison to normoxic controls. The hypoxia-mediated upregulation of CTR1 seemed to be mediated by a HIF-1α-dependent mechanism because downregulation of HIF-1α significantly attenuated the hypoxia-mediated CTR1 upregulation. The upregulated CTR1 was functionally associated with an increased Cu uptake in PASMC exposed to hypoxia, and the increased intracellular Cu contributed to augmenting PASMC proliferation, survival and migration during hypoxia.

Our data also showed that hypoxia upregulated the Cu export pump ATP7A and the Cu-dependent enzyme LOX in lung tissue homogenates, isolated pulmonary arteries and cultured PASMC. The hypoxia- (or $CoCl_2$-) mediated increase in expression of ATP7A was, however, due to a HIF-1α-independent mechanism because downregulation of HIF-1α had negligible effect on hypoxia-mediated ATP7A upregulation. Upregulated LOX expression and increased Cu-LOX activity usually lead to crosslink of collagen and elastin in extracellular matrix and increase in pulmonary arterial stiffness (or PASMC stiffness) which, in combination with the increased PASMC proliferation and migration, further contributes to the development and progression of HPH. By identifying upregulation of the entire Cu transport cascade (CTR1, ATOX1, ATP7A, and LOX), the data from this study demonstrate that Cu and Cu-dependent enzymes may play an important role in HPH and the Cu transporters may be good targets to develop therapeutic approaches for pulmonary hypertension.

Since the identification and cloning of CTR1 [44], various studies have characterized the kinetics of CTR1-mediated Cu transport and the structural properties of CTR1, such as topology, mapping of glycosylation sites, identifying amino acids essential for transport, and determining the 3D structure using cryoelectron microscopy [19,30,45,46]. Despite this knowledge, information is still very limited regarding the cellular regulation of Cu homeostasis and transport in mammalian cells. Recently, White et al. reported a novel regulatory mechanism of Cu homeostasis in a mammalian macrophage cell line (RAW 264.7) that was dependent on hypoxia [47].

Similar to macrophages, PASMC are uniquely equipped to sense O_2 tension and orchestration of cellular responses to hypoxia is mediated in mammals by two isoforms of hypoxia-inducible factors, HIF-1α and HIF-2α. HIF-1α mediates primarily an acute response to hypoxia, while HIF-2α is most often thought to require a chronic stimulus to accumulate, and becomes more important during the late phases of hypoxia [48]. In the present study, we were able to knockdown both HIF-1α and HIF-2α with respective siRNA, but only HIF-1α-siRNA attenuated CTR1 mRNA levels in PASMC exposed to 3% O_2 for 48 hrs. Examination of the promoter region of the CTR1 gene found the presence of the putative hypoxia-responsive element (HRE) (5′-cgtg-3′), a recognition binding site for HIF-1α/2α [49]. More extensive studies are needed to investigate whether and how HIF-1α transcriptionally regulates the CTR1 gene in PASMC.

It has recently been shown that excess Cu stabilizes HIF-1α [50,51]. Together with the data mentioned above that HIF-1α is involved in hypoxia-mediated upregulation of CTR1 and, subsequently, increase in intracellular Cu, we speculate that a positive feedback loop or chain reaction exists in hypoxic PASMC. Hypoxia activates HIF-1α and upregulates CTR1 expression via HIF-1α, and then increases intracellular Cu which may subsequently stabilize HIF-1α and further potentiate the HIF-1α-mediated upregulation of CTR1. This scenario may not occur physiologically, as the intracellular Cu concentration capable of exerting a positive effect on HIF-1α activation is 50–125 μM, which is much higher than the normal physiological intracellular Cu concentration (less than 5 μM). During hypoxia (or when HIF-1-α is activated and CTR1 is upregulated), intracellular Cu concentration may rise to the level that can exert the positive effect on HIF-1α leading to sustained activation of HIF-1α and maintain a prolonged effect of hypoxia on PASMC proliferation and migration. A previous study demonstrated that that Cu depletion using a Cu-chelation decreased the binding of HIF-1α to its downstream HRE domain-containing target genes, by inhibiting the formation of complexes between HIF-1α and DNA [51].

In rats with severe pulmonary hypertension (induced by Sugen and hypoxia), Bogaard et al. [25] recently showed that Cu chelation with TTM or Cu-restricted diet caused regression of established pulmonary vascular intimal lesions and prevented formation of new intimal lesions through inhibition of pulmonary arterial endothelial cell (PAEC) proliferation. Their histological examination, however, showed that Cu restriction had no effect on pulmonary vascular thickening attributable to the medial hypertrophy (due mainly to excessive PASMC proliferation). These observations suggest that Cu is mainly involved in stimulating PAEC proliferation causing intimal lesions, but has little effect on stimulating PASMC proliferation. By determining BrdU incorporation and PCNA expression, we showed in our in vitro study that Cu chelation led to a dramatic inhibition of PASMC proliferation, while knockdown of CTR1 with siRNA also resulted in attenuation of PASMC proliferation (and migration) during hypoxia. Furthermore, inhibition of LOX has been proposed to treat hypertensive and fibrotic disorders [52,53] and metastatic cancers [54]. In PASMC cultured in hypoxia, inhibition of LOX activity with βAPN also significantly attenuated proliferation indicating that increased Cu-dependent LOX activity is involved in stimulating PASMC proliferation.

In summary, the data from this study imply that increased Cu transport due to upregulated CTR1 (and ATP7A) contribute to the increase in PASMC proliferation and migration, which subsequently cause pulmonary vascular remodeling characterized by medial and adventitial hypertrophy. The enhanced Cu uptake and elevated ATP7A expression in PASMC may also contribute to increasing pulmonary arterial stiffness by potentiating Cu-LOX activity and collagen/elastin crosslink. Development of drugs targeting the Cu-CTR1-LOX signaling axis may be a novel strategy to develop more efficient therapeutic approaches for pulmonary hypertension associated with hypoxia.

Acknowledgments

The authors thank Drs. Goufei Zhou and Tohru Fukai for their critical review and constructive suggestions for the manuscript.

Author Contributions

Conceived and designed the experiments: AMZ JXY. Performed the experiments: AMZ HT QG FKK MO JW JC MSRC. Analyzed the data: AMZ JXY. Contributed reagents/materials/analysis tools: JC KAS DRF IL RFM JHK. Wrote the paper: AMZ KAS DRF JXY.

References

1. Firth AL, Mandel J, Yuan JX (2010) Idiopathic pulmonary arterial hypertension. Dis Model Mech 3: 268–273.
2. Stamm JA, Risbano MG, Mathier MA (2011) Overview of current therapeutic approaches for pulmonary hypertension. Pulm Circ 1: 138–159.
3. Wang Z, Chesler NC (2011) Pulmonary vascular wall stiffness: An important contributor to the increased right ventricular afterload with pulmonary hypertension. Pulm Circ 1: 212–223.
4. Durmowicz AG, Stenmark KR (1999) Mechanisms of structural remodeling in chronic pulmonary hypertension. Pediatr Rev 20: e91–e102.
5. van Suylen RJ, Smits JF, Daemen MJ (1998) Pulmonary artery remodeling differs in hypoxia- and monocrotaline-induced pulmonary hypertension. Am J Respir Crit Care Med 157: 1423–1428.
6. Morrell NW, Adnot S, Archer SL, Dupuis J, Jones PL, et al. (2009) Cellular and molecular basis of pulmonary arterial hypertension. J Am Coll Cardiol 54: S20–31.
7. Pak O, Aldashev A, Welsh D, Peacock A (2007) The effects of hypoxia on the cells of the pulmonary vasculature. Eur Respir J 30: 364–372.
8. Tian L, Chesler NC (2012) In vivo and in vitro measurements of pulmonary arterial stiffness: A brief review. Pulm Circ 2: 505–517.
9. Budhiraja R, Tuder RM, Hassoun PM (2004) Endothelial dysfunction in pulmonary hypertension. Circulation 109: 159–165.
10. Malenfant S, Neyron AS, Paulin R, Potus F, Meloche J, et al. (2013) Signal transduction in the development of pulmonary arterial hypertension. Pulm Circ 3: 278–293.
11. Turski ML, Thiele DJ (2009) New roles for copper metabolism in cell proliferation, signaling, and disease. J Biol Chem 284: 717–721.
12. Kaplan JH, Lutsenko S (2009) Copper transport in mammalian cells: special care for a metal with special needs. J Biol Chem 284: 25461–25465.
13. Cross JB, Currier RP, Torraco DJ, Vanderberg LA, Wagner GL, et al. (2003) Killing of bacillus spores by aqueous dissolved oxygen, ascorbic acid, and copper ions. Appl Environ Microbiol 69: 2245–2252.
14. Gaetke LM, Chow CK (2003) Copper toxicity, oxidative stress, and antioxidant nutrients. Toxicology 189: 147–163.
15. Durand MJ, Lombard JH (2013) Low-dose angiotensin II infusion restores vascular function in cerebral arteries of high salt-fed rats by increasing copper/zinc superoxide dimutase expression. Am J Hypertens 26: 739–747.
16. Gabrielli LA, Castro PF, Godoy I, Mellado R, Bourge RC, et al. (2011) Systemic oxidative stress and endothelial dysfunction is associated with an attenuated acute vascular response to inhaled prostanoid in pulmonary artery hypertension patients. J Card Fail 17: 1012–1017.
17. Schaefer M, Gitlin JD (1999) Genetic disorders of membrane transport. IV. Wilson's disease and Menkes disease. Am J Physiol 276: G311–314.
18. Rucker RB, Romero-Chapman N, Wong T, Lee J, Steinberg FM, et al. (1996) Modulation of lysyl oxidase by dietary copper in rats. J Nutr 126: 51–60.
19. Eisses JF, Kaplan JH (2002) Molecular characterization of hCTR1, the human copper uptake protein. J Biol Chem 277: 29162–29171.
20. Eisses JF, Stasser JP, Ralle M, Kaplan JH, Blackburn NJ (2000) Domains I and III of the human copper chaperone for superoxide dismutase interact via a cysteine-bridged Dicopper(I) cluster. Biochemistry 39: 7337–7342.
21. Kim BE, Nevitt T, Thiele DJ (2008) Mechanisms for copper acquisition, distribution and regulation. Nat Chem Biol 4: 176–185.
22. Barnes N, Bartee MY, Braiterman L, Gupta A, Ustiyan V, et al. (2009) Cell-specific trafficking suggests a new role for renal ATP7B in the intracellular copper storage. Traffic 10: 767–779.
23. Linz R, Barnes NL, Zimnicka AM, Kaplan JH, Eipper B, et al. (2008) Intracellular targeting of copper-transporting ATPase ATP7A in a normal and ATP7B$^{-/-}$ kidney. Am J Physiol Renal Physiol 294: F53–61.
24. White C, Kambe T, Fulcher YG, Sachdev SW, Bush AI, et al. (2009) Copper transport into the secretory pathway is regulated by oxygen in macrophages. J Cell Sci 122: 1315–1321.
25. Bogaard HJ, Mizuno S, Guignabert C, Al Hussaini AA, Farkas D, et al. (2012) Copper dependence of angioproliferation in pulmonary arterial hypertension in rats and humans. Am J Respir Cell Mol Biol 46: 582–591.
26. Erler JT, Bennewith KL, Nicolau M, Dornhofer N, Kong C, et al. (2006) Lysyl oxidase is essential for hypoxia-induced metastasis. Nature 440: 1222–1226.
27. Schermuly RT, Dony E, Ghofrani HA, Pullamsetti S, Savai R, et al. (2005) Reversal of experimental pulmonary hypertension by PDGF inhibition. J Clin Invest 115: 2811–2821.
28. Byfield FJ, Aranda-Espinoza H, Romanenko VG, Rothblat GH, Levitan I (2004) Cholesterol depletion increases membrane stiffness of aortic endothelial cells. Biophys J 87: 3336–3343.
29. Hochachka PW, Buck LT, Doll CJ, Land SC (1996) Unifying theory of hypoxia tolerance: molecular/metabolic defense and rescue mechanisms for surviving oxygen lack. Proc Natl Acad Sci U S A 93: 9493–9498.
30. Eisses JF, Chi Y, Kaplan JH (2005) Stable plasma membrane levels of hCTR1 mediate cellular copper uptake. J Biol Chem 280: 9635–9639.
31. Yuan Y, Hilliard G, Ferguson T, Millhorn DE (2003) Cobalt inhibits the interaction between hypoxia-inducible factor-alpha and von Hippel-Lindau protein by direct binding to hypoxia-inducible factor-alpha. J Biol Chem 278: 15911–15916.
32. Xie L, Collins JF (2011) Transcriptional regulation of the Menkes copper ATPase (ATP7A) gene by hypoxia-inducible factor (HIF-2alpha) in intestinal epithelial cells. Am J Physiol Cell Physiol 300: C1298–1305.
33. Molloy SA, Kaplan JH (2009) Copper-dependent recycling of hCTR1, the human high affinity copper transporter. J Biol Chem 284: 29704–29713.
34. Ashino T, Sudhahar V, Urao N, Oshikawa J, Chen GF, et al. (2010) Unexpected role of the copper transporter ATP7A in PDGF-induced vascular smooth muscle cell migration. Circ Res 107: 787–799.
35. Song M, Song Z, Barve S, Zhang J, Chen T, et al. (2008) Tetrathiomolybdate protects against bile duct ligation-induced cholestatic liver injury and fibrosis. J Pharmacol Exp Ther 325: 409–416.
36. Rae TD, Schmidt PJ, Pufahl RA, Culotta VC, O'Halloran TV (1999) Undetectable intracellular free copper: the requirement of a copper chaperone for superoxide dismutase. Science 284: 805–808.
37. Maryon EB, Molloy SA, Kaplan JH (2013) Cellular glutathione plays a key role in copper uptake mediated by human copper transporter 1. Am J Physiol Cell Physiol 304: C768–779.
38. Levental KR, Yu H, Kass L, Lakins JN, Egeblad M, et al. (2009) Matrix crosslinking forces tumor progression by enhancing integrin signaling. Cell 139: 891–906.
39. Sun M, Northup N, Marga F, Huber T, Byfield FJ, et al. (2007) The effect of cellular cholesterol on membrane-cytoskeleton adhesion. J Cell Sci 120: 2223–2231.
40. Shentu TP, Titushkin I, Singh DK, Gooch KJ, Subbaiah PV, et al. (2010) oxLDL-induced decrease in lipid order of membrane domains is inversely correlated with endothelial stiffness and network formation. Am J Physiol Cell Physiol 299: C218–229.
41. Byfield FJ, Tikku S, Rothblat GH, Gooch KJ, Levitan I (2006) OxLDL increases endothelial stiffness, force generation, and network formation. J Lipid Res 47: 715–723.
42. Sato M, Theret DP, Wheeler LT, Ohshima N, Nerem RM (1990) Application of the micropipette technique to the measurement of cultured porcine aortic endothelial cell viscoelastic properties. J Biomech Eng 112: 263–268.
43. Oh MJ, Kuhr F, Byfield F, Levitan I (2012) Micropipette aspiration of substrate-attached cells to estimate cell stiffness. J Vis Exp.
44. Zhou B, Gitschier J (1997) hCTR1: a human gene for copper uptake identified by complementation in yeast. Proc Natl Acad Sci U S A 94: 7481–7486.
45. Maryon EB, Molloy SA, Kaplan JH (2007) O-linked glycosylation at threonine 27 protects the copper transporter hCTR1 from proteolytic cleavage in mammalian cells. J Biol Chem 282: 20376–20387.
46. De Feo CJ, Aller SG, Siluvai GS, Blackburn NJ, Unger VM (2009) Three-dimensional structure of the human copper transporter hCTR1. Proc Natl Acad Sci U S A 106: 4237–4242.
47. White C, Lee J, Kambe T, Fritsche K, Petris MJ (2009) A role for the ATP7A copper-transporting ATPase in macrophage bactericidal activity. J Biol Chem 284: 33949–33956.
48. Patel SA, Simon MC (2008) Biology of hypoxia-inducible factor-2alpha in development and disease. Cell Death Differ 15: 628–634.
49. Benita Y, Kikuchi H, Smith AD, Zhang MQ, Chung DC, et al. (2009) An integrative genomics approach identifies Hypoxia Inducible Factor-1 (HIF-1)-target genes that form the core response to hypoxia. Nucleic Acids Res 37: 4587–4602.
50. Martin F, Linden T, Katschinski DM, Oehme F, Flamme I, et al. (2005) Copper-dependent activation of hypoxia-inducible factor (HIF)-1: implications for ceruloplasmin regulation. Blood 105: 4613–4619.
51. Feng W, Ye F, Xue W, Zhou Z, Kang YJ (2009) Copper regulation of hypoxia-inducible factor-1 activity. Mol Pharmacol 75: 174–182.
52. Alcudia JF, Martinez-Gonzalez J, Guadall A, Gonzalez-Diez M, Badimon L, et al. (2008) Lysyl oxidase and endothelial dysfunction: mechanisms of lysyl oxidase down-regulation by pro-inflammatory cytokines. Front Biosci 13: 2721–2727.
53. Rodriguez C, Martinez-Gonzalez J, Raposo B, Alcudia JF, Guadall A, et al. (2008) Regulation of lysyl oxidase in vascular cells: lysyl oxidase as a new player in cardiovascular diseases. Cardiovasc Res 79: 7–13.
54. Siddikuzzaman, Grace VM, Guruvayoorappan C (2011) Lysyl oxidase: a potential target for cancer therapy. Inflammopharmacology 19: 117–129.

Permissions

All chapters in this book were first published in PLOS ONE, by The Public Library of Science; hereby published with permission under the Creative Commons Attribution License or equivalent. Every chapter published in this book has been scrutinized by our experts. Their significance has been extensively debated. The topics covered herein carry significant findings which will fuel the growth of the discipline. They may even be implemented as practical applications or may be referred to as a beginning point for another development.

The contributors of this book come from diverse backgrounds, making this book a truly international effort. This book will bring forth new frontiers with its revolutionizing research information and detailed analysis of the nascent developments around the world.

We would like to thank all the contributing authors for lending their expertise to make the book truly unique. They have played a crucial role in the development of this book. Without their invaluable contributions this book wouldn't have been possible. They have made vital efforts to compile up to date information on the varied aspects of this subject to make this book a valuable addition to the collection of many professionals and students.

This book was conceptualized with the vision of imparting up-to-date information and advanced data in this field. To ensure the same, a matchless editorial board was set up. Every individual on the board went through rigorous rounds of assessment to prove their worth. After which they invested a large part of their time researching and compiling the most relevant data for our readers.

The editorial board has been involved in producing this book since its inception. They have spent rigorous hours researching and exploring the diverse topics which have resulted in the successful publishing of this book. They have passed on their knowledge of decades through this book. To expedite this challenging task, the publisher supported the team at every step. A small team of assistant editors was also appointed to further simplify the editing procedure and attain best results for the readers.

Apart from the editorial board, the designing team has also invested a significant amount of their time in understanding the subject and creating the most relevant covers. They scrutinized every image to scout for the most suitable representation of the subject and create an appropriate cover for the book.

The publishing team has been an ardent support to the editorial, designing and production team. Their endless efforts to recruit the best for this project, has resulted in the accomplishment of this book. They are a veteran in the field of academics and their pool of knowledge is as vast as their experience in printing. Their expertise and guidance has proved useful at every step. Their uncompromising quality standards have made this book an exceptional effort. Their encouragement from time to time has been an inspiration for everyone.

The publisher and the editorial board hope that this book will prove to be a valuable piece of knowledge for researchers, students, practitioners and scholars across the globe.

List of Contributors

Han Zheng
Department of Surgery, University of Pittsburgh School of Medicine, Pittsburgh, Pennsylvania, United States of America

Eileen M. Bauer and Michael T. Lotze
Department of Surgery, University of Pittsburgh School of Medicine, Pittsburgh, Pennsylvania, United States of America
University of Pittsburgh Cancer Institute, University of Pittsburgh School of Medicine, Pittsburgh, Pennsylvania, United States of America

Philip M. Bauer
Department of Surgery, University of Pittsburgh School of Medicine, Pittsburgh, Pennsylvania, United States of America
University of Pittsburgh Cancer Institute, University of Pittsburgh School of Medicine, Pittsburgh, Pennsylvania, United States of America
Department of Pharmacology and Chemical Biology, University of Pittsburgh School of Medicine, Pittsburgh, Pennsylvania, United States of America
Vascular Medicine Institute, University of Pittsburgh School of Medicine, Pittsburgh, Pennsylvania, United States of America

Lina Qiao, Liang Xie, Tongfu Zhou, Yimin Hua and Hanmin Liu
Department of Pediatric Cardiology, West China Second University Hospital, Sichuan University, Chengdu, China
Key Laboratory of Obstetric and Gynecologic and Pediatric Diseases and Birth Defects of Ministry of Education, West China Second University Hospital, Sichuan University, Chengdu, China,

Kun Shi
Department of Cardiology, Chengdu Women and Children Center Hospital, Chengdu, China

Rolf Rossaint
Department of Anaesthesiology, Institute of Pharmacology and Toxicology, Medical Faculty Aachen, RWTH-Aachen, Aachen, Germany

Annette D. Rieg
Department of Anaesthesiology, Institute of Pharmacology and Toxicology, Medical Faculty Aachen, RWTH-Aachen, Aachen, Germany
Institute of Pharmacology and Toxicology, Medical Faculty Aachen, RWTH-Aachen, Aachen, Germany

Stefan Uhlig and Christian Martin
Institute of Pharmacology and Toxicology, Medical Faculty Aachen, RWTH-Aachen, Aachen, Germany

Stephen F. Vatner and You-Tang Shen
CV Dynamics, Inc., North Brunswick, New Jersey, United States of America,
Cardiovascular Research Institute, University of Medicine and Dentistry of New Jersey, New Jersey Medical School, Newark, New Jersey, United States of America

David Ho, Li Chen, Xin Zhao and Dorothy E. Vatner
Cardiovascular Research Institute, University of Medicine and Dentistry of New Jersey, New Jersey Medical School, Newark, New Jersey, United States of America

Nicquanna Durham, Malar Pannirselvam, David J. Morgans, Fady I. Malik
Cytokinetics, Inc., South San Francisco, California, United States of America

Qiang Wang, Yan-Zhe Yu, Hui Wang, Li-Qing Bi, Wei-Ping Xie and Hong Wang
Department of Respiratory Medicine, The First Affiliated Hospital of Nanjing Medical University, Nanjing, Jiangsu, People's Republic of China

Xiang-Rong Zuo
Department of Respiratory Medicine, The First Affiliated Hospital of Nanjing Medical University, Nanjing, Jiangsu, People's Republic of China

Quan Cao
Department of Critical Care Medicine, The First Affiliated Hospital of Nanjing Medical University, Nanjing, Jiangsu, People's Republic of China

Ying Wang
Beijing Key Laboratory of Respiratory and Pulmonary Circulation Disorders, Beijing Chao-Yang Hospital, Capital Medical University, Beijing, P.R. China,

Lijuan Guo, Yuanhua Yang, Lei Wang and Jifeng Li
Beijing Key Laboratory of Respiratory and Pulmonary Circulation Disorders, Beijing Chao-Yang Hospital, Capital Medical University, Beijing, P.R. China

Beijing Institute of Respiratory Medicine, Capital Medical University, Beijing, P.R. China

Chen Wang
Beijing Key Laboratory of Respiratory and Pulmonary Circulation Disorders, Beijing Chao-Yang Hospital, Capital Medical University, Beijing, P.R. China
Beijing Institute of Respiratory Medicine, Capital Medical University, Beijing, P.R. China
Department of Beijing Hospital, Ministry of Health, Beijing, P.R. China

Jie Liu
Department of Physiology, Capital Medical University, Beijing, P.R. China

Yan Liu, Song Gu and Jun Cai
Department of Cardiology, Beijing Chao-Yang Hospital, Capital Medical University, Beijing, P.R. China,

Huili Gan
Department of Cardiac Surgery, Beijing Anzhen Hospital, Capital Medical University, Beijing, P.R. China
Beijing Institute of Heart, Lung and Vessel Disease, Capital Medical University, Beijing, P.R. China

Jason X.-J. Yuan
Department of Medicine, University of Illinois at Chicago, Chicago, Illinois, United States of America

Sung-Hyun Park, Wen-Chi Chen and Carol Hoffman
Department of Environmental Medicine, New York University School of Medicine, Tuxedo, New York, United States of America

Gabriele Grunig
Department of Environmental Medicine, New York University School of Medicine, Tuxedo, New York, United States of America
Division of Pulmonary Medicine, Department of Medicine, New York University School of Medicine, New York, New York, United States of America

Leigh M. Marsh
Ludwig Boltzmann Institute for Lung Vascular Research, Graz, Austria

James West
Division of Allergy, Pulmonary, and Critical Care Medicine, Department of Medicine, Vanderbilt University Medical Center, Nashville, Tennessee, United States of America

Christoph Hammerstingl, Robert Schueler, Lisa Bors, Diana Momcilovic, Stefan Pabst and Georg Nickenig, Dirk Skowasch
Department of Internal Medicine II, Cardiology/Pneumology, University of Bonn, Bonn, Germany

Hui Cao, Xinhua Hu, Qiang Zhang, Jun Li, Junpeng Wang, Yang Shao, Bing Liu and Shijie Xin
Department of Vascular and Thyriod Surgery, the First Affiliated Hospital of China Medical University, Shenyang, China

Marilyn Gwen Connell
Division of Child Health, Institute of Translational Medicine, The University of Liverpool, Liverpool, United Kingdom

Harriet Jane Corbett, Paul Damion Losty and Edwin Chitran Jesudason
Division of Child Health, Institute of Translational Medicine, The University of Liverpool, Liverpool, United Kingdom
Department of Paediatric Surgery, Alder Hey Children's National Health Service (NHS) Foundation Trust, Liverpool, United Kingdom

David Garth Fernig
Department of Chemical and Structural Biology, Institute of Integrative Biology, The University of Liverpool, Liverpool, United Kingdom

Benoît Gore, Mohamed Izikki, Marc Humbert and Gerald Simonneau
INSERM U999, Le Plessis-Robinson, France

Saadia Eddahibi
INSERM U999, Le Plessis-Robinson, France,
Centre Chirurgical Marie Lannelongue, Le Plessis-Robinson, France

Laurence Dewachter and Robert Naeije
Laboratory of Physiology, Faculty of Medicine, Free University of Brussels, Brussels, Belgium

Olaf Mercier, Philippe Dartevelle and Elie Fadel
Centre Chirurgical Marie Lannelongue, Le Plessis-Robinson, France

Franck Lebrin
INSERM U833, Collège de France, Paris, France

Skevi Neofitidou, Thomas Kirschning and Manuel Christian Hofstetter
Department of Anesthesiology and Critical Care Medicine, University Hospital Mannheim, Faculty of Medicine, University of Heidelberg, Heidelberg, Germany

Marc Revermann
Department of Anesthesiology and Critical Care Medicine, University Hospital Mannheim, Faculty of Medicine, University of Heidelberg, Heidelberg, Germany

Institute for Cardiovascular Physiology, Medical Faculty of the Goethe-University Frankfurt, Frankfurt, Germany

Schloss and Ralf P. Brandes
Institute for Cardiovascular Physiology, Medical Faculty of the Goethe-University Frankfurt, Frankfurt, Germany

Daniel J. Kass, Rehan Kahloon and Liyang Yu
Division of Pulmonary, Allergy, and Critical Care Medicine, Department of Medicine, University of Pittsburgh School of Medicine and the Dorothy P. and Richard P. Simmons Center for Interstitial Lung Disease, Pittsburgh, Pennsylvania, United States of America

Asaf Savir
Division of Pulmonary, Allergy, and Critical Care Medicine, Department of Medicine, University of Pittsburgh School of Medicine and the Dorothy P. and Richard P. Simmons Center for Interstitial Lung Disease, Pittsburgh, Pennsylvania, United States of America
Division of Pulmonary, Allergy, and Critical Care Medicine, Department of Medicine, Columbia University College of Physicians and Surgeons, New York, New York, United States of America

Hunter C. Champion
Division of Pulmonary, Allergy, and Critical Care Medicine, Department of Medicine, University of Pittsburgh School of Medicine and the Dorothy P. and Richard P. Simmons Center for Interstitial Lung Disease, Pittsburgh, Pennsylvania, United States of America
Department of Medicine, Cardiovascular Institute, University of Pittsburgh School of Medicine, Pittsburgh, Pennsylvania, United States of America
Vascular Medicine Institute, University of Pittsburgh School of Medicine, Pittsburgh, Pennsylvania, United States of America

Eileen Rattigan
Department of Cardiology, Geisinger Health System, Wilkes-Barre, Pennsylvania, United States of America

Katrina Loh and Mark Markowski
Division of Pulmonary, Allergy, and Critical Care Medicine, Department of Medicine, Columbia University College of Physicians and Surgeons, New York, New York, United States of America

Anjali Saqi
Department of Pathology, Columbia University College of Physicians and Surgeons, New York, New York, United States of America

Revathi Rajkumar
Department of Medicine, Cardiovascular Institute, University of Pittsburgh School of Medicine, Pittsburgh, Pennsylvania, United States of America

Ferhaan Ahmad
Department of Medicine, Cardiovascular Institute, University of Pittsburgh School of Medicine, Pittsburgh, Pennsylvania, United States of America
Vascular Medicine Institute, University of Pittsburgh School of Medicine, Pittsburgh, Pennsylvania, United States of America

Piotr Sklepkiewicz, Xia Tian, Hossein Ardeschir Ghofrani, Norbert Weissmann, Friedrich Grimminger and Soni Savai
Medical Clinic II/V, University Hospital, Giessen, Germany

Ralph Theo Schermuly, Werner Seeger and Pullamsetti
Max-Planck-Institute for Heart and Lung Research, Bad Nauheim, Germany

Daniel Sedding
Medical Clinic I, University Hospital, Giessen, Germany

Tarek Kashour
King Fahad Medical City, Riyadh, Saudi Arabia

Clark Undem, Eon J. Rios, Julie Maylor and Larissa A. Shimoda
Division of Pulmonary and Critical Care Medicine, Department of Medicine, Johns Hopkins School of Medicine, Baltimore, Maryland, United States

Eileen M. Bauer, Han Zheng and Timothy R. Billiar
Department of Surgery, University of Pittsburgh School of Medicine, Pittsburgh, Pennsylvania, United States of America

Philip M. Bauer
Department of Surgery, University of Pittsburgh School of Medicine, Pittsburgh, Pennsylvania, United States of America
Department of Pharmacology and Chemical Biology, University of Pittsburgh School of Medicine, Pittsburgh, Pennsylvania, United States of America

Vascular Medicine Institute, University of Pittsburgh School of Medicine, Pittsburgh, Pennsylvania, United States of America

Suzy Comhair and Serpil Erzurum
Department of Pathobiology, Lerner Research Institute, Cleveland Clinic, Cleveland, Ohio, United States of America
Respiratory Institute, Cleveland Clinic, Cleveland, Ohio, United States of America

Abbas Bitar
Department of Medicine, Internal Medicine Residency Program, Krannert Institute of Cardiology, Indiana University, Indianapolis, Indiana, United States of America

Mona Selej
Department of Medicine, Division of Pulmonary, Allergy, Critical Care, Occupational and Sleep Medicine, Krannert Institute of Cardiology, Indiana University, Indianapolis, Indiana, United States of America

Tim Lahm
Department of Medicine, Division of Pulmonary, Allergy, Critical Care, Occupational and Sleep Medicine, Krannert Institute of Cardiology, Indiana University, Indianapolis, Indiana, United States of America
Richard L. Roudebush Veterans Affairs Medical Center, Indianapolis, Indiana, United States of America

Islam Bolad
Department of Medicine, Krannert Institute of Cardiology, Indiana University, Indianapolis, Indiana, United States of America
Richard L. Roudebush Veterans Affairs Medical Center, Indianapolis, Indiana, United States of America

Rebecca Colman and John Granton
Pulmonary hypertension program, Toronto General Hospital, Division of Respirology, Faculty of Medicine, University of Toronto, Toronto, Ontario, Canada

Heather Whittingham
Department of Critical Care Medicine, Hamilton General Hospital, McMaster University, Hamilton, Ontario, Canada

George Tomlinson
Department of Medicine, Mount Sinai Hospital and University Health Network, Faculty of Medicine, University of Toronto, Toronto, Ontario, Canada

Partha Sen, Avinash V, Mahmoud A. Mohammad and Stephen Welty
Department of Pediatrics, Baylor College of Medicine, Houston, Texas, United States of America

John Belmont
Department of Pediatrics, Baylor College of Medicine, Houston, Texas, United States of America
Department of Molecular and Human Genetics, Baylor College of Medicine, Houston, Texas, United States of America

Sundararajah Thevananther
Department of Pediatrics, Baylor College of Medicine, Houston, Texas, United States of America
Interdepartmental Program in Translational Biology and Molecular Medicine, Baylor College of Medicine, Houston, Texas, United States of America

Przemyslaw Szafransk
Department of Molecular and Human Genetics, Baylor College of Medicine, Houston, Texas, United States of America

Dharmadhikari, Monica J. Justice and Pawel Stankiewicz
Department of Molecular and Human Genetics, Baylor College of
Medicine, Houston, Texas, United States of America
Interdepartmental Program in Translational Biology and Molecular Medicine, Baylor College of Medicine, Houston, Texas, United States of America

Hannah M. Brown
Department of Molecular and Human Genetics, Baylor College of Medicine, Houston, Texas, United States of America
Robinson Research Institute, School of Pediatrics and Reproductive Health, University of Adelaide, Adelaide, Australia

Tadeusz Majewski
Department of Pathology, University of Texas MD Anderson Cancer Center, Houston, Texas, United States of America

Xiaomeng Ren, Tanya V. Kalin and Vladimir V. Kalinichenko
Division of Pulmonary Biology, Cincinnati Children's Hospital Research Foundation, Cincinnati, Ohio, United States of America

Joanna Zabielska
Institute of Informatics, University of Warsaw, Warsaw, Poland

Anna Gambin
Institute of Informatics, University of Warsaw, Warsaw, Poland
Mossakowski Medical Research Center, Polish Academy of Sciences, Warsaw, Poland

Molly Bray
Department of Epidemiology, University of Alabama at Birmingham, Birmingham, Alabama, United States of America

Claire Langston
Department of Pathology, Baylor College of Medicine, Houston, Texas, United States of America

Matthew J. Campen, Michael L. Paffett, E. Sage Colombo and Selita N. Lucas
Department of Pharmaceutical Sciences, College of Pharmacy, University of New Mexico Health Sciences Center, Albuquerque, New Mexico, United States of America

Tamara Anderson, Monique Nysus ans Jeffrey P. Norenberg
Radiopharmaceutical Sciences Program, College of Pharmacy, University of New Mexico Health Sciences Center, Albuquerque, New Mexico, United States of America

Ben Gershman, Jacob Hesterman and Jack Hoppin
inviCRO, LLC., Boston, Massachusetts, United States of America

Monte Willis
McAllister Heart Institute and Department of Pathology and Laboratory Medicine, University of North Carolina, Chapel Hill, North Carolina, United States of America

Bernhard Moser, Anna Megerle, Stefan Janik Shahrokh Taghavi and Walter Klepetko
Department of Thoracic Surgery, Division of Surgery, Medical University Vienna, Vienna, Austria

Christine Bekos and Hendrik Jan Ankersmit
Christian Doppler Laboratory for the Diagnosis and Regeneration of Cardiac and Thoracic Diseases, Medical University Vienna, Vienna, Austria

Tamás Szerafin
Department of Cardiac Surgery, University of Debrecen, Debrecen, Hungary

Peter Birner and Ana-Iris Schiefer
Department of Pathology, Medical University Vienna, Vienna, Austria

Michael Mildner
Department of Dermatology, Medical University Vienna, Vienna, Austria

Irene Lang, Nika Skoro-Sajer and Roela Sadushi-Kolici
Department of Internal Medicine II, Division of Cardiology, Medical University Vienna, Vienna, Austria

Nicolás Molano-González, Monica Rodríguez-Jiménez and Yeny Acosta-Ampudia
Center for Autoimmune Diseases Research (CREA), School of Medicine and Health Sciences, Universidad del Rosario, Bogotá, Colombia

Juan-Sebastian Franco, Rubén D. Mantilla, Jenny Amaya-Amaya, Adriana Rojas-Villarraga and Juan-Manuel Anaya
Center for Autoimmune Diseases Research (CREA), School of Medicine and Health Sciences, Universidad del Rosario, Bogotá, Colombia
Mederi, Hospital Universitario Mayor, Bogotá, Colombia

Lara Zafrani, Virginie Lemiale, Benoît Schlemmer and Elie Azoulay
Medical Intensive Care Unit, Saint-Louis University Hospital, Paris, France

Nathanael Lapidus
Biostatistics Department, Saint-Louis University Hospital, Paris, France

Gwenael Lorillon
Pulmonology Department, Saint-Louis University Hospital, Paris, France

Akira Naito, Toshihiko Sugiura, Seiichiro Sakao and Koichiro Tatsumi
Department of Respirology, Graduate School of Medicine, Chiba University, 1-8-1 Inohana, Chuo-Ku, Chiba 260-8670, Japan

Nobuhiro Tanabe, Takayuki Jujo and Ayako Shigeta
Department of Advanced Medicine in Pulmonary Hypertension, Graduate School of Medicine, Chiba University, 1-8-1 Inohana, Chuo-Ku, Chiba 260-8670, Japan

Keiichi Ishida
Department of Cardiovascular Surgery, Graduate School of Medicine, Chiba University, 1-8-1 Inohana, Chuo-Ku, Chiba 260-8670, Japan

Takumi Inami, Hideaki Yoshino and Toru Satoh
Division of Cardiology, Second Department of Internal Medicine, Kyorin University School of Medicine, Tokyo, Japan

Masaharu Kataoka
Division of Cardiology, Second Department of Internal Medicine, Kyorin University School of Medicine, Tokyo, Japan
Department of Cardiology, Keio University School of Medicine, Tokyo, Japan

Keiichi Fukuda
Department of Cardiology, Keio University School of Medicine, Tokyo, Japan

Motomi Ando
Department of Cardiovascular Surgery, Fujita Health University, Aichi, Japan

Yidan Zhao, Jenny Peng, Catherine Lu, Michael Hsin, Marco Mura, Licun Wu, Lei Chu, Ricardo Zamel, Tiago Machuca, Thomas Waddell, Mingyao Liu, Shaf Keshavjee, John Grantonand Marc de Perrot
Latner Thoracic Surgery Research Laboratories and Division of Thoracic Surgery, Toronto General Hospital, University Health Network, University of Toronto, Toronto, Ontario, Canada

Adriana M. Zimnicka, Haiyang Tang, Qiang Guo, Frank K. Kuhr, Jun Wan, Jiwang Chen, Kimberly A. Smith, Dustin R. Fraidenburg, Moumita S. R. Choudhury and Roberto F. Machado
Department of Medicine, Section of Pulmonary, Critical Care, Sleep and Allergy Medicine, University of Illinois at Chicago, Chicago, Illinois, United States of America

Irena Levitan and Myung Jin Oh
Department of Medicine, Section of Pulmonary, Critical Care, Sleep and Allergy Medicine, University of Illinois at Chicago, Chicago, Illinois, United States of America
Department of Pharmacology, University of Illinois at Chicago, Chicago, Illinois, United States of America

Jason X.-J. Yuan
Department of Medicine, Section of Pulmonary, Critical Care, Sleep and Allergy Medicine, University of Illinois at Chicago, Chicago, Illinois, United States of America
Department of Pharmacology, University of Illinois at Chicago, Chicago, Illinois, United States of America
Center for Cardiovascular Research, University of Illinois at Chicago, Chicago, Illinois, United States of America

Jack H. Kaplan
Department of Biochemistry and Molecular Genetics, University of Illinois at Chicago, Chicago, Illinois, United States of America

Index